FETAL AND NEONATAL SECRETS

FETAL AND NEONATAL SECRETS

Richard A. Polin, MD

Professor of Pediatrics
College of Physicians and Surgeons
Columbia University
Chief, Division of Neonatology
Children's Hospital of New York
New York, New York

Alan R. Spitzer, MD

Professor of Pediatrics
Chief, Division of Neonatology
State University of New York at Stony Brook
Health Sciences Center
Stony Brook, New York

HANLEY & BELFUS, INC./Philadelphia

Publisher: HANLEY & BELFUS, INC.
                  Medical Publishers
                  210 South 13th Street
                  Philadelphia, PA 19107
                  (215) 546-7293; 800-962-1892
                  FAX (215) 790-9330
                  Web site: http://www.hanleyandbelfus.com

Note to the reader: Although the information in this book has been carefully reviewed for correctness of dosage and indications, neither the authors nor the editors nor the publisher can accept any legal responsibility for any errors or omissions that may be made. Neither the publisher nor the editors make any warranty, expressed or implied, with respect to the material contained herein. Experimental compounds and off-label uses of approved products are discussed. Before prescribing any drug, the reader must review the manufacturer's current product information (package inserts) for accepted indications, absolute dosage recommendations, and other information pertinent to the safe and effective use of the product described. This is especially important when drugs are given in combination or as an adjunct to other forms of therapy.

Library of Congress Cataloging-in-Publication Data

Fetal and neonatal secrets / |edited by| Richard A. Polin, Alan R. Spitzer.
     p. ; cm.—(The Secrets Series®)
   Includes index.
   ISBN 1-56053-424-9 (alk. paper)
    1. Infants (Newborn)—Diseases—Examinations, questions, etc. 2.
   Fetus—Diseases—Examinations, questions, etc. I. Polin, Richard A. (Richard Alan),
   1945- II. Spitzer, Alan R. III. Series
    |DNLM: 1. Fetal Diseases—Examination Questions. 2. Infant, Newborn,
   Diseases—Examination Questions. WQ 18.2 F419 2001|
   RJ254.F48 2001
   618.3'2'0076—dc21
                                                              00-069522

FETAL AND NEONATAL SECRETS   ISBN 1-56053-424-9

Last digit is the print number: 9 8 7 6 5 4 3 2

CONTENTS

1. Fetal Development and Growth 1

2. Obstetric Issues, Labor, and Delivery 7

3. General Neonatology 19

4. Cardiology 31

5. Dermatology 77

6. Endocrinology and Metabolism 87

7. Fluid, Electrolytes, and Renal Disorders 115

8. Gastroenterology and Nutrition 143

9. Genetics and Gene Therapy 205

10. Hematology 227

11. Infection and Immunity 261

12. Neurology 315

13. Orthopaedics and Neonatal Pain Management 341

14. Pulmonology 349

INDEX 401

CONTRIBUTORS

Linda J. Addonizio, M.D.
Associate Professor of Pediatrics, Columbia University College of Physicians and Surgeons; Presbyterian Hospital, New York, New York

Francis Akita, M.B., Ch.B.
Assistant Professor of Clinical Pediatrics, Division of Neonatology, Columbia University College of Physicians and Surgeons; Attending, Children's Hospital of New York, New York, New York

Maureen Andrew, M.D.
Professor, Department of Pediatrics, Division of Hematology/Oncology, University of Toronto Faculty of Medicine; The Hospital for Sick Children, Toronto, Ontario, Canada

Richard Auten, M.D.
Associate Professor of Pediatrics, Department of Pediatrics, Duke University Medical College; Duke University Medical Center, Durham, North Carolina

Steven Bachrach, M.D.
Associate Professor of Pediatrics, Jefferson Medical College of Thomas Jefferson University, Philadelphia, Pennsylvania; Director, Division of General Pediatrics, Alfred I. duPont Hospital for Children, Wilmington, Delaware

Jeanne Marie Baffa, M.D.
Clinical Associate Professor of Pediatrics, Jefferson Medical College of Thomas Jefferson University; Thomas Jefferson University Hospital, Philadelphia, Pennsylvania; Alfred I. duPont Hospital for Children, Wilmington, Delaware

H. Scott Baldwin, M.D.
Associate Professor of Pediatrics, Division of Cardiology, University of Pennsylvania School of Medicine; Children's Hospital of Philadelphia, Philadelphia, Pennsylvania

Doreen Balmer, R.D., M.A.
Registered Dietitian, Jefferson Medical College of Thomas Jefferson University, Philadelphia, Pennsylvania

David A. Bateman, M.D.
Associate Professor of Clinical Pediatrics, Columbia University College of Physicians and Surgeons; Director, Division of Neonatology, Allen Pavilion of New York Presbyterian Hospital, New York, New York

Stephen Baumgart, M.D.
Professor of Pediatrics, State University of New York at Stony Brook Health Sciences Center, Stony Brook, New York

Louis M. Bell, M.D.
Associate Professor of Pediatrics and Division Chief, General Pediatrics, University of Pennsylvania School of Medicine; Director, Infection Control, Children's Hospital of Philadelphia, Philadelphia, Pennsylvania

A.G. Christina Bergqvist, M.D.
Assistant Professor of Neurology and Pediatrics, University of Pennsylvania School of Medicine; Children's Hospital of Philadelphia, Philadelphia, Pennsylvania

Judy C. Bernbaum, M.D.
Professor of Pediatrics, University of Pennsylvania School of Medicine, Philadelphia, Pennsylvania

Gerard T. Berry, M.D.
Professor of Pediatrics, University of Pennsylvania School of Medicine; Attending, Children's Hospital of Philadelphia, Philadelphia, Pennsylvania

Vinod K. Bhutani, M.D.
Clinical Professor of Pediatrics, University of Pennsylvania School of Medicine, Philadelphia, Pennsylvania

Thomas Biancaniello, M.D.
Professor of Pediatrics; Associate Dean for Medical Affairs; Director, Division of Pediatric Cardiology; Medical Director, State University of New York at Stony Brook Health Sciences Center, Stony Brook, New York

Ronald J. Bolognese, M.D.
Professor and Chairman, Department of Obstetrics and Gynecology, Jefferson Medical College of Thomas Jefferson University, Philadelphia, Pennsylvania

Delma Bouchard, M.D.
Department of Pediatrics, University of Pennsylvania School of Medicine, Philadelphia, Pennsylvania

Sarah Bouchard, M.D.
Department of Pediatrics, University of Pennsylvania School of Medicine; Children's Institute for Surgical Science, Children's Hospital of Philadelphia, Philadelphia, Pennsylvania

Scott Boulanger, M.D.
Department of Surgery, State University of New York at Buffalo School of Medicine and Biomedical Sciences, Buffalo, New York

J. Richard Bowen, M.D.
Professor of Orthopedic Surgery, Jefferson Medical College of Thomas Jefferson University, Philadelphia, Pennsylvania; Director, Orthopedic Surgery, Alfred I. duPont Hospital for Children, Wilmington, Delaware

James B. Bussel, M.D.
Associate Professor of Pediatrics, Cornell University Weill Medical College, New York, New York

Joan Caddell, M.D.
Research Professor of Pediatrics, Jefferson Medical College of Thomas Jefferson University, Philadelphia, Pennsylvania

Gary G. Carpenter, M.D.
Associate Professor of Pediatrics, Division of Pediatric Endocrinology, Jefferson Medical College of Thomas Jefferson University; Thomas Jefferson University Hospital, Philadelphia, Pennsylvania

Joanne Carroll, R.D., M.S.
Registered Dietitian, Columbia University College of Physicians and Surgeons; Children's Hospital of New York, New York, New York

Timothy Centongo, M.D.
Department of Pediatrics, University of Pennsylvania School of Medicine, Philadelphia, Pennsylvania

Stephen T. Chasen, M.D.
Assistant Professor of Obstetrics and Gynecology, Department of Obstetrics and Gynecology, Cornell University Weill Medical College, New York, New York

Frank A. Chervenak, M.D.
Professor and Chairman, Department of Obstetrics and Gynecology, Cornell University Weill Medical College, New York, New York

Tina Chou, M.D.
Assistant Professor of Ophthalmology, Department of Ophthalmology, State University of New York at Stony Brook Health Sciences Center, Stony Brook, New York

Robert D. Christensen, M.D.
Professor of Pediatrics, University of Florida College of Medicine; Shands Hospital, Gainesville, Florida

Robert R. Clancy, M.D.
Professor of Neurology and Pediatrics, Division of Neurology, University of Pennsylvania School of Medicine; Children's Hospital of Philadelphia, Philadelphia, Pennsylvania

Bernard J. Clark III, M.D.
Associate Professor of Pediatrics, University of Pennsylvania School of Medicine; Medical Director, Heart Transplantation Program, Children's Hospital of Philadelphia, Philadelphia, Pennsylvania

Reese H. Clark, M.D.
Director of Research, Pediatrix Medical Group, Fort Lauderdale, Florida

Alan R. Cohen, M.D.
Professor of Pediatrics and Chief, Division of Hematology, University of Pennsylvania School of Medicine; Chairman, Department of Pediatrics, Children's Hospital of Philadelphia, Philadelphia, Pennsylvania

C. Michael Cotton, M.D.
Associate Professor of Pediatrics, Department of Pediatrics, Duke University Medical College; Duke University Medical Center, Durham, North Carolina

Irina Cuzino, M.D.
Neonatology Specialist, Hospital for Obstetrics and Gynecology, Bucharest, Romania

Steven M. Donn, M.D.
Professor of Pediatrics, Division of Neonatal-Perinatal Medicine, Department of Pediatrics, University of Michigan Medical School; Director, Intensive Care Nursery, C.S. Mott Children's Hospital, University of Michigan Medical Center, Ann Arbor, Michigan

David Edwards, M.D.
Professor of Neonatal Medicine and Chairman, Division of Pediatrics and Obstetrics and Gynecology, Imperial College of Medicine, London, United Kingdom

Lawrence F. Eichenfield, M.D.
Associate Clinical Professor, Departments of Pediatrics and Medicine; Chief, Division of Dermatology, Department of Pediatrics, University of California, San Diego, School of Medicine; Chief, Pediatric Dermatology and Dermatology Laser Surgery, Children's Hospital and Health Center, San Diego, California

Jacquelyn Evans, M.D.
Associate Clinical Professor of Pediatrics, Division of Neonatology, University of Pennsylvania School of Medicine; Children's Hospital of Philadelphia, Philadelphia, Pennsylvania

Karen Fairchild, M.D.
Assistant Professor of Pediatrics, University of Maryland School of Medicine, Baltimore, Maryland; Jefferson Medical College of Thomas Jefferson University, Philadelphia, Pennsylvania

T. Ernesto Figueroa, M.D.
Assistant Professor of Urology and Chief, Division of Pediatric Urology, Jefferson Medical College of Thomas Jefferson University; Thomas Jefferson University Hospital, Philadelphia, Pennsylvania; Alfred I. duPont Hospital for Children, Wilmington, Delaware

Michael Fisher, M.D.
Department of Pediatrics, University of Pennsylvania School of Medicine, Philadelphia, Pennsylvania

Alan W. Flake, M.D.
Associate Professor of Surgery, University of Pennsylvania School of Medicine; Attending Surgeon and Director, The Children's Institute for Surgical Science, Children's Hospital of Philadelphia, Philadelphia, Pennsylvania

John W. Foreman, M.D.
Professor of Pediatrics and Chief, Division of Pediatric Nephrology, Duke University Medical College; Duke University Medical Center, Durham, North Carolina

David F. Friedman, M.D.
Assistant Professor of Hematology and Clinical Pathology, University of Pennsylvania School of Medicine; Children's Hospital of Philadelphia, Philadelphia, Pennsylvania

Maria C. Garzon, M.D.
Assistant Professor, Departments of Dermatology and Pediatrics; Director, Division of Pediatric Dermatology, Columbia University College of Physicians and Surgeons; Children's Hospital of New York, New York, New York

Michael Georgieff, M.D.
Professor of Pediatrics and Child Development, University of Minnesota-Duluth School of Medicine, Duluth, Minnesota

Jeffrey S. Gerdes, M.D.
Associate Clinical Professor of Pediatrics, University of Pennsylvania School of Medicine, Philadelphia, Pennsylvania

Anne A. Gershon, M.D.
Professor of Pediatrics and Director, Division of Pediatric Infectious Disease, Columbia University College of Physicians and Surgeons; Children's Hospital of New York, New York, New York

Welton M. Gersony, M.D.
Alexander S. Nadas Professor of Pediatrics and Director, Division of Pediatric Cardiology, Columbia University College of Physicians and Surgeons; Children's Hospital of New York, New York, New York

Eric Gibson, M.D.
Assistant Professor of Pediatrics; Director, Infant Apnea Program, Jefferson Medical College of Thomas Jefferson University; Thomas Jefferson University Hospital, Philadelphia, Pennsylvania; Alfred I. duPont Hospital for Children, Wilmington, Delaware

Marie Gleason, M.D.
Clinical Associate Professor of Pediatrics, University of Pennsylvania School of Medicine; Attending Cardiologist, Children's Hospital of Philadelphia, Philadelphia, Pennsylvania

Philip Glick, M.D.
Professor, Departments of Surgery, Pediatrics, and Obstetrics and Gynecology; Surgeon-in-Chief, State University of New York at Buffalo School of Medicine and Biomedical Sciences, Buffalo, New York

Ronald N. Goldberg, M.D.
Professor of Pediatrics and Chief, Division of Neonatology, Department of Pediatrics, Duke University Medical College; Duke University Medical Center, Durham, North Carolina

Michael Goodman, M.D.
Assistant Professor of Pediatrics and Neurology, Jefferson Medical College of Thomas Jefferson University, Philadelphia, Pennsylvania; Alfred I. duPont Hospital for Children, Wilmington, Delaware

Richard A. Greene, M.D.
Assistant Professor of Obstetrics and Gynecology, Jefferson Medical College of Thomas Jefferson University, Philadelphia, Pennsylvania

Jay S. Greenspan, M.D.
Professor of Pediatrics and Chief, Division of Neonatology, Department of Pediatrics, Jefferson Medical College of Thomas Jefferson University, Philadelphia, Pennsylvania

Frank Greer, M.D.
Professor of Pediatrics, University of Wisconsin Medical School; Meriter Hospital, Madison, Wisconsin

George W. Gross, M.D.
Professor of Radiology and Director, Pediatric Radiology, University of Maryland School of Medicine, Baltimore, Maryland

Anju Gupta-Modak, M.D.
Attending Neonatologist, Maimonides Medical Center, Brooklyn, New York

Barbara A. Haber, M.D.
Assistant Professor of Pediatrics, Division of Gastroenterology and Nutrition, University of Pennsylvania School of Medicine; Attending, Children's Hospital of Philadelphia, Philadelphia, Pennsylvania

Elizabeth Hailu, M.D.
Attending Neonatologist, St. Vincent's Hospital, New York, New York

Louis P. Halamek, M.D.
Associate Professor of Pediatrics and Obstetrics and Gynecology, Stanford University School of Medicine; Stanford University Medical Center, Palo Alto, California

Catherine Hansen, M.D.
Assistant Clinical Professor of Pediatrics, Division of Infectious Disease, Columbia University College of Physicians and Surgeons; Children's Hospital of New York, New York, New York

Mary Catherine Harris, M.D.
Associate Professor, Department of Pediatrics, Division of Neonatology, University of Pennsylvania School of Medicine; Attending, Children's Hospital of Philadelphia, Philadelphia, Pennsylvania

Constance J. Hayes, M.D.
Professor of Clinical Pediatrics, Division of Cardiology, Columbia University College of Physicians and Surgeons; Attending, Children's Hospital of New York, New York, New York

Andre Hebra, M.D.
Associate Professor, Departments of Surgery and Pediatrics, Medical University of South Carolina, Charleston, South Carolina

Terry W. Hensle, M.D.
Professor of Urology and Director, Division of Pediatric Urology, Columbia University College of Physicians and Surgeons; Children's Hospital of New York, New York, New York

Daniel Hershey
University of California, San Diego, School of Medicine, San Diego, California

Susan R. Hintz, M.D.
Assistant Professor of Pediatrics, Department of Pediatrics, Stanford University School of Medicine; Stanford University Medical Center, Palo Alto, California

Alan J. Hordof, M.D.
Professor of Clinical Pediatrics, Columbia University College of Physicians and Surgeons; Attending Cardiologist, Children's Hospital of New York, New York, New York

Daphne T. Hsu, M.D., Ph.D.
Associate Professor of Clinical Pediatrics, Columbia University College of Physicians and Surgeons; Attending Cardiologist, Children's Hospital of New York, New York, New York

Hallum Hurt, M.D.
Director, Division of Neonatology, Albert Einstein Medical Center, Philadelphia, Pennsylvania

Sudarshan R. Jadcherla, M.D.
Assistant Professor of Pediatrics, Medical College of Wisconsin, Milwaukee, Wisconsin

Lucky Jain, M.D.
Associate Professor of Pediatrics, Emory University School of Medicine, Atlanta, Georgia

Lois Johnson-Hamerman, M.D.
Professor of Pediatrics, University of Pennsylvania School of Medicine, Philadelphia, Pennsylvania

Bernard S. Kaplan, M.B., B.Ch.
Professor of Pediatrics and Director, Division of Pediatric Nephrology, University of Pennsylvania School of Medicine; Children's Hospital of Philadelphia, Philadelphia, Pennsylvania

Paige Kaplan, M.B., B.Ch.
Professor of Pediatrics, Division of Genetics, University of Pennsylvania School of Medicine; Attending, Children's Hospital of Philadelphia, Philadelphia, Pennsylvania

Sudha Kashyap, M.D.
Associate Professor of Pediatrics, Division of Neonatology, Columbia University College of Physicians and Surgeons; Attending, Children's Hospital of New York, New York, New York

Kent R. Kelley, M.D.
Assistant Professor of Clinical Neurology and Clinical Pediatrics, Northwestern University Medical School; Children's Memorial Hospital, Chicago, Illinois

Andrea Kelly, M.D.
Department of Pediatrics, Division of Endocrinology, University of Pennsylvania School of Medicine, Philadelphia, Pennsylvania

Martin Keszler, M.D.
Associate Professor of Pediatrics, Georgetown University School of Medicine; Georgetown University Medical Center, Washington, D.C.

Joel D. Klein, M.D.
Clinical Associate Professor of Pediatrics, Jefferson Medical College of Thomas Jefferson University, Philadelphia, Pennsylvania; Chief, Division of Infectious Disease, Alfred I. duPont Hospital for Children, Wilmington, Delaware

Robert M. Kliegman, M.D.
Professor and Leslie Muma Chair, Department of Pediatrics and Pediatrician-in-Chief, Medical College of Wisconsin; Children's Hospital of Wisconsin, Milwaukee, Wisconsin

Mary Kumar, M.D.
Professor, Departments of Pediatrics and Pathology, Case Western Reserve University School of Medicine, Cleveland, Ohio

Satyan Laksminrusimha, M.D.
Assistant Professor of Pediatrics, State University of New York at Buffalo School of Medicine and Biomedical Sciences, Buffalo, New York

Eric L. Lazar, M.D.
Assistant Professor of Surgery, Columbia University College of Physicians and Surgeons; Assistant Attending Surgeon, Children's Hospital of New York, New York, New York

H. Robin Lee, M.D.
Instructor in Clinical Pediatrics, Division of Neonatology, Columbia University College of Physicians and Surgeons; Children's Hospital of New York, New York, New York

Lenore Levine, M.D.
Professor of Pediatrics, Division of Pediatric Endocrinology, Columbia University College of Physicians and Surgeons, New York, New York

Joseph Levy, M.D.
Professor of Clinical Pediatrics (in Surgery), Columbia University College of Physicians and Surgeons, New York, New York

Chris A. Liacouras, M.D.
Assistant Professor of Pediatrics, Division of Gastroenterology and Nutrition, University of Pennsylvania School of Medicine; Children's Hospital of Philadelphia, Philadelphia, Pennsylvania

Ronald Librizzi, D.O.
Professor of Obstetrics and Gynecology, Department of Obstetrics and Gynecology, Jefferson Medical College of Thomas Jefferson University, Philadelphia, Pennsylvania

Richard Lin, M.D.
Assistant Professor of Anesthesia and Pediatrics, Division of Critical Care Medicine, University of Pennsylvania School of Medicine; Children's Hospital of Philadelphia, Philadelphia, Pennsylvania

John M. Lorenz, M.D.
Professor of Clinical Pediatrics, Columbia University College of Physicians and Surgeons; Director of Network Nurseries, New York Presbyterian Health Network, New York, New York

Peter Mamula, M.D.
Department of Pediatrics, Division of Gastroenterology and Nutrition, University of Pennsylvania School of Medicine, Philadelphia, Pennsylvania

Gerald A. Mandell, M.D.
Professor of Radiology, Jefferson Medical College of Thomas Jefferson University; Thomas Jefferson University Hospital, Philadelphia, Pennsylvania; Alfred I. duPont Hospital for Children, Wilmington, Delaware

Catherine S. Manno, M.D.
Associate Professor of Pediatrics, University of Pennsylvania School of Medicine; Director, Transfusion Service, Children's Hospital of Philadelphia, Philadelphia, Pennsylvania

Zvi S. Marans, M.D.
Associate Clinical Professor of Pediatrics, Columbia University College of Physicians and Surgeons; Attending Cardiologist, Children's Hospital of New York, New York, New York

Jonathan E. Markowitz, M.D.
Instructor of Pediatrics, Division of Gastroenterology and Nutrition, University of Pennsylvania School of Medicine; Attending, Children's Hospital of Philadelphia, Philadelphia, Pennsylvania

Mary J. Marron-Corwin, M.D.
Associate Professor of Clinical Pediatrics, New York Medical College, Valhalla, New York

Maria Mascarenas, M.D.
Assistant Professor of Pediatrics, University of Pennsylvania School of Medicine, Philadelphia, Pennsylvania

Peter Mattei, M.D.
Assistant Professor of Surgery, Jefferson Medical College of Thomas Jefferson University; Thomas Jefferson University Hospital, Philadelphia, Pennsylvania; Alfred I. duPont Hospital for Children, Wilmington, Delaware

Charles P. McKay, M.D.
Assistant Professor of Pediatrics and Director, Bone and Mineral Program, Jefferson Medical College of Thomas Jefferson University; Pediatric Nephrologist, Thomas Jefferson University Hospital, Philadelphia, Pennsylvania; Alfred I. duPont Hospital for Children, Wilmington, Delaware

Steven E. McKenzie, M.D., Ph.D.
Professor of Medicine and Pediatrics, Jefferson Medical College of Thomas Jefferson University; Thomas Jefferson University Hospital, Philadelphia, Pennsylvania; Alfred I. duPont Hospital for Children, Wilmington, Delaware

T. Allen Merritt, M.D., M.H.A.
Adjunct Professor of Pediatrics, University of Oregon Health Sciences Center, Portland, Oregon; Director, Neonatology, St. Charles Medical Center, Bend, Oregon

Sonya Misra, M.D.
Attending Neonatologist, Santa Clara Valley Hospital, San Jose, California

John Moore, M.D.
Professor of Pediatrics, Medical College of Pennsylvania and Hahnemann University School of Medicine, Philadelphia, Pennsylvania

Kimberly D. Morel, M.D.
Department of Dermatology, Columbia University College of Physicians and Surgeons; New York Presbyterian Hospital, New York, New York

Peter Morelli, M.D.
Assistant Professor of Clinical Pediatrics, Department of Pediatrics, State University of New York at
Stony Brook Health Sciences Center, Stony Brook, New York

Frederick C. Morin III, M.D.
Professor of Pediatrics and Physiology and Chairman, Department of Pediatrics, State University of
New York at Buffalo School of Medicine and Biomedical Sciences; Pediatrician-in-Chief, Kaleida
Health-Children's Hospital of Buffalo, Buffalo, New York

Kenneth A. Murdison, M.D.
Clinical Associate Professor of Pediatrics, Jefferson Medical College of Thomas Jefferson University,
Philadelphia, Pennsylvania; Nemours Cardiac Center, Alfred I. duPont Hospital for Children,
Wilmington, Delaware

John Murphy, M.D.
Clinical Professor of Pediatrics, Jefferson Medical College of Thomas Jefferson University; Thomas
Jefferson University Hospital; Methodist Hospital, Philadelphia, Pennsylvania; Alfred I. duPont
Hospital for Children, Wilmington, Delaware

Martin A. Nash, M.D.
Professor of Clinical Pediatrics and Director, Division of Pediatric Nephrology, Columbia University
College of Physicians and Surgeons; Children's Hospital of New York, New York, New York

Susan Nasser-Sharif, M.D., FRCS(C)
Division of Orthopedic Surgery, Alfred I. duPont Hospital for Children, Wilmington, Delaware

Martha Nelson, M.D.
Clinical Assistant Professor of Pediatrics, Division of Neonatal-Perinatal Medicine, Department of
Pediatrics, University of Michigan Medical School; C.S. Mott Children's Hospital, University of
Michigan Medical Center, Ann Arbor, Michigan

John Nicholson, M.D.
Associate Professor of Pediatrics and Pathology, Columbia University College of Physicians and
Surgeons, New York, New York

Doug Nordli, M.D.
Associate Professor of Clinical Neurology and Clinical Pediatrics, Northwestern University Medical
School, Chicago, Illinois

William I. Norwood, Jr., M.D., Ph.D.
Professor of Surgery, Jefferson Medical College of Thomas Jefferson University, Philadelphia, Pennsylvania; Director, Nemours Cardiac Center, Alfred I. duPont Hospital for Children, Wilmington, Delaware

Sharon Oberfield, M.D.
Professor of Pediatrics, Columbia University College of Physicians and Surgeons; Presbyterian
Hospital, New York, New York

Bernadette O'Hare, M.D.
Department of Pediatrics, Division of Pediatric Infectious Diseases, University of Toronto Faculty of
Medicine, Toronto, Ontario, Canada

Robin K. Ohls, M.D.
Associate Professor of Pediatrics, University of New Mexico School of Medicine, Albuquerque, New
Mexico

Elvira Parravacini, M.D.
Department of Pediatrics, Division of Neonatology, Columbia University College of Physicians and
Surgeons, New York, New York

David A. Paul, M.D.
Assistant Professor of Pediatrics, Jefferson Medical College of Thomas Jefferson University,
Philadelphia, Pennsylvania; Christiana Care Medical Center, Wilmington, Delaware

Richard H. Pearl, M.D.
Professor, Departments of Surgery and Pediatrics, University of Illinois College of Medicine, Peoria, Illinois

Stephen A. Pearlman, M.D.
Associate Professor of Pediatrics, Jefferson Medical College of Thomas Jefferson University, Philadelphia, Pennsylvania; Associate Director, Neonatology, Christiana Medical Center, Newark, Delaware

James B. Pelegano, M.D.
Assistant Clinical Professor of Pediatrics, Columbia University College of Physicians and Surgeons, New York, New York

Gilberto R. Pereira, M.D.
Professor of Pediatrics, Division of Neonatology, University of Pennsylvania School of Medicine; Attending, Children's Hospital of Philadelphia, Philadelphia, Pennsylvania

Sergio Piomelli, M.D.
James A. Wolff Professor of Pediatrics and Director, Division of Pediatric Hematology, Columbia University College of Physicians and Surgeons; Children's Hospital of New York, New York, New York

Richard A. Polin, M.D.
Professor of Pediatrics, Columbia University College of Physicians and Surgeons; Chief, Division of Neonatology, Children's Hospital of New York, New York, New York

Alice Prince, M.D.
Professor of Pediatrics (in Pharmacology), Columbia University College of Physicians and Surgeons, New York, New York

Roy Proujansky, M.D.
Robert L. Brent Professor and Chairman, Department of Pediatrics, Jefferson Medical College of Thomas Jefferson University; Thomas Jefferson University Hospital, Philadelphia, Pennsylvania; Alfred I. duPont Hospital for Children, Wilmington, Delaware

Elizabeth B. Rand, M.D.
Assistant Professor of Pediatrics, University of Pennsylvania School of Medicine; Medical Director, Liver Transplant Program, Children's Hospital of Philadelphia, Philadelphia, Pennsylvania

Shantanu Rastogi, M.D.
Attending Neonatologist, Maimonides Medical Center, Brooklyn, New York

Albert E. Reece, M.D.
The Abraham Roth Professor and Chairman, Department of Obstetrics, Gynecology, and Reproductive Sciences, Temple University School of Medicine, Philadelphia, Pennsylvania

Joan A. Regan, M.D.
Associate Professor of Clinical Pediatrics, Columbia University College of Physicians and Surgeons; Director, Well Baby Nursery, Children's Hospital of New York, New York, New York

Ted S. Rosenkrantz, M.D.
Professor, Departments of Pediatrics and Obstetrics and Gynecology, University of Connecticut School of Medicine, Farmington, Connecticut

Judith L. Ross, M.D.
Professor of Pediatrics, Jefferson Medical College of Thomas Jefferson University; Thomas Jefferson University Hospital, Philadelphia, Pennsylvania; Alfred I. duPont Hospital for Children, Wilmington, Delaware

Philip Roth, M.D.
Associate Professor of Pediatrics, State University of New York at Stony Brook Health Sciences Center, Stony Brook, New York

S. David Rubenstein, M.D.
Professor of Clinical Pediatrics, Columbia University College of Physicians and Surgeons; Director, Neonatal Intensive Care Unit, Children's Hospital of New York, New York, New York

Rakesh Sahni, M.D.
Assistant Professor of Clinical Pediatrics, Columbia University College of Physicians and Surgeons; Attending, Children's Hospital of New York, New York, New York

Lisa Saiman, M.D.
Associate Professor of Clinical Pediatrics, Columbia University College of Physicians and Surgeons; Children's Hospital of New York, New York, New York

Richard Schanler, M.D.
Professor, Section of Neonatology and Children's Nutrition, Department of Pediatrics, Baylor University College of Medicine, Houston, Texas

Adele Schneider, M.D.
Department of Pediatrics, Albert Einstein Medical Center, Philadelphia, Pennsylvania

Seth Lewis Schulman, M.D.
Associate Professor of Pediatrics and Surgery, University of Pennsylvania School of Medicine; Assistant Division Chief, Division of Urology, Children's Hospital of Philadelphia, Philadelphia, Pennsylvania

Karl F. Schulze, M.D.
Associate Professor of Clinical Pediatrics, Columbia University College of Physicians and Surgeons; Children's Hospital of New York, New York, New York

Marshall Z. Schwartz, M.D.
Professor of Surgery and Pediatrics; Vice Chairman, Department of Surgery, Jefferson Medical College of Thomas Jefferson University; Thomas Jefferson University Hospital, Philadelphia, Pennsylvania; Alfred I. duPont Hospital for Children, Wilmington, Delaware

Robert Seigle, M.D.
Assistant Professor of Clinical Pediatrics, Columbia University College of Physicians and Surgeons; Attending, Children's Hospital of New York, New York, New York

Istvan Seri, M.D., Ph.D.
Assistant Professor of Pediatric Neonatology, University of Pennsylvania School of Medicine; Clinical Director, Newborn/Infant Center, Children's Hospital of Philadelphia, Philadelphia, Pennsylvania

Shailen S. Shah, M.D.
Assistant Professor of Obstetrics and Gynecology, Department of Obstetrics and Gynecology, Jefferson Medical College of Thomas Jefferson University, Philadelphia, Pennsylvania

Sujit Sheth, M.D.
Assistant Professor, Department of Pediatrics, Division of Hematology, Columbia University College of Physicians and Surgeons; Children's Hospital of New York, New York, New York

Michael L. Spear, M.D.
Associate Professor of Pediatrics, Jefferson Medical College of Thomas Jefferson University, Philadelphia, Pennsylvania; Clinical Director, Neonatal Intensive Care Unit and Medical Director, Infant Apnea Team, Alfred I. duPont Hospital for Children, Wilmington, Delaware

Alan R. Spitzer, M.D.
Professor of Pediatrics and Chief, Division of Neonatology, State University of New York at Stony Brook Health Sciences Center, Stony Brook, New York

Charles A. Stanley, M.D.
Professor of Pediatrics and Chief, Division of Endocrinology, University of Pennsylvania School of Medicine; Children's Hospital of Philadelphia, Philadelphia, Pennsylvania

Thomas J. Starc, M.D.
Professor of Clinical Pediatrics, Columbia University College of Physicians and Surgeons; Attending Cardiologist, Children's Hospital of New York, New York, New York

Robert Stanton, M.D.
Director of the Musculoskeletal Tumor Service, Alfred I. duPont Hospital for Children, Wilmington, Delaware

Stuart E. Starr, M.D.
Professor of Pediatrics and Chief, Division of Immunologic and Infectious Diseases, University of Pennsylvania School of Medicine; Children's Hospital of Philadelphia, Philadelphia, Pennsylvania

John Stefano, M.D.
Associate Professor of Pediatrics, Jefferson Medical College of Thomas Jefferson University, Philadelphia, Pennsylvania; Section Chief, Division of Neonatology, Alfred I. duPont Hospital for Children, Wilmington, Delaware

David K. Stevenson, M.D.
Chief, Division of Neonatal and Developmental Medicine; Vice Chairman, Department of Pediatrics, Stanford University Medical Center, Palo Alto, California

Charles J. H. Stolar, M.D.
Professor of Surgery and Pediatric Surgery (in Pediatrics); Surgeon-in-Chief, Columbia University College of Physicians and Surgeons; Children's Hospital of New York, New York, New York

Barbara J. Stoll, M.D.
Professor and Vice-Chairman for Research, Emory University School of Medicine, Atlanta, Georgia

Steven Stylianos, M.D.
Associate Professor of Clinical Surgery and Clinical Pediatric Surgery (in Pediatrics), Columbia University College of Physicians and Surgeons; Director, Pediatric Trauma Program, Children's Hospital of New York, New York, New York

Jorge E. Tolosa, M.D.
Assistant Professor of Obstetrics and Gynecology; Director, Division of Research and International Health, Jefferson Medical College of Thomas Jefferson University, Philadelphia, Pennsylvania

Helen M. Towers, MBBCh
Assistant Professor of Pediatrics, Columbia University College of Physicians and Surgeons; Attending, Children's Hospital of New York, New York, New York

Edouard J. Trabulsi, M.D.
Department of Urology, Jefferson Medical College of Thomas Jefferson University, Philadelphia, Pennsylvania

Melissa Tsai, M.D.
Attending Neonatologist, Northern Westchester Hospital, Mount Kisco, New York

Elaine E. L. Wang, M.D., C.M.
Associate Professor, Department of Pediatrics, Division of Infectious Diseases, University of Toronto Faculty of Medicine; The Hospital for Sick Children, Toronto, Ontario, Canada

Ronald J. Wapner, M.D.
Professor of Obstetrics and Gynecology and Director, The Center for Genetics and Fetal Medicine, MCP Hahnemann University, Philadelphia, Pennsylvania

Michael Weiner, M.D.
Professor of Clinical Pediatrics and Director, Division of Pediatric Oncology, Columbia University College of Physicians and Surgeons; Children's Hospital of New York, New York, New York

Gil Wernovsky, M.D.
Associate Professor of Pediatrics, University of Pennsylvania School of Medicine; Medical Director, Cardiac Intensive Care Unit, Children's Hospital of Philadelphia, Philadelphia, Pennsylvania

Valerie E. Whiteman, M.D.
Assistant Professor of Obstetrics and Gynecology; Director of Obstetrical Services, Department of Obstetrics, Gynecology, and Reproductive Sciences, Temple University School of Medicine, Philadelphia, Pennsylvania

Delbert R. Wigfall, M.D.
Assistant Professor, Department of Pediatrics, Division of Nephrology, Duke University Medical College; Duke University Medical Center, Durham, North Carolina

Gloria D. Wiseman, M.D.
Associate Professor of Pediatrics, Columbia University College of Physicians and Surgeons; Director of Nurseries and Director of Neonatal-Perinatal Medicine, Holy Name Hospital, New York, New York

Thomas E. Wiswell, M.D.
Professor of Pediatrics and Director of Neonatal Research, State University of New York at Stony Brook Health Sciences Center, Stony Brook, New York

Philip J. Wolfson, M.D.
Professor of Surgery and Director of Undergraduate Education, Jefferson Medical College of Thomas Jefferson University; Thomas Jefferson University Hospital, Philadelphia, Pennsylvania; Alfred I. duPont Hospital for Children, Wilmington, Delaware

Jen-Tien Wung, M.D.
Professor of Clinical Anesthesia (in Pediatrics), Columbia University College of Physicians and Surgeons, New York, New York

Mervin C. Yoder, M.D.
Professor of Pediatrics, Biochemistry, and Molecular Biology, University of Indiana School of Medicine, Indianapolis, Indiana

Elaine H. Zackai, M.D.
Professor of Pediatrics and Genetics, University of Pennsylvania School of Medicine; Director, Clinical Genetics Center, Children's Hospital of Philadelphia, Philadelphia, Pennsylvania

Theoklis Zaoutis, M.D.
Division of Infectious Diseases, Children's Hospital of Philadelphia, Philadelphia, Pennsylvania

Stephen A. Zderic, M.D.
Assistant Professor of Urology, University of Pennsylvania School of Medicine; Attending Urologist, Children's Hospital of Philadelphia, Philadelphia, Pennsylvania

PREFACE

From the time we become physicians until the time we retire from medicine, we are guided by the phrase widely attributed to Hippocrates: *primum non nocere*, "first do no harm." Although the origins of that exact phrase are unclear, Hippocrates certainly conveyed that meaning in his oath: "I will prescribe regimen for the good of my patients according to my ability and my judgment and never do harm to anyone." Fundamental to the concept of "doing good" is the acquisition of medical knowledge that allows each of us to practice according to the highest possible standards. In the first two years of medical school, knowledge is transferred predominantly by large group lectures and required readings. Once we enter the clinical years, the process of acquiring new information begins to change. We continue to read textbooks, but journal articles become increasingly important sources of the newest information, and much information is transmitted to us through "personal communications" by individuals who are further along in their training. For the medical student, that often means an intern or resident, and for the senior resident, a fellow or an attending. This apprenticeship aspect of medicine has been an intrinsic part of the field since its inception. Even in this era of rapidly intensifying technologic advances, "see one, do one, teach one" remains a cornerstone of bedside medical education.

With this concept in mind, *Fetal and Neonatal Secrets* is designed to serve as a primer for the bedside teaching that remains such an important part of medical education. While it can be read from cover to cover (e.g., to prepare for a certifying examination), we believe that the information in the book should be shared wherever health care providers congregate to provide care (inpatient service, clinics, operating room) to the fetus and newborn infant. Although the word *secrets* connotes a sense of privacy, we hope that this book reveals rather than obscures secrets, and that the cumulative wisdom shared by the many experienced contributors serves to enlighten the reader. Furthermore, we would love to see these secrets used by the youngest members of the health care team to challenge those more experienced, as well as by professors to make their residents and students think. We fear that we may need to tote around a copy of this book on rounds ourselves, as our house staff, fellows, and nurse practitioners may throw down the gauntlet to test us on a daily basis! Although we have tried to make this book as comprehensive and practical as possible, the reader will encounter many facts that might be considered trivial (e.g., what is the ductus of Botallo?), but we hope that the reader is forgiving in this respect. The retention of important information has always seemed to be enhanced by its association with interesting, but less essential information (the Mary Poppins approach—"a spoonful of sugar helps the medicine go down"). Where would medicine be without mnemonics? In any event, we hope you find this book useful in your daily practice, but more importantly, we want you to have some fun along the way.

Richard A. Polin, M.D.
Alan R. Spitzer, M.D.

ACKNOWLEDGMENTS

In my development as a physician, I have been exposed to many wonderful teachers, scientists, and clinicians. However, because of the enormous influence they have had on my career, I would like to acknowledge five individuals by name: Bill Speck (my lifelong friend; no one has ever cared more about resident and student education), David Cornfield (the consummate general pediatrician who helped shape my career in academic medicine), John Driscoll (the person who first excited me about neonatology and my role model for the warm, caring physician), Bill Fox (my coeditor for *Fetal and Neonatal Physiology*, who shared with me his infectious excitement about research), and Mark Ditmar (my coeditor for *Pediatric Secrets*, whose combination of humor, knowledge, and compassion has allowed me to achieve a balance in medicine and who has shown me how "academic" and wonderful the practice of general pediatrics can be). I am indebted to all of them.

I also want to thank my wonderful family: my wife, Helene, and my children, Allison, Mitchell, Jessica, and Gregory. Without their love and support I could not have accomplished nearly as much as I have as a physician and teacher.

Finally, I would like to thank my publisher, Linda Belfus, for hooking me on The Secrets Series® and allowing me to put my love of education into print.

RAP

Because this book is designed to foster the teaching of neonatology, the great teachers that I have been exposed to in my career remain role models for the clinician-educator and have inspired my efforts in teaching. Lewis Barness, Frank Oski, David Cornfeld, C. Everett Koop, and William Schwartz were highly influential during my student and residency years. As I embarked on my career in neonatal medicine, the incredible group of neonatologists during my fellowship training at the University of California in San Francisco, Roderic Phibbs, William Tooley, George Gregory, and Joseph Kitterman, had a profound influence on my development as a physician and a teacher in neonatal medicine. As a faculty member at several great institutions in Philadelphia, I was deeply influenced by my daily exposure to some of the finest neonatologists in the country, including Maria Delivoria-Papadopoulos, William Fox, and my coeditor of this book, Richard Polin. Several people who have remained close friends throughout long stretches of my career have also been great role models for me. In particular, Stephen Baumgart and Thomas Wiswell, now colleagues at SUNY-Stony Brook, are two of the finest teachers I have ever seen. Leonard Graziani, former Chief of Child Neurology at Thomas Jefferson University, remains a model of the academic clinician and researcher. His insights into the neurology of the newborn have greatly improved our understanding of these infants. I would also like to thank my current Chairman, Richard Fine, for his friendship and strong support since I joined the faculty at SUNY-Stony Brook.

I most emphatically hope that future neonatologists now in training will continue to build on my efforts and the efforts of those individuals who truly developed the field of neonatology. Several of my current fellows, Vladimir Burdjalov, Sudhish Chandra, Munir Kapasi, and Pinchi Srinivasan, proofed and critiqued much of the manuscript, adding immeasurably to the quality of the book. It has been a pleasure to work with them and many other neonatology fellows over the years. Many of these individuals will unquestionably become great teachers and academicians in the years ahead, and they represent a very strong future for neonatal-perinatal medicine.

Lastly, no effort would be realized without the support of my wife, Elaine. She and my children, Stephen (and new daughter-in-law Jennifer), Sara, and Lauren, are the reasons why everything I do is worthwhile.

ARS

1. FETAL DEVELOPMENT AND GROWTH

1. What features constitute the biophysical profile?

The biophysical profile is a scoring system that assesses fetal well-being before birth. Five variables are assessed: fetal breathing movements, gross body movements, fetal tone, reactive fetal heart rate, and qualitative amniotic fluid volume. Normal results equate to 2 points per variable with a maximum possible total of 10 points.

2. Can one really detect breathing movements before birth?

The use of fetal ultrasound has made it simple to assess many different forms of fetal activity. For some time, it has been possible to show that fetuses of many species demonstrate breathing movements before birth. These movements appear to tone the respiratory muscles for assumption of breathing at the time of birth and also to assist in the movement of fetal lung fluid into the amniotic cavity. There may be other reasons for fetal breathing as well.

In both experimental animal models and human fetus observations, hypoxemia appears to decrease fetal breathing significantly. In addition, exposure of the fetus to maternal smoking in utero decreases fetal breathing movements. The effects of hypoxemia on fetal breathing appear to be mediated through central nervous system (CNS) dysfunction. As a result, fetal breathing appears to be an important indicator of fetal well-being and therefore is included in the fetal biophysical profile.

3. Why are fetal heart rate reactivity and gross bodily movements part of the biophysical profile?

The acute response of the fetus to hypoxemic events is a centrally mediated suppression of a series of biophysical activities. By decreasing these activities, the fetus can significantly reduce oxygen requirements by up to 19% and raise the fetal venous Po_2 by as much as 30%. Consequently, assessment of the decrease in events such as bodily movements, fetal breathing, and reactive fetal heart rate permits the observer to make important judgments about the state of fetal health, especially with regard to hypoxemia.

4. Is the fetal biophysical profile applicable in cases of chronic intrauterine hypoxemia, or is it just applied in acute events?

Chronic hypoxemia is actually the more common form of fetal hypoxemia. Most cases of fetal exposure to decreasing concentration of oxygen occur over a more protracted period of time than just minutes or hours. The biophysical profile is equally helpful in chronic hypoxemia because many of the changes that occur with acute events also begin to appear with chronic exposure to decreasing oxygen. In addition, factors such as measurement of amniotic fluid volume provide the obstetrician and perinatologist with valuable information about chronic intrauterine hypoxemia.

5. How does one know that fetal breathing movements are absent because the observation was made during fetal sleep periods?

To account for the possibility of fetal sleep during an observation period, the observer must scan the mother for a minimum of 30 minutes. It is exceedingly rare for the fetus to go beyond 30 minutes with no fetal breathing movements, no gross fetal activity, or abnormal fetal tone activity as assessed by at least one episode of hand-opening with finger and thumb extension. Fetal tone may also be normal, however, with the fetal hand remaining in a fist or flexed formation for the entire 30-minute period of observation.

6. How does the biophysical profile relate to the umbilical venous pH?

The following graph reveals the relationship between the fetal biophysical profile and mean umbilical venous pH:

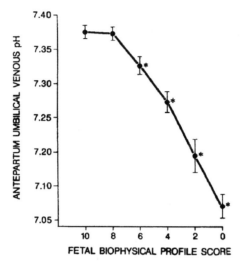

7. What is the relationship between the fetal biophysical profile score and neonatal outcome?

The work of Frank Manning has been instrumental in developing and establishing the biophysical profile's value in neonatal outcome. Manning has shown that the risk of perinatal morbidity increases significantly with a decreasing biophysical profile score (BPS). The incidence of meconium aspiration also rises with a decreasing score.

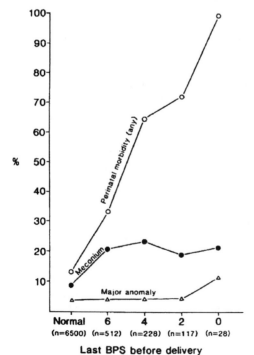

Relationship between perinatal mortality (PNM), either total or corrected for major anomaly, and the last biophysical profile score (BPS). (From Manning FA, et al: Fetal assessment based on fetal biophysical profile scoring: IV. An analysis of perinatal morbidity and mortality. Am J Obstet Gynecol 162:703, 1990, with permission.)

8. What is the first bone in the human fetus to ossify?

The clavicle. In the long bones, the process of ossification occurs in the primary centers of ossification in the diaphysis during the embryonic period of fetal development. Although the femurs are the first long bones to show traces of ossification, the clavicles, which develop initially by intramembranous ossification, begin to ossify before any other bones in the body.

9. At which gestational age does pupillary reaction to light develop?

Pupillary reaction to light may appear as early as 29 weeks' gestation but is not consistently present until approximately 32 weeks.

10. At which gestational age does a sense of smell develop?

By 32 weeks' gestation, normal premature infants respond to concentrated odor.

11. How does postmaturity differ from dysmaturity?

An infant born of a post-term pregnancy (> 42 weeks' gestation) is referred to as postmature. The baby is dysmature if features of placental insufficiency are present. These include loss of subcutaneous fat and muscle mass, as well as meconium staining of the amniotic fluid, skin, and nails.

12. What is the normal rate of head growth in the preterm infant?

During the first 2–4 months of life, the normal rate is 0.5–1.0 cm per week. An increase in the circumference of the head of > 2.0 cm in 1 week should raise suspicion of CNS pathology, such as hydrocephalus. However, some premature infants may experience rapid "catch-up" head growth following significant early stress or illness. During these periods, the picture is confused even further by the fact that additional dilation of the ventricular system occasionally appears on head ultrasound examination. The ratio of body length to head circumference may be used to distinguish normal from abnormal head growth. A ratio of 1.42–1.48 is reportedly normal, whereas a low ratio of 1.12–1.32 indicates relative or absolute macrocephaly.

13. What is meant by growth retardation? What is the difference between growth retardation and growth restriction?

Intrauterine growth retardation describes a fetus or child whose weight for gestational age is less than the 10th percentile. Because of the pejorative nature of the term *retardation*, the term *restriction* has been substituted. Growth potential needs to be assessed with precision because of the risk it poses for the fetus. Low birth weight in its broadest definition (< 2500 gm) includes prematurity and accounts for 75% of poor perinatal outcomes. There is no essential difference between growth retardation and growth restriction.

14. What issue is paramount in separating the growth-retarded from the low–birth-weight fetus?

When assessing gestational age in utero, one is measuring the relative size of the fetus compared to known normative values. The size of the fetus is most consistent with the age of the fetus in utero during early gestation. Early ultrasound (i.e., measuring the fetus in the first trimester of pregnancy using crown–rump length) is most accurate in assessing gestational age. Later in pregnancy, various factors make ultrasound assessment of size somewhat less accurate in evaluating the possibility of growth retardation. Gestational age is important in defining the potential long-term outcome for the fetus. An appropriately grown fetus that is delivered prematurely has significantly different hurdles and long-term potential than the fetus of the same birth weight that is more advanced in gestation. A 26-week-old, 600-gm neonate born to a mother with a previously uncomplicated history who developed idiopathic premature labor is a very different infant than the 30-week-old, 600-gm neonate born to a mother with significant renal disease due to longstanding diabetes mellitus. In general, infants at every gestational age after 26 weeks appear to do better when they are of normal size than if they are either small or large for gestational age.

15. What measurements are used in the assessment of fetal growth?

With ultrasound, head size or biparietal diameter was one of the first measurements to assess growth. This approach, however, often produced large errors because the head size was often spared when the fetus was growth restricted. Crown–rump length is much more precise but needs to be determined early in gestation. Other measurements of fetal growth and well-being that have been used include the abdominal circumference, amniotic fluid volume, fetal activity, and cardiovascular adjustments.

16. What factors increase risk for fetal growth restriction?

- Prior maternal history of fetal growth restriction
- Maternal history of immunologic or collagen vascular disease
- Maternal TORCH infection—toxoplasmosis, other (congenital syphilis and viruses), rubella, cytomegalovirus, and herpes simplex virus
- Maternal hypertension or preeclampsia
- Genetic syndromes in the fetus—trisomy 21, 18, 13; Turner syndrome
- Teratogens—cigarette smoking, retin-A, warfarin, alcohol
- Advanced maternal diabetes
- Placental insufficiency
- Placental infarction
- Idiopathic

17. How should one follow a fetus at risk for growth retardation?

If intrauterine growth restriction (IUGR) is suspected, follow the fetus closely with nonstress testing and biophysical profiles at regular intervals to evaluate fetal well-being. Amniotic fluid levels give an estimate on a more chronic basis. With the marginally viable fetus, there is always controversy about whether the fetus is better off in utero or out. Signs of jeopardy require one to respond quickly and decisively with delivery to ensure neonatal survival. Electronic fetal monitoring in labor is essential for the fetus lagging in growth. Fetal acid/base status is another indicator that can be used in labor to confirm findings from electronic fetal monitoring. Evaluation of placental blood flow by Doppler is also helpful in evaluating the fetus in jeopardy. The important issue is not to deal with acidosis and asphyxia, but to prevent these changes.

18. What are the delivery implications for the growth-restricted fetus?

Growth-restricted fetuses do not tolerate labor as well as appropriately grown fetuses. In addition, they are at higher risk for necrotizing enterocolitis (NEC), intraventricular hemorrhage (IVH), metabolic problems, and thermoregulatory problems. The liberal use of cesarean section affords the best potential for these children. Fetuses with IUGR who are born asphyxiated have less ability to withstand insults and have greater morbidity when exposed to the same insult as an appropriately grown fetus.

19. What short-term and long-term morbidities are known to occur more frequently in growth-retarded babies?

- Short-term morbidities include perinatal asphyxia, meconium aspiration, fasting hypoglycemia, alimented hypoglycemia, polycythemia-hyperviscosity, and immunodeficiency
- Long-term morbidities include poor developmental outcome and altered postnatal growth.

Most studies demonstrate normal intelligence and developmental quotients in infants who are small for gestational age (SGA), although there seems to be a higher incidence of behavioral and learning problems. The presence or absence of severe perinatal asphyxia is extremely important in predicting later intellectual and neurologic function.

20. What are the current prenatal and postnatal approaches to a child with a congenital diaphragmatic hernia?

The care of the infant with a congenital diaphragmatic hernia (CDH) remains complex, and survival is still only approximately 65%, even at the most complete neonatal centers. CDH occurs in about 1/2500 deliveries and is characterized by the herniation of the bowel into the chest, which compresses both ipsilateral and contralateral lung, producing pulmonary hypoplasia to varying degrees. Recently, cardiac hypoplasia has been raised as an issue, which also helps to explain the poor prognosis. Many of these children also have associated abnormalities in feeding, developmental problems, and skeletal anomalies.

Prenatal approaches have included direct attempts at surgical repair of the CDH to reduce the degree of lung hypoplasia. Such efforts, however, have not been highly successful, often resulting in fetal death from compromised umbilical venous flow when the liver is brought back into the abdomen. Tracheal occlusion to allow retention of fetal lung fluid and greater lung growth has been used with some success, but is still highly experimental.

Postnatal treatment can include any and all of the following at various times:
- Conventional mechanical ventilation with or without permissive hypercapnia
- Surfactant replacement
- Inhalational nitric oxide
- High-frequency ventilation
- Extracorporeal membrane oxygenation
- Partial liquid ventilation

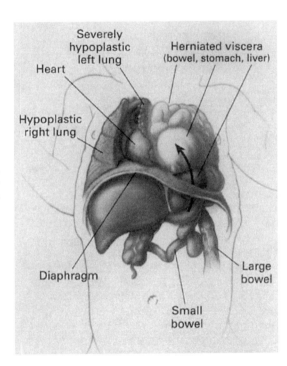

Congenital diaphragmatic hernia. (From Adzick NS, Nance ML: Pediatric surgery. N Engl J Med 342:1652, 2000, with permission.)

21. What should one consider in assessing the potential value of fetal surgical intervention?
- The nature and history of the disease being treated should be amenable to fetal intervention.
- In utero correction has appeared to be efficacious in animal models.
- Maternal risk is low.
- Prenatal repair appears to offer advantages above and beyond postnatal correction.
- Failure to intervene is likely to result in permanent injury or death to the fetus.

22. What management considerations become critical with fetal surgical intervention?
- In utero vs. postnatal repair success rates
- Fetal diagnosis capabilities

- Monitoring of fetus and mother during surgery
- Maternal risks
- Timing of surgery
- Uterine irritability postoperatively
- Tocolytic therapy
- Timing of delivery
- Mode of delivery (cesarean section vs. vaginal birth)
- Ethical dilemmas

23. What disease entities have been approached with fetal surgical intervention? How successful have they been?

FETAL SURGICAL INTERVENTION	DEGREE OF SUCCESS
Congenital diaphragmatic hernia	+/–
Congenital cystic adenomatoid malformation	+
Fetal hydronephrosis	+
Posterior urethral valve decompression	+
Myelomeningocele	+/–
Congenital hydrothorax/chylothorax	+
Sacrococcygeal teratoma	+/–
Airway obstruction from neck masses	+
Twin-to-twin transfusion syndrome	+
Congenital hydrocephalus	–
Cleft palate	+/–

+ = usually successful; +/– = occasionally successful; – = not successful.

BIBLIOGRAPHY

1. Manning FA: Fetal biophysical profile. Obstet Gynecol Clin North Am 25:557–577, 1999.
2. Manning FA, et al: Fetal biophysical profile scoring: Correlation with antepartum umbilical venous fetal pH. J Obstet Gynecol 169:755, 1993.
3. Rurak DW, Cooper C: The effect of relative hypoxemia on the pattern of breathing movements in fetal lambs. Respir Physiol 55:23–37, 1984.

2. OBSTETRIC ISSUES, LABOR, AND DELIVERY

1. What is amniocentesis?

Amniocentesis is a procedure that involves the aspiration of amniotic fluid from the amniotic sac during pregnancy. It is generally carried out with a spinal needle (20–22 gauge) in a transabdominal approach, using a sterile technique under ultrasound guidance.

2. How is amniocentesis classified?

Amniocentesis is classified by the time in the pregnancy when it is done and by its indication. Early amniocentesis is performed before 15 weeks in the pregnancy, and 1 ml of amniotic fluid per week of gestation is obtained. About 15–20 ml of fluid is removed at mid-trimester amniocentesis, and the 1–2 ml obtained initially is discarded to avoid maternal cell contamination. Liters of fluid can be removed during therapeutic amniocentesis. A small amount of amniotic fluid (between 5 and 10 ml) is obtained for fetal lung maturity testing.

3. What are the indications for amniocentesis?

The indications can be classified as diagnostic and therapeutic.

Diagnostic indications
- Prenatal diagnosis—genetic conditions, amniotic fluid alpha-fetoprotein levels
- Detection of congenital and intra-amniotic infection
- Definitive diagnosis of ruptured membranes (using injection of indigo carmine)
- Fetal lung maturity testing of preterm gestations, or if an elective cesarean section is to be performed (e.g., in patients with insulin-dependent diabetes)
- Monitoring OD450 as a marker for hemolytic anemia in rhesus isoimmunization

Therapeutic indications
- Amniotic fluid reduction in acute polyhydramnios (excessive amount of fluid)
- Amniotic fluid reduction in the treatment of twin-to-twin transfusion

4. When is genetic amniocentesis performed?

Genetic amniocentesis can be performed after 9 weeks up to term. The most common time for genetic amniocentesis is during the mid-trimester at 15–20 weeks' gestation. At this time, there is about 150–300 ml of amniotic fluid from which one can remove 15–20 ml.

5. If genetic studies are indicated, how quickly can the results be obtained?

Immediate and preliminary (1–3 day) results can be obtained for cytogenetics using fluorescence in situ hybridization (FISH). Definitive chromosome studies require cultured amniocytes (cells from amniotic fluid) and, therefore, usually require 10–14 days.

6. What are the complications of amniocentesis?
- Miscarriage and fetal loss occurring in 0.5–1.0% of cases above the background rate of spontaneous loss (1.5–3.0%)
- Premature rupture of the membranes
- Neonatal respiratory distress (probably related to chronic amniotic fluid leak)
- Infection
- Fetal trauma (rare)
- Failure to achieve diagnosis (i.e., cell culture failure, which occurs in 1% of cases)
- Increased rhesus isoimmunization, especially if the placenta is transversed (give anti-D immunoglobulin if this complication occurs in an Rh negative patient)

7. Why not use early amniocentesis more frequently if it could give the patient an answer earlier in the pregnancy?

Early amniocentesis is performed between 9 and 14 weeks' gestation. It has been associated with a higher pregnancy loss rate (2% vs. 0.5% above background miscarriage rates) when compared with mid-trimester amniocentesis. Early amniocentesis is associated with an increase in the rate of fetal talipes equinovarus (FTE) (0.56–3.1%). In a study comparing early amniocentesis (defined as 11–13 weeks) with transabdominal chorionic villus sampling (CVS), 7 cases of FTE were identified in 527 live births after early amniocentesis, whereas no cases were seen in the group that has CVS. There is a higher rate of vaginal bleeding, and failure to obtain an adequate sample occurs in 1–2% of procedures. This failure is related to the increased technical difficulties of the procedure at the earlier gestation. CVS performed between 11 and 13 weeks can also provide information on fetal karyotype. In view of the safety considerations, early amniocentesis is being abandoned for safer alternatives such as mid-trimester amniocentesis or chorionic villus sampling.

8. How is third trimester hemorrhage defined and classified? What is its incidence?

Third trimester hemorrhage refers to any bleeding from the genital tract during the third trimester of pregnancy. In practice it refers to any bleeding that occurs from the time of viability, i.e., 23–24 weeks' gestation. The common causes are classified as placenta previa (7%), placental abruption (13%), and other bleeding (80%), including local lesions of the lower genital tract, vasa previa, early labor, trauma, neoplasia, and marginal placental separation. Such bleeding complicates about 6% of pregnancies.

9. How is placenta previa diagnosed?

Ultrasound visualization is the method of choice for this diagnosis in modern obstetrics. Multiple reports show a transvaginal approach to be safe and superior in its accuracy when compared with transabdominal ultrasound.

10. Should a vaginal examination be performed if there is vaginal bleeding?

Vaginal examination should be avoided when bleeding occurs until placenta previa is excluded by performing an ultrasound examination. *Clinical pearl:* If ultrasound is not available in late pregnancy, a useful approach is the double set-up examination in which two teams with anesthesiology are in the operating room. A vaginal examination is performed. Should bleeding occur from a placenta previa, an emergency cesarean section is performed by the second team.

11. How is placenta previa classified?

- **Complete**—where the placenta symmetrically covers the entire internal os of the cervix
- **Partial**—where the placenta lies asymmetrically toward one wall of the uterus and crosses part of the internal os
- **Marginal**—where the placental edge just reaches the edge of the internal cervical os

If the lower margin on ultrasound scan is > 2–3 cm from the internal os, it is not a placenta previa but a low-lying placenta.

12. What are the incidence and cause of placenta previa?

Placenta previa occurs in 1 in 200 deliveries at term. Complete placenta previa is detected in 5% of second trimester gestations, with 90% resolving by term; partial placenta previa is seen in 45% and resolves in more than 95% of cases. This apparent resolution is most likely related to the development of the lower uterine segment in late pregnancy, so the placenta appears to move upward with the hypertrophied uterine upper segment. The most likely etiologic factor is endometrial damage.

13. What are the risk factors for placenta previa?

- Previous placenta previa (8-fold risk)
- Previous uterine surgery (1.5–15-fold risk)

- Multiparity (1.7-fold risk)
- Advanced age > 35 years (4.7-fold risk)
- Advanced age > 40 years (9-fold risk)
- Cigarette smoking (1.4–3.0-fold risk)
- Multiple birth pregnancy

14. What are the complications of placenta previa?
- Life-threatening maternal hemorrhage
- Cesarean delivery
- Placenta accreta—when the placenta infiltrates the uterine wall (1–5%; 25% with one previous uterine surgery; 45% if more than one previous surgery)
- Increased risk of postpartum hemorrhage
- Perinatal mortality (27–32 weeks, 19.7%; after 36 weeks, 2.6%)
- Fetal growth restriction (16%)
- Increased fetal malformations (2-fold risk)
- Increased neurodevelopment abnormalities at 2 years that are possibly related to fetal hypoxia

15. What is placental abruption? How often does it occur?

Placental abruption is the separation of the normally implanted placenta before the birth of the fetus. It results from bleeding from a small arterial vessel into the decidua basalis. It is termed a *revealed* abruption when vaginal bleeding is present (90%) and a **concealed** abruption if there is no bleeding visible (10%). It is uniquely dangerous to the fetus and the mother because of its serious pathophysiologic sequelae. The incidence varies but averages about 0.83% or 1 in 120 deliveries. Abruption severe enough to cause fetal death is less common (approximately 1 in 420 deliveries).

16. What are the main risk factors for a placental abruption? Is placental abruption a recurrent disease?
- Maternal hypertension and preeclampsia
- Increasing maternal age and parity
- Cigarette smoking
- Cocaine use
- Trauma
- Uterine anomalies/fibroids
- Premature rupture of the membranes
- Spontaneous or artificial rupture of the membranes

The risk of placental abruption is between 6 and 16.6%; after two consecutive abruptions, the subsequent risk is 25%. Women who have a placental abruption severe enough to cause fetal death have a 7% risk of a similar outcome in a subsequent pregnancy.

17. What maternal and fetal complications occur with placental abruption?

Maternal complications	Fetal and neonatal complications
• Hypovolemic shock	• Intrauterine growth restriction, especially in preterm deliveries
• Maternal mortality (< 1%)	• Increased congenital malformations (4.4%)
• Acute renal failure	• Neonatal anemia
• Disseminated intravascular coagulation	• Increased abnormal neurodevelopment at 2 years
• Postpartum hemorrhage	• Perinatal mortality 14.4–67%—higher rates occur at earlier gestations; 50% are stillbirths. Normally grown term babies have a perinatal mortality rate of less than 2%.
• Severe rhesus isoimmunization unless adequate treatment with anti-D immunoglobulin	

18. What is vasa previa? What is its main complication?

Vasa previa is a velamentous insertion of the umbilical cord in the lower uterine segment with the cord vessels coursing unsupported within the membranes in advance of the presenting part. The vessels are prone to tearing at spontaneous/artificial rupture of the membranes with fetal exsanguination. Compression from the presenting part can also lead to extreme compromise of placental circulation. Fetal mortality rates are as high as 75–80% with rupture of the vessels and 60% with compression. Diagnosis is most often made after delivery. Fetal death and neurologic damage are the rule rather than the exception with this condition. It occurs in 1 in 3000 deliveries.

19. A 32-year-old, G2P1001 woman at term gestation presents in labor. Her membranes are intact; she is afebrile; and the fetal heart tracing is reassuring. Upon review of her prenatal records, you notice that she had a positive group B streptococcal culture obtained at 34 weeks' gestation. She is allergic to penicillin and "had difficulty breathing and swelled up" when she received it many years ago. What therapy is appropriate?

The Centers for Disease Control and Prevention (CDC) protocol, as well as the American Academy of Pediatrics (AAP) and American College of Obstetricians and Gynecologists (ACOG) guidelines, recommends prophylactic treatment with penicillin or ampicillin for women in labor who are positive for group B streptococci (GBS). Erythromycin or clindamycin are appropriate alternatives for penicillin-allergic patients. Recent in vitro data demonstrate an 18% rate of resistance to erythromycin (compared to 1/85 from isolates before the CDC recommendations). Of 100 isolates tested for antibiotic resistance, 5 were resistant to both erythromycin and clindamycin. The clinical implications of this remain unclear. One point that is notable is the 50% reduction in the rate of neonatal GBS infection in institutions following the CDC protocols, which underscores the usefulness of appropriate chemoprophylaxis.

20. What are the major risk factors for preterm labor?
- Low socioeconomic status
- Smoking
- Chorioamnionitis
- Prior preterm birth
- Preterm premature rupture of membranes
- Diethylstilbestrol (DES) exposure
- Uterine anomalies
- Hemorrhage
- Congenital anomalies
- Fetal demise
- Abruptio placentae
- Placenta previa
- Advanced maternal age
- Maternal age < 18 years
- Urinary tract infection
- Bacterial vaginosis
- Polyhydramnios
- Prior cervical surgery
- Poor nutritional status

21. What are absolute contraindications to tocolysis?
- Severe pregnancy induced hypertension
- Acute abruptio placentae
- Chorioamnionitis
- Fetal death
- Severe fetal growth restriction (especially with reversed umbilical venous flow)

22. What is fetal fibronectin?

Fetal fibronectin is an extracellular matrix protein, the presence of which in cervicovaginal secretions is a predictor of preterm labor. This predictor has a high negative predictive accuracy (99%), but only a mediocre positive predictive accuracy.

23. Is sedation or hydration of any benefit in the treatment of preterm labor?

No!

24. What are the common pharmacologic agents used for the inhibition of preterm labor and their mechanisms of action?

Inhibition of Preterm Labor

PHARMACOLOGIC AGENT	MECHANISM OF ACTION
Beta-adrenergic agonists (e.g., terbutaline, ritodrine)	Suppression of uterine activity
Magnesium sulfate	Uncertain—magnesium suppresses muscle contraction of myometrial strips in vitro, decreases intracellular calcium, and affects acetylcholine release
Prostaglandin synthase inhibitors (indomethacin)	Inhibition of the cyclooxygenase enzyme responsible for prostaglandins that promote uterine contractions
Calcium antagonists (nifedipine)	Inhibition of influx of calcium through the cell membrane

25. What are the main adverse effects of tocolytic agents on the fetus and neonate?

Adverse Effects of Tocolytic Agents

PHARMACOLOGIC AGENT	ADVERSE EFFECTS
Beta-adrenergic agonists	Fetal tachycardia; neonatal hypoglycemia, hypocalcemia, and hypotension
Magnesium	Fetal demineralization with prolonged use; neonatal respiratory and motor depression at higher serum levels
Prostaglandin synthase inhibitors	Constriction of fetal ductus arteriosus leading to pulmonary hypertension, oligohydramnios, decreased fetal urine production, and spontaneous intestinal perforation
Calcium antagonists	No known human effects—decreases fetal arterial Po_2 and pH in animal studies

26. Is tocolysis effective?

There is no question that tocolysis is effective over short-term intervals; however, clinical trials have not consistently demonstrated that gestation can be prolonged significantly or respiratory distress uniformly prevented.

27. A patient makes inquiries regarding multiple courses of steroids to enhance fetal lung maturity. What should you tell her about this approach?

Multiple doses of antenatal steroids (> 3) are associated with neonatal cortisol levels of 5.8 ± 1.0 µg/dl compared with 20.1 ± 3.4 µg/dl in neonates exposed to only one course of antenatal steroids. The suppression of the fetal adrenal gland and the subsequent response to stress in the critically ill neonate are a major concern with repeated doses of cortisol. In addition, animal data suggest smaller brain growth after multiple doses of steroids. The implications of this finding for humans are presently under investigation.

Exposure to more than three courses of antenatal steroids has not been associated with an additional reduction in the incidence of respiratory distress syndrome, regardless of the gestational age at the time of delivery, compared with exposure of neonates to one course. In one study, neonates exposed to more than 3 courses of antenatal steroids had a significantly increased risk of chronic lung disease or death (odds ratio = 2.0). Birth weight was reduced by 39 gm on the average after one course of antenatal steroids. Infants who were exposed to more than 2 courses had a reduction in birth weight of 80 gm. Correction for gestational age at delivery and multifetal pregnancies did not change this difference in birth weight. It appears, therefore, that there are significant risks to multiple steroid courses during preterm labor. Although lung maturation may be helped by a course of corticosteroids, repeated use of this therapy may have major risks to the neonate.

28. During a review of the perinatal outcomes for premature infants at your hospital, the nurse manager for the intensive care nursery inquires if there is an effective method to detect women at risk for premature delivery before they present in active preterm labor. What do current data indicate?

Levels of amniotic fluid interleukin-6 are markedly elevated in pregnancies destined for preterm labor and delivery, possibly indicating an inflammatory marker for such occurrences. The modified Creasy score, using patient history and other findings, detects only 7% of patients destined to develop preterm labor and delivery as compared with the 87% detection rate associated with two elevated salivary estriol levels. The Creasy score looks at a series of variables (see table) in an attempt to define clinical indicators that are likely to result in preterm labor. Other factors that appear to have some predictive value for prematurity include fetal fibronectin levels (women with higher levels are more likely to have cervical shortening before term) and cervical lactoferrin concentration (more likely to be elevated with lower genital tract infection). Granulocyte colony-stimulating factor also appears to have some predictive value for identifying which mother will deliver prematurely during the subsequent 4 weeks of gestation. The optimal mode of management for such pregnancies, however, has not been determined at this time, and prevention of premature birth remains an elusive goal. Consequently, there is no truly effective way of predicting premature labor ahead of the event itself.

Risk Factors in the Prediction of Spontaneous Preterm Labor
(The Modified Creasy Score)

Major risk factors	Minor risk factors
Multiple gestation	Febrile illness
DES exposure	Bleeding after 12 weeks
Hydramnios	History of pyelonephritis
Uterine anomaly	Cigarette smoking > 10/day
Cervix dilated > 1 cm at 32 weeks	Second trimester abortion × 1
Second trimester abortion × 2	More than 2 first trimester abortions
Previous preterm delivery	
Previous preterm labor, term delivery	
Abdominal surgery during pregnancy	
History of cone biopsy	
Cervical shortening < 1 cm at 32 weeks	
Uterine irritability	
Cocaine abuse	

29. What are some of the increased risks of twin pregnancies?

- Premature birth
- Intrauterine growth retardation, including discordant growth (which may occur in up to one-third of twin pregnancies)
- Increased perinatal mortality, especially for premature, monozygotic, and discordant twins
- Spontaneous abortion
- Birth asphyxia
- Fetal malposition
- Placental abnormalities (abruptio placentae, placenta previa)
- Polyhydramnios
- Twin-to-twin transfusion syndrome

30. Why are monozygotic twins considered to be at higher risk than dizygotic twins?

Monozygotic twins (identical twins) arise from the division of a single fertilized egg. Depending on the timing of the division of the single ovum into separate embryos, the amnionic and chorionic membranes can be shared (if division occurs > 8 days after fertilization), separate (if < 72 hours after fertilization), or mixed (separate amnion, shared chorion if 4–8 days after fertilization). Sharing of the chorion and/or amnion is associated with potential problems of vascular anastomoses (and possible twin–twin transfusions), cord entanglements, and congenital anomalies. These problems increase the risk of intrauterine growth retardation and intrauterine death. Dizygotic twins, however, result from two separately fertilized ova and, as such, usually have a separate amnion and chorion.

31. Who is higher risk, the first- or second-born twin?

The second-born twin has a 2–4-fold increased risk of developing respiratory distress syndrome (RDS) and is more likely to be asphyxiated. The exact reason for this difference in outcome is not entirely clear. Although is is assumed that placental separation and diminishing function play a role, that concept has never been well substantiated, especially in dizygotic twins. It may be that circulating vasoactive substances are released upon delivery of the first fetus that subsequently impair circulation to the remaining twin. As acidosis progresses, surfactant release is decreased, leading to an enhanced likelihood of RDS. It should be noted, however, that the risks for sepsis and necrotizing enterocolitis may be increased in first-born twins.

32. What are the varieties of conjoined twins?

Conjoined twins are classified according to the degree and nature of their union. These are listed below in order of decreasing frequency:

Thoracopagus	Joined at the thorax
Xiphopagus	Joined at the anterior abdominal wall
	Joined from the xiphoid to the umbilicus
Pygopagus	Joined at the buttocks or rump
Ischiopagus	Joined at the ischium
Craniopagus	Joined at the head

33. Who were Chang and Eng?

Chang and Eng were the original conjoined twins from whom the misnomer *Siamese twins* arose.

34. What is the treatment for conjoined twins? What problems are likely to arise?

The treatment of conjoined twins is a highly technical surgical exercise that should only be attempted at institutions with complete surgical subspecialty expertise and the ability to perform highly technical vascular evaluation preoperatively. Because of the entangled anatomies and circulations of the involved twins, it is sometimes not possible to separate the babies without sacrificing one infant. Many conjoined twins share a single vital organ, such as the liver, or have a single kidney. In such cases, normal survival for one of the conjoined twins may necessitate the sacrifice of the other twin. The incidence of conjoined twins is approximately 1:50,000 to 1:100,000. Of these, it appears that stillbirth occurs in nearly 50% of cases. In the surviving 50%, approximately 33–50% share a common vital organ, which can be divided in a certain percentage of cases, depending on organ involvement.

The ethical considerations in such cases test the limits of all concerned, especially of the parents, who are often emotionally distraught and unable to make the kinds of decisions that are often necessary. Substantial psychosocial support is crucial for both parents and medical staff during the care and separation of conjoined twins.

35. What is the clinical significance of fetal decelerations?

The character or pattern of decelerations often seen during fetal heart rate monitoring can be a valuable indicator of fetal well-being or the need for intervention. Fetal heart rate monitoring, however, is not infallible, and an occasional infant with a normal fetal heart rate tracing can have serious neonatal problems. Conversely, some infants with frightening heart rate patterns may be entirely fine at birth. Abnormal decelerations have a poor positive-predictive value, with only 15–25% being associated with a significantly compromised fetus. Normal studies, however, have a much higher predictive value of ongoing fetal well-being. The fetal heart rate tracing is simply an assessment of fetal well-being that needs to be weighed in conjunction with other information, such as fetal acidosis and the biophysical profile. The following are some common patterns of fetal heart rate:

- **Early decelerations** are associated with head compression. These are usually of no consequence.
- **Variable decelerations** are observed with cord compression. They may indicate fetal distress when prolonged, frequent, and associated with bradycardia.
- **Late decelerations** may indicate uteroplacental insufficiency and the presence of fetal distress. Both variable and late decelerations may be associated with acidosis and fetal compromise.

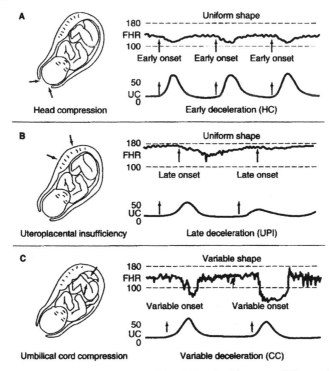

Examples of fetal heart rate monitoring abnormalities. FHR = fetal heart rate; UC = uterine contraction; HC = head compression; UPI = uteroplacental insufficiency; CC = cord compression. (From Gomella T: Neonatology, 4th ed. Stamford, CT, Appleton and Lange, 1999, p 4, with permission.)

36. What is a nonstress test?

The fetal heart rate accelerates in response to fetal activity, contractions of the uterus, or various other stimuli. This responsiveness forms the basis of one of the most widely used assessments of fetal well-being, the nonstress test (NST). In the NST, normal fetal intrauterine activity is examined to evaluate the fetal heart rate pattern. The NST is usually performed in an outpatient setting, and the patient is connected to a standard tocodynamometer while the fetal heart rate is monitored, usually by the Doppler ultrasound transducer. In general, one looks for at least two accelerations of the fetal heart rate of > 15 bpm amplitude lasting at least 15 seconds in a 20-minute period of monitoring. If reactivity standards are not met, the tracing is considered nonreactive, although a second period of 20 minutes may be observed to eliminate the possibility of fetal sleep.

If the study is deemed nonreactive, it should be followed by a contraction stress test or a biophysical profile to further assess fetal well-being.

37. What is a contraction stress test?

A contraction stress test (CST), or oxytocin challenge test, was one of the earliest techniques to assess fetal well-being. In this test, the mother receives an infusion of oxytocin until adequate uterine contractions have started, while being monitored on a tocodynamometer and a fetal ultrasound transducer. In a negative test, there are three uterine contractions within 10 minutes with no late decelerations of the fetal heart rate. In a positive test, in which there are late decelerations, the risk of mortality and morbidity for the fetus increases, with some reports of mortality as high as 15%. There are, however, many false-positive instances of CSTs, and the obstetrician often faces a difficult decision of how aggressively to proceed to delivery of the fetus, because the cervix may not be favorable at that time and a cesarean section may be required. If the test is equivocal, it may be reasonable to wait for an additional 24 hours to repeat the test.

An alternative to the use of oxytocin is the use of nipple stimulation by the mother. With this approach, the test may be over more rapidly, with no intravenous infusion required. Results are similarly interpreted.

38. What is an acceptable scalp pH in the fetus?

Fetal scalp sampling to measure blood pH is used in conjunction with electronic fetal heart rate monitoring to assess fetal well-being during labor. The range of acceptable values for fetal pH is broad. A pH > 7.25 is considered normal. Values between 7.20 and 7.25 are often referred to as pre-acidotic and may be associated with increased incidence of depression at delivery. As labor progresses, repeat testing is warranted. A pH < 7.20 may indicate significant fetal compromise.

Normal Fetal Scalp Blood Values in Labor

	EARLY FIRST STAGE	LATE FIRST STAGE	SECOND STAGE
pH	7.33 ± 0.03	7.32 ± 0.02	7.29 ± 0.03
pCO_2 (mmHg)	44 ± 4.05	42 ± 5.1	46.3 ± 4.2
pO_2 (mmHg)	21.8 ± 2.6	19.1 ± 2.1	17.2 ± 3.1
Base deficit (mmol/L)	3.9 ± 1.9	4.1 ± 2.5	6.4 ± 1.8

Adapted from Boylan PC, Parisi VM: Fetal acid-base balance. In Creasy RK, Resnik R (eds): Maternal-Fetal Medicine, 3rd ed. Philadelphia, W.B. Saunders, 1994, p 352.

39. Is length of labor the same for male and female babies?

No. Labor length for boys is about 1 hour longer than for girls on the average. As usual, boys prove to be a bigger pain than girls right from the start!

40. What is perinatal asphyxia?

Few terms evoke more trepidation from obstetricians and neonatologists (particularly in a court room, not to mention the delivery room) than perinatal asphyxia. The term *perinatal asphyxia*, however, is so vague and so arbitrarily applied that it is virtually meaningless. Nevertheless, it contains such a charged implication that ACOG has suggested it not be used, except when all of the following criteria are clearly met:
- An arterial cord pH sample < 7.0
- Apgar scores of 4 or less for at least 5 minutes
- Evidence of altered neurological status (e.g., obtundation, seizures, altered level of consciousness)
- Multisystem organ injury or failure

Our personal experience has indicated that the best way to assess a fetus and subsequent newborn is simply to describe the factual difficulties that exist and to avoid the use of vague terms. By describing the infant's physical examination, any abnormal findings, and objective laboratory data, one can avoid categorizing the infant as asphyxiated, yet convey the necessary information to the caregivers of the child.

41. Which drugs that cross the placenta can produce problems in the neonate?

Virtually all drugs cross the placenta to some degree, but few produce any significant problems for either the fetus or the neonate. Large organic ions such as heparin and insulin do not cross the placenta and are therefore safe. There are some drugs taken by the mother, however, with which one does occasionally need to contend in the newborn period:

• **Anticonvulsants.** Infants of mothers using anticonvulsants have twice the risk of malformations compared with the general population, especially cleft lip and palate and congenital cardiac defects. Valproic acid may cause neural tube defects, and diphenylhydantoin is associated with fetal hydantoin syndrome (microcephaly, developmental delay, growth failure, mental retardation, dysmorphic facies, and nail hypoplasia). Carbamazepine may also produce dysmorphism.

• **Psychoactive medications.** Lithium has been associated with a slightly increased risk of cardiac defects. In addition, lithium can produce polyhydramnios and fetal diabetes insipidus. Hypotonia, lethargy, and feeding problems are also seen in some infants. The effects of other psychotropic agents upon the fetus appear minimal, but some cases of teratogenesis have been reported, especially with some benzodiazepines. The critical issue that remains unresolved, however, is whether these drugs alter the development of the maturing fetal central nervous system.

• **Anticoagulants.** Warfarin is known to produce teratogenic effects in the fetus. About 5% of pregnancies result in fetal warfarin syndrome (mental retardation, bone stippling, dysmorphic characteristics, ophthalmologic abnormalities). If necessary, warfarin should be replaced by heparin during pregnancy.

• **Antihypertensive medications.** Angiotensin-converting enzyme inhibitors may cause fetal renal failure in later stages of gestation, leading to oligohydramnios, pulmonary hypoplasia, and fetal deformities.

• **Thyroid drugs.** Propylthiouracil (PTU) and methimazole (Tapazole) cross the placenta and can cause a fetal goiter and fetal hypothyroidism. Thyroid hormone use itself appears generally to be safe. Maternal Graves disease can result in neonatal thyroid storm and hyperthyroidism in rare cases.

• **Acne medications.** Isoretinoin (Accutane) is a significant human teratogen that should be avoided in women planning to become pregnant. It is associated with a high risk of both structural abnormalities and mental retardation. The use of topical tretinoin (Retin-A) appears to be safe.

• **Antineoplastic drugs.** The anticancer drugs that appear to have the greatest significance for teratogenesis are methotrexate and cyclophosphamide. Both can cause malformations of the skull and bones, as well as mental retardation.

• **Steroids.** The value of steroids for lung maturation is well established. Chronic exposure to steroids has been reported to inhibit neuronal development. Prednisone and prednisolone appear to cross the placenta to a small degree and therefore are the drugs of choice during gestation.

• **Antibiotics.** Tetracycline is the most notorious drug for producing both skeletal and dental abnormalities in pregnant women. Sulfa drugs may accentuate hyperbilirubinemia during the neonatal period by displacing bilirubin from binding sites. Sulfamethoxazole/trimethoprim has been associated with congenital cardiac defects. Kanamycin and streptomycin (rarely used today) have produced congenital deafness. It is unclear whether gentamicin has the same potential, but it does produce deafness in some neonates when used at high levels. Careful drug monitoring appears to reduce the likelihood of hearing loss. Some cephalosporins (cefaclor, cephalexin, and cephradine) have been associated with congenital defects, but the association is weak. Most other antibiotics appear to be safe for use during pregnancy, including acyclovir.

• **Prostaglandin synthase inhibitors.** Aspirin, ibuprofen, and naproxen may cause in utero closure of the ductus arteriosus in rare cases and probably should be avoided if possible. Indomethacin has been used frequently as a tocolytic agent and is also reported to produce ductal closure, but appears to be reasonably safe with careful fetal monitoring. These drugs do not appear to be teratogens, however. Platelet aggregation is also reduced by many of these agents and may increase the potential for bleeding.

• **Alcohol.** Fetal alcohol syndrome may occur with even minimal ingestion of alcohol. Symptoms include mental retardation, craniofacial abnormalities, and growth failure. Fetal alcohol syndrome contains many of the same features as full fetal alcohol syndrome but with fewer physical stigmata.

• **Narcotics.** The use of narcotics results in significant problems for the neonate, of which the most classic is neonatal drug withdrawal. Withdrawal typically begins in the immediate newborn period and lasts for days to weeks. With some narcotics, such as methadone, withdrawal may not be seen for several days. There appears to be an increased risk of abortion, prematurity, and growth failure in babies of mothers who use narcotics.

• **Cocaine.** Cocaine use appears to result in a higher risk of abortion and stillbirth. Birth weight is generally slightly lower than normal, and there is an increased risk of prematurity. Microcephaly does occur in rare instances with cocaine use during pregnancy. Fetal infarction to various organs may also occur and lead to bowel atresia, porencephaly from cerebral infarcts, and limb maldevelopment.

• **Smoking.** Exposure to cigarette smoke in utero reduces birth weight by an average of 300 grams if the mother consistently smokes throughout gestation. The risk of apnea and sudden infant death syndrome (SIDS) is increased. The incidence of abruptio placenta also increases.

Although this list is relatively complete for many of the drugs known to produce significant fetal problems, the practitioner should always review the most recent medical literature for any updates that might reflect changes in awareness of potential risks of drugs during pregnancy. As was demonstrated by the maternal DES story, the full teratogenic potential of some medications may not be known for many years and may not appear until the next generation.

42. Which drugs should be used with caution in nursing mothers?

The amount of drug that enters breast milk is rarely more than 1–2% of the maternal dose. In general, the level is so trivial that it can be ignored because the effects on the neonate are negligible. Some medications, however, should be used with caution:

Lithium	Cyclosporine	Methotrexate
Tetracycline	Cyclophosphamide	Sulfonamides in the first week of life

Most other medications do not concentrate sufficiently in breast milk and cause few neonatal problems, even those such as narcotics or anticonvulsants, which cause significant damage during fetal stages.

BIBLIOGRAPHY

1. Ananth CV, Berkowitz GS, Savitz DA, Lapinski RH: Placental abruption and adverse perinatal outcome. JAMA 17:1646–1651, 1999.
2. Ananth CV, Savitz DA, Luther ER: Maternal cigarette smoking as a risk factor for placental abruption, placental previa and uterine bleeding in a pregnancy. Am J Epidemiol 144:881–887, 1996.
3. Banks BA, Cnaan A, Morgan MA, et al, and North American Thyrotropin-Releasing Hormone Study Group: Multiple courses of antenatal steroids and the outcome of premature neonates. Am J Obstet Gynecol 181:709–717, 1999.
4. The Canadian Early and Mid-trimester Amniocentesis Trial (CEMAT) Group: Randomised trial to assess safety and fetal outcome of early and mid-trimester amniocentesis. Lancet 351:242–247, 1998.
5. Clarke SL: Placenta previa and abruptio placenta. In Creasy RK, Resink R (eds): Maternal-Fetal Medicine. Philadelphia, W.B. Saunders, 1999, pp 616–631.
6. El-Sayed YY, Holbrook RH Jr, Gibson R, et al: Diltiazem for maintenance tocolysis of preterm labor: Comparison to nifedipine in a randomized trial. J Maternal Fetal Med 7:217–221, 1998.
7. El-Sayed YY, Riley ET, Holbrook RH Jr, et al: Randomized comparison of nitroglycerin and magnesium sulfate for treatment of preterm labor. Obstet Gynecol 93:79–83, 1999.
8. Farine D, Peisner DB, Timor-Tritch IE: Placenta previa: Is the traditional diagnostic approach satisfactory? J Clin Ultrasound 18:328, 1990.
9. Ghidini A, Salafia CM, Minior VK: Repeated courses of steroids in preterm membrane rupture do not increase the risk of histologic chorioamnionitis. Am J Perinatol 14:309–313, 1997.
10. Goldenberg RL, Andrews WW, Guerrant RL, et al: The preterm prediction study: Cervical lactoferrin concentration, other markers of lower genital tract infection, and preterm birth. National Institute of Child Health and Human Development Maternal-Fetal Medicine Units Network. Am J Obstet Gynecol 182:631–635, 2000.
11. Goldenberg RL, Andrews WW, Mercer BM, et al: The preterm prediction study: Granulocyte colony-stimulating factor and spontaneous preterm birth. National Institute of Child Health and Human Development Maternal-Fetal Units Network. Am J Obstet Gynecol 182:625–630, 2000.

12. Goldenberg RL, Iams JD, Das A, et al: The preterm prediction study: Sequential cervical length and fetal fibronectin testing for the prediction of spontaneous preterm birth. National Institute of Child Health and Human Development Maternal-Fetal Medicine Units Network. Am J Obstet Gynecol 182:636–643, 2000.

13. Guinn DA, Goepfert AR, Owen J, et al: Terbutaline pump maintenance therapy for prevention of preterm delivery: A double blind trial. Am J Obstet Gynecol 179:874–878, 1998.

14. Hamersley SL, Landy HJ, O'Sullivan MJ: Fetal bradycardia secondary to magnesium sulfate therapy for preterm labor. A case report. J Reprod Med 43:206–210, 1998.

15. Hammerman C, Glaser J, Kaplan M, et al: Indomethacin tocolysis increases postnatal patent ductus arteriosus severity. Pediatrics 102:E56, 1998.

16. Heine RP, McGregor JA, Dullien VK: Accuracy of salivary estriol testing compared to traditional risk factor assessment in predicting preterm birth. Am J Obstet Gynecol 180:5214–5218, 1999.

17. Huang WL, Beazley LD, Quinlivan JA, et al: Effect of corticosteroids on brain growth in fetal sheep. Obstet Gynecol 94:213–218, 1999.

18. Joffe GM, Jacques D, Bernis-Heys R, et al: Impact of the fetal fibronectin assay on admissions for preterm labor. Am J Obstet Gynecol 180:581–586, 1999.

19. Konje JC, Walley RJ: Bleeding in late pregnancy. In James DK, Steer PJ, Weiner CP, Gonik B (eds): High Risk Pregnancy: Management Options. Philadelphia, W.B. Saunders, 1994, pp 119–136.

20. Medical Research Council: An assessment of the hazards of amniocentesis. Br J Obstet Gynaecol 85:1–41, 1978.

21. Morales WJ, Dickey SS, Bornick P, Lim DV: Change in antibiotic resistance of group B streptococcus: Impact on intrapartum management. Am J Obstet Gynecol 181:310–314, 1999.

22. National Institutes of Child Health and Human Development National Registry for Amniocentesis Study Group: Amniocentesis for prenatal diagnosis: Safety and accuracy. JAMA 236:1471–1476, 1976.

23. Pearlman MD, Pierson CL, Faix RG: Frequent resistance of clinical group B streptococci isolates to clindamycin and erythromycin. Obstet Gynecol 92:258–261, 1998.

24. Ramsay PA, Fisk NM: Amniocentesis. In James DK, Steer PJ, Weiner CP, Gonik B (eds): High Risk Pregnancy: Management Options. Philadelphia, W.B. Saunders, 1994, pp 19–136.

25. Sameshima H, Ikenoue T, Kamitomo M, Sakamoto H: Effects of 4 hours magnesium sulfate infusion on fetal heart rate variability and reactivity in a goat model. Am J Perinatol 15:535–538, 1998.

26. Sanchez-Ramos L, Kaunitz AM, Gaudier FL, Delke I: Efficacy of maintenance therapy after acute tocolysis: A meta-analysis. Am J Obstet Gynecol 181:484–490, 1999.

27. Schorr SJ, Ascarelli MH, Rust OA, et al: A comparative study of ketorolac (Toradol) and magnesium sulfate for arrest of preterm labor. South Med J 91:1028–1032, 1998.

28. Schuchat A, Whitney C, Zangwill K: Prevention of perinatal group B streptococcal disease: A public health perspective. MMWR Morb Mortal Wkly Rep 45:1–24, 1996.

29. Scioscia AL: Prenatal genetic diagnosis. In Creasy RK, Resink R (eds): Maternal-Fetal Medicine. Philadelphia, W.B. Saunders, 1999, pp 735–744.

30. Simpson NE, Dallaire L, Miller JR, et al: Prenatal diagnosis of genetic disease in Canada: Report of a collaborative study. Can Med Assoc J 115:739–746, 1976.

31. Sundberg K, Bang J, Smidt-Jensen S, et al: Randomised study of risk of fetal loss related to early amniocentesis versus chorionic villus sampling. Lancet 350:697–703, 1997.

32. Wenstrom KD, Andrews WW, Hauth JC, et al: Elevated second-trimester amniotic fluid interleukin-6 levels predict preterm delivery. Am J Obstet Gynecol 178:546–550, 1998.

33. Wright JW, Ridgway LE, Wright BD, et al: Effect of $MgSO_4$ on heart rate monitoring in the preterm fetus. J Repro Med 41:605–608, 1996.

3. GENERAL NEONATOLOGY

1. What are Spitzer's laws of neonatology?

1. The more stable a baby appears to be, the more likely he will "crump" that day.

2. The nicer the parents, the sicker the baby.

3. The likelihood of BPD (bronchopulmonary dysplasia) is directly proportional to the number of physicians involved in the care of that baby.

4. The longer a patient is discussed on rounds, the more certain it is that no one has the faintest idea of what's going on or what to do.

5. The sickest infant in the nursery can always be discerned by the fact that she is being cared for by the newest, most inexperienced nursing orientee.

6. The surest way to have an infant linger interminably is to inform the parents that death is imminent.

7. The more miraculous the "save," the more likely that you'll be sued for something totally inconsequential.

8. If they're not breathin', they may be seizin'.

9. Antibiotics should always be continued for _____ days. (Fill in the blank with any number from 1 to 21)

10. If you can't figure out what's going on with a baby, call the surgeons. They won't figure it out either, but they'll sure as hell do something about it.

From Spitzer A: Spitzer's laws of neonatology. Clin Pediatr 20:733, 1981, with permission.

2. How does the handling of the umbilical cord at birth affect neonatal hemoglobin concentrations?

At the time of birth, the placental vessels may contain up to 33% of the fetal-placental blood volume. Constriction of the umbilical arteries limits blood flow from the infant, but, if there is perinatal hypoxemia, the vessels may remain somewhat dilated for a period and blood may be pumped away from the infant. The umbilical vein remains dilated, and the the extent of drainage from the placenta to the infant via the umbilical vein is dependent on gravity. The recommendation is to keep the baby at least 20 cm below the placenta for approximately 30 seconds before clamping the cord. More elevated positioning or rapid clamping can minimize the placental transfusion and decrease red cell volume. The old practice of "stripping the cord," still used by some obstetricians, is best avoided. It only makes the baby plethoric, and we have had to perform partial exchange transfusions on a number of infants treated in this manner.

3. Describe the best method of umbilical cord care in the immediate neonatal period.

No single method of cord care has been determined to be superior in preventing colonization and infections. Antimicrobial agents such as bacitracin or triple dye are commonly used. Alcohol accelerates drying of the cord, but it has not been shown to reduce the rates of colonization or omphalitis.

Parents (and especially grandparents) often ask if there is any way to determine whether their child will have an "innie" or an "outie" belly-button when the cord ultimately does fall off. It is best to leave such discussions to the great philosophers, but taping quarters or half-dollars over the umbilicus will definitely not influence the outcome. To date, there have been no studies looking at whether the new gold dollar coin will prove more effective in this regard.

4. Which way does the umbilical cord twist?

Usually counterclockwise. Coiling of the umbilical cord occurs in approximately 95% of newborns, and most are twisted in a sinistral manner. Because this helical arrangement is absent in species in which fetuses are arranged longitudinally in a bicornuate uterus, spiraling may result from the mobility of the primary fetus. Noncoiled cords may be associated with an increased likelihood of anomalies.

5. When should a parent begin to worry if an umbilical cord has not fallen off?

The umbilical cord generally dries up and sloughs by 2 weeks of life. Delayed separation can be normal up to 45 days. Because neutrophilic and/or monocytic infiltrations appear to play a major role in autodigestion, however, persistence of the cord beyond 30 days should prompt consideration of an underlying functional abnormality of neutrophils (leukocyte adhesion deficiency) or neutropenia.

6. What are some good sites for venous access in the neonate?

The neonate is not so difficult to get blood from as one thinks. In addition to the peripheral sites shown in the figure below, access to the central circulation through the umbilical vessels is a great advantage. The increased use of percutaneous lines has also helped a great deal in recent years, although one must be cautious of infection with the prolonged use of indwelling lines in neonates.

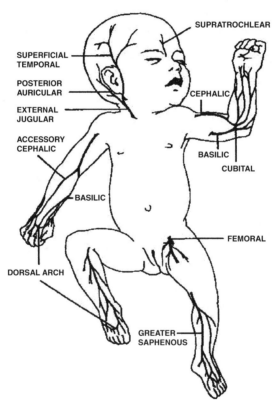

Sites for venous access in neonates. (From Bollinger E, Karp T, Ruth-Sanchez V, et al: Nursing care. In Goldsmith JP, Karotkin EH (eds): Assisted Ventilation of the Neonate. Philadelphia, W.B. Saunders, 1996, p 128, with permission.)

7. How do you estimate the insertion distance necessary for umbilical catheters?

Measuring the distance from the umbilicus to the shoulder (lateral end of clavicle) allows an estimation of the desired length.

Insertion Distance for Umbilical Catheters

SHOULDER TO UMBILICUS (cm)	AORTIC CATHETER TO DIAPHRAGM (cm)	AORTIC CATHETER TO AORTIC BIFURCATION (cm)	VENOUS CATHETER TO RIGHT ATRIUM (cm)
9	11	5	6
10	12	5	6–7
11	13	6	7
12	14	7	8
13	15	8	8–9
14	16	9	9
15	17	10	10
16	18	10–11	11
17	20	11–12	11–12

Adapted from Dunn PM: Localization of umbilical catheters by post mortem measurement. Arch Dis Child 41:69, 1966.

8. What are the risks of umbilical catheters?
Short-term risks
• Perforation and development of retroperitoneal hemorrhage (umbilical artery [UA] catheter)
• Decreased femoral pulses and blanching of limbs and/or buttocks (UA catheter)
• Accidental hemorrhage (both UA and umbilical vein [UV] catheters)
• Infection (both UA and UV catheters)
• Cardiac rhythm disturbances (usually UV catheters, if catheter enters the right atrium)
• Hemopericardium (extremely rare, usually right atrial perforation from UV catheter)
• Air embolus (both UA and UV catheters)
Long-term risks
• Embolization and infarcts (both UA and UV catheters)
• Thrombosis of hepatic vein (UV catheter)
• Liver necrosis (UV catheter)
• Aortic thrombi (UA catheter)
• Renal artery thrombosis (UA catheter)
• Mesenteric thrombosis and necrotizing enterocolitis (UA catheter)
• Infection (both UA and UV catheters)

9. Should palpable lymph nodes in a newborn be considered pathologic?
No. Up to 25% of newborns have palpable nodes, particularly in the inguinal and cervical regions. By 1 month of age, the prevalence is nearly 40%.

10. How loud is the noise inside an infant's isolette? Should you ever pound on the isolette to rouse a child during an apnea spell?
The noise usually ranges from about 50–90 db. With the slamming of an isolette door, the level can approach 100 db. By comparison, room conversation is 60–70 db, and louder rock music is 100–120 db. The American Academy of Pediatrics (AAP) recommends no more than 70 db because (1) > 70 db disrupts or awakens sleeping infants, (2) > 70 db is associated with cardiovascular changes (e.g., increased heart rate), and (3) ototoxicity secondary to use of aminoglycoside antibiotics may be potentiated by constant loud noise. Hence, do not pound the isolette!

11. In infants, why is it dangerous to use an intravenous flush containing benzyl alcohol as a bacteriostatic agent?
In an association first recognized in 1982, intravenous (IV) fluids containing benzyl alcohol can result in central nervous system (CNS) depression, increasing respiratory distress with gasps

(the gasping syndrome), severe metabolic acidosis, thrombocytopenia, hepatic and renal failure, cardiovascular collapse, and death. Benzyl alcohol may also increase the risk of kernicterus by facilitating passage of bilirubin into the CNS. It may be said, "look before you flush."

12. How valuable is the footprinting of newborns for the permanent medical record?
This time-honored tradition is, alas, of minimal benefit. Although the AAP recommended discontinuing the practice in 1983 because of the fact that in nearly 80% the quality was so poor as to render the print useless, up to 80% of U.S. hospitals continue to use footprinting as a means of identification. Of note, footprinting is legally mandated only in New York State. It is highly likely that footprinting will be replaced in the near future by a simple genetic screen done on a drop of blood.

13. What are the most common causes of fetal death?
Chromosomal abnormalities (especially in early pregnancy) and congenital malformations.

14. Is "catch-up" growth good for low–birth-weight infants?
Catch-up growth is a phenomenon often seen in low–birth-weight infants. Because of their intrauterine and subsequent neonatal problems, the growth in both premature and small-for-gestational-age babies is often limited during the first weeks and months of life. Subsequently, they commonly exhibit a rapid growth phase that brings them back to their expected, genetically determined growth potential. Catch-up growth has always been viewed as a relatively important phenomenon associated with good health and recovery from early neonatal problems. Recently, however, a study by Ong and colleagues has suggested that it may be associated with a significantly higher risk of childhood obesity and, potentially, adult obesity with its attendant illnesses—hypertension, diabetes, and heart disease. Our enthusiasm about catch-up growth may need to be tempered if this data holds true in other collaborative investigations.

BRAIN DEATH

15. How is brain death diagnosed in the neonate?
• Absence of a reversible cause (e.g., drugs, hypotension, hypothermia)
• Absence of neocortical function (e.g., spontaneous movements, response to stimuli, and awareness of environment)
• Complete absence of brainstem function (including nonresponsive midposition or fully dilated pupils), no spontaneous or reflexive eye movements on oculovestibular testing (Doll's eyes and calorics), no bulbar function (e.g., corneal, gag, cough, sucking, and rooting reflexes), and absence of respirations
• Examination that remains unchanged over time

16. What other supportive testing is recommended?
• An electroencephalogram (EEG) must be performed to demonstrate electrocerebral silence (ECS).
• Because hypotension, hypothermia (32.2°C for adults), and medications (including phenobarbital level > 25 μg/ml) may suppress the EEG, the patient must have a stable temperature and blood pressure and appropriate drug levels. Absence of cerebral blood flow (by vessel arteriography or radionuclide study) is also supportive of ECS.
• Other tests that may be helpful include transcranial Doppler to demonstrate an absence of intracranial flow and testing for bilateral absence of N20-22 responses.
• Further supportive testing is always recommended in the infant. For example, a child with Guillain-Barré syndrome might mistakenly appear to satisfy the criteria for brain death.

17. What are the technical EEG recommendations for the determination of ECS?
The guidelines published by the American Electroencephalographic Society recommend (1) a minimum of 8 scalp electrodes; (2) interelectrode impedances less than 10,000 ohms, but over

100; (3) testing of the integrity of the entire system by touching each electrode; (4) interelectrode distances of at least 10 cm; (5) sensitivity of at least 2 μV/mm for at least 30 minutes; (6) low frequency filter less than 1 and high frequency filter greater than 30; (7) consideration of artifact from surrounding equipment or monitors; (8) no EEG reactivity to intense somatosensory, auditory, or visual stimuli; (9) recordings made only by a qualified technologist; and (10) repeat EEG if any doubt about ECS.

18. What are the AAP task force recommendations for the duration of observation for infants and children?

The task force recommends that no determination of brain death be made in neonates less than 7 days old. In infants 7 days to 2 months of age, two examinations and EEGs separated by at least 48 hours are recommended. In infants 2 months to 1 year of age, two examinations and EEGs separated by at least 24 hours are recommended. A repeat examination and EEG are not required if cerebral blood flow (CBF) study shows absence of flow. In children older than 1 year, if the cause is irreversible, laboratory testing is not required, and a 12-hour period of observation is recommended. If the condition is potentially reversible (e.g., hypoxic-ischemic encephalopathy), then at least a 24-hour period of observation is recommended.

19. Why is there an exception for the first week of life?

The most controversial group is the youngest, and the task force recommends that the "determination of brain death not be made in neonates less than 1 week of age." Very young infants are different because they have lower CBF and oxygen requirements and greater cranial compliance. The lower blood flow requirements may explain why some neonates may transiently demonstrate EEG activity in the face of no discernable cerebral blood flow. Indeed, retrospective review of preterm and term infants less than 1 month of age showed that EEG or radionuclide study confirmed the clinical criteria for brain death in only one-half to two-thirds of patients. Even though the determination of brain death cannot be made formally in neonates less than 7 days old, retrospective review of the validity of brain death criteria suggests that if all clinical criteria are fulfilled, the chance of neurologic survival is nil.

20. What are the ethical, religious, and legal concerns about the formulation of brain death criteria for infants and children?

The Ad Hoc Committee of the Harvard Medical School to Examine the Definition of Brain Death considered that their task in 1968 was to define a new criterion for death. They perceived a conflict arising from the ability, on the one hand, to support the heart and lungs indefinitely and the potential for organ transplantation on the other. Individual and societal concerns regarding the determination of brain death include the possibility of diagnostic error and the conceptual difficulty of a definition of death, the mind-body question. In a 1957 address, "The Prolongation of Life," Pope Pius XII stated that it was not "within the competence of the church," but was rather that of the physician to make the determination of death. Legislation and court rulings in the United States have concluded that it is lawful for the medical profession to diagnose brain death according to their own established criteria. It is the responsibility and the right of the physician to make the determination of death by the absence of either cardiac or cerebral activity.

FOLLOWUP OF THE PRETERM INFANT

21. How does one calculate adjusted (corrected) age? When is it appropriate to use this calculation instead of chronologic age?

Chronologic age – number of weeks born prematurely = adjusted age

For example, a preterm infant of 32-weeks' gestational age (GA) at 6 months' chronologic age has an adjusted age of 4 months. Adjusted age is used for plotting growth parameters and for assessing developmental milestones until 2½–3 years of age.

22. What is the typical daily caloric requirement needed to promote optimal growth in a healthy preterm infant and in a preterm infant with chronic lung disease?

A healthy infant requires 110–130 kcal/kg/day, and a preterm infant with chronic lung disease requires 120–150 kcal/kg/day.

23. What should be considered in the differential for a preterm infant who presents to the office with ongoing problems with inadequate oral intake?

Hypoxia

Oral-motor dysfunction

Gastroesophageal reflux (GER)

Upper airway compromise

Chronic microaspiration

Chronic lung disease

Mechanical: feedings not flowing adequately through nipple or inappropriate nipple for child's sucking abilities (e.g., using a fast-flowing nipple for a child with a strong suck, which may result in child trying to limit formula flow to avoid choking)

Caregiver limiting volume of formula offered

24. What are the guidelines for scheduling routine immunizations of preterm infants?

Preterm infants should be immunized according to the guidelines developed by the AAP Advisory Committee on Immunization Practices. Immunizations should be given according to chronologic age.

25. Which additional inoculations beyond those given routinely should be considered for the preterm infant?

Influenza vaccine and palivizumab (Synagis).

Influenza should be given each fall to preterm infants with chronic lung disease (CLD) so long as their chronologic age is more than 6 months. Other family members and caretakers should be immunized as well. The first year that a child is immunized, 2 doses are given, 1 month apart. During subsequent years, if still necessary, only 1 dose is required.

RSV prophylaxis (Synagis) is given intramuscularly monthly throughout the respiratory syncytial virus (RSV) season to the following categories of infants:

• Chronic lung disease in a child of less than 2 years' chronologic age who required medical therapy for CLD within 6 months before the onset of RSV season.

• Preterm infants without CLD as follows:

GESTATIONAL AGE (GA)	CHRONOLOGIC AGE AT START OF RSV SEASON
< 28 weeks	Until 12 months
29–32 weeks	Until 6 months
32–35 weeks	Until 6 months*

* Only if additional risk factors exist, e.g., exposure to smoke, attendance at day care, one of a multiple birth, or other siblings at home.

26. What visual abnormalities are common sequelae of mild-to-moderate stages of retinopathy of prematurity?

Refractive errors, strabismus, and amblyopia are the most common abnormalities.

27. What is the incidence of cerebral palsy in the low–birth-weight (< 1500 gm) population?

The incidence of cerebral palsy in the low–birth-weight population is 7–8%.

28. What is the most common type of cerebral palsy seen in this population?

Spastic diplegia (legs affected more than upper extremities) is the most common. Most of the children with cerebral palsy are affected to a mild–moderate degree and are ambulatory.

Hemiplegia is seen less commonly, most frequently in an infant with a history of a lateralizing brain insult (e.g., unilateral periventricular leukomalacia [PVL] with cysts, infarct, unilateral grade 4 intraventricular hemorrhage [IVH]).

29. Why should the diagnosis of mild or moderate cerebral palsy usually be delayed until after 12–18 months?

Preterm infants frequently exhibit mild tonal abnormalities in the first year of life that are transient in nature and gradually resolve by 12-18 months' adjusted age. However, cerebral palsy can be diagnosed earlier if there are significant abnormalities on the neurologic examination that correlate with a known CNS insult during the neonatal period.

30. What is the most common risk factor for cerebral palsy in the preterm infant?

PVL with white matter damage (WMD). WMD encompasses various pathologic entities that tend to target developing white matter. PVL involves either unilateral or bilateral focal necrosis in the periventricular region, sometimes resulting in multiple small cavities or cysts. Other forms of WMD include porencephalic cysts and ischemic or hemorrhagic infarctions.

31. What is the difference between developmental delay and mental retardation?

The term *developmental delay* is used for all preschoolers who exhibit any degree of delay. It is the preferred term for younger children because it does not indicate that the delay will be permanent. The diagnosis of mental retardation (MD) is restricted to children (and later adults) who demonstrate delays based on standardized assessments of intelligence and adaptive skills. MR is generally not used until the child approaches school age and it is apparent that the delays are not transient.

32. How do infants less than 24 weeks' gestation fare developmentally?

Infants less than 24 weeks' gestation are at high risk for delay. The incidence of sensory impairment, specifically visual impairment, occurs in 25–30%. Approximately 30% of infants will have mental retardation, some of whom will be multihandicapped. Approximately 30% show mild lags in learning and learning disabilities. Roughly a third, however, do well developmentally.

33. At what age are early intervention services available for children? What are the indications for and the laws that govern referral?

Early intervention services are available from birth. Federal Law 99-457 has mandated that each state provide therapeutic and educational services for affected children from childbirth through 2 years, 11 months. Eligibility varies from state to state but typically includes developmental delays greater than 25–33% of the child's age. In some states, a child is eligible because of an "at risk status," i.e., by virtue of a medical diagnosis that places the child at risk for a delay.

34. How does one counsel a family about the probable outcome for a preterm infant weighing less than 1500 grams in terms of major disabilities or school-related problems?

The healthy 1500-gm infant is likely to be free of major disabilities. Progress in school should be monitored closely to detect the presence of learning disabilities. The lower the birth weight of the child, the higher the illness indexes and the higher the risk for more significant delay.

35. What are some of the school-age sequelae of prematurity that can be seen despite the achievement of normal IQ?

It has been documented that even low–birth-weight children with IQs in the normal range make greater use of special education services than full-term infants. Such services address learning disabilities, attention deficit disorder, and academic delays.

36. What are some of the possible stresses experienced by the family of a preterm infant after hospital discharge?

The stresses are more dramatic for families of infants with ongoing medical issues and home care needs than for families of healthy preterm infants. The following are some common stresses:

1. Insecurity with parenting abilities
2. Marital stress and possible discord
3. Bonding and attachment issues due to prolonged hospitalization
4. Financial stress, especially when there is a loss of income because one parent needs to remain home with the infant
5. Inadequate or lack of insurance coverage for home care needs, e.g., nursing, equipment, special formulas and therapies
6. Isolation, reduced contact with family and friends due to concerns about exposure to infection (especially during winter months)
7. Resentment felt by siblings because of parent's attention and time spent with new infant

CIRCUMCISION

37. Is there a benefit to male circumcision in the newborn period?

Potential medical benefits of male circumcision include a possible reduction in the incidence of urinary tract infection, penile cancer, and sexually transmitted disease.

38. Are there risks to male circumcision?
- Complications occur in approximately 0.2–0.6% of cases.
- The most frequent complication of bleeding is seen in about 0.1% of circumcisions.
- Infection, recurrent phimosis, urinary retention, meatitis, metal stenosis, chordee, wound separation, inclusion cysts, and unsatisfactory cosmesis have been reported.
- Other rare complications include scalded skin syndrome, necrotizing fasciitis, sepsis and meningitis, urethral fistula, partial amputation of the glans penis, and penile necrosis.

39. What are the 5 Ms of circumcision?

Cultural, religious, and ethnic traditions, in addition to medical factors, may influence parents to request male circumcision of their newborn. A useful mnemonic is the **5 Ms: M**oses, **M**ohammad, **M**other, **M**oney, and **M**edicine. Both Jewish and Muslim religions routinely circumcise males. The rate of circumcision has been directly linked to the maternal socioeconomic group. In many instances, parents choose to have their son circumcised because the father is circumcised. Newborn circumcision can certainly generate a medical bill. Finally, there are occasional medical indications for circumcision, such as recurrent balanitis or secondary phimosis.

40. What are the current recommendations for circumcision in the newborn male?

According to the 1999 American Academy of Pediatrics Task Force Policy Statement, the benefits of circumcision are not compelling enough to recommend it as a routine procedure.

41. Is analgesia for circumcision necessary?

It is essential that pain relief be provided to newborns undergoing circumcision. Considerable evidence shows that newborns who undergo circumcision without analgesia experience pain and stress, which are measured by changes in heart rate, blood pressure, oxygen saturation, and cortisol levels. Furthermore, lack of analgesia for circumcision may influence later responses to pain.

42. What analgesia should be used for circumcision?
- Application of 1–2 gm of eutectic mixture of local anesthetics (EMLA) to the distal half of the penis. EMLA, which contains 2.5% lidocaine and 2.5% pilocaine, lessens pain if applied 60–90 minutes before the procedure.
- The dorsal penile nerve block is effective in reducing the behavioral and physiologic indicators of pain. A 27-gauge needle is used to inject the 0.4 ml of 1% lidocaine at both the 10- and 12-o'clock positions at the base of the penis. Peak concentrations are achieved at 60 minutes. Bruising at the site is the most frequent complication.

- A subcutaneous ring block of 0.8 ml of 1% lidocaine without epinephrine administered at the midshaft of the penis has also been effective in reducing a pain response.
- The administration of sucrose on a pacifier or acetaminophen is insufficient for the operative pain.

CATHETERIZATION AND INTUBATION

43. Is there a good way to sample blood from a small vein?
- Apply a tourniquet, and clean the skin over the site.
- Puncture the vein with a small needle or catheter in the opposite direction of venous flow (i.e., opposite of usual venous cannulation). When blood is seen, release the tourniquet. In this way, blood flows toward the needle and is not occluded by the needle.
- Attach a syringe and gently aspirate the blood.

44. How is a peripheral artery cannulated percutaneously?
- Locate the artery to be cannulated. Arteries in the extremity can be visualized with a trans-illuminator. If the scalp is used, shave the area, palpate the artery, and place the index finger over the artery, compressing it with a side-to-side rolling motion to push tissue fluid aside.
- Clean the skin using Betadine solution and alcohol swab.
- Insert a 24-gauge or 22-gauge angiocatheter slowly (aiming at the artery in the direction against the arterial blood flow at an angle as parallel to the skin as possible) until a "give" is felt.
- When blood is observed in the lumen of the catheter, hold the stylet and advance the catheter farther into the artery. Withdraw the stylet.
- Attach the tubing with a three-way stopcock prefilled with heparinized normal saline or 5% dextrose in water (D5W).
- Aspirate blood and repeatedly flush the catheter and tubing with 0.05 ml aliquots
- Tape the catheter securely in place with Tegaderm and tape. Leave the skin over the tip of the catheter exposed to enable observation of blanching, discoloration, or induration.

45. How is nasotracheal intubation done?
- Suction the nasal cavity, mouth, and stomach.
- Position the infant supine with the intubator at the head end of the infant.
- Place the infant's head in the "sniffing" position (i.e., the head slightly extended with the jaw thrust forward). Flexion of the neck is not required because of the neonate's occipital prominence.
- Use an oxyscope (a laryngoscope with a built-in oxygen port), or tape a catheter to the top of the laryngoscope blade (Miller #0) and connect to oxygen flow at 2–3 lpm to provide oxygen supplementation during laryngoscopy to prevent hypoxia.
- Select the endotracheal tube (2.5-mm inside diameter [ID], 3.0-mm ID, and 3.5-mm ID for < 1000-gm, 1000–2000-gm, and > 2000-gm infants, respectively), and mark the length of insertion with tape according the the chart that follows (see next page).
- A right-handed person should hold the laryngoscope in the left hand and insert the right thumb and forefinger into the mouth to open it. Insert the blade in the right side of the mouth and move the blade to the midline, keeping the tongue to the left of the blade. Place the tip of the blade in the valecula and lift the blade superiorly with a motion from the shoulder. Do not bend the wrist, because this causes a levering motion, forcing the blade against the gum and pushing the larynx anteriorly out of the line of vision. As the blade is lifted, the larynx should be visualized.
- Lubricate the outside of the endotracheal tube with Surgilube, and gently advance through the nose with steady pressure perpendicular to the floor. If the tube fails to pass, it is usually because of an incorrect direction rather than a small nostril. A 5-Fr feeding tube inserted into the nostril can serve as a guide.

- Once the tube is seen in the oropharynx, insert the alligator forceps under direct vision from the right side of the mouth. The tube is grasped with the alligator forceps, 1 cm proximal to the tip, and gently inserted through the vocal cords and advanced until the premarked tape is at the nare. If the tube passes the cords but cannot be advanced, it is usually because of hyperextension of the neck, not because the tube is too big. The tube will generally pass when the head is flexed.
- Once the tube is in place, ventilate the patient. Check the position of the tube by auscultation over the stomach and both axillary areas, looking for mist inside the tube, chest wall excursion, and improvement in oxygenation.
- Secure the tube.
- Obtain a stat chest roentgenogram with the infant's head in the neutral position to check the tube position. The tip should be 1 cm above the carina for < 1000-gm infants and 2 cm for > 2000-gm infants.

CROWN HEEL LENGTH (cm)	NASOTRACHEAL LENGTH (cm)
30	6.50
32	7.00
34	7.50
36	8.00
38	8.25
40	8.75
42	9.25
44	9.50
46	10.00
48	10.25
50	10.50
52	11.00
54	11.50
56	12.00
58	12.50

Adapted from Coldiron JS: Estimation of nasotracheal tube length in neonates. Pediatrics 41:823–828, 1968.

46. How is endotracheal tube suctioning performed?

1. Check that wall suction is in working order. The suction pressure should be 100–200 cm H_2O.
2. Increase oxygen by 20%. If the intermittent mechanical ventilation (IMV) rate is < 20/min, increase to 20/min.
3. Disconnect the respirator between the endotracheal tube and the connector.
4. Instill a few drops of normal saline into the endotracheal tube for lubrication. If secretions are loose, normal saline is not needed.
5. If necessary, reconnect the infant to the respirator and ventilate several times until oxygen saturation recovers.
6. Don disposable sterile gloves. Handle the sterile part of the catheter with the gloved hand only.
7. Turn the infant's head to one side (to the right to suction left main bronchus and to the left to suction right main bronchus).
8. Disconnect the respirator as in step 3.
9. Insert the suction catheter quickly but gently. The depth of catheter insertion should be the endotracheal tube length plus 3 cm, 4 cm, or 5 cm for an infant weighing < 1000 gm, 1000–2000 gm, or > 2000 gm, respectively. Use a 6.0-Fr suction catheter for a 2.5-mm ID endotracheal tube and 8.0-Fr catheter for a 3.0-mm or 3.5-mm ID endotracheal tube.

10. Close the suction catheter's vent with a finger intermittently, and withdraw the catheter while twisting it slightly. Keep suction time as short as possible.

11. Ventilate the infant for 10–30 seconds using a bag capable of supplying 100% oxygen attached directly to the endotracheal tube. Allow sufficient time for the oxygen saturation to recover.

12. Turn the head to the other side. Disconnect the respirator as in step 3, repeat suction is in steps 9 and 10, and then reconnect the respirator. (*Note:* If the saturation remains depressed, remove the infant from the ventilator, and ventilate the infant with a bag as in step 11.)

13. Change chest position after suctioning.

14. Decrease oxygen and IMV rate to presuction settings.

47. How should a chest tube be placed in the newborn infant?

1. Place the infant in a semisupine position with the side for chest tube placement facing up; restrain and give appropriate sedation.

2. The site for chest tube placement is at the third (usually at the nipple level) or fourth intercostal space in the anterior axillary line for evacuation of the pneumothorax and in the posterior axillary line to drain pleural effusion.

3. Prepare the skin with Betadine solution, and drape the area.

4. Use 1% xylocaine for local anesthesia.

5. Use a no. 11 surgical blade to make a small incision, not larger than the outside diameter of the chest tube, through the full thickness of the skin.

6. Premeasure the length of the chest tube to be inserted from the intended placement site to the sternal notch.

7. Insert the tip of 10-Fr chest tube with trocar (Argyle, Sherwood, St. Louis, MO) through the skin until the pleural "pop" is felt. Hold the trocar and advance the chest tube to the premeasured length.

8. Withdraw the trocar and connect the chest tube to Pleur-evac (Deknatel, Inc., Fall River, MA). Apply continuous suction at 10 cm H_2O.

9. Observe for respiratory fluctuations in the water-seal chamber indicating that the tube is patent and in the pleural cavity.

10. Secure the tube with air-tight dressing (Vaseline gauze) and tapes (Tegaderm by 3M Health Care, St. Paul, MN, and airproof tape), leaving adequate chest exposure for observation of chest wall excursion.

11. Obtain a chest roentgenogram immediately after the tube is secured to confirm the chest tube position.

BIBLIOGRAPHY

1. The Ad Hoc Committee of the Harvard Medical School to Examine the Definition of Brain Death: A definition of irreversible coma. JAMA 205:337–340, 1968.
2. American Academy of Pediatrics: Circumcision policy statement. Pediatrics 103:686–693, 1999.
3. Ashwal S: Brain death in the newborn. Pediatrics 84:429–437, 1989.
4. Bamji M, et al: Palpable lymph nodes in healthy newborns and infants. Pediatrics 78:573–575, 1986.
5. Beresford HR: Brain death. Neurol Clin 17:295–306, 1999.
6. Bollinger E, Karp T, Ruth-Sanchez V, et al: Nursing care. In Goldsmith JP, Karotkin EH (eds): Assisted Ventilation of the Neonate. Philadelphia, W.B. Saunders, 1996, p 128.
7. Coldiron JS: Estimation of nasotracheal tube length in neonates. Pediatrics 41:423–828, 1968.
8. Committee on Environmental Hazards: Noise pollution: Neonatal aspects. Pediatrics 54:483–486, 1974.
9. Dunn PM: Localization of umbilical catheters by post mortem measurement. Arch Dis Child 41:69, 1966.
10. Fishman MA: Validity of brain death criteria in infants. Pediatrics 96(3 Pt 1):513–515, 1995.
11. Guideline Three: Minimum technical standards for EEG recording in suspected cerebral death. J Clin Neurophys 11:10–13, 1994.
12. Kemp AS, Lubitz L: Delayed cord separation in alloimmune neutropenia. Arch Dis Child 68:52–53, 1993.
13. Ong KKL, Ahmed ML, Emmett PM, et al: Association between postnatal catch-up growth and obesity in childhood: Prospective cohort study. BMJ 320:967–971, 2000.

14. Peter G (ed): 1997 Red Book: Report of the Committee on Infectious Diseases, 24th ed. Elk Grove Village, IL, American Academy of Pediatrics, 1997.
15. Pius XII: The prolongation of life. Pope Speaks 4:393–398, 1958.
16. President's Commission for the Study of Ethical Problems in Medicine and Biomedical and Behavioral Research: Guidelines for the determination of death. JAMA 246:2184–2186, 1981.
17. Report of Special Task Force: Guidelines for the determination of brain death in children. Pediatrics 80:298–300, 1987.
18. Spitzer A: Spitzer's laws of neonatology. Clin Pediatr 20:733, 1981.
19. Strong TH, et al: Antepartum diagnosis of noncoiled umbilical cords. Am J Obstet Gynecol 170:1729–1733, 1994.

4. CARDIOLOGY

HISTORY

1. What is the ductus of Botallo?

Leonardo Botallo was an Italian surgeon working at the French royal court in the 16th century. Perhaps because of a too superficial interpretation of Botallo's text, his name became attached to the ductus arteriosus that had already been described in the 2nd century by Galeno. In fact, in his *Opera Cinema*, Botallo aimed to show that blood passes by means of a "duct" between the right and left atria. Therefore, he actually described the foramen ovale.

PHYSIOLOGIC VARIABLES IN FETAL AND PERINATAL LIFE

2. What three shunts are present in the fetal circulation?

1. Ductus venous: allows placental blood flow to bypass the liver
2. Fossa ovalis: allows venous return to bypass the right heart
3. Patent ductus arteriosus: allows right ventricular blood to bypass the pulmonary circulation

3. How is the systemic venous return directed in fetal circulation?

Oxygenated blood from the placenta is preferentially directed from the inferior vena cava toward the fossa ovalis by a venous valve located at the junction of the inferior vena cava (IVC) and the right atrium. As a result, blood entering the left side of the heart and supplying the head vessels is relatively well oxygenated. Superior vena caval blood is preferentially directed through the right atrium to the right ventricle and from there to the ductus arteriosus and the descending aorta. Thus, the fetal heart and brain are perfused with more highly oxygenated blood than the abdomen and lower extremities.

4. Why does the fossa ovalis close shortly after birth?

The fossa ovalis is comprised of the septum primum overlying the septum secundum in the left atrium. In fetal life, right atrial pressure is greater than left atrial pressure; thus the septum primum is held open and there is a right-to-left shunt. Once pulmonary blood flow increases following birth, left atrial pressure rises with the marked increase in pulmonary venous return. The increase causes the septum primum to flatten against the septum secundum, closing the fossa ovalis.

5. What are the determinants of pulmonary vascular resistance (PVR)? How does PVR change after birth?

$$\text{Total PVR} = \frac{\text{Pulmonary artery pressure}}{\text{Pulmonary blood flow}}$$

In fetal life, PVR is is high and falls initially as the nonmuscular pulmonary arteries dilate and small muscular arteries are recruited into the circulation. PVR continues to fall as the arterial wall thins and remodels, leading to normal PVR by age 6–8 weeks.

6. What is the most important determinant of cardiac output in the neonate?

$$\text{Cardiac output} = \text{Heart rate} \times \text{Stroke volume}$$

Stroke volume is relatively fixed by low ventricular compliance and a high degree of ventricular inotropy secondary to the stress of birth. Thus, heart rate is an important determinant of cardiac output in the neonate.

NONINVASIVE ASSESSMENT OF VENTRICULAR FUNCTION
AND PULMONARY HYPERTENSION

7. Name three scenarios in which a right-to-left shunt is seen in the ductus arteriosus.

1. A right-to-left shunt in the ductus can be seen in a normal newborn within the first 24 hours of life. Usually, this right-to-left shunt occurs in early systole and is brief in duration.

2. Infants with left heart obstructive lesions such as coarctation of the aorta, interrupted aortic arch, or hypoplastic left heart syndrome typically have a right-to-left ductal shunt in systole and a left-to-right shunt beginning in late systole and extending through diastole. The right-to-left shunt in this scenario helps to bypass the region of obstruction and supplies the systemic circulation with blood.

3. Infants with a high pulmonary vascular resistance (i.e., persistent pulmonary hypertension of the newborn or congenital heart disease complicated by severe elevation of pulmonary vascular resistance) tend to have continuous right-to-left flow in the ductus arteriosus.

8. Is right-to-left shunting through a foramen ovale diagnostic of pulmonary artery hypertension?

No. Shunting at the atrial level is determined by the relative compliance of the two ventricles. If the right ventricle is noncompliant or stiff, there is often a right-to-left shunt or bidirectional flow across the foramen ovale. Infants with pulmonary artery hypertension usually, but not always, have right-to-left shunting at the atrial level. Patients with certain types of congenital heart disease without pulmonary artery hypertension can also have right-to-left shunting across the foramen ovale, i.e., tricuspid atresia, Ebstein anomaly of the tricuspid valve, right ventricular hypoplasia, or pulmonary valvar stenosis/atresia.

9. What finding on fetal echocardiography indicates an increased risk for persistent pulmonary hypertension postnatally?

Premature constriction of the ductus arteriosus may be a precursor to persistent pulmonary hypertension postnatally.

10. A neonate with hypoxemia undergoes echocardiography. The report indicates tricuspid valve regurgitation with a peak velocity of 4.0 m/sec. There are no congenital heart abnormalities detected. What do the findings imply about pulmonary artery pressure?

Peak velocity measured on Doppler echocardiography is used to estimate pressure difference between two chambers or across a site of stenosis. The difference is calculated using a modification of the Bernoulli equation:

$$\Delta P = (2 \times Vmax)^2$$

where ΔP = pressure difference and Vmax = maximal or peak velocity.

A jet of tricuspid regurgitation is used to determine the difference between the right ventricle pressure (RVp) and the right atrial pressure (RAp) during ventricular systole.

$$RVp - RAp = (2 \times Vmax)^2$$
$$RVp = (2 \times Vmax)^2 + RAp$$

Entering the tricuspid regurgitation velocity of 4.0 m/sec into this equation, you learn that RVp = 64 mmHg + RAp. The right atrial pressure can be estimated or measured directly with a central venous catheter located in the right atrium. *In the absence of right ventricular outflow tract disease, the RV systole pressure is equal to the pulmonary artery systolic pressure.* Thus, this neonate clearly has pulmonary artery hypertension.

11. What are some additional methods of assessing right ventricular and/or pulmonary artery pressure with echocardiography?

In a patient with a ventricular septal defect (VSD), measurement of peak velocity across the VSD allows estimation of the pressure difference between the RV and the LV.

$$RVp = LVp - (2 \times Vmax)^2$$

Since systolic blood pressure (SBP) is equal to the LVp in the absence of left ventricular outflow tract obstruction,

$$RVp = SBP - (2 \times Vmax)^2$$

This measurement is inaccurate in the presence of either right ventricular outflow tract obstruction or left ventricular outflow tract obstruction.

Measurement of flow velocity across a patent ductus arteriosus (PDA) is another method of estimating pulmonary artery (PA) pressure. Low flow velocity implies high PA pressure; high flow velocity implies low PA pressure. This method has several technical limitations and, therefore, is less accurate for assessing PA pressure.

Measurement of the end-diastolic velocity of pulmonary valve insufficiency, when present, allows estimation of pulmonary artery diastolic pressure relative to the right ventricular diastolic pressure.

The position of the ventricular septum in a short axis view allows a qualitative, not quantitative, assessment of RV pressure relative to LV pressure. Normally, the LV appears rounded and the septum bulges into the crescent-shaped RV. If RV pressure is close to systemic pressure, the septum will be flattened. If RV pressure is suprasystemic, the septum bulges into the LV.

12. Does shortening fraction measure contractility of the heart?

No. Shortening fraction is a measure of the percentage of change in diameter of the left ventricle that occurs during the cardiac cycle. Preload, afterload, heart rate, and contractility influence the shortening fraction. Only one echocardiographic technique (measurement of the velocity of circumferential fiber shortening-wall stress relationship) measures the contractility of the LV. This evaluation is technically difficult to perform in neonates.

13. How is the shortening fraction measured? What is the normal range?

$$\% \text{ Shortening fraction (SF)} = \frac{\text{LV diastolic diameter} - \text{LV systolic diameter}}{\text{LV diastolic diameter}} \times 100$$

The normal range is 28–44%, with a mean of 33%, varying slightly with the patient's size.

14. How does ejection fraction differ from shortening fraction? Can ejection fraction be measured with echocardiography?

Ejection fraction (EF) measures a change in *volume* as opposed to a change in diameter of the left ventricle during the cardiac cycle.

$$\% \text{ EF} = \frac{\text{LV diastolic volume} - \text{LV systolic volume}}{\text{LV diastolic volume}} \times 100$$

Ejection fraction can be measured on echocardiography by measuring ventricular volumes in two orthogonal views with acceptable accuracy. ***Caution:*** EF measurements reported on many echocardiographic reports frequently are obtained purely from a mathematical calculation derived from the shortening fraction number rather than the more cumbersome method of measuring volumes.

15. How do the resistances in the pulmonary vascular bed and in the systemic vascular bed change with the transition from fetal to neonatal circulation?

Pulmonary vascular resistance decreases because of mechanical expansion of the lungs with the first breath and inspiration of oxygen, which is a potent pulmonary vasodilator. Systemic vascular resistance increases because of removal of the low-resistance placenta from the circuit.

16–19. A newborn is found to have a large ventricular septal defect. His echocardiographic evaluation demonstrates mild tricuspid insufficiency with a peak instantaneous velocity of 4 m/sec. There is no obstruction to right ventricular outflow.

16. What is the estimated right ventricular pressure?
RVp = $(2 \times 4)^2$ + RAp → 64 mmHg + RAp

17. How does this relate to the pulmonary arterial systolic pressure?
RVp = PAp (because it is stated that there is no obstruction to right ventricular outflow)

18. Does this imply a large left-to-right shunt? Why or why not?
Not necessarily. The magnitude of the shunt is not simply reflected by the pulmonary artery pressure; it is also inversely related to pulmonary vascular resistance.

$$\text{Pulmonary blood flow (PBF)} = \frac{\Delta P \text{ across the pulmonary vascular bed}}{\text{Pulmonary vascular resistance}}$$

And shunt is related to PBF as follows:

$$\text{PBF} = \text{systemic venous return} + \text{left-to-right shunt}$$

Therefore, in the face of high PVR, high pulmonary arterial pressures can exist with normal PBF, e.g., with minimal or no left-to-right shunt.

19. Assuming that the normal circulatory transitions occur, what changes can be expected with respect to the pulmonary arterial pressure at 6 weeks of age? What changes can be expected in the magnitude of the left-to-right shunt?
The principal circulatory change during the transitional circulation is an exponential decrement in PVR over the first 6–8 weeks of life. With a large ventricular septal defect, the right ventricular and pulmonary artery pressures remain high (must be equal to the LVP in a nonrestrictive ventricular septal defect). The volume of the left-to-right shunt increases because there is an inverse relationship between PBF and PVR.

INNOCENT MURMURS

20. What is the incidence of innocent murmurs?
Innocent murmurs occur in approximately 50% of the pediatric population. They are commonly described in children over 2 years old, are systolic in timing, and are transient. The occurrence is even higher in the neonate or premature infant, with some reported incidences > 75%.

21. What are the common innocent murmurs heard in the newborn period?
- Peripheral pulmonary stenosis (PPS), which is also called branch pulmonary stenosis (most common)
- Transient systolic murmur of a closing PDA
- Transient systolic murmur of tricuspid regurgitation (TR)

22. What is the cause of PPS?
PPS is caused by flow acceleration at the acute angle of the bifurcation of the pulmonary artery into right and left branches. This angle becomes less acute with growth, and the murmur usually disappears by 2 months of age.

23. What are the clinical findings of PPS?
- A short grade 2/6 midsystolic murmur is heard at the cardiac base with radiation to axillae and back.
- No cardiac symptoms are involved.

24. What type of murmur is associated with a patent foramen ovale?
None.

DISTINGUISHING CARDIAC FROM PULMONARY DISEASE IN THE CYANOTIC NEONATE

25. With a cyanotic newborn, what information from the maternal, prenatal, and perinatal history is likely to increase one's suspicion for congenital heart disease?
The incidence of congenital or acquired heart problems increases in the following situations:

MATERNAL OR PERINATAL CONDITION	HEART ABNORMALITY
Maternal diabetes, cocaine	Dextro-transposition of great arteries (d-TGA)
Maternal congenital heart disease	5–10% incidence of congenital heart disease in child
Maternal use of	
Lithium	Ebstein malformation
Phenytoin, valproate	Atrial septal defect (ASD), ventricular septal defect (VSD), tetralogy of Fallot (TOF)
Ethanol	Septal defects
Maternal lupus erythematosus	Heart failure from bradycardia, third degree atrioventricular block
Omphalocele	TOF
Imperforate anus, esophageal atresia	TOF, complex single ventricle
Perinatal stress/asphyxia	Tricuspid or mitral regurgitation, ventricular dysfunction

26. What oxygen saturation should be considered abnormal in a neonate?
A transcutaneous oxygen saturation less than 93–94% in room air is abnormal.

27. At what level of desaturation is cyanosis detectable at physical examination in most neonates?
Because of the high content of fetal hemoglobin in neonatal blood, which shifts the oxygen-hemoglobin dissociation curve to the left, an infant may not become visibly cyanotic until the saturation drops to the mid-80s. Cyanosis may be especially difficult to appreciate in children of color, whose mucous membranes and tongue must be looked at carefully.

28. What is differential cyanosis?
Differential cyanosis occurs when there is either a visible color difference or discrepant oxygen saturations between the upper and lower portions of the body.

29. What is the implication of differential cyanosis?
The implication is that desaturated blood is perfusing one portion of the body while oxygen-saturated blood perfuses the other portion.
Differential cyanosis occurs in two ways:
- **Pink upper body with blue lower body** occurs when blood shunts from right to left (PA to aorta) at the level of the ductus arteriosus.
    Examples: Cardiac: left heart obstructive lesions: critical aortic stenosis, aortic coarctation, or interrupted aortic arch
                 Pulmonary: high pulmonary vascular resistance
The pO_2 and pCO_2 of a preductal arterial blood gas (ABG) sample gives further information about whether there is underlying heart or lung disease.
- **Blue upper body with pink lower body** occurs **only** when there is dextro-transposition of the great arteries (d-TGA) with pulmonary hypertension or d-TGA with aortic coarctation or interruption. In this situation, the oxygenated blood from the left ventricle enters the

pulmonary artery, and with a right-to-left ductal shunt, pink blood perfuses to the lower body. The aorta carries deoxygenated blood from the right ventricle.

30. What is a hyperoxia test? How is it used in differentiating pulmonary and cardiac causes of cyanosis?

A hyperoxia test attempts to differentiate between pulmonary disease with ventilation/perfusion mismatch and cyanotic congenital heart disease. In both situations, the patient's saturation is low in room air. After being exposed to 100% FiO_2, the patient with pulmonary disease shows an increase in pO_2 (variable degree), whereas the patient with a fixed intracardiac mixing lesion does not change significantly.

- An ABG is obtained in room air from the right radial artery (preductal sample) *and* either an umbilical or lower extremity artery (postductal sample).
- The procedure is repeated after the patient has been placed in 100% FiO_2 for at least 10 minutes. *Note:* Some infants with pulmonary disease do not increase their pO_2 unless they are ventilated with 100% oxygen.

In pulmonary disease, the preductal arterial pO_2 in 100% FiO_2 exceeds 150 mmHg. If the ductus arteriosus is patent and a right-to-left ductal shunt occurs as a result of high pulmonary vascular resistance, the postductal pO_2 is lower than the preductal pO_2. In addition, the arterial pCO_2 is elevated relative to the patient's respiratory effort.

In cyanotic congenital heart disease, the pO_2 in room air is < 70 mmHg (usually < 50 mmHg) and does not change significantly in 100% O_2. Typically, the arterial pCO_2 is normal or low, related to hyperventilation as a response to hypoxia. Acidosis is typically of a metabolic nature because of abnormal systemic perfusion and/or tissue hypoxia.

31. Which critical cyanotic heart defects are excluded if the hyperoxia test yields a pO_2 after 10 minutes > 150 torr?

The following cyanotic heart defects are excluded:
- Pulmonary valve atresia with intact ventricular septum
- Pulmonary valve atresia with ventricular septal defect
- Transposition of the great arteries

32. Which cyanotic lesions may not be excluded if the hyperoxia test yields a a pO_2 after 10 minutes > 150 torr?

Common mixing lesions such as the following may not be excluded:
- Total anomalous pulmonary venous return
- Tetralogy of Fallot with predominant left-to-right shunt
- Hypoplastic left heart

33. What cyanotic heart lesion typically does not have an associated murmur?

A common but lethal congenital heart abnormality is d-TGA, which has an incidence of 20–30 per 100,000 live births. There is a strong male predominance (60–70%). Approximately 60% of cases are simple, with no associated cardiac anomalies, so **no murmur is audible**. The ABG does not reflect CO_2 retention or a pulmonary cause. In addition, the electrocardiogram (ECG) and chest radiograph are relatively normal for a neonate.

34. Under what circumstances can information from an ECG in a cyanotic neonate rapidly indicate the presence of congenital heart disease?

The key is an abnormal frontal plane electrical axis.
- A **leftward** axis for a newborn (i.e., left superior axis –90 to 0° or between 0 and 60°) implies a structural anomaly of the heart. This anomaly is often accompanied by dominant left ventricular forces. The differential diagnosis includes tricuspid valve atresia, pulmonary valve atresia with intact ventricular septum, critical pulmonary stenosis, or complex single left ventricle.

• A **right superior/northwest axis** (i.e., –90 to –180°) suggests a complete atrioventricular canal or single right ventricle, in which a right-to-left intracardiac shunt may occur.

35. A chest radiograph is essential to the workup of cyanosis. What should be evaluated to differentiate between a pulmonary problem and a congenital heart problem?

Pulmonary. Rule out the following:
- Pneumothorax
- Effusions
- Infiltrates
- Space occupying lesions: diaphragmatic hernia, cystic malformations of the lung
- Lung hypoplasia/chest cavity deformities

Cardiac. Remember the Ts:

LESION	HEART SIZE	PULMONARY VESSELS	MURMUR
Transposition of the great arteries	Normal or ↑	Normal or ↑	Absent
Tetralogy of Fallot*	Normal or ↑	↓	Present
Truncus arteriosus*	Normal or ↑	Normal or ↑	Present
Total anomalous pulmonary veins (unobstructed)	Normal or ↑	Normal or ↑	Variable
Total anomalous pulmonary veins (obstructed)	Normal or ↓	↑	Absent
Tricuspid or pulmonary atresia	Normal or ↑	↓	Variable
Ebstein malformation	↑↑	Normal or ↓	Present
Hypoplastic left heart syndrome	↑	↑↑	Variable

* A right aortic arch strongly suggests heart disease.

36. One is evaluating a newborn with cyanosis and tachypnea during the first few hours of life. While waiting for the portable chest radiograph, one performs a preductal ABG in room air: pH 7.1, pCO_2 80, pO_2 20, base deficit –10. What cardiac condition must be suspected?

The overall picture is one of respiratory insufficiency with severely altered ventilation and oxygenation, and a combined respiratory and metabolic acidosis. One must think about **obstructed total anomalous pulmonary venous connection** (TAPVC), where blood enters the lungs but cannot adequately exit because of obstruction in the draining vessel that directs the anomalous pulmonary venous return to the right side of the heart. This condition results in severe pulmonary venous congestion, CO_2 retention, hypoxia, and metabolic acidosis due to limited cardiac output. The diagnosis should be suspected if the chest radiograph shows a **normal or small cardiac silhouette with bilateral pulmonary venous congestion** (ground glass).

Affected neonates require extraordinary airway and circulatory support. Echocardiography will show both right-to-left atrial shunting and right-to-left ductal shunting with right ventricular enlargement, which are similar to the findings in persistent pulmonary hypertension. Therefore, careful assessment of the pulmonary venous connections is mandatory.

37. In the evaluation of an infant with cyanosis, after ensuring that the airway, respirations, heart rate, and blood pressure are adequate or supported, what must one do next?

Perform a good physical exam!

CONGESTIVE HEART FAILURE

38. What is heart failure?

Heart failure is a condition in which the cardiac output cannot meet the metabolic needs of the body without compensatory mechanisms. Clinical symptoms result from the compensatory responses.

39. What are the symptoms of heart failure?

The symptoms reflect the insufficiency of cardiac output as well as the adverse effects of the body's basic compensatory mechanisms:

• **Tachycardia.** Mediated by the autonomic nervous system in response to a fall in cardiac output.

• **Cardiomegaly.** Associated with increased diastolic volume resulting in cardiac dilatation.

• **Tachypnea.** Decreased pulmonary compliance secondary to interstitial congestion and/or pulmonary edema leads to rapid shallow respirations.

• **Hepatomegaly.** In infants with low cardiac output, fluid retention is reflected by enlargement of the liver, which is soft and has a distensible capsule. In older patients, fluid retention is seen as peripheral edema.

• **Failure to thrive.** A greater than normal caloric intake is needed to sustain the higher demands on the body. However, intake is reduced because of fatigue and dyspnea during feedings. Weight gain is decreased although height remains normal.

40. What is high output failure?

High output failure is the development of the signs and symptoms of congestive heart failure when increased demands for cardiac output exceed the ability of the system to respond.

41. Name the major causes of heart failure in the fetus.

• Severe anemia
• Arrhythmias
• Infection
• Large systemic AV fistulae
  (e.g., vein of Galen AV malformation)
• Severe AV valve insufficiency

42. Name the major causes of congestive heart failure within the first week of life.

• Hypoplastic left heart syndrome
• Interrupted aortic arch
• Coarctation with VSD, critical aortic stenosis
• Truncus arteriosus
• Total anomalous pulmonary venous return
• Atrioventricular canal
• Single ventricle complex

Infants with large left-to-right shunts (e.g., VSD) without significant valvular abnormalities do not usually develop congestive heart failure in the first month of life because the decline in pulmonary vascular resistance is delayed.

43. Why does the newborn heart have a reduced ability to adapt to stress?

The newborn heart has fewer myofilaments with which to generate the force of contraction. In addition, the newborn ventricle has decreased compliance compared with the older adult ventricle. Therefore, the newborn heart generates less augmentation in stroke volume for a given increase in diastolic volume. Furthermore, the O_2 consumption and cardiac output/m^2 are much higher in the newborn, and there is very little systolic reserve.

TREATMENT OF HYPOTENSION IN THE NEONATE

44. What is the most frequent primary cause of hypotension in the preterm neonate in the immediate postnatal period?

Disturbance of peripheral vasomotor regulation is the most frequent primary cause of hypotension in the preterm neonate. In cases with sepsis, the decrease in the peripheral vascular resistance is caused by the release of inflammatory mediators induced by infectious agents and/or endotoxins. However, in most cases of hypotension in the preterm neonate, there is no evidence of infection. In these patients, oxidant stress and other noninfectious stimuli initiate a nonspecific systemic inflammatory response resulting in a decrease in peripheral vascular resistance and systemic blood pressure. In addition, in over one-third of hypotensive preterm neonates, impaired myocardial function may contribute to the cardiovascular compromise.

Finally, unlike the hypovolemia in the pediatric patient population, absolute hypovolemia in the sick preterm neonate is infrequently the primary cause of hypotension during the immediate postnatal period.

45. What evidence supports the notion that absolute hypovolemia is infrequently the primary cause of shock in the preterm neonate during the immediate postnatal period?

The lack of any relationship between intravascular volume and blood pressure has repeatedly been documented in the preterm neonate. Thus, factors other than intravascular volume are the primary causes for the development of systemic hypotension in this patient population. In addition, administration of dopamine without volume supplementation is effective in 90% of preterm neonates, whereas volume supplementation alone is effective in only 40% during the first day of life. This finding again suggests that peripheral vasodilation with or without myocardial dysfunction is the most frequent primary causative factor in the pathophysiology of hypotension in the sick preterm neonate.

46. Should normal saline or 5% albumin be used for fluid resuscitation in preterm and term neonates with hypotension in the immediate postnatal period?

The volume of resuscitation fluid, and not its protein content, determines the efficacy of the fluid bolus in raising the blood pressure in preterm neonates. Isotonic saline is as effective as 5% albumin in increasing blood pressure in hypotensive preterm neonates and, importantly, causes less fluid retention. The beneficial effect of normal saline on total body fluid homeostasis may be especially significant for the sick preterm neonate because colloid administration during the first few days after birth may increase the incidence of and worsen the severity of bronchopulmonary dysplasia. Finally, based on recent findings in adults with shock, administration of albumin may be associated with increased morbidity and mortality. However, randomized controlled trials are needed in hypotensive and term neonates before final conclusions can be drawn concerning the use of albumin as a volume expander in the neonatal patient population.

47. What are the sites of expression and the function of the cardiovascular adrenoreceptors?

TYPES OF RECEPTORS	PERIPHERAL VASCULAR	FUNCTION	CARDIAC	FUNCTION
Alpha adrenoreceptors	Relatively evenly distributed	Vasocon-striction	Present	↑ contractility
Beta adrenoreceptors	Relatively evenly distributed	Vasodilation	Present	↑ rate ↑ conduction velocity ↑ contractility
Dopaminergic receptors	Primarily in the renal mesenteric and coronary circulation	Vasodilation	Present	↑ contractility

48. What are the sites of expression and the function of the renal adrenoreceptors?

TYPES OF RECEPTORS	GLOMERULI	FUNCTION	TUBULES	FUNCTION
Alpha adrenoreceptors	Present	Vasoconstriction	Present	↑ sodium retention ↑ phosphorus retention ↑ free water retention
Beta adrenoreceptors	Present	Vasodilation	Present	Unclear
Dopaminergic receptors	Present	Vasodilation	Present	↑ sodium excretion ↑ phosphorus excretion ↑ free water excretion ↑ bicarbonate losses

49. What are the mechanisms of action of the cardiovascular effects of dopamine in the preterm neonate?

In the preterm neonate, dopamine **increases systemic blood pressure** by increasing total peripheral vascular resistance (afterload) and myocardial contractility. Dopamine also increases the effective circulating blood volume (preload) by decreasing venous capacitance, which may also contribute to the beneficial cardiovascular effects of the drug. Thus, the most important physiologic determinants of cardiac function and systemic blood pressure are all affected by dopamine. Dopamine **increases total renal blood flow** by inducing selective vasodilation of the renal artery in the preterm neonate. Finally, dopamine **has no direct effect on the cerebral and mesenteric circulation** in this population.

50. What are the mechanisms of action of the renal vascular and tubular effects of dopamine in the preterm neonate?

Activation of the **renal vascular dopaminergic receptors** results in increases in total renal blood flow, renal cortical and medullary blood flow, and glomerular filtration rate. Activation of the **renal tubular dopaminergic receptors** causes increases in renal sodium, phosphorus, bicarbonate, and free water excretion through the drug-induced inhibition of the tubular sodium-potassium-adenosine triphosphatase (Na^+-K^+-ATPase) enzyme, the Na^+-inorganic phosphate (P_i) cotransporter, the Na^+/hydrogen (H^+) countertransporter, and the antidiuretic hormone (ADH)-induced activation of water channels, respectively. Both the vascular and tubular actions of dopamine are present in the immediate postnatal period in the human preterm neonate as early as the 23rd to 24th weeks of gestation.

51. What are the adrenergic receptor-mediated pharmacodynamic actions of the most frequently used cardiovascular agents?

AGENT	ADRENERGIC RECEPTOR					
	$\alpha1$	β_1	α_2	β_2	DOPAMINE	
	CARDIAC	CARDIAC	VASCULAR	VASCULAR	CARDIAC	VASCULAR
	↑ contractility	↑ rate ↑ conduction ↑ contractility	Peripheral vaso-constriction	Peripheral vaso-dilation	↑ contractility	Vasodilation in the renal, mesenteric, and coronary circulation
Norepinephrine	+++	++++	++++	0	0	0
Epinephrine	+++	++++	++++	++	0	0
Dopamine*	+++	++++	++++	++	++++	++++
Dobutamine	+++	++++	+	++	0	0
Isoprenaline	0	++++	0	+++	0	0
Amrinone, milrinone, and others	Type III Phosphodiesterase Inhibitors					

0 = no effect; + = minimal effect; ++++ = maximum effect.
* Dopamine stimulates the α- and β-adrenergic and dopaminergic receptors in a dose-dependent manner. In children and adults, low doses (0.5–4 µg/kg/min) preferentially activate the dopaminergic receptors, whereas medium doses (4–8 µg/kg/min) induce a primarily β-adrenergic cardiovascular response in addition to the cardiovascular and renal dopaminergic effects. Finally, at higher dopamine doses (> 8 µg/kg/min) the cardiovascular effects of α-adrenoreceptor stimulation gradually become predominant. However, in neonates, especially in the preterm infant, as long as adrenoreceptor downregulation has not taken place, the order of adrenoreceptor sensitivity is different from that seen in the older age groups with the cardiovascular effects of α-adrenoreceptor stimulation preceding those of the β-adrenoreceptors. This difference is believed to result primarily from the developmentally-regulated enhanced expression of α-adrenoreceptors during early development.

52. Why is dopamine superior to dobutamine in the treatment of hypotension in the preterm neonate?

Dopamine is more effective than dobutamine in the treatment of systemic hypotension in the preterm neonate because the most frequent cause of hypotension in this patient population is abnormal regulation of the peripheral vascular tone with or without associated myocardial dysfunction. Because dopamine increases both total peripheral vascular resistance and myocardial contractility, it corrects the major underlying pathophysiologic abnormalities causing systemic hypotension in the preterm neonate. Dobutamine, on the other hand, effectively increases myocardial contractility; however, it also frequently causes peripheral vasodilation. Thus, although cardiac output significantly increases with dobutamine, blood pressure may not increase at all because of the dobutamine-induced decrease in the afterload. Indeed, several randomized controlled trials have demonstrated the superiority of dopamine over dobutamine in increasing systemic blood pressure in the preterm neonate. Because cerebral blood flow in the neonatal period is determined primarily by the systemic blood pressure (and not the cardiac output), dobutamine administration alone may not result in an improvement of cerebral blood flow in the hypotensive preterm neonate unless blood pressure is normalized. Finally, dobutamine lacks the beneficial renal vascular and tubular actions of dopamine, which may contribute to the recovery of the abnormal cardiovascular status and fluid homeostasis in the hypotensive preterm neonate.

53. What is the maximum dose of dopamine in the neonate?

Neonatology and pharmacology textbooks recommend a dose range of 2–20 µg/kg/min for the use of dopamine in the preterm and term neonate. However, there are no data supporting the recommendation that the maximum dose of dopamine be limited to 20 µg/kg/min. Because there is no evidence that dopamine is more harmful at doses beyond 20µg/kg/min than at lower doses, the cardiovascular response to the drug should determine its dosing schedule rather than a dosing limit. Indeed, a few descriptive studies have indicated that doses in the 30–50 µg/kg/min range (or even higher in some reports) have been used successfully to increase blood pressure and urine output in neonates unresponsive to dopamine in the 10–20 µg/kg/min dose range. However, it is important to note that these studies were not designed to investigate potential toxicity of high-dose dopamine treatment.

54. What is the difference between the mechanisms of the myocardial effects of dobutamine and dopamine in the hypotensive neonate?

Dobutamine selectively stimulates the myocardial β- and α-adrenergic receptors and is an extremely potent inotrope. On the other hand, only approximately one-half of the positive inotropic effects of dopamine result from the direct stimulation of the myocardial β- and α-adrenergic receptors. The remainder of the positive inotropic effects of dopamine is indirect and results from the drug-induced release of stored norepinephrine from the sympathetic nerve endings in the heart. Because norepinephrine stores are rapidly (within a few hours) depleted from the neonatal myocardium, neonates whose hypotension is primarily caused by myocardial dysfunction, such as cases with asphyxia or viral myocarditis, may benefit from the addition of dobutamine to dopamine. It is also important to remember that dobutamine tends to decrease peripheral vascular resistance, whereas medium to high doses of dopamine increase the afterload. Therefore, to achieve an appropriate balance between cardiac output and peripheral vascular resistance, one must carefully titrate the dose of dopamine in hypotensive neonates with primary myocardial dysfunction receiving combined dopamine and dobutamine treatment. Finally, dobutamine tends to maintain a better balance between myocardial oxygen delivery and consumption than does dopamine.

55. What is the difference between a pressor and an inotrope?

A cardiovascular agent with a significant peripheral vasoconstrictive (α_2 adrenoreceptor-stimulatory) effect is referred to as a **pressor** regardless of its action on myocardial contractility. Pressor medications increase systemic blood pressure by both increasing peripheral vascular resistance (afterload) and enhancing myocardial contractility. Because of the elevation in the afterload, the positive inotropic effect of such agents may not result in an increase in the stroke volume. The positive inotropic effect, however, contributes to the ability of the myocardium to maintain an appropriate cardiac output despite the higher afterload, which explains the effectiveness of these agents in raising the systemic blood pressure. Dopamine, epinephrine, and norepinephrine are the pressor agents used most frequently.

A cardiovascular agent without a notable peripheral vasoconstrictive (α_2 adrenoreceptor-stimulatory) action but with a significant inotropic effect is usually referred to as an **inotrope**. Dobutamine is one of the inotropes that effectively increase blood pressure in neonates in whom the hypotension results primarily from a decrease in myocardial contractility associated with normal or increased peripheral vascular resistance.

56. Why is steroid administration effective in most cases of pressor-resistant hypotension in the neonate?

Sick preterm neonates, especially the extremely low–birth-weight infants with a history of long-term (> 1–2 weeks) steroid treatment, may not be able to respond to stress appropriately because of the insufficiency of the hypothalamic-pituitary-adrenal axis or that of the adrenal gland itself. In these patients, steroid administration supplements insufficient endogenous steroid production. However, prolonged activation of the sympathetic nervous system and the administration of high doses of exogenous catecholamines (dopamine, epinephrine) also result in the down-regulation of the cardiovascular adrenergic receptors and second messenger systems leading to desensitization of the cardiovascular system to catecholamines. Because the genes of the adrenergic receptors and some components of the second messenger systems contain a steroid-responsive element, administration of steroids increases the expression and membrane assembly of these proteins within 8–12 hours of administration. Restoration of adrenergic receptor expression and function results in increased sensitivity of the cardiovascular system to catecholamines with improved myocardial function and vascular reactivity.

In addition to these genomic effects, steroids also exert certain nongenomic cardiovascular actions. Nongenomic steroidal actions are rapid in onset (within minutes) and do not affect gene regulation. The nongenomic cardiovascular actions of steroids include the inhibition of catecholamine metabolism and the rapid increase in cytosolic calcium availability in myocardial and vascular smooth muscle cells (mineralocorticoid-mediated). These nongenomic steroidal actions may then lead to a more rapid improvement in cardiovascular status. The results of a few recent descriptive and two randomized studies suggest that the combined genomic and nongenomic steroidal actions may have the potential to restore the responsiveness of the myocardial and vascular smooth muscle cells to inotrope/pressor treatment in subjects with pressor-resistant hypotension.

57. Is steroid administration contraindicated in the treatment of hypotension in a neonate with shock caused by bacterial sepsis?

Based on the findings of a few recent studies, administration of a single dose or a short course of steroids in neonates with pressor-resistant hypotension associated with bacterial sepsis may be beneficial in restoring the sensitivity of the cardiovascular system to catecholamines and does not appear to be associated with adverse effects. These findings are contrary to those seen in older age groups with hypotension and bacterial sepsis treated with high-dose steroids.

CYANOTIC CONGENITAL HEART DISEASE

58. What are the five Ts of cyanotic congenital heart disease?

1. Transposition of the great arteries	4. Total anomalous pulmonary venous return
2. Tetralogy of Fallot	5. Tricuspid atresia
3. Truncus arteriosus	

The rule of Ts can be stretched to include pulmonary atresia and aortic atresia (hypoplastic left heart syndrome).

59. If the hemoglobin level is normal, how much does the oxygen saturation need to decrease before cyanosis results?

The perception of cyanosis occurs when there is 5 gm of reduced hemoglobin in the capillaries. In the infant with a normal hemoglobin level, perception of cyanosis occurs at an oxygen saturation of 70%. The experienced observer can sometimes detect cyanosis when the saturation falls to 80–85%.

60. How can cyanosis occur if the arterial saturation is normal?

Cyanosis can occur in states of low cardiac output, even when the arterial saturation is normal. When the cardiac output is low, the arteriovenous difference widens, leading to an increased amount of reduced hemoglobin in the capillaries. Low-output cyanosis is commonly referred to as acrocyanosis.

Polycythemia can also cause cyanosis because of the formation of reduced hemoglobin in capillaries.

61. What is the most common cyanotic heart lesion presenting in the newborn period?

Transposition of the great arteries is the most common form of cyanotic congenital heart disease in the neonate and comprises 6–10% of infants with congenital heart disease. In older children, tetralogy of Fallot is most common and represents 7–9% of cardiac cases.

62. What cardiac lesions should one consider when the radiologist says the infant has a right aortic arch?

- Tetralogy of Fallot   13–34%
- Truncus arteriosus   36%
- Double-outlet right ventricle 20%
- Tricuspid atresia   5–8%
- Transposition of the great vessels 3%
- Ventricular septal defect   2–6%

63. Transposition of the great vessels can be associated with other cardiac defects such as ventricular septal defect and atrial septal defect. How do these defects affect the age at which the infant's disease will be recognized?

In transposition of the great vessels (TGV), the aortic arch rises from the right ventricle, and the pulmonary artery comes off the left ventricle. Unless mixing of the pulmonary and systemic circulation occurs, the infant will become hypoxic and acidotic and die in the first few days of life. The more mixing between the chambers, the later the children are recognized. The majority of infants with TGV have an intact ventricular septum and patent foramen ovale. They present in the first 6–24 hours of life with profound cyanosis and, depending on the size of the foramen ovale, need intervention in the first few days of life. Infants with TGV and a large ASD can present at 24–48 hours of life with moderate cyanosis and usually do not develop acidosis. Children with TGV and a large VSD may present between 2 and 6 weeks of life with signs of congestive heart failure and minimal-to-moderate cyanosis.

64. What chromosomal deletion is common in truncus arteriosus, tetralogy of Fallot, and interrupted aortic arch?

Truncus arteriosus, tetralogy of Fallot, and interrupted aortic arch are often associated with "CATCH-22", i.e., syndromes with a deletion of chromosome 22.

65. Tetralogy of Fallot consists of three findings: pulmonary stenosis, overriding of the aorta across the ventricular septal defect, and right ventricular hypertrophy. Which of these are critical for the tetralogy physiology?

The findings that are critical for the tetralogy physiology are pulmonary stenosis and a large VSD with equalization of the right and left ventricular pressures.

66. What are the manifestations of tetralogy of Fallot at birth?
- The most common manifestation is murmur due to obstruction of the right ventricular in-fundibulum. *Note:* the murmur often sounds like a VSD, but in the first few days of life VSDs do not produce a murmur because ventricular pressures are equal.
- Cyanosis is uncommon unless there is pulmonary atresia. *Note:* With closure of the ductus, cyanosis appears.
- Congestive heart failure is almost never seen. Because pulmonary stenosis is progressive, congestive heart failure is seen in early infancy.
- "Spells" are rarely seen in neonates.

67. Who was the first person to describe an individual with tetralogy of Fallot?
Stensen was the first person to describe the condition.

68. Name the four types of anomalous pulmonary venous return.
1. **Supracardiac.** The pulmonary veins connect with the innominate vein or the superior vena cava.
2. **Cardiac.** The pulmonary veins connect with the right ventricle or the coronary sinus.
3. **Infracardiac.** The pulmonary veins connect with the inferior vena cava or the portal or hepatic veins.
4. **Mixed.** A combination of types contribute to the anomaly.

69. What are the manifestations of anomalous pulmonary venous return in the neonate?
- With obstructed veins, cyanosis and respiratory distress are common.
- With unobstructed veins, tachypnea develops gradually.
- A systolic ejection murmur along the upper left sternal border (due to increased flow) is commonly heard.

70. What are the clinical signs of truncus arteriosus in neonates?
- The presentation is subtle, often with only mild tachypnea or cyanosis.
- If the truncal valve is abnormal, there is a systolic ejection murmur.
- The second heart sound is single.
- The pulses are bounding, and the pulse pressure is wide.
- There occasionally may be signs of congestive heart failure.

ACYANOTIC CONGENITAL HEART DISEASE

71. Name the common causes of left-to-right shunts.
- Ventricular septal defect (VSD)
- Atrioventricular canal (AV canal)
- Patent ductus arteriosus (PDA)
- Atrial septal defect (ASD)

72. The most common cause of heart failure in infants is a ventricular septal defect, and af-fected infants are often identified between 2 and 6 weeks of age. Why do they escape detec-tion in the newborn period?
Infants with a VSD are usually identified after they leave the hospital because both the heart murmur of a VSD and the symptoms of heart failure do not appear in the first few days of life. In the immediate postnatal period, pulmonary vascular resistance is still elevated, thereby limiting the shunting of blood from the left ventricle to the right ventricle and into the lungs. As the pul-monary vascular resistance falls, an increased volume flows through the defect, which leads to a louder murmur, increased pulmonary blood flow, and congestive heart failure.

73. What heart defects are associated with coarctation of the aorta?
Infants with neonatal coarctation syndrome often have a VSD or AV canal that complicates the hemodynamic picture. Newborn infants with isolated coarctation of the aorta typically have

normal ventricles, but often have anomalies of the aortic valve, such as bicuspid aortic valve, aortic stenosis, or some degree of mitral valve stenosis. Both types of heart defect may have severe narrowing of the preductal aorta.

74. Name three conditions associated with persistent patency of the ductus arteriosus.
  1. Prematurity
  2. Hypoxia (pulmonary disease/high altitude)
  3. Congenital rubella infection

75. What kinds of acyanotic congenital heart disease are typically seen in children with Down syndrome?
  • AV canal (the AV canal can be either complete, with ventricular and atrial components, or partial, with a defect principally in the septum primum)
  • VSD

76. Which syndromes are associated with a common atrium?
  • Ellis-van Creveld syndrome
  • Ivemark's syndrome

77. What is the typical ECG finding in an infant with an endocardial cushion defect?
  The typical ECG finding in an infant with an endocardial cushion defect is left axis deviation with normal right ventricular forces.

78. What is a pink tet?
  A pink tet is a patient with a VSD, pulmonary stenosis, and adequate pulmonary blood flow. Infants with tetralogy of Fallot commonly have predominantly left-to-right shunting during the first few months of life, which can be severe enough to lead to congestive heart failure but often is not severe. With increasing age, the pulmonary outflow tract becomes narrow at the pulmonary valve level and the infundibular level (subvalvar region), leading to cyanosis and typical findings of tetralogy of Fallot.

79. When was the first report of a successful ligation of a patent ductus arteriosus?
  The first successful ligation of a PDA was by Gross and Hubbard in 1938.

80. What is the differential diagnosis of heart failure in the first few hours of life?
  • Altered rhythm (congenital heart block, SVT, or flutter)
  • Altered preload (arteriovenous malformation)
  • Altered afterload (aortic atresia, aortic stenosis, coarctation of the aorta)
  • Altered contractility (asphyxia, cardiomyopathy, sepsis)
  Note: Many other lesions present with heart failure a few days later, after the pulmonary vascular resistance starts to fall (VSD, truncus arteriosus).

81. If the apex of the heart is on the opposite side of the patient from the stomach, what is the likelihood that the patient has congenital cardiac disease?
  The likelihood that the patient has congenital cardiac disease is high, probably in excess of 90–95%. This condition, referred to as cardiac dextroversion if the cardiac apex is on the right and the stomach is on the left, is nearly always associated with cardiac disease.

DUCTUS ARTERIOSUS

82. What is the purpose of the ductus arteriosus in the fetus?
  The purpose of the ductus arteriosus in the fetus is diversion of right ventricular blood away from the fluid-filled lungs toward the descending aorta and placenta. In the fetus, 90% of the

right ventricular output shunts in this fashion through the ductus arteriosus, and only 10% flows through the pulmonary vascular bed.

83. When does the ductus arteriosus normally close after birth?

The ductus arteriosus is patent in all neonates at the time of birth. In the vast majority of term infants, physiologic closure occurs by 12–15 hours of life. Similarly, the ductus arteriosus undergoes spontaneous closure in 90% of infants between 30 and 37 weeks' gestation. However, in infants of < 30 weeks' gestation, the ductus closes in < 50%. Although anatomic obliteration of the ductus arteriosus usually is not complete for several months, a ductus that is functionally open beyond 72 hours postnatally can be considered a persistently patent ductus arteriosus (PDA).

84. Name the major risk factors for the development of a symptomatic PDA?
• Prematurity
• Respiratory distress syndrome
• Excessive fluid administration in the first few days after birth
• Surfactant therapy
• Perinatal asphyxia

85. What are the potential deleterious effects of a symptomatic PDA in the premature infant?
• Pulmonary **overperfusion** resulting in an increased risk of pulmonary hemorrhage and bronchopulmonary dysplasia
• Cerebral, mesenteric, and renal **hypoperfusion** resulting in an increased incidence of metabolic acidosis, intracranial hemorrhage, periventricular leukomalacia, necrotizing enterocolitis, and oliguria

86. What are the clinical manifestations of a PDA?
• Cardiac murmur (usually systolic)
• Apnea
• Increased pulse volume and widened pulse pressure (bounding pulses and presence of palmar pulses)
• Worsening pulmonary status as evidenced by tachypnea, a need for increased ventilator settings, and failure to wean from the ventilator
• Congestive heart failure (a late sign of PDA)

87. What murmurs are associated with a PDA?

Although the classic murmur of a PDA is a continuous systolic and diastolic "machinery" murmur, this type of murmur is heard infrequently in the neonatal period. Instead, there is usually only a systolic murmur, which is best heard in the pulmonic area. In 50% of ventilated preterm infants, the ductus may be silent with no murmur heard at all.

88. When should an echocardiogram be performed in evaluating for a PDA?

Two-dimensional echocardiographic visualization of the ductus with either pulsed, continuous wave, or color Doppler is both sensitive and specific in identifying ductal patency. Therefore, echocardiography is very useful in the determination of ductal patency in the low–birth-weight, ventilated infant who may have few, if any, clinical signs. Much to the chagrin of the cardiology fellow, all mechanically ventilated infants of < 1000-gm birth weight should have a cardiac echocardiogram performed within the first 3–4 days after birth to allow early detection and treatment of a PDA. Larger premature infants should have a cardiac echocardiogram if symptoms compatible with a PDA develop, both to confirm the diagnosis and to rule out other cardiac pathology. A cardiac echocardiogram performed 24–48 hours after indomethacin therapy is also the best way to document treatment failure and to allow alternative interventions to occur without delay.

89. Why is a patent ductus not usually symptomatic in the first few days after birth?

Symptoms of a PDA result from left-to-right ductal shunting of blood away from the systemic circulation into the pulmonary vascular bed; however, blood does not shunt in this direction until the normal decrease in high pulmonary vascular resistance occurs over the first few days after birth. For similar reasons, in infants with pulmonary disease, the patent ductus becomes symptomatic only when the lung disease begins to improve.

90. How should a persistent PDA in the premature infant be treated?

Treatment options for a PDA include indomethacin and surgical ligation. Temporizing measures such as fluid restriction, digitalis, diuretics, packed red cell transfusions, and increased positive end expiratory pressure, although sometimes warranted while awaiting surgery or the effect of indomethacin, should not be used as the primary means of treatment. In most nurseries, indomethacin is the first-line treatment of choice for the patent ductus; however, surgical ligation of the ductus remains an important therapy for the infant whose ductus fails to close with indomethacin or for whom a contraindication to indomethacin therapy exists. The goal is to begin treatment once the diagnosis is made and to achieve permanent closure of the ductus by 10–12 days after birth.

In the premature infant who does not require mechanical ventilation, there is less urgency in affecting closure of the ductus. In many of these infants, the ductus closes spontaneously over the first few weeks after birth; however, if signs of significant left-to-right ductal shunting develop, such infants should also be treated.

91. What are the indications for surgical ligation when a PDA is present?

Surgical ligation of a PDA is generally indicated in infants who have failed two courses of indomethacin treatment or who have a contraindication to indomethacin treatment such as renal failure. Surgical ligation may also be indicated as the primary therapy in infants who already have serious sequelae of left-to-right ductal shunting such as pulmonary hemorrhage or necrotizing enterocolitis; infants with ductal patency beyond a postnatal age of 10–12 days; and infants who have shown minimal to no ductal constriction after a single course of indomethacin, particularly infants with an extremely low birth weight (< 750 gm).

92. Describe the side effects of indomethacin treatment.

Indomethacin affects platelet and neutrophil function in premature infants; however, clinically apparent adverse effects are not well documented. Indomethacin decreases mesenteric perfusion, and spontaneous gastrointestinal perforation is associated with indomethacin use. A decreased renal perfusion results in decreased glomerular filtration rates, oliguria, increased serum creatine levels, fluid retention, and hyponatremia. Indomethacin decreases cerebral blood flow, decreases reactive postasphyxial hyperemia, and accelerates maturation of the germinal matrix microvasculature. The beneficial effect of indomethacin in preventing intraventricular hemorrhage is controversial.

93. What are the common radiographic findings in a newborn infant with a PDA and a left-to-right shunt?

Infants with a PDA exhibit a number of important radiographic findings, which include a diffuse increase in lung density (opacity) that is homogeneous, an increase in heart size, and, occasionally, increased prominence of the pulmonary vasculature. Perihilar congestion may also be increased. Rarely, pleural effusions may be noted.

94. Describe the two most common chest radiographic findings that indicate a neonate has had surgical ligation of a PDA?

Most cardiac surgeons use a lateral thoracotomy on the side of the aortic arch, which almost always means a left thoracotomy. It is usually easy to identify an infant who has had a ductal ligation from the routine chest radiograph because many of these infants have a radio-opaque clip in the area of the ligation. In addition, the radiograph commonly shows deformity of two left-sided ribs, usually the 4th and 5th ribs, where the chest has been entered.

PREOPERATIVE STABILIZATION

95. What are the principles of preoperative management in the neonate with critical congenital heart disease?

In critical congenital heart lesions, the ultimate outcome depends on timely and accurate assessment of the structural anomaly and on the evaluation and resuscitation of secondary organ damage. The principles of preoperative management are as follows:

1. Initial stabilization: airway management, the establishment of vascular access, maintenance of a PDA with prostaglandin E_1, when necessary

2. Delineation of the anatomic defect(s) by echocardiography

3. Evaluation and treatment of additional organ system dysfunction, particularly of the pulmonary, renal, hepatic, and central nervous systems

4. Evaluation for additional congenital defects

5. Genetic evaluation, if indicated

6. Cardiac catheterization, if indicated

7. Surgical management, if indicated, when cardiac, pulmonary, renal, hepatic, and central nervous system functions are optimized.

96. How does the neonate with critical congenital heart disease typically present?

The timing of presentation with the accompanying symptomatology depends on the nature and severity of the anatomic defect; the in utero effects, if any, of the structural lesion; and, following birth, the alterations in cardiovascular physiology secondary to the effects of the closure of the ductus arteriosus and the fall in pulmonary vascular resistance.

In the first few weeks of life, the many heterogeneous forms of heart disease present in a surprisingly limited number of ways, which include the following signs and symptoms:

1. Cyanosis

2. Congestive heart failure or shock

3. Asymptomatic heart murmur

4. Arrhythmia

Although an increasing number of neonates with congenital heart disease are diagnosed before delivery by fetal echocardiography, the majority of neonates with congenital heart anomalies are not discovered until after birth. Frequently, the clinician is diverted from the diagnosis of congenital heart disease because of the report of a normal prenatal ultrasound performed for screening purposes. Conversely, the diagnosis of heart disease should not deter the clinician from performing a complete noncardiac evaluation to search for additional medical problems such as sepsis.

97. When do congenital heart defects present during the neonatal period?

Presentation of Congenital Heart Defects

AGE ON ADMISSION	DIAGNOSIS	PATIENTS (%)
0–6 days (n = 537)	D-transposition of the great arteries	19
	Hypoplastic left heart syndrome	14
	Tetralogy of Fallot	8
	Coarctation of the aorta	7
	Ventricular septal defect	3
	Others	49
7–13 days (n = 195)	Coarctation of the aorta	16
	Ventricular septal defect	14
	Hypoplastic left heart syndrome	8
	D-transposition of the great arteries	7
	Tetralogy of Fallot	7
	Others	48

(Table continued on next page.)

Presentation of Congenital Heart Defects (Continued)

AGE ON ADMISSION	DIAGNOSIS	PATIENTS (%)
14–28 days (n = 177)	Ventricular septal defect	16
	Coarctation of the aorta	12
	Tetralogy of Fallot	7
	D-transposition of the great arteries	7
	Patent ductus arteriosus	5
	Others	53

Adapted from Flanagan MF, Fyler DC: Cardiac disease. In Avery GB, Fletcher MA, MacDonald M, eds: Neonatology: Pathophysiology and Management of the Newborn. Philadelphia, J.B. Lippincott, 1994, p 524.

98. What does the initial evaluation of a neonate with suspected congenital heart disease include?

The initial evaluation of the neonate with suspected congenital heart disease includes a thorough history, a physical examination with four extremity blood pressures, a chest radiograph, an electrocardiogram, preductal and postductal oxygen saturations, a hyperoxia test, and an echocardiogram, if indicated.

Blood pressure measurement, manually or with an automated blood pressure machine, should be performed on all four extremities if there is a suspicion of congenital heart disease. A systolic pressure that is more than 10 mmHg higher in the upper body relative to the lower body is abnormal and suggests coarctation of the aorta, aortic arch hypoplasia, or interrupted aortic arch. It should be noted that testing for a systolic blood pressure gradient is quite specific for an arch abnormality but not very sensitive; a systolic blood pressure gradient will not be present in the neonate with an arch abnormality in whom the ductus arteriosus is patent and nonrestrictive. *Therefore, the lack of a systolic blood pressure gradient in the newborn does not conclusively rule out coarctation or other arch abnormalities, but the presence of a systolic pressure gradient is diagnostic of an aortic arch abnormality.*

99. What is differential cyanosis and reverse differential cyanosis?

Measuring oxygen saturations at both preductal and postductal sites is part of the initial evaluation for congenital heart disease. If the preductal saturation is higher than the postductal saturation, there is **differential cyanosis**, which results when the great arteries are normally related and deoxygenated blood from the pulmonary circulation enters the descending aorta through a patent ductus arteriosus.

Differential cyanosis is seen in the following conditions:

1. Persistent pulmonary hypertension of the newborn (PPHN)

2. Left ventricular outflow tract obstruction (aortic arch hypoplasia, interrupted aortic arch, critical coarctation, and critical aortic stenosis)

There are also rare cases of **reverse differential cyanosis** in which the postductal saturation is higher than the preductal saturation. This occurs only in children with transposition of the great arteries when oxygenated blood from the pulmonary circulation enters the descending aorta through a patent ductus arteriosus.

Reverse differential cyanosis is seen in the following conditions:

1. Transposition of the great arteries with coarctation of the aorta or interrupted aortic arch

2. Transposition of the great arteries and pulmonary hypertension. In this circumstance the descending aorta is filled with oxygenated blood from the pulmonary system, and the lower extremities have a higher oxygen saturation than the upper extremities.

100. When is a hyperoxia test indicated? How is it performed and interpreted?

A hyperoxia test should be carried out in neonates with a resting pulse oximetry reading less than 95%, visible cyanosis, or circulatory collapse. The hyperoxia test consists of obtaining a baseline right radial (preductal) arterial blood gas measurement with the child breathing room air, $FiO_2 = 0.21$, and then repeating the measurement with the child inspiring 100% oxygen, FiO_2 = 1.00. Pulse oximetry should be documented at preductal and postductal sites to assess for differential or reverse differential cyanosis. In some instances, the hyperoxia test must be performed using positive pressure ventilation because neonates with severe pulmonary disease may not be able to raise their PaO_2 unless they are ventilated.

The arterial partial pressure of oxygen (pO_2) should be measured directly through arterial puncture, although properly acquired transcutaneous oxygen monitor (TCOM) values for pO_2 are also acceptable. *Pulse oximetry should not be used for interpretation of the hyperoxia test* because a neonate given 100% inspired oxygen may have an arterial pO_2 of 80 mmHg with a pulse oximeter reading of 100% (abnormal) or an arterial pO_2 greater than 300 mmHg with a pulse oximeter reading of 100% (normal). Interpretation of the hyperoxia test is delineated below:

Interpretation of the Hyperoxia Test

	$FiO_2 = 0.21$ PaO_2 (% saturation)		$FiO_2 = 1.00$ PaO_2 (% saturation)	$PaCO_2$
Normal	70 (95)		> 300 (100)	35
Pulmonary disease	50 (85)		> 150 (100)	50
Neurologic disease	50 (85)		> 150 (100)	50
Methemoglobinemia	70 (95)		> 200 (100)	35
Cardiac disease				
Parallel circulation*	< 40 (< 75)		< 50 (< 85)	35
Mixing with restricted PBF[†]	< 40 (< 75)		< 50 (< 85)	35
Mixing without restricted PBF[‡]	50–60 (85–93)		< 150 (< 100)	35
	Preductal	*Postductal*		
Differential cyanosis[§]	70 (95)	< 40 (< 75)	Variable	35–50
Reverse differential cyanosis[//]	< 40 (< 75)	70 (95)	Variable	35–50

PBF = pulmonary blood flow.
* D-transposition of the great arteries with intact ventricular septum, D-transposition of the great arteries with ventricular septal defect.
[†] Tricuspid atresia with pulmonary stenosis or atresia, pulmonary atresia or critical pulmonary stenosis with intact ventricular septum, or tetralogy of Fallot.
[‡] Truncus arteriosus, total anomalous pulmonary venous return, single ventricle, hypoplastic left heart syndrome.
[§] Persistent pulmonary hypertension of the newborn (PPHN), left ventricular outflow tract obstruction (aortic arch hypoplasia, interrupted aortic arch, critical coarctation, and critical aortic stenosis).
[//] D-transposition of the great arteries with coarctation of the aorta or interrupted aortic arch, D-transposition of the great arteries and pulmonary hypertension.
Adapted from Barone, MA (ed): The Harriet Lane Handbook, 14th ed. St. Louis, Mosby, 1996, p 155.

101. When should prostaglandin E₁ be used? What are its side effects?

Prostaglandin E_1 (PGE_1) should be used in the following situations:

1. The neonate who fails a hyperoxia test, which indicates that the child is highly likely to have congenital heart disease with ductal-dependent systemic or pulmonary blood flow or that a lesion exists that requires a patent ductus arteriosus for intercirculatory mixing.

2. The neonate diagnosed by fetal echocardiography with a congenital heart defect that is ductal-dependent for systemic flood flow, pulmonary blood flow, or intercirculatory mixing.

3. The neonate who presents with shock or congestive heart failure in the first or second week of life.

PGE_1 administered as a continuous intravenous infusion has adverse reactions that must be anticipated. Adverse cardiovascular, respiratory, and infectious side effects are more common in premature and/or low–birth-weight infants. The incidence of the most common side effects is listed in the following table:

SIDE EFFECTS	> 2.0 kg (%)	< 2.0 kg (%)
Cardiovascular (hypotension, rhythm disturbance, peripheral vasodilation	16	36
Central nervous system (seizure, temperature elevation)	16	16
Respiratory (apnea, hypoventilation)	10	42
Metabolic (hypoglycemia, hypocalcemia)	3	5
Infectious (sepsis, wound infections)	3	10
Gastrointestinal (diarrhea, necrotizing enterocolitis)	4	10
Hematologic (DIC, hemorrhage, thrombocytopenia)	3	5
Renal (renal failure, renal insufficiency)	1	3

DIC = disseminated intravascular coagulopathy.
Adapted from Lewis AB, Freed MD, Heymann MA, et al: Side effects of therapy with prostaglandin E_1 in infants with critical congenital heart disease. Circulation 64:893–898, 1981.

Rarely, the patient with congenital heart disease may become progressively more unstable after the institution of PGE_1 therapy. This clinical deterioration after institution of PGE_1 is an important diagnostic finding that identifies the congenital heart defect as one that has obstructed blood flow out of the pulmonary veins or left atrium. The following are lesions that have impaired blood flow out of the left atrium:

1. Hypoplastic left heart syndrome with restrictive or intact foramen ovale
2. Mitral atresia with restrictive foramen ovale
3. Transposition of the great arteries with an intact ventricular septum and restrictive foramen ovale
4. Total anomalous pulmonary venous return with obstruction.

If there is clinical deterioration from PGE_1 therapy, emergent plans for echocardiography and interventional catheterization or cardiac surgery must be urgently undertaken.

102. How is hypoxemia resulting from D-transposition of the great arteries managed?

Treatment of the severely hypoxemic patient with transposition of the great arteries involves ensuring adequate mixing between the two parallel circuits and maximizing the mixed venous oxygen saturation.

Ensuring **adequate mixing** is accomplished by the following:

1. Maintaining patency of the ductus arteriosus with PGE_1.
2. Providing mild hyperventilation and increased FiO_2 to decrease pulmonary vascular resistance and increase pulmonary blood flow.
3. In patients who do not have an adequate pO_2 (> 30 torr) after opening the ductus arteriosus, encouraging pulmonary blood flow with PGE_1, hyperventilation, and increased FiO_2; and enlarging the foramen ovale emergently with balloon atrial septostomy.

Balloon atrial septostomy remains an elective procedure in patients with adequate oxygen delivery. Many find it helpful to perform a balloon atrial septostomy, even in the stable patient on prostaglandin, so that PGE_1 can be discontinued and surgery can take place on a more elective basis.

Maneuvers that **maximize the mixed venous oxygen saturation** include the following:

1. Decreasing oxygen consumption through sedation, paralysis, and mechanical ventilation.
2. Improving oxygen delivery by increasing cardiac output with inotropic agents.
3. Increasing oxygen-carrying capacity by treating anemia.
4. Removing coexisting causes of pulmonary venous desaturation (e.g., pneumothorax).

It is important to note that increasing the fraction of inspired oxygen to 100% has little effect on the arterial pO_2 unless the increase lowers pulmonary vascular resistance and increases total pulmonary blood flow.

103. What is a tet spell? How is it managed?

The classic tetralogy of Fallot "spell" includes the following symptoms: agitation/irritability, hyperpnea, profound cyanosis, and syncope. Auscultation during the spell frequently reveals an absent murmur due to minimal flow across the right ventricular outflow tract. If frequent or inadequately managed, these spells can, in rare cases, result in death. Initial treatment typically consists of the following:

1. Supplemental oxygen
2. Sedation (subcutaneous or intravenous morphine 0.1 mg/kg)
3. Volume expansion

Some have advocated the knee-chest position for these children to increase both systemic venous return and systemic vascular resistance. In some irritable children, this positioning tends to worsen the situation because it can be very upsetting and increase the irritability. It is particularly important for the physicians and nurses at the bedside to keep the patient calm. Frequently, the most effective position for such children is to be held by their parent across the shoulder, with their knees bent and with supplemental oxygen being given by an additional person. In the case of persistent cyanosis despite these maneuvers, agents to increase systemic afterload, such as phenylephrine (5–20 µg/kg/dose intravenously every 10 min), can reverse the spell in some cases. Emergency intubation and mechanical ventilation, as well as surgery or extracorporeal membrane oxygenation (ECMO), are occasionally, but rarely, needed.

POSTOPERATIVE MANAGEMENT

104. What information is needed to care for the neonate with congenital heart disease after cardiothoracic surgery?

Ideal postoperative care of the neonate following either reparative or palliative operations requires a thorough understanding and systemic evaluation of the following:

1. The underlying anatomic defect
2. The pathophysiology of the preoperative state
3. The anesthetic regimen used during surgery
4. The duration of cardiopulmonary bypass, aortic cross-clamp time, and circulatory arrest time
5. The details of the operative procedure and any concerns of the surgeon regarding the potential for residual defects
6. The data available from monitoring catheters, physical examination, radiographs, and echocardiography

105. Discuss the most common noncardiac causes of respiratory compromise after cardiothoracic surgery.

Noncardiac causes of respiratory failure can be broadly grouped into central nervous system disorders, neuromuscular disorders, isolated neuropathies, airway abnormalities proximal to the alveoli, alveolar disease, extrinsic compression of the lungs, and chest wall abnormalities. Such derangements of the respiratory system may result in impaired gas exchange, poor lung compliance, and/or ventilation/perfusion mismatch. The most common noncardiac causes of respiratory compromise are listed below:

Noncardiac Causes of Respiratory Compromise after Cardiothoracic Surgery

Central nervous system	Neuromuscular
1. General anesthesia	1. Residual neuromuscular blockade
2. Administration of analgesics or sedative/hypnotics	2. Respiratory muscle weakness—from disuse and/or malnutrition
3. Hypoxic-ischemic encephalopathy	
4. Apnea of prematurity	

(Table continued on next page.)

Noncardiac Causes of Respiratory Compromise after Cardiothoracic Surgery (Continued)

Isolated neuropathies	Alveolar disease
1. Hemidiaphragmatic paresis or paralysis—phrenic nerve injury	1. Acute lung injury from cardiopulmonary bypass
2. Vocal cord paralysis—recurrent laryngeal nerve injury	2. Increased lung fluid—from left-to-right shunt lesions
Airway abnormalities proximal to the alveoli	3. Atelectasis
1. Tracheostomy or endotracheal tube obstruction	4. Pneumonia
2. Postextubation subglottic edema	5. Pulmonary hemorrhage
3. Laryngotracheomalacia	6. Pulmonary hypoplasia
4. Left mainstem bronchomalacia—from long-standing left atrial or left pulmonary artery enlargement	Extrinsic lung compression
	1. Pleural effusion (transudate vs. exudate)
	2. Pneumothorax, hemothorax, chylothorax
	Chest wall
	1. Midsternal, thoracotomy, or "clam shell" chest incisions

Adapted from Newth CJL, Hammer J: Pulmonary issues. In Chang AC, Hanley FL, Wernovsky G, Wessel DL (eds): Pediatric Cardiac Intensive Care. Baltimore, Williams & Wilkins, 1998, p 352.

106. What is deep hypothermic circulatory arrest? What are the neurologic sequelae associated with it?

Deep hypothermic circulatory arrest (DHCA) has been increasingly used in centers with expertise in neonatal and infant cardiac surgery. The major surgical advantage of this technique is the absence of perfusion cannulae and blood from the operative field. The use of DHCA assumes that there is a safe duration that is inversely related to body temperature. The organ with the shortest safe period is the brain. A recent randomized study has suggested that a period of DHCA > 45 minutes is associated with a significantly greater incidence of perioperative neurologic abnormalities.

Follow-up studies focusing on neurologic sequelae after DHCA have primarily emphasized the incidence of seizures, choreoathetosis, and long-term development of abnormalities. Seizures are the most frequently observed neurologic consequence of cardiac surgery using DHCA, with a reported incidence of 4–25%. Both focal and generalized seizures have been described, usually occurring during postoperative days 1–4. Although the long-term prognosis after hypoxic-ischemic seizures in the normothermic neonate may be guarded, it appears that long-term seizure disorders are rare. Patients with postoperative seizures are more likely to have neurologic and developmental abnormalities at midterm follow-up.

107. What are the most common causes of phrenic nerve injury?

The most common isolated neuropathy after surgery is phrenic nerve injury resulting in hemidiaphragmatic paresis or paralysis. Hemiparesis is defined as incomplete paralysis. Mechanisms of injury include nerve transection, nerve stretch, electrocautery heat trauma, or cold injury from topical cardiac hypothermia. The postoperative incidence of phrenic nerve injury has been estimated to be as high as 10% in children under 2 years of age.

Phrenic nerve injury may be noted after a patient fails ventilator weaning or extubation. The physical examination may reveal asymmetric movement of the chest and upper abdomen, whereas chest radiograph may show the affected hemidiaphragm to be higher than the unaffected hemidiaphragm. Fluoroscopy may demonstrate a hemidiaphragm with minimal movement (paresis) or no movement (paralysis). The procedures associated with phrenic injury are listed below:

Procedures Associated with Phrenic Nerve Injury

Arch reconstruction:	Norwood palliation
	Interrupted aortic arch repair
	Coarctation repair

(Table continued on next page.)

Procedures Associated with Phrenic Nerve Injury (Continued)

Hilar Dissection:	Arterial switch operation
	Tetralogy of Fallot
	TOF/APV repair: PA plication
	TOF/PA: unifocalization
	Truncus arteriosus repair
	PDA ligation
Systemic-to-pulmonary artery shunt	

TOF/APV = tetralogy of Fallot with absent pulmonary valve, TOF/PA = tetralogy of Fallot with pulmonary atresia, PDA = patent ductus arteriosus.
Adapted from Marino BS, Wernovsky G: Preoperative and postoperative care of the infant with critical congenital heart disease. In Avery GB, Fletcher MA, MacDonald MG (eds): Neonatology: Pathophysiology and Management of the Newborn. Philadelphia, Lippincott Williams & Wilkins, 1999, p 664.

108. When during the postoperative period is low cardiac output most likely? How is it addressed?

In neonates and infants studied after the arterial switch operation, the cardiac index falls predictably by 25% from baseline 6–12 hours postoperatively, while pulmonary and systemic vascular resistance increases. In particular, neonates may have a severely decreased cardiac index; 15–25% of patients may have a cardiac index < 2.0 L/min/m^2. Infants or neonates suffering from low output are generally tachycardic, cool peripherally, and oliguric, and they have a decreased mixed venous saturation. In severe cases, the child may be hypotensive and anuric and have a significant metabolic acidosis. Factors implicated in low output include the following:

1. The effects of myocardial ischemia from aortic cross clamping
2. Hypothermia
3. Reperfusion injury
4. Inadequate myocardial protection
5. Ventriculotomy, when performed
6. Acute changes in loading conditions

Anticipation of this reproducible phenomenon greatly reduces the associated morbidity and potential mortality. Volume therapy to increase preload and the appropriate use of inotropic and afterload-reducing agents have been shown to oppose this phenomenon.

109. What are the early and late postoperative sequelae of the common neonatal reparative and palliative operations?

See table on following three pages.

INTERVENTIONAL CARDIOLOGY

110. Which kinds of congenital heart disease may benefit from a cardiac catheterization interventional procedure?

- **Transposition of the great arteries with intact ventricular septum:** Rashkind's balloon atrial septostomy
- **Critical aortic stenosis:** Aortic balloon valvuloplasty
- **Critical pulmonary stenosis:** Pulmonary balloon valvuloplasty
- **Restrictive atrial septum:** Balloon atrial septostomy/atrial septoplasty/blade atrial septectomy

Right heart lesions:	Tricuspid atresia
	Pulmonary atresia with intact ventricular septum
Left heart lesions:	Total anomalous pulmonary venous return
	Mitral atresia/hypoplastic left heart syndrome

- **Scimitar syndrome:** Coil embolization of systemic to pulmonary collateral vessels

Common Neonatal Operations and Their Early and Late Postoperative Sequelae

LESION	SURGICAL REPAIR (EPONYM)	EARLY POSTOPERATIVE SEQUELAE		LATE POSTOPERATIVE SEQUELAE	
		COMMON	RARE	COMMON	RARE
COA	Subclavian flap repair (Waldhausen) *or* Resection with end-to-end or end-to-side anastomosis *or* Patch augmentation	Systemic hypertension Absent left arm pulse (if subclavian flap repair)	Ileus Hemidiaphragm paresis Vocal cord paresis Chylothorax Residual obstruction	Systemic hypertension (if repaired as adolescent) Recoarctation (if repaired as neonate)	Aortic aneurysm formation
TOF	Patch closure of VSD via ventriculotomy, right atriotomy, or pulmonary arteriotomy Englargement of RVOT with infundibular patch +/– Pulmonary valvotomy +/– Transannular RV to PA patch +/– RV to PA conduit	Pulmonary regurgitation (if transannular patch, valvotomy, or nonvalved conduit) Transient RV dysfunction Right-to-left shunt via PFO, which usually resolves 2–4 days postoperatively as RV function improves	Residual left-to-right shunt at VSD patch Residual RVOTO JET Complete heart block Pleural effusions Chylothorax	Conduit obstruction PVCs	Branch PA obstruction Aortic regurgitation Ventricular arrhythmias Ventricular dysfunction Sudden death
PDA	Ligation (+/– division) of PDA using open thoracotomy and direct visualization or VATS		Hemidiaphragm paresis Vocal cord paresis Chylothorax Interruption of LPA or descending aorta		Residual PDA (if ligation used without division)
VSD	Repair via transatrial/transventricular or pulmonary arteriotomy approach	Small residual VSD Right bundle branch block (50%) or bifascicular block (50%)	Complete heart block JET Large residual VSD Pulmonary hypertension		Ventricular arrhythmia Ventricular dysfunction (especially if ventriculotomy)
CAVC	"Single patch" technique *or* "Double patch" technique	Small residual VSD Mild MR Right bundle branch block Sinoatrial node dysfunction	Complete heart block JET Large residual VSD Pulmonary hypertension Severe MR Subaortic stenosis	Mild MR	Mitral valvuloplasty or replacement

(Table continued on next page.)

Common Neonatal Operations and Their Early and Late Postoperative Sequelae (Continued)

LESION	SURGICAL REPAIR (EPONYM)	EARLY POSTOPERATIVE SEQUELAE		LATE POSTOPERATIVE SEQUELAE	
		COMMON	RARE	COMMON	RARE
Truncus arteriosus	Closure of VSD; baffling LV to truncus (neo-aorta) Removal of PAs from truncus Conduit placement from RV to PAs	Reactive pulmonary hypertension Transient RV dysfunction with right-to-left shunt via PFO Hypocalcemia (DiGeorge syndrome)	Truncal valve stenosis or regurgitation Residual VSD JET Complete heart block	Conduit obstruction	Significant AS or AI
TGA	*Arterial switch operation (Jatene)* Division and reanastomosis of pulmonary artery and aorta to anatomically correct ventricle Translocation of coronary arteries Closure of septal defects if present	Transient decrease in cardiac output 6–12 hours after surgery	Coronary ostial stenosis or occlusion Sudden death Hemidiaphragm paresis Chylothorax	Supravalvular PS Aortic regurgitation	Coronary ostial stenosis or occlusion Sudden death Supravalvar AS SVT Sick sinus syndrome
	Atrial switch operation (Senning or Mustard) Intra-atrial baffling of the systemic venous return to the left ventricle (to PA) and pulmonary venous return to the right ventricle (to aorta) Closure of septal defects if present	SVT Sick sinus syndrome Tricuspid regurgitation	Pulmonary or systemic venous obstruction	SVT Sick sinus syndrome Tricuspid regurgitation Mild sub-PS	Pulmonary or systemic venous obstruction Ventricular arrhythmias Ventricular dysfunction Sudden death Severe sub-PS
TAPVC	Reanastomosis of pulmonary venous confluence to posterior aspect of left atrium Division of connecting vein	Pulmonary hypertension Transient low cardiac output	Residual pulmonary venous obstruction		SVT Sick sinus syndrome Residual pulmonary venous obstruction

(Table continued on next page.)

Common Neonatal Operations and Their Early and Late Postoperative Sequelae (Continued)

LESION	PALLIATIVE PROCEDURES	EARLY POSTOPERATIVE SEQUELAE		LATE POSTOPERATIVE SEQUELAE	
		COMMON	RARE	COMMON	RARE
HLHS*	Stage I (Norwood) Connection of MPA to aorta with reconstruction of aortic arch Systemic to pulmonary shunt Atrial septectomy	Low systemic cardiac output due to excessive PBF Ventricular dysfunction Tricuspid regurgitation	Aortic arch obstruction Restrictive atrial septal defect	Progressive cyanosis	Sudden death LPA distortion Aortic arch obstruction Restrictive atrial septum
Complex lesions with decreased PBF*	Systemic to pulmonary shunt (Blalock-Taussig shunt) Classic—subclavian artery is ligated and directly anastomosed to the ipsilateral pulmonary artery Modified—placement of a gortex tube graft between the subclavian or innominate artery to the ipsilateral pulmonary artery	Excessive PBF and mild congestive heart failure	Hemidiaphragm paresis Vocal cord paralysis Chylothorax	PA distortion	Vertebral artery "steal" syndrome Decreased limb growth (classic)
Complex lesions with excessive PBF*	Pulmonary artery band (prosthetic or silastic constriction of MPA)		Pulmonary artery distortion Aneurysm of MPA	PA distortion	

AI = aortic insufficiency; AS = aortic stenosis; CAVC = common atrioventricular canal; COA = coarctation of the aorta; HLHS = hypoplastic left heart syndrome; JET = junctional ectopic tachycardia; LPA = left pulmonary artery; LV = left ventricle; MPA = main pulmonary artery; MR = mitral regurgitation; PA = pulmonary artery; PBF = pulmonary blood flow; PDA = patent ductus arteriosus; PFO = patent foramen ovale; PS = pulmonary stenosis; PVC = premature ventricular contraction; RV = right ventricle; RVOT = right ventricular outflow tract; RVOTO = right ventricular outflow tract obstruction; SVT = supraventricular tachycardia; TAPVC = total anomalous pulmonary venous connection; TGA = transposition of the great arteries; TOF = tetralogy of Fallot; VATS = video-assisted thoracoscopic surgery; VSD = ventricular septal defect.
* In patients with a single ventricle, the goal is to separate pulmonary and systemic venous return, creating cavopulmonary anastomoses to route systemic venous return directly to the pulmonary arteries (bidirectional Glenn shunt, hemi-Fontan, modified Fontan operation).
Adapted from Wernovsky G, Erickson LC, Wessel DL: Cardiac emergencies. In May HL (ed): Emergency Medicine. Boston, Little Brown, 1992.

111. What are the indications for a diagnostic cardiac catheterization in a neonate with congenital heart disease?

- **Tetralogy of Fallot with or without pulmonary atresia:** Delineation of segmental pulmonary blood flow, coronary and pulmonary artery anatomy
- **Truncus arteriosus:** Delineation of pulmonary artery/branch pulmonary artery origin
- **Pulmonary atresia/intact ventricular septum:** Evaluation of right ventricular–dependent coronary circulation
- **Vascular rings/slings**
- **Scimitar syndrome:** Identification of anomalous pulmonary veins, systemic collateral vessels, and assessment of pulmonary hypertension

112. Name the sites of arterial and venous access for diagnostic and interventional cardiac catheterization procedures.

For diagnostic procedures:
- Arterial access—femoral artery and umbilical artery
- Venous access—femoral vein, umbilical vein, internal jugular vein, and subclavian vein

For interventional procedures:
- Balloon atrial septostomy—femoral vein and umbilical vein
- Aortic balloon valvuloplasty—femoral artery, carotid artery, umbilical artery, femoral vein with transseptal access to the left atrium, and anterograde placement of balloon dilation catheter across the aortic valve from the left ventricle
- Pulmonary balloon valvuloplasty—femoral vein, umbilical vein, internal jugular vein, and subclavian vein

113. Which anomaly of the systemic veins prevents access to the right heart from the femoral veins?

An **interrupted inferior vena cava** (IVC) prevents access to the right heart from the femoral veins. The interruption, however, is usually below the level of the hepatic veins. Therefore, the umbilical vein remains an alternative way to access the right heart. (The umbilical vein drains into the portal vein, which empties through the ductus venosus into the hepatic veins. The hepatic veins connect directly to the undersurface of the right atrium in the case of an interrupted IVC).

114. How do prostaglandins work in transposition of the great arteries?

By maintaining patency of the ductus arteriosus, poorly oxygenated blood from the aorta flows across the ductus arteriosus into the pulmonary artery. Therefore, pulmonary blood flow and venous return to the left atrium are both increased. The resultant higher left atrial pressure and volume enhance flow across the patent foramen ovale, thus improving mixing of well-saturated blood with the poorly oxygenated blood in the right atrium. Because of mixing in the right atrium, better-oxygenated blood is expected to enter the aorta from the right ventricle.

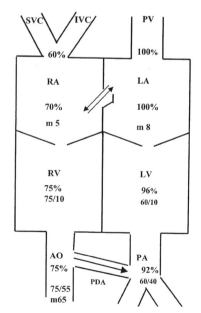

From Rudolph AM: Aortopulmonary transposition. In Rudolph AM: Congenital Disease of the Heart. Chicago, Year Book, 1974, p 475, with permission.

115. In infants with transposition of the great arteries, how does a balloon atrial septostomy improve systemic oxygen saturation?

The balloon atrial septostomy permits unrestricted bidirectional mixing of fully saturated blood in the left atrium with desaturated blood in the right atrium so as to achieve a higher net saturation of blood in the systemic circulation. Patency of the ductus is no longer essential. Variations in oxygen saturations from 50–80% are usual, although mixing is excellent.

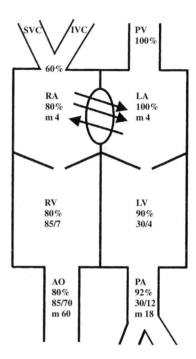

From Rudolph AM: Aortopulmonary transposition. In Rudolph AM: Congenital Disease of the Heart. Chicago, Year Book, 1974, p 485, with permission.

116. What is the current preoperative management of transposition of the great arteries with intact ventricular septum?

- Neonates with transposition of the great arteries with intact ventricular septum are started on prostaglandins. If the oxygen saturation on PGE_1 is acceptable (> 70%), then a balloon septostomy is not done, and an early arterial switch operation is done.
- [a] If the oxygen is less than acceptable (< 70%), a ballon atrial septostomy is undertaken to improve mixing in the atria (PGE_1 is no longer essential). The septostomy is followed by an early arterial switch.
- If delays are expected for the arterial switch operation, a balloon atrial septostomy is undertaken for more reliable mixing of oxygenated and deoxygenated blood.

117. Is there an interventional approach to treating a patent ductus arteriosus in a premature newborn?

No. Indomethacin or surgical ligation are the only two options.

118. What is critical aortic stenosis?

Aortic stenosis in a neonate that results in congestive cardiac failure with circulatory shock is termed **critical aortic stenosis**. In affected infants, the systemic circulation is dependent on patency of the ductus arteriosus with flow from the pulmonary artery into the descending aorta. Therefore, prostaglandin therapy is required.

Intravenous pressor support is usually necessary for hypotension and poor left ventricular function. Supportive therapy may include ventilation, volume replacement, and correction of acidosis. Most of the infants can be palliated by an aortic balloon valvuloplasty.

119. What are the clinical and laboratory findings in infants with critical aortic stenosis?

Echocardiography is diagnostic. The aortic valve is abnormal and often unicuspid. Severity of stenosis cannot be judged by the derived pressure gradient across the aortic valve. The left ventricular function is depressed. The following table lists clinical and laboratory findings:

CLINICAL FINDINGS	CHEST RADIOGRAPH	ELECTROCARDIOGRAM
Tachycardia	Cardiomegaly	Right ventricular hypertrophy
Tachypnea	Pulmonary edema	ST–T changes
Reduced distal pulses (symmetrical)		
Poor peripheral perfusion		
Gallop		
Murmur +/–, almost never heard		

120. What are the indications and contraindications to aortic balloon valvuloplasty in critical aortic stenosis?

The left ventricular size and shape influence the outcome. Effective intermediate term palliation is expected by aortic balloon valvuloplasty if the left ventricle is elliptical, apex forming, and normal in size. A globular, nonapex-forming, shortened left ventricle is associated with poor outcome after aortic balloon valvuloplasty, and patients with critical aortic stenosis are best served by the staged surgical Norwood approach as in hypoplastic left heart syndrome.

121. What is the access used for aortic balloon valvuloplasty?

For aortic balloon valvuloplasty the approach is retrograde through the umbilical artery or the femoral artery. Entry into the left ventricle through the stenotic aortic valve can be difficult, but in experienced hands is usually successful. Once the pressure in the left ventricle and the ascending aorta is measured, an aortic/left ventricular angiogram is done. The aortic valve annulus is measured on the angiogram, and a balloon dilation catheter with a balloon size 0.8 to 1 times the size of the aortic annulus is positioned with the balloon across the aortic valve. The balloon is inflated to stretch the aortic valve. Larger balloon sizes are associated with development of significant aortic regurgitation and should be avoided.

122. What are the hemodynamics in a neonate with truncus arteriosus and congestive heart failure?

The infant with truncus arteriosus develops congestive heart failure when the pulmonary vascular resistance falls. The increased pulmonary blood flow results in an increase in left atrial pressure (a16, v15, m10). Therefore, the patent foramen ovale closes. There is a small increase in left ventricular end diastolic pressure (10 mmHg), and an increase occurs in left ventricular stroke volume as well. The right and left ventricular pressures are equal because of a nonrestrictive ventricular septal defect. The increase in pulmonary flow is larger than the increase in systemic flow; therefore, systemic arterial saturations are higher. Because of the runoff into the pulmonary arteries, the truncal diastolic pressure may be lower with impairment of coronary blood flow. The infant is therefore at risk for development of myocardial ischemia. Truncal insufficiency may worsen the clinical picture, and some infants may develop congestive heart failure before the fall in pulmonary vascular resistance occurs.

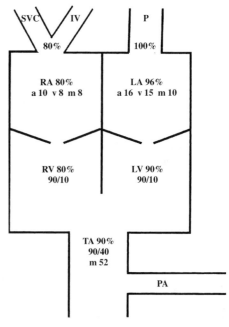

From Rudolph AM: Truncus arteriosus. In Rudolph AM: Congenital Disease of the Heart. Chicago, Year Book, 1974, p 527, with permission.

123. What is critical pulmonary stenosis?

Pulmonary stenosis in a neonate severe enough to cause cyanosis and acidosis (rare) with signs of right heart failure (also rare) is defined as **critical pulmonary stenosis**. Ductal patency is essential for maintaining pulmonary blood flow. Essential diagnostic features are the presence of forward flow through the stenotic pulmonary valve, excluding pulmonary atresia, and a right-to-left flow across the patent foramen ovale because of stenosis severe enough to cause right ventricular diastolic hypertension. Pulmonary balloon valvuloplasty is undertaken to relieve the stenosis after stabilization of the infant.

124. What is scimitar syndrome?

Scimitar syndrome is another name for the hypogenetic right lung syndrome, which involves the following conditions:
- Anomalous connection of the right pulmonary veins to the inferior vena cava
- Right pulmonary artery hypoplasia
- Right lung hypoplasia
- Anomalous systemic arterial supply to the right lung
- Bronchial anomalies
- Dextrocardia reflecting the hypogenetic right lung

The term *scimitar syndrome* derives from a feature on the chest radiograph: the right pulmonary veins cast a shadow like the handle of a scimitar in the right lower zone as they drain anomalously into the IVC.

125–128. A female term infant (weight 2.66 kg) is diagnosed to have hypoplastic left heart syndrome.

125. Which valves are expected to be atretic?

The left atrioventricular valve (mitral atresia) and the left aortic valve (aortic atresia).

126. What is the most pressing clinical issue?

Signs of impaired systemic blood flow and pulmonary overcirculation.

127. The infant was started on PGE$_1$. Despite an improvement of systemic blood flow, however, she exhibited poor weight gain. What is the next course of action?

The infant needs a reevaluation by cardiology. In this case, the chest radiograph demonstrated pulmonary venous congestion, and the echocardiogram demonstrated a restrictive atrial septum. There was poor egress of blood from the left heart because the atrial septal defect was the only exit for blood from the left atrium.

128. What should be done to relieve the problem of poor egress of blood?

Cardiac catheterization and balloon atrial septoplasty. In this case, there was evidence of left atrial hypertension (a 24, v 16, m 18) and a pressure gradient of 17 mmHg from the left atrium to the right atrium confirming a restrictive atrial septum. The infant had a successful balloon atrial septoplasty. A balloon dilation catheter was advanced across the atrial septum, and the balloon was positioned across the atrial septum and inflated several times. After septoplasty the pressure gradient across the atrial septum was reduced to 3 mmHg with relief of the obstructed left atrium and improved cardiac output.

INTERPRETING ELECTROCARDIOGRAMS IN THE NEONATAL PERIOD

129. What is characteristic in the normal newborn electrocardiogram?

Compared with the ECG of an older infant or child, the newborn ECG is remarkable for (1) right axis deviation, +60° to +180°; (2) right ventricular dominance, tall R wave in V1, and deep S wave in V6; (3) a positive T wave in the right precordial leads V4r and V1; and (4) a longer QT$_C$ interval up to 0.46 sec.

At birth, the right ventricle has slightly greater mass than the left ventricle, and the pulmonary artery pressure is initially as high as the systemic blood pressure. For this reason, the normal newborn ECG shows evidence of increased right ventricular forces, namely a tall R wave in V4r and V1, a positive T wave in V4r and V1, and an S wave greater than the R wave in V6. Evidence of increased right ventricular forces decreases over the first 6 months of life.

130. What ECG finding is always abnormal in a newborn?

The normal ECG in a newborn shows a preponderance of right ventricular forces because the right and left ventricle are of equal mass at birth. The normal QRS axis for a newborn is +30° to +200°. The **left axis deviation** (< +30°) is always abnormal. Downward forces in the QRS in lead avF and upward forces in lead I indicate a left axis deviation. Leads I and avL may show a Q wave or negative deflection, which is known as **left axis deviation with a counterclockwise loop**. This finding is seen in congenital heart disease including complete AV canal or in defects that have a canal-type VSD. A newborn suspected of having trisomy 21 who has left axis deviation on ECG should be assumed to have cardiac disease until proved otherwise and most often has a complete AV canal. The figure below shows Q waves in leads I and avL and a deep S wave in avF.

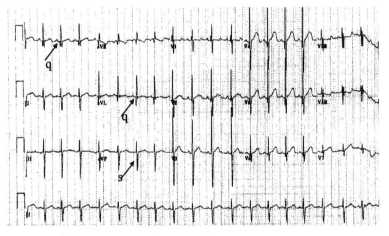

Left axis deviation.

131. What is the common differential diagnosis of bradycardia in a newborn?

- Complete heart block
- Blocked premature atrial contractions
- Sinus bradycardia

Complete heart block is often diagnosed in utero and can be associated with maternal lupus erythematosus and with severe forms of congenital heart disease. Infants with bradycardia can have hydrops as part of the presentation. Urgent evaluation with placement of a pacemaker is often necessary to maintain cardiac output. Emergent use of isoproterenol can increase ventricular heart rate, but generally the rate increases only 10–15%. In complete heart block, the P wave on ECG is at a rate two to three times faster than that of the ventricular rate and can be seen marching through the slower QRS rate. Higher atrial rates in excess of 160/min, secondary to increased sympathetic tone, may indicate distress. The figure (top of next page) shows disassociation between the P waves and QRS.

It may occasionally be necessary to differentiate blocked premature atrial contraction (PAC) from sinus bradycardia. Sinus bradycardia is almost always due to secondary causes, which include respiratory illness, sepsis, or metabolic or electrolyte abnormalities. In a sinus rhythm, each QRS should be preceded by a P wave. Premature atrial contractions are the most common arrhythmia in infancy and can be blocked, leading to a decreased heart rate. Look at the

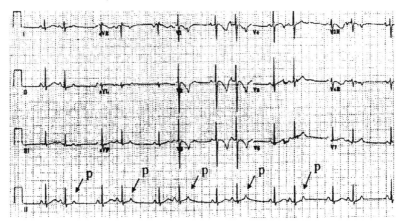

Congenital complete heart block.

T wave in several leads for evidence of a P wave superimposed on the T wave, which is a sign of a blocked PAC. Look also to see if the heart rate is at all irregular to see if, at times, the PAC is conducted. Generally, PACs are transient and do not require treatment. Occasionally, PACs are associated with supraventricular tachycardia. In the rare case in which bradycardia is persistent secondary to blocked PACs, the use of digoxin can often suppress the PACs and restore normal heart rates. The figure below shows a P wave following a QRS, but the P wave is not conducted, which accounts for the bradycardia.

Blocked premature atrial contractions.

132. What is the most common abnormal tachycardia in the term newborn or premature infant?

Supraventricular tachycardia (SVT) is the most common tachycardia in the term newborn and premature infant. It is usually a narrow complex tachycardia at rates of 300/minute. The mechanism is usually a reentrant type of tachycardia. Initially it can be treated with intravenous adenosine, 100–250 µg/kg, given as a rapid push. Adenosine blocks conduction through the AV node, resulting in transient bradycardia and interruption of the reentrant circuit. Once converted to normal sinus rhythm, the infant should have a 12-lead ECG to rule out a delta wave and the presence of Wolff-Parkinson-White (WPW)–type SVT. The following figure shows a narrow complex tachycardia without identifiable P waves.

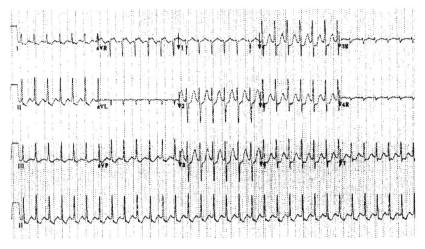

Supraventricular tachycardia.

133. What is a delta wave? What is its importance?

A **delta wave** is a slurring in the up-stroke of the QRS seen together with a short PR interval. It is a sign of Wolff-Parkinson-White syndrome, occurring as atrial depolarization proceeds down a bypass tract to the ventricle. A bypass tract is a special group of cells that allow direct conduction from the atria to the ventricle. Normally, atrial depolarization goes down through the AV node to the ventricle. Because conduction is slower through the AV node, the delta wave is that part of the QRS or ventricular depolarization occurring first from the bypass tract. Once the depolarization gets through the AV node, the depolarization of the ventricle is through the normal pathway. Thus, the short PR interval and delta wave are indications of the presence of a bypass tract that potentially places an infant at risk for supraventricular tachycardia.

When infants have SVT on the basis of WPW syndrome, they usually require medications other than digoxin to treat the SVT. Patients with WPW are usually treated with beta blockers such as propranolol. Digoxin slows conduction through the AV node and, therefore, can enhance the conduction through the bypass tract, producing a rapid tachycardia that can degenerate to ventricular fibrillation. The figure shows the delta wave at the commencement of the QRS.

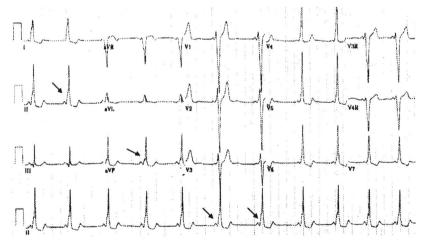

Wolff-Parkinson-White syndrome with delta wave.

134. When is the QT$_C$ abnormally prolonged in infants?

The normal range for the QT$_C$ for infants is shown below and varies with age. The youngest infants can have a QT$_C$ up to 0.48 seconds.

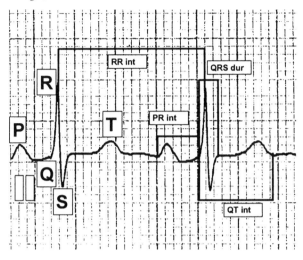

The QT$_C$ is calculated with the Bazett equation, which divides the measured QT by the square root of the RR interval measured in seconds. This equation allows a correction for heart rate.

$$QTC = \frac{QT \text{ interval}}{\sqrt{RR \text{ interval}}}$$

Top normal for infants (0.46 sec) is longer than that for children and adults (0.44 sec). Newborns with a prolonged QT$_C$ on the first day of life should have a repeat ECG in 1–2 days.

ELECTROLYTES AND THE ELECTROCARDIOGRAM

135. What are the ECG abnormalities observed in infants with hyperkalemia?

The earliest change in hyperkalemia is the development of tall, peaked T waves in the precordial leads. With further elevation of the serum potassium concentration, there are a reduction in the R wave, a widening of the QRS complex, ST-segment elevation or depression and PR prolongation. Ultimately, there is further widening of the QRS complex and cardiac arrest.

136. What are the ECG abnormalities in infants with hypokalemia?
- Depression of the ST segment with flattening of the T wave
- Development of prominent U waves with QTU prolongation
- Development of ventricular arrhythmias (torsades de pointes)

137. Describe the treatment for hyperkalemia.
- Intravenous calcium (antagonizes the cardiotoxic effects of potassium)
- NaHCO$_3$ (acutely reduces serum potassium levels)
- Glucose and insulin (acutely reduce serum potassium in the intravascular compartment)
- Kayexalate (a chelating agent that slowly removes potassium from the body)

138. What electrolyte disturbance mimics the ECG findings in hypokalemia?
Hypomagnesemia

139. Name the ECG abnormality in infants with hypocalcemia?
Prolongation of the QT interval

FETAL AND NEONATAL ARRHYTHMIAS

140. When is the conduction system of the fetal heart fully mature?

The conduction system is fully mature by the 16th week of gestation.

141. Name the most common fetal arrhythmia requiring treatment and its hemodynamic consequences.

The most common fetal arrhythmia requiring treatment is reentrant supraventricular tachycardia due to the presence of a bypass tract, which is called Wolff-Parkinson-White syndrome (WPW). The hemodynamic consequences depend on the rate and duration of the tachycardia. The most serious complication is fetal hydrops.

142. How is supraventricular tachycardia treated in the fetus?

Digoxin is the drug of choice. Placental transfer is excellent except in the hydropic fetus. In the presence of hydrops, relatively high maternal levels are needed to obtain adequate fetal levels. Second-line drugs in the past have been procainamide and verapamil. However, flecainide and sotalol have recently become the second-line drugs of choice.

143. Which maternal illnesses are associated with congenital complete heart block?

- Maternal systemic lupus erythematosus (SLE) has been associated with congenital complete heart block. Approximately 1% of pregnancies in women with SLE have fetuses with complete heart block. However, 5% of those who are anti-Ro positive have fetuses with complete heart block. Heart block develops from transplacental transfer of antibody resulting in an immune-mediated destruction of the AV node.
- Collagen vascular disease in the mother is often associated with complete heart block in the newborn.

144. What is the most common form of congenital heart disease associated with congenital complete heart block?

The most common form of congenital heart disease associated with complete heart block is atrioventricular discordance associated with L-transposition of the great vessels ("corrected" transposition of the great vessels).

145. Name the three most common causes of sinus bradycardia in newborns.

1. Hypoventilation
2. Central nervous system disorders
3. Hypothyroidism (watch out for this in trisomy 21)

146. What is the most common benign dysrhythmia seen in newborns?

The most common benign dysrhythmia seen in newborns is premature atrial contractions (PACs). This benign dysrhythmia is commonly detected during fetal monitoring; blocked PACs often cause what appears to be a pause on the monitoring strips, and they occur when the ventricle is refractory and not conducted.

147. Name the common fetal arrhythmias that may result in distress.

Premature beats account for 80–90% of fetal arrhythmias but are generally benign. Reentrant supraventricular tachycardia accounts for 5% of fetal arrhythmias; complete heart block, 2.5%; and atrial flutter 1–2%. Ventricular arrhythmias are rare.

148. How long should a neonate be treated with antiarrhythmic drugs?

In the majority of infants, treatment can be stopped after 6–12 months. Most of the infants have bypass tracts, one-third of which resolve. Approximately one-third of the initial group of patients will develop supraventricular arrhythmias during preadolescence or adolescence.

COR PULMONALE

149. What is cor pulmonale?
Cor pulmonale is a severe abnormality in right ventricular function that is secondary to lung pathology. The common denominator in all cases is significantly elevated pulmonary vascular resistance (PVR) and right ventricular hypertension. The right ventricular dysfunction is manifested as a combination of right ventricular hypertrophy with decreased ventricular compliance and right ventricular dilatation with decreased systolic function. By definition, cor pulmonale excludes all cases of right ventricular pathology due to congenital heart disease.

150. Identify the causes of cor pulmonale in the neonate and infant.
PVR is high in the fetus and normally decreases substantially within the first few days of life. Cor pulmonale may be the result of any process that causes PVR to remain significantly elevated following birth. By far, the most common cause of cor pulmonale in the infant is bronchopulmonary dysplasia (BPD). Other categories of lung disease include upper airway obstruction, neuromuscular disease, restrictive lung disease, thoracic cage abnormalities, and other forms of parenchymal lung disease.

151. If PVR is elevated in the fetus, why does the fetus *not* develop cor pulmonale?
Right ventricular pathology develops when the right ventricle "sees" the full effect of the high PVR. In the fetus, a large patent ductus arteriosus (PDA) with right-to-left shunting decompresses the right ventricle. Right ventricular physiology is therefore normal, and cor pulmonale does not develop. Of interest, in rare cases of intrauterine premature closure of the ductus arteriosus, the fetal right ventricle begins to develop signs of cor pulmonale.

152. Does cor pulmonale occur if the neonate has a large PDA and high PVR?
Cor pulmonale usually does not occur if there is a large PDA. Instead, the fetal circulation persists with right-to-left shunting through the PDA and differential cyanosis in the lower extremities. In addition, a large patent foramen ovale or atrial septal defect also decompresses the right ventricle.

153. What are the signs and symptoms of cor pulmonale?
- Poor feeding—inability to substantially increase cardiac output with exercise
- Signs and symptoms of the underlying pulmonary pathology—oxygen requirement, tachypnea and retractions, and rales and wheezes
- Heaving right ventricular impulse, loud S2 (due to pulmonary hypertension), and murmur of tricuspid insufficiency
- Hepatosplenomegaly

154. Discuss the typical noninvasive laboratory findings of cor pulmonale.
ECG
- Persistent frontal QRS right axis deviation in full-term baby; development of right axis deviation in premature infant
- Right ventricular hypertrophy

Chest radiograph
- Generalized cardiomegaly, prominent main pulmonary artery segment
- Prominent right heart border reflecting right atrial enlargement

Echocardiogram
- Right ventricular hypertrophy, right ventricular dilatation, decreased right ventricular systolic function, right atrial dilatation, prominent pulmonary arteries
- Findings of significantly increased right ventricular pressure, such as systolic flattening of the interventricular septum and a high pressure tricuspid valve regurgitant jet

155. What is the treatment for cor pulmonale?
- The underlying pulmonary abnormality is treated.
- Cardiac function is improved with standard medications for heart failure (i.e., digoxin and furosemide).

156. What is the prognosis?

The prognosis depends greatly on the severity of the pulmonary hypertension and the reversibility of the underlying pulmonary abnormality. The right ventricle initially responds to pulmonary hypertension with hypertrophy resulting in decreased wall stress. As the pulmonary hypertension progresses, however, the right ventricle begins to fail and dilates, with a concomitant significant increase in wall stress. The more severe the pulmonary hypertension, the worse the right ventricular failure.

The infant ventricle has an extraordinary capacity to recover from significant stress, provided that the high PVR decreases. If the underlying pulmonary process can be reversed, one can anticipate a drop in PVR and improvement in right ventricular function. Unfortunately, many of the causes of cor pulmonale are not significantly reversible, and for infants with irreversible causes, the prognosis is poor.

ENDOCARDITIS

157. True or false: Traditional neonatal pathogens including group B *Streptococcus*, *Escherichia coli*, and *Listeria monocytogenes* are often associated with bacterial endocarditis in neonatal patients.

False. *Staphylococcus* spp. predominate in this group as well as in older children; however, *Candida* spp. and unusual gram-negative organisms including *Acinetobacter* spp., *Serratia* spp., *Enterobacter* spp., and *Klebsiella* spp. are described with increasing frequency. Traditional neonatal pathogens are rare causes of endocarditis.

158. What are the risk factors for neonatal endocarditis?

Although no prospective trials have been performed, case reports suggest that children with underlying congenital heart disease, including premature infants with normal intracardiac anatomy and a PDA, and children in whom central venous catheters (UVCs) have been used are at risk for acquiring neonatal endocarditis.

159. Describe the signs of endocarditis in the neonate.

In a recent retrospective review of 16 cases, heart murmurs, skin abscesses, and hepatomegaly were the most frequent signs found in the neonatal patients. Less commonly associated were petechiae, arthritis, and splenomegaly. The common signs in the neonate contrast with those in the older child for whom splenomegaly, petechiae, and splinter hemorrhages are considered findings in subacute bacterial endocarditis.

160. A 28-week-old premature infant now 1 month old has been on several courses of broad-spectrum antibiotics for possible sepsis and to rule out necrotizing enterocolitis. Two days after the removal of antibiotic therapy, the infant has an increasing frequency of apnea and bradycardia, and he appears dusky. Cultures are obtained and antibiotics are reinstituted. The infant subsequently grows the same organism from three blood cultures. The diagnosis of endocarditis is entertained, and an echocardiogram reveals a vegetation on the tricuspid valve close to the tip of a previously removed, peripherally inserted central catheter (PICC) line. What is the likely pathogen?

Fungal endocarditis with *Candida* spp. has traditionally been a rare diagnosis in the neonatal age group. A recent case report with literature review found a total of 17 reported cases. Almost universally, infants were premature and required central venous access for total parenteral nutrition (TPN). Most patients had received broad-spectrum antibiotics before the diagnosis. The authors postulate that the infants acquire the organism at delivery and that because of the reduced integrity of low–birth-weight infants' skin, they are at risk for inoculation during procedures and routine care.

CARDIOMYOPATHY AND MYOCARDITIS

161. Define the three types of cardiomyopathy in the neonate.

1. In **dilated cardiomyopathy**, the left ventricle is globular and poorly contracting; right ventricular size and contractility may be normal or similarly depressed.

2. **Hypertrophic cardiomyopathy** involves marked ventricular hypertrophy with normal systolic function. Asymmetric septal hypertrophy may or may not be present.

3. **Restrictive cardiomyopathy** is marked by normal ventricular size and contractility with abnormal diastolic filling and markedly decreased ventricular compliance.

162. Hypertrophic cardiomyopathy, short PR interval, and huge QRS voltage are found in which metabolic disease?

Pompe disease (glycogen storage disease type II or acid maltase deficiency)

163. What is the most common cause of dilated cardiomyopathy?

The most common cause of dilated cardiomyopathy is idiopathic.

164. What is the most common syndrome associated with cardiomyopathy?

Of patients with Noonan syndrome, 10–20% have an associated hypertrophic cardiomyopathy. Most patients are symptomatic.

165. What treatment is available to an infant with myocarditis?

Treatment for myocarditis is supportive, to maintain cardiac output and decrease volume overload. Although many studies have been undertaken to study immunosuppressive agents or immunoglobulin in the treatment of myocarditis, no agent has proved to be efficacious.

CARDIAC TRANSPLANTATION

166. A 5-week-old infant was about to be discharged from the hospital after cardiac transplantation when the following electrocardiogram was obtained. What is the arrhythmia?
   a. Mobitz type I
   b. Atrial bigeminy
   c. Normal sinus rhythm with residual native P waves
   d. Sinus exit block

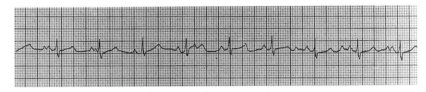

The ECG shows sinus rhythm with residual native P waves. During heart transplantation, the back half of the patient's left and right atria are left in place with the venae cavae and pulmonary veins attached. The donor atria are then anastomosed to the recipient's atria. Because the recipient's native sinus node remains at the junction of the superior vena cava (SVC) and right atrium, a nonconducted P wave can be seen marching through the electrocardiogram without any relationship to the new donor sinus rate. Many surgeons, when anatomically possible, now perform transplantation using a bicaval anastomosis, which removes the recipient's native sinus node and thereby eliminates this confounding finding of extra P waves on the surface ECG.

167. In the first few days following heart transplantation in the neonate, changes in cardiac output are directly proportional to which of the following?
   a. Amount of fluid given
   b. Heart rate
   c. Dow Jones factor
   d. Stroke volume

During cardiac transplantation, all nerves to the heart are severed so that the patient's donor heart is **denervated**; i.e., there is no direct sympathetic or parasympathetic control of heart rate. Concomitantly, during the first few postoperative days, the stroke volume of the transplanted heart is relatively fixed, and the contractility of the heart is diminished secondary to the ischemic time at harvest and implantation. Therefore, the cardiac output is directly proportional to changes in the heart rate in the early postoperative period. Many surgeons strive to keep the heart rate in the neonate from 110–120 bpm, as needed, during this time, either by using chronotropic agents such as isoproterenol or by atrial pacing.

168. What is the average length of time that immunosuppressive therapy is necessary following neonatal heart transplantation if the patient has had no rejection?
   a. 6 months
   b. 1 year
   c. 3 years
   d. None of the above

With present immunologic knowledge and tools, no long-term tolerance has been achieved in any pediatric heart transplant recipient. Lifelong immunosuppression is required to prevent rejection. Some infants, however, can be maintained on monotherapy or with low levels of immunosuppressants for many years.

169. What are the major long-term complications that can occur following heart transplantation? More than one answer may be applicable.
   a. Rejection   d. Hypertension
   b. Infection   e. Renal dysfunction
   c. Coronary artery disease   f. Tumors

All of the major long-term complications in cardiac transplant patients are directly related to the side effects of the immunosuppressive drugs or from ineffective immunosuppressive protection of the graft. Therefore, all of the answers above are correct. Graft coronary artery disease is believed to be the single most important limitation to longevity in cardiac transplant recipients, accounting for the majority of deaths after the first postoperative year.

170. Rejection in a neonate may present with all of the following except:
   a. Fever   d. Low serum sodium
   b. Tachycardia   e. Loss of appetite
   c. Gallop rhythm

Most rejection episodes in the era of cyclosporine immunosuppression are relatively asymptomatic, especially in the older child. The neonatal recipient, however, can often have the nonspecific findings of fever, tachycardia, loss of appetite, and an S3 gallop on exam. The parents often describe the child as "just not being right" or irritable. The serum sodium is usually normal in children with rejection.

CARDIAC TUMORS

171. Which are the most frequent histologic types of primary cardiac tumors in infants and newborns?

Rhabdomyomas are by far the most common cardiac tumors in newborns and infants (overall reported incidence at pediatric age is over 50%, most frequently diagnosed in newborn infants). Such tumors involve the myocardium in numerous areas, the most common of which is the ventricular septum. Although they are usually multiple and intramural, they can occur as single, intracavitary masses as well. Rhabdomyomas have the potential for spontaneous regression.

Fibromas are the second most common primary cardiac tumors in infants and young children, comprising 25% of such tumors. They are predominantly single and intramural, and they involve the left ventricular free wall and/or intraventricular septum. Fibromas are often located at the left ventricular apex.

Intrapericardial teratomas have been reported by some authors to be a more frequent pathologic finding than fibromas in patients less than 1 year old.

Atrial myxomas can occur in neonates, but they are seen more often in older children and adolescents.

172. What is the most frequent disease associated with primary cardiac tumors?

Approximately 50% of patients with cardiac rhabdomyomas have **tuberous sclerosis (Bourneville disease).** Multiple rhabdomyomas are more consistent with the diagnosis of tuberous sclerosis than a solitary tumor. Neonates with this syndrome may have no clinical manifestation other than cardiac tumors or cutaneous and ophthalmic lesions. Seizures and mental retardation usually become evident later in life.

173. Describe the conditions through which intracardiac tumors can cause perinatal or neonatal death.

Depending on size and location, cardiac tumors have been demonstrated to cause death because of the following conditions:
- Severe, intractable dysrhythmias
- Nonimmune hydrops
- Decreased cardiac output due to complete intracardiac inflow or outflow obstruction
- Myocardial infarction due to large coronary embolization
- Acute rupture of intrapericardial cysts into the pericardial space and tamponade
- Severe encroachment by intrapericardial teratomas on the heart and great vessels

174. When is surgery indicated for cardiac tumor?

Surgery is recommended in cases with symptoms of cardiac failure and/or ventricular arrhythmias refractory to medical treatment and in patients with inlet or outlet obstruction. Intrapericardial teratomas and atrial myxoma should be removed upon diagnosis.

CARDIAC SURGERY

175. Name the major shunt operations for congenital heart disease (CHD).

Shunt operations between a systemic artery and pulmonary artery are used to improve oxygen saturation in patients with cyanotic CHD and diminished pulmonary blood flow. Venoarterial shunts, which connect a systemic vein and the pulmonary artery, are also used for similar purposes.

1. The **Blalock-Taussig** shunt consists of an anastomosis between a subclavian artery and the ipsilateral pulmonary artery. The subclavian artery can be divided, and the distal end anastomosed to the pulmonary artery (classic BT shunt), or a prosthetic graft can be interposed between the two arteries (modified BT shunt).

2. The **Waterston** shunt is an anastomosis between the ascending aorta and right pulmonary artery.

3. The **Potts** shunt is an anastomosis between the descending aorta and left pulmonary artery.

4. The **Glenn** anastomosis is a connection between the distal right pulmonary artery and the superior vena cava, which is ligated below the site of the anastomosis.

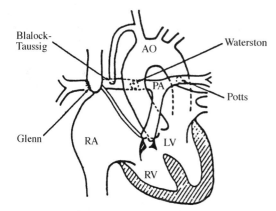

From Park MK: Pediatric Cardiology for Practitioners, 3rd ed. St. Louis, Mosby-Year Book, 1995, with permission.

176. Which factors are associated with more favorable outcomes with the Fontan procedure?

The Fontan procedure, initially done in 1971 for tricuspid atresia, establishes a direct continuity between the systemic venous channels (right atrium/superior vena cava/inferior vena cava) and pulmonary arteries. It thus bypasses the need for a functioning ventricle to pump blood to the lungs and also minimizes the need for conduits and valves. Favorable outcomes are more likely under the following conditions:

1. Pulmonary artery pressure is normal.
2. Pulmonary vascular resistance is normal.
3. Pulmonary arteries are of adequate size.
4. End-diastolic pressure is low.
5. The lesion is tricuspid atresia.

From Park MK: Pediatric Cardiology for Practitioners, 3rd ed. St. Louis, Mosby-Year Book, 1995, with permission.

177. For which congenital heart disorder is the "switch operation" done?

Transposition of the great vessels (TGV). Also known as the Jatene operation, the procedure involves reimplantation of the coronary arteries, bisection of the pulmonary artery and aorta, and resuturing of the two great vessels into their correct anatomic positions. This operation, first done in 1976, has become the treatment of choice for TGV over others which use intra-atrial baffles to redirect blood along more proper anatomic paths (i.e., Senning and Mustard procedures). Because these baffles have been associated with much higher incidences of RV failure and dysrhythmias, they are no longer performed in most major academic centers, except in unusual circumstances. For physicians who cared for children who had undergone the earlier approach to TGV of a Rashkind procedure (balloon pulled through the atrial septum to create a large ASD), followed by a Mustard procedure, an arterial switch appears remarkable. With the former approach, infants were ill and hospitalized for weeks or months. Many infants now are discharged from the hospital within a week following a switch.

178. What are the indications for surgical repair of ASD and VSD?

Ventricular septal defect: Infants with a large VSD refractory to medical therapy, causing failure to thrive and/or repeated lower respiratory tract infections, should be referred for surgery.

If there is intractable congestive heart failure that interferes with feeding and growth, early repair is indicated. Pulmonary hypertension is another indication for surgery, although the surgery should ideally be performed before pulmonary hypertension becomes significant or fixed. In older children with normal pulmonary artery pressure, but with pulmonary blood flow near or equal to twice systemic blood flow, surgical closure is advised.

Atrial septal defect: Symptomatic infants with an ASD should undergo surgery at the time of diagnosis. Surgical results usually are excellent. Asymptomatic children should be scheduled for repair during the first 5 years of life.

179. Is there any surgical therapy for hypoplastic left heart syndrome?

In hypoplastic left heart syndrome (HLHS), severe underdevelopment of the left ventricle, mitral valve, aortic valve, and ascending aortic arch occurs. This entity may present with variable degrees of hypoplasia of any of the structures on the left side of the heart. Newborns usually develop signs of severe congestive heart failure (CHF). In most infants, the diagnosis becomes apparent immediately, but some neonates may have a persistently patent ductus arteriosus that allows sufficient blood flow to the systemic circulation for some period of time. When the ductus finally closes, acute, profound CHF ensues. For many years, the diagnosis of HLHS carried with it a fatal prognosis. Until the last 15 years, neonates diagnosed with HLHS were simply made comfortable and allowed to die. In recent years, however, two surgical procedures have become available: heart transplantation and the Norwood procedure.

The **Norwood procedure**, reported initially in 1983, is performed in three stages. In stage I, the proximal main pulmonary artery is transected, and with additional homograft material, it is used to help rebuild the aorta. This creates a univentricular systemic pumping chamber and changes the physiology from aortic atresia to pulmonic atresia. The distal main pulmonary artery is oversewn, and a systemic-to-pulmonary shunt is created between the innominate artery and right pulmonary artery to correct pulmonary flow.

Stage II (performed at about age 6 months) seeks to regulate pulmonary blood flow by changing to a bidirectional Glenn anastomosis (superior vena cava to distal right pulmonary artery). One to 2 years later, a Fontan procedure (Stage III Norwood) is performed (right atrium to pulmonary artery), which ultimately separates the venous and arterial sides. The learning curve for this procedure is steep, and it takes many years for even the best cardiac surgeons to become comfortable with the complexity of this surgery. Even in the most skilled hands, there is still about a 10–30% mortality rate associated with each stage of the procedure.

Long-term survival is significantly better with heart transplantation; however, a shortage of donors is a major problem, and many ethical issues have arisen with the use of hearts from neurologically damaged infants. Thus 20–30% of infants die awaiting transplant.

BIBLIOGRAPHY

1. Adams J: Neonatalogy. In Garson A, Bricker JT, McNamara DG (eds): The Science and Practice of Pediatric Cardiology. Philadelphia, Lea & Febiger, 1990.
2. Addonizio LJ: Late complications of pediatric cardiac transplantation. Am Col Cardiol Curr J Rev, 23–25, 1994.
3. Allen HD, et al: Pediatric therapeutic cardiac catheterization: A statement for healthcare professionals from the council on cardiovascular disease in the young. Circulation 97:609–625, 1998.
4. Anderson PW: Myocardial Development. In Long WA: Fetal and Neonatal Cardiology. Philadelphia, W.B. Saunders, 1990.
5. Barone, MA (ed): The Harriet Lane Handbook, 14th ed. St. Louis, Mosby, 1996.
6. Boucek MM, Faro A, Novick RJ, et al: The Registry of the International Society for Heart and Lung Transplantation: Third Official Pediatric Report—1998. J Heart Lung Transplant 18:1151–1172, 1998.
7. Brook MM, Heymann MA: Patent ductus arteriosus. In Emmanouilides GC, et al (eds): Heart Disease in Infants, Children, and Adolescents, 5th ed. Baltimore, Williams & Wilkins, 1995, pp 746–764.
8. Chinnock RE, Larsen RL, Emery JR, Bailey LL: Pretransplant risk factors and causes of death or graft loss after heart transplantation during early infancy. J Heart Lung Transplant 2:206–209, 1995.
9. Clyman RI: Patent ductus arteriosus in the premature infant. In Taeusch HW, Ballard RA: Avery's Diseases of the Newborn, 7th ed. Philadelphia, W.B. Saunders, 1998, pp 699–710.

10. Clyman RI: Recommendations for the postnatal use of indomethacin: An analysis of four separate treatment strategies. J Pediatr 128:601–607, 1996.

11. Colan SD, Borow KM, Neumann A: Left ventricular end-systolic wall stress-velocity of fiber shortening relation: A load-independent index of myocardial contractility. J Am Coll Cardiol 4:715–724, 1984.

12. Doyle TP, Hellenbrand WE: The role of cardiac catheterization in the evaluation and treatment of neonates with congenital heart disease. Semin Perinatol 17:122–134, 1993.

13. Emmanouilides GC, Allen HD, Riemenschneider TA, Gutgesell HP (eds): Moss and Adams' Heart Disease in Infants, Children and Adolescents Including the Fetus and Young Adult, 5th ed. Baltimore, Williams & Wilkins, 1994.

14. Feldt RH, Porter CJ, Edwards WD, et al: Defects of the atrial septum and atrioventricular canal. In Adams FH, Emmanouilides GC, Riemenschneider TA (eds): Moss' Heart Disease in Children and Adolescents, 4th ed. Baltimore, Williams & Wilkins, 1989.

15. Flanagan MF, Fyler DC: Cardiac disease. In Avery GB, Fletcher MA, MacDonald M, eds: Neonatology: Pathophysiology and Management of the Newborn. Philadelphia, J.B. Lippincott, 1994.

16. Franco K (ed): Pediatric Cardiopulmonary Transplantation. Armonk, NY, Futura, 1997.

17. Freedom RM: Abnormalities of the pulmonary venous connections including subdivided left atrium. In Freedom RM, Mawson JB, Yoo SJ, Benson LN: Congenital Heart Disease: Textbook of Angiocardiography. Armonk, NY, Futura, 1997.

18. Fyler DC (ed): Nadas' Pediatric Cardiology. Philadelphia, Hanley & Belfus, 1992.

19. Gaissmaier RE, Pohlandt F: Single-dose dexamethasone treatment of hypotension in preterm infants. J Pediatr 134:701–705, 1999.

20. Garson A, Bricker JT, McNamara T (eds): The Science and Practice of Pediatric Cardiology, 2nd ed. Baltimore, Williams & Wilkins, 1997.

21. Gest AL, Moise AA: Fetal circulation and changes occurring at birth. In Garson A, Bricker JT, McNamara DG (eds): The Science and Practice of Pediatric Cardiology, Philadelphia, Lea & Febiger, 1990.

22. Gewitz MH: Cor pulmonale–pulmonary heart disease. In Emmanouilides GC, et al: Moss and Adams' Heart Disease in Infants, Children and Adolescents, 5th ed. Baltimore, Williams & Wilkins, 1995, pp 1717–1719.

23. Graham TP, Bender HW, Spach MS: Ventricular septal defect. In Adams FH, Emmanouilides GC, Riemenschneider TA (eds): Moss' Heart Disease in Children and Adolescents, 4th ed. Baltimore, Williams & Wilkins, 1989.

24. Haworth SG: Pulmonary vasculature. In Anderson RH, et al: Paediatric Cardiology. New York, Churchill Livingstone, 1987, pp 152–153.

25. Hrodmar H, et al: Balloon dilation of the aortic valve: Studies in normal lambs and in children with aortic stenosis. J Am Coll Cardiol 9:816–822, 1987.

26. Huhta JC, Moise KJ, Fisher DJ, et al: Detection and quantitation of constriction of the fetal ductus arteriosus by Doppler echocardiography. Circulation 75:406–412, 1987.

27. Huhta JC, Strassburger JF, Carpenter RJ, et al: Pulsed Doppler fetal echocardiography. J Clin Ultrasound 13:247, 1985.

28. Keren A, Popp RL: Assignment of patients into the classification of cardiomyopathies. Circulation 86:1622–1633, 1992.

29. Lewis AB, Freed MD, Heymann MA, et al: Side effects of therapy with prostaglandin E1 in infants with critical congenital heart disease. Circulation 64:893–898, 1981.

30. Marino BS, Wernovsky G: Preoperative and postoperative care of the infant with critical congenital heart disease. In Avery GB, Fletcher MA, MacDonald MG (eds): Neonatology: Pathophysiology and Management of the Newborn. Philadelphia, Lippincott Williams & Wilkins, 1999.

31. Mercier JC, DiSessa TG, Jarmekani JM, et al: Two-dimensional echocardiographic assessment of left ventricular volumes and ejection fraction in children. Circulation 65:962, 1982.

32. Moes CAF, Freedom RM: Rings, slings, and other things: Vascular structures contributing to a neonatal "noose." In Freedom RM, Benson LN, Smallhorn JF: Neonatal Heart Disease. New York, Springer-Verlag, 1992, pp 731–749.

33. Morrow WR, Naftel D, Chinook R, et al, and the Pediatric Heart Transplantation Study Group: Outcome of listing for transplantation in infants younger than six months: predictors of death and interval to transplantation. J Heart Lung Transplant 16:1255–1266, 1997.

34. Mosca RS, et al: Critical aortic stenosis in the neonate. A comparison of balloon valvuloplasty and transventricular dilation. J Thorac Cardiovasc Surg 109:147–154, 1995.

35. Moss AJ, Adams FH, Emmanouilides GC: Heart Disease in Infants, Children and Adolescents. Baltimore, Williams & Wilkins, 1995.

36. Murphy DJ: Doppler echocardiography. In Garson A, Bricker JT, McNamara DG (eds): The Science and Practice of Pediatric Cardiology. Philadelphia, Lea & Febiger, 1990.

37. Newth CJL, Hammer J: Pulmonary issues. In Chang AC, Hanley FL, Wernovsky G, Wessel DL (eds): Pediatric Cardiac Intensive Care. Baltimore, Williams & Wilkins, 1998.

38. Park M: Pediatric Cardiology for Practitioners, 3rd ed. St. Louis, Mosby, 1996.
39. Perry SB: Manual techniques of cardiac catheterization: Vessel entry and catheter manipulation. In Lock JE, Keane JF, Perry SB (eds): Diagnostic and Interventional Catheterization in Congenital Heart Disease, 2nd ed. Boston, Kluwer Academic Publishers, 2000, pp 13–21.
40. Roze JC, Tohier C, Maingureneau C, et al: Response to dobutamine and dopamine in the hypotensive very preterm infant. Arch Dis Child 69:59–63, 1993.
41. Rudolph AM: Aortopulmonary transposition. In Rudolph AM: Congenital Disease of the Heart. Chicago, Year Book, 1974.
42. Rudolph AM: Truncus arteriosus. In Rudolph AM: Congenital Disease of the Heart. Chicago, Year Book, 1974.
43. Schwartz ML, Cox GF, Lin AE, et al: Clinical approach to genetic cardiomyopathy in children. Circulation 94:2021–2038, 1996.
44. Schowengerdt KO, Naftel DC, Seib PM, et al, and the Pediatric Heart Transplant Study Group: Infection after pediatric heart transplantation: Results of a multi-institutional study. J Heart Lung Transplant 16:1207–1216, 1997.
45. See DM, Tiles JG: Viral Myocarditis. Rev Infect Dis 13:951–956, 1991.
46. Seri I: Cardiovascular, renal, and endocrine actions of dopamine in neonates and children. J Pediatr 126:333–344, 1995.
47. Seri I, Abbasi S, Wood DC, Gerdes JS: Effect of dopamine on regional blood flows in sick preterm neonates. J Pediatr 133:728–734, 1998.
48. Sigfusson G, Fricker FJ, Bernstein D, et al: Long term survivors of pediatric heart transplantation: A multicenter report of 68 children who have survived greater than five years. J Pediatr 130:851–853, 1997.
49. Silverman NH, Snider AR: Two-dimensional echocardiography in congenital heart disease. Norwalk, CT, Appleton-Century-Crofts, 1982.
50. Simsic J, et al: Critical care management of critical aortic stenosis. J Am Coll Cardiol 35(2 Suppl A): 520A, 2000.
51. Snider AR, Serwer GA, Ritter SB: Echocardiography in Pediatric Heart Disease, 2nd ed. St. Louis, Mosby, 1997.
52. So KW, Fok TG, Ng PC, et al: Randomized controlled trial of colloid or crystalloid in hypotensive preterm infants. Arch Dis Child 76:F43–F46, 1997.
53. Weber HS, et al: Transcarotid balloon valvuloplasty with continuous transesophageal echocardiographic guidance for neonatal critical aortic valve stenosis: An alternative to surgical palliation. Pediatr Cardiol 19:212–217, 1998.
54. Wernovsky G, Erickson LC, Wessel DL: Cardiac emergencies. In May HL (ed): Emergency Medicine. Boston, Little Brown, 1992.
55. Zeevi B, Keane JF, Castaneda AR, et al: Neonatal critical valvar aortic stenosis: A comparison of surgical and balloon dilation therapy. Circulation 80:831–839, 1989.

5. DERMATOLOGY

1. Name three forms of epidermal inclusion cysts that are commonly found in the neonate.

1. **Milia:** tiny cysts usually found on the face in up to 40% of newborns
2. **Epstein pearls:** cysts found on the palate of approximately 64% of newborns
3. **Bohn nodules:** alveolar cysts

All three forms represent cystic retention of keratin, appear and resolve in the first month, and can be present at birth. They are white 1–2-mm papules that can be found singularly or in clusters.

2. What is the standard treatment for milia, sebaceous gland hyperplasia, transient neonatal pustular melanosis, erythema toxicum, and sucking blisters?

The treatment is the same for all—e.g., no treatment other than reassuring the family that they will resolve with time.

CONDITION	ONSET	RESOLUTION	TREATMENT
Milia	Can be at birth, < 1 mo old	Usually < 1mo	None
Sebaceous gland hyperplasia	Can be at birth, < 1 mo old	Usually < 1mo	None
Transient neonatal pustular melanosis (TNPN)	Usually present at birth	Vesicopustules < 5 days Pigment macules < 3 mo	None
Erythema toxicum	24–48 hr, new lesions < 10 days old	Each lesion < 5 days All lesions < 2 wk	None
Sucking blisters	Present at birth	Days	None

3. What are neonatal acne and transient cephalic neonatal pustulosis? How do these entities differ from infantile acne?

There is some degree of controversy regarding the cause and nomenclature of these conditions. Neonatal acne-like lesions typically are not distinct pimples (comedones) but superficial pustules.

Neonatal acne usually begins at a few weeks of life and resolves over several months. Affected infants exhibit multiple inflammatory erythematous papules and pustules. Treatment is rarely needed.

Transient cephalic neonatal pustulosis (TCNP) has been proposed as a subset of neonatal acne caused by *Malassezia* species rather than by elevation in androgen levels, which occurs in infantile or classic acne. Others have proposed that there is no true neonatal acne and that the term TCNP should be used as a substitute. Like neonatal acne, TCNP usually begins at a few weeks of life and resolves in several months. Affected infants demonstrate multiple inflammatory erythematous papules and pustules. Comedonal lesions are rare, and treatment is rarely needed, although some experts believe that topical anti-yeast agents speed resolution.

Infantile acne is truly an acneiform condition, with open and closed comedones as well as papules and pustules. It presents later, usually beyond the age of 2–3 months, and generally resolves between the ages of 6 and 12 months. That time sequence parallels decreases in fetal adrenal pubertal androgen levels and male testosterone levels (one possible reason males are more commonly affected). Unlike neonatal acne or TCNP, infantile acne may persist and cause scarring. For this reason, like adolescent acne, it is treated with topical antibiotics and occasionally with retinoids or systemic agents.

4. What is prickly heat? Which bacteria is believed to contribute to its cause?

Prickly heat is the term for **miliaria rubra**, which is caused by obstruction of the eccrine ducts. The extracellular polysaccharide substance from *Staphylococcus epidermidis* has been implicated in its pathogenesis.

5. How are miliaria crystallina and rubra differentiated? How are they treated?

Miliaria is found in up to 15% of newborns. Both forms are caused by eccrine duct obstruction and resultant sweat leakage to different levels of skin (crystallina under the stratum corneum and rubra at the upper dermis). Miliaria is more common in hot, humid environments and is distributed to the forehead, upper trunk, or other covered surfaces. Don't sweat about the treatment—just keep the baby from being overheated. The removal of excess layers of clothing (or moving the infant to Alaska) is helpful. Air conditioning may also be helpful.

6. Is erythema toxicum toxic? In which kind of infant is it rarely seen?

Erythema toxicum (ET) is a benign condition. ET is no alien to the nursery; it is present in 50% of full-term newborns. It is much less prevalent, however, in premature infants, occurring in only approximately 5%.

7. When do the lesions of ET occur? What do they look like?

ET usually begins between 24 and 48 hours of life and spontaneously resolves in 4–5 days; however, new lesions can occur up to day 10 of life. All lesions should resolve by 2 weeks. ET lesions are irregularly bordered, erythematous macules, 2–3 cm in diameter, with central yellowish vesicopustules. They are mostly discrete, but some erythematous macules become confluent. Lesions do not involve the palms or soles.

8. Which type of cells is seen on microscopic examination of pustules scraped from erythema toxicum lesions?

Wright-Giemsa stain of pustule scrapings show mostly eosinophils. Up to 15% of affected infants demonstrate peripheral eosinophilia as well.

9. What is harlequin color change?

Harlequin color change (HCC) is a demarcated erythema forming on the dependent half of the body of newborns. The more superior half of the body appears pale. This appearance can occur in any position and commonly lasts from seconds up to 20 minutes. It is rarely seen after 10 days of life. HCC is explained by immature autonomic vasomotor control because it is more common in premature infants and is reversible. If the baby is flipped over during an episode, the newly dependent portion will become erythematous.

10. What are the modes of inheritance of neurofibromatosis 1 and 2? What protein mutations are involved in these genetic diseases?

Both diseases are autosomal dominant, but spontaneous mutations account for approximately half of cases. The incidence of neurofibromatosis 1 (NF1) is 1/2500; the mutated gene product is neurofibromin, a protein involved in tumor suppression. Neurofibromatosis 2 (NF2) has a reported incidence of 1/33,000; the involved gene product is Merlin, which mediates cytoskeleton and extracellular movement.

11. When should NF1 be suspected in a newborn?

NF1 should be suspected in any infant with multiple café-au-lait spots, congenital glaucoma, a plexiform neurofibroma, or pseudoarthrosis. Without a positive family history, it can be difficult to diagnose neurofibromatosis in the first months of life. The diagnosis requires two or more of the following criteria: ≥ 6 café-au-lait macules (CALM) of 0.5 cm before puberty (1.5 cm post-puberty), ≥ 2 neurofibromas or plexiform neurofibromas, axillary freckles or inguinal freckles, ≥ 2 Lisch nodules (iris hamartomas), osseous lesions, or a first-degree relative with NF1. Other features that are associated with neurofibromatosis but unlikely to be found in neonates include learning disability, macrocephaly, short stature, juvenile xanthogranulomas, angiomas, mental retardation, impaired coordination, seizures, cerebral tumors (i.e., optic gliomas), increased risk of malignancy, and hypertension.

12. What is the most common cutaneous finding in neonates with tuberous sclerosis?

Hypopigmented macules, known as ash-leaf spots, are the most common skin finding of tuberous sclerosis in infants. Connective tissue nevi, known as shagreen patches, may also be present at birth. Adenoma sebaceum (facial angiofibromas) generally appear at age 3 and older; periungual or gum fibromas appear in early adulthood. During the first months of life, hypopigmented macules may be recognizable only with Wood's lamp because of the general lack of pigmentation in the skin.

13. Are hypopigmented macules always a sign of tuberous sclerosis?

No! Most hypopigmented macules are a variant of normal. However, multiple ash-leaf–like macules, a family history of tuberous sclerosis, neonatal seizures, cardiac rhabdomyomas, or renal cysts may alert you to the diagnosis of tuberous sclerosis.

14. At which ages are the most common cutaneous lesions of tuberous sclerosis found?

Hypopigmented (ash-leaf) macules can be found at birth, but more likely in infancy. These are the most likely encountered lesions in the newborn period.

Collagenomas (shagreen patch) can occur in newborns, but are more likely in later childhood.

Angiofibromas (adenoma sebaceum) usually appear after the age of 3 years. They can be confused with acne.

15. Tuberous sclerosis is inherited in an autosomal dominant fashion. What is peculiar about the genetic abnormalities associated with the TS phenotype?

Two distinct chromosomal complexes on two different chromosomes are implicated as areas of mutation that result in tuberous sclerosis. Tuberous sclerosis complex 1 (TSC1) is due to mutations in the gene hamartin on chromosome 9, located at 9q34.3. Tuberous sclerosis complex 2 (TSC2) is caused by mutations in the tuberin gene on chromosome 16 at 16p13.3

16. What is a collodion baby?

Collodion baby is a term used to describe neonates born with a yellow, shiny membrane, which resembles collodion.

17. Collodion baby is associated most commonly with which type of ichthyosis?

Of newborns with collodion membrane, the most common ichthyosis that develops is non-bullous ichthyosiform erythroderma, also called congenital ichthyosiform erythroderma (CIE). Lamellar ichthyosis is another rare form of ichthyosis that may present initially with collodion membrane. Approximately 10% of babies with collodion membrane do not go on to have clinically significant skin disease. Furthermore, not all patients with ichthyotic skin disease have a collodion membrane at birth.

18. How should one care for a baby with collodion membrane?

Supportive care is important until the collodion membrane sheds. Affected newborns have difficulty with temperature regulation, are prone to sepsis, and have increased fluid and nutritional requirements. Therefore, temperature should be controlled in an incubator, and any signs of infection should be promptly investigated and treated. Ectropion occurs as a result of taut skin everting eyelid margins, which leaves patients at risk for corneal ulceration. Topical ocular lubricants should be instituted early. Eclabium occurs by a similar mechanism of taut skin everting the lips. Nasogastic tube feedings may be required for poor suck and feeding difficulties.

19. What is a harlequin baby?

The term *harlequin baby* is used to describe neonates born with massive shiny plates of stratum corneum with deep, red fissures that form geometric patterns resembling a harlequin costume. As in neonates with collodion membrane, temperature regulation is defective; fluid requirements are increased; and there is a high risk of infection. The skin defect is usually restrictive, and respiratory insufficiency results. Harlequin babies rarely survive beyond the neonatal period.

20. What is KID syndrome, and how does it present in kids?

KID syndrome is a rare disorder characterized by **k**eratitis, **i**chthyosis and congenital neurosensory **d**eafness. Newborns have erythematous, thickened skin that eventually peels. The face and extremities then become ichthyotic; scaly keratoconjunctivitis usually develops during infancy.

21. Are newborns with epidermolytic hyperkeratosis hyperkeratotic?

Epidermolytic hyperkeratosis (EH) is also called bullous congenital ichthyosiform erythroderma. Newborns most often have blisters or bullae along with denuded skin. Although subtle hyperkeratosis appears in some newborns, it usually develops over time as the blistering subsides.

22. What is subcutaneous fat necrosis of the newborn?

Subcutaneous fat necrosis of the newborn usually presents within the first month of life with red to violaceous mobile plaques, especially on the back, thighs, and cheeks. The cause of subcutaneous fat necrosis is not definitively known.

23. In which clinical situations may subcutaneous fat necrosis of the newborn occur?

Subcutaneous fat necrosis may occur in cases of prematurity, fetal distress, birth trauma, infection, or cold stress.

24. How should newborns with subcutaneous fat necrosis be monitored?

Although the disorder is most often benign and self-limited, in some cases subcutaneous fat necrosis of the newborn may be associated with hypercalcemia and death. Therefore, serum calcium levels must be monitored, and caregivers must be vigilant for clinical signs and symptoms of hypercalcemia.

25. What is a blueberry muffin baby?

Blueberry muffin baby is a term used to describe neonates whose skin resembles a blueberry muffin; i.e., the skin shows diffuse, dark blue to violaceous purpuric macules and papules. The spots represent dermal hematopoiesis and are a sign of serious systemic disease, most often congenital infection.

26. Which diseases may cause blueberry muffin syndrome?

Congenital Infections	Hemolytic disease of the newborn
Toxoplasmosis	Neoplastic Disease
Rubella	Leukemia
Cytomegalovirus	Neuroblastoma
Herpes	Langerhans' cell histiocytosis
Coxsackie B2	Congenital rhabdomyosarcoma with
Parvovirus B19	cutaneous metastases

27. What is the clinical presentation of sclerema neonatorum?

Findings usually appear in the first two weeks of life, but can begin as late as four months. Infants who are poorly nourished, dehydrated, hypothermic, or septic are most commonly affected. Sclerema neonatorum begins in the lower extremities with the appearance of hard, cool skin and decreased mobility and subsequently involves the trunk and face. Palms, soles, and genitalia are not involved. Joints become immobile, and the face appears mask-like. Sclerema may be associated with necrotizing enterocolitis, pneumonia, intracranial hemorrhage, hypoglycemia, and electrolyte disturbances.

28. What is the cause of sclerema? Why is it more common in infants with infection, hypothermia, or other stressors?

Sclerema is likely a result of lipoenzyme dysfunction and occurs in infants who are stressed with severe illnesses. More specifically, dysfunction of enzymes regulating the conversion of saturated fatty acids to unsaturated fatty acids results in excess saturated fatty acids. This dysfunction allows fat solidification. The incidence of sclerema has decreased significantly because events such as malnutrition, dehydration, and hypothermia occur less commonly in modern nurseries. Treating the underlying condition can result in resolution of sclerema. Some authors also propose systemic steroids or therapy with exchange transfusions.

29. Why is presence of pruritus a poor way to differentiate atopic dermatitis and seborrheic dermatitis in infants?

Hope you are itching for the answer! Although atopic dermatitis (AD) classically includes pruritus, infants and especially newborns may not have the coordination to scratch. However, occipital alopecia can occur as a result of excessive rubbing of the back of the head against the bed sheets. In this situation, hair may fall out or break off due to friction.

30. Describe the usual distributions of the rash caused by atopic dermatitis and that caused by seborrheic dermatitis in neonates.

If dermatitis involves the axillae or groin, it is more likely to be seborrheic dermatitis (SD). If extensor surfaces such as forearms and shins are involved, AD is more likely. Both AD and SD involve scalp and posterior auricular areas, although SD has large, yellowish scale and, when severe, characteristically extends down to the forehead and eyebrow areas.

31. What is scalded skin syndrome?

Staphylococcal scalded skin syndrome (SSSS) is caused by toxins released by *Staphylococcus aureus* that lead to blistering and desquamation of the skin. Nikolsky sign is positive; simply rubbing the skin causes a blister to form. Outbreaks of such blistering have been reported in newborn nurseries. Remember, however, that scalding thermal burns have been reported in neonates bathed in overly hot water—another "scalding skin syndrome."

32. What is aplasia cutis congenita?

Aplasia cutis congenita occurs as a result of failure of development of the normal layers of skin. It occurs most often on the scalp and may present clinically as an ulcer, healed erosion, or well-formed scar. Therefore, it is often mistaken for trauma due to a scalp pH probe. In cases of large lesions or lesions overlying the midline neurocranial axis, imaging should be considered because aplasia cutis congenita may be associated with underlying malformations of bone or extend deeply to the meninges.

33. What is the significance of preauricular skin tags?

Preauricular skin tags, also called accessory tragi, are embryonic remnants of the first branchial arch. The formation of the first branchial arch occurs during the 4th week of fetal development. The kidneys and heart also develop during this time. Renal ultrasound has been recommended in patients with preauricular skin tags because they can be associated with urinary tract abnormalities (8.6% of cases according to a recent prospective study).

34. What are accessory nipples? Where are they located?

Accessory nipples, also called supernumerary nipples, are embryonic remnants of the mammary line, which extend from the axilla to the inner thigh. They appear as pink or brown papules, with or without surrounding areola, anywhere along the mammary line. There have been conflicting reports about an association with urinary tract abnormalities.

35. What are the risk factors for development of hemangiomas?

Hemangiomas are common vascular tumors that arise during the neonatal period. One study found that 10% of Caucasian children had hemangiomas when examined at 1 year of age. Hemangiomas occur more frequently in female children, with an incidence of 2–5:1. In addition, they arise more commonly in premature infants and in infants whose mothers underwent chorionic villus sampling.

36. What do strawberries and caverns have to do with hemangiomas?

In the older and lay literature superficial hemangiomas have been called strawberry birthmarks because the color and texture of the skin is somewhat reminiscent of a strawberry. Deep hemangiomas have been called cavernous hemangiomas, but the term is particularly confusing because it has also been used to describe venous malformations, which are a completely different kind of vascular birthmark. So it is prudent to avoid both terms and to use the terms superficial, deep, or mixed hemangiomas to describe a particular type of hemangioma.

37. Explain the difference between a hemangioma and a vascular malformation.

The classification of vascular birthmarks has historically been a problematic issue. The most commonly accepted classification was introduced almost 20 years ago and has been modified slightly. It divides vascular birthmarks into two broad categories: **vascular tumors** and **vascular malformations**. Vascular tumors include the most common birthmark, the hemangioma of infancy, and other rare childhood-onset vascular tumors. The lesions are proliferating lesions composed of blood vessels. Hemangiomas have a characteristic natural history. They are usually noted in the first few weeks of life, undergo rapid proliferation that may last for several months, and then slowly regress over several years. At the end of the period of spontaneous regression, they may be undetectable or leave a residual mass or textural changes. Hemangiomas are distinct histologically and show increased endothelial turnover.

Vascular malformations include various lesions, e.g., capillary malformations (port-wine stains). They are classified according to the type of vessels that compose them. They are often noted in the immediate newborn period. Vascular malformations grow with the child, although they may become more prominent as the child matures. They do not show a marked increase in proliferation and differ histologically from tumors. Most importantly, they do not regress spontaneously, and they persist throughout the patient's lifetime. Therefore, management is significantly different from that for a hemangioma.

38. In which situations should you worry about coexistent internal hemangiomas?

Infants who present with multiple cutaneous hemangiomas may have underlying internal hemangiomas. The liver, gastrointestinal tract, central nervous system, eyes, and lungs are the most common sites of extracutaneous involvement. Not all children with multiple skin hemangiomas have underlying systemic involvement; conversely, children with visceral hemangiomas may have no skin lesions. Children with hemangiomas located on the lower face in a "beard" pattern often have laryngeal hemangiomas that may not become detectable until they compromise breathing. Therefore, a pediatric otolaryngologist should evaluate these children early in life.

39. What are some of the complications that can occur with a large hemangioma?

Large hemangiomas may impair vital functions. Even smaller lesions in problematic locations can lead to complications. Hemangiomas located around the eye may obstruct the visual axis or lead to astigmatism by deforming the shape of the globe, which leads to visual impairment. Large lesions with high flow may cause congestive heart failure. Large facial hemangiomas have been seen in association with underlying congenital anomalies including cardiac and central nervous system malformations. Finally, large hemangiomas may lead to significant disfigurement even as they regress spontaneously. Ulceration may complicate large or small hemangiomas.

40. What treatments have been used for problematic hemangiomas?

Problematic hemangiomas include those that compromise vital functions, cause significant distortion or disfigurement of normal underlying structures, and have ulcerated and become infected. Treatment strategy varies depending on the clinical situation. Oral prednisone or prednisolone is the most commonly used treatment for problematic hemangiomas; the duration of treatment varies according to the age of the patient and the lesion. Intralesional injection of other types of corticosteroids may also be indicated. Interferon-α has been used to treat some patients with life-threatening hemangiomas; however, its use has been complicated by neurotoxicity (spastic diplegia). Other treatments for problematic hemangiomas include laser therapy, surgery, embolization, and cryotherapy.

41. How should a child with a hemangioma located over the lumbosacral spine be evaluated?

Hemangiomas in this location may be associated with underlying spinal cord anomalies (such as a tethered spinal cord), underlying bony defects, and anomalies of the genitourinary and gastrointestinal systems. For detection of tethered cord, magnetic resonance imaging (MRI) is the study of choice.

42. What is Kasabach-Merritt phenomenon? With which tumors is it associated?

Kasabach-Merritt phenomenon (syndrome) is a rare complication that occurs in infants with large vascular tumors. Patients present in the first few months of life with a rapidly enlarging vascular mass associated with profound thrombocytopenia and coagulopathy. It is a life-threatening condition. In the past, this phenomenon was thought to be a complication of "garden variety" hemangiomas, but recent evidence indicates an association with rare vascular tumors such as the kaposiform hemangioendothelioma and the congenital tufted angioma.

43. What is a lymphangioma?

A lymphangioma is a vascular malformation composed of lymphatic tissue. The lesions are sometimes noted in the immediate newborn period or may become more prominent as a child grows. They do not regress spontaneously. A cystic hygroma is one type of lymphatic malformation that is composed of larger cystic spaces. It usually is apparent in the immediate newborn period and is located on the head and neck. Some patients with cystic hygroma have underlying genetic abnormalities such as Turner syndrome.

44. How is a port-wine stain capillary malformation treated?

A port-wine stain is a malformation composed of small capillary and venular-sized vessels. As a child matures, the lesion may darken, thicken, and develop blebs. Pulsed dye laser therapy is the preferred method of treatment and may lead to significant lightening in many patients. Multiple treatments are usually required.

45. When should Sturge-Weber syndrome be considered in a child with facial port-wine stain? What are the characteristic findings in Sturge-Weber syndrome?

Approximately 10% of children with a port-wine stain in the distribution of the ophthalmic branch of the trigeminal nerve have findings of Sturge-Weber syndrome (SWS). SWS is characterized by seizures (onset usually < 2 years old), hemiplegia, mental retardation, and glaucoma. However, in infancy many of these findings may not be present or may be difficult to discern. Similarly, a computed tomography (CT) or MRI scan in infancy may not show the characteristic calcification, cerebral atrophy, or abnormalities of the cortex and white matter. However, an enlarged choroid plexus or increased myelination may be present early in the course of SWS. Neonates with a port-wine stain in that distribution should have an urgent eye examination to assess for possible glaucoma.

46. What is epidermolysis bullosa?

Epidermolysis bullosa (EB) is a heterogeneous group of inherited disorders characterized by skin fragility and blistering. The majority of patients develop symptoms in the newborn period. The most common types are epidermolysis bullosa simplex, junctional epidermolysis bullosa, and dystrophic epidermolysis bullosa. Within each subset there are different clinical phenotypes. It is now understood that these diseases are caused by an inability to synthesize proteins that play an important role in maintaining the skin's integrity. EB simplex is caused by mutations in keratins located in the basal layer of the epidermis; junctional EB is caused by defects in the protein laminin 5 and other proteins at the dermal-epidermal junction; and dystrophic EB is caused by a defect in collagen VII. There is no cure for these conditions, and treatment is supportive.

47. What are the basic principles of skin care for children with epidermolysis bullosa?

Skin trauma (rubbing, chafing) should be avoided because the skin will likely blister at the site. Tape should not be applied directly to the skin. New skin blisters should be ruptured with a sterile needle or lancet to prevent them from enlarging and dressed with a topical antibiotic and nonadherent dressing such as plain petrolatum gauze. The blisters need to be monitored closely because superinfection may be a complication. Infants with severe forms of epidermolysis bullosa are at risk for nutritional deficiencies, poor weight gain, and anemia.

48. Define congenital melanocytic nevus.

A congenital melanocytic nevus is usually defined as a melanocytic lesion that is present at birth. The incidence is reported between 0.5 and 2%.

49. What are some complications of congenital melanocytic nevi?

Congenital melanocytic nevi are often subdivided according to their size. Melanoma has been reported to arise within congenital lesions, but the exact risk for this complication is controversial. It is known that large lesions carry the greatest risk and that melanoma, when it occurs, does so earlier in life. The incidence is reported between 4.6% and 14%. One prospective study reported a 5-year cumulative risk of 4.5% compared with that in the general population. Leptomeningeal melanosis is a rare complication that may occur in association with a giant congenital nevus located over the head, neck, or spine or multiple (> 3) congenital nevi.

50. An infant is born at 29 weeks' gestation. Name five clinical problems that may be related to immature skin barrier function?

The skin of premature infants is immature and has compromised barrier function. Clinical consequences include increased transepidermal water loss, fluid and electrolyte disturbances, temperature instability, infection (cutaneous and systemic), absorption of substances applied to the skin, and susceptibility to mechanical, chemical, and thermal stresses.

51. Approximately when will an infant born at 30 weeks' gestation have skin barrier function equivalent to that of an adult?

Most premature infants exhibit rapid maturation of skin barrier function over the first 2–3 weeks of life. In infants of < 25 weeks' gestation, skin barrier function may require 8 weeks following birth to mature.

52. Two weeks into a neonatal intensive care unit (ICU) course, an infant born at 27 weeks' gestation develops two superficial erosions on the anterior trunk. Subsequently, these heal with a brownish, wrinkled appearance. What is the diagnosis ? What is the cause?

Skin injury may accompany routine care of very premature infants. *Anetoderma of prematurity* is the term for focal depressions or outpouchings, which are presumed to be a response to mechanical or thermal injury to the skin.

BIBLIOGRAPHY

1. Eichenfield LF, Frieden IJ, Esterly NB: Textbook of Neonatal Dermatology. Philadelphia, W.B. Saunders, 2001
2. Fine J, Eady RAJ, Bauer EA, et al: Revised classification system for inherited epidermolysis bullosa: Report of the second international consensus meeting on diagnosis and classification of epidermolysis bullosa. J Am Acad Dermatol 42:1051–1066, 2000.
3. Harper J, Oranje A, Prose N (eds): Textbook of Pediatric Dermatology. Oxford, Blackwell Science, 2000.
4. Niamba P, Weill FX, Sarlangue J, et al: Is neonatal cephalic pustulosis (neonatal acne) triggered by *Malassezia sympodialis*? Arch Dermatol 134:995, 1998.
5. Resnick SD: Staphylococcal and streptococcal skin infections: Pyodermas and toxin-mediated syndromes. In Harper J, Oranje A and Prose N (eds): Textbook of Pediatric Dermatology. Oxford, Blackwell Science, 2000, pp 369–383.

6. ENDOCRINOLOGY AND METABOLISM

HYPOCALCEMIA

1. How is calcium transported across the placenta? What is the relationship between maternal and fetal calciotropic hormones?

Because maternal calcium is always lower than fetal calcium, placental calcium transport is an active process. Parathyroid hormone (PTH), calcitonin (CT), and PTH-related peptide (PTH-rp) do not cross the placenta, whereas 25-hydroxy (25-OH) vitamin D crosses the placenta readily from mother to fetus. Very little, if any, 1,25-dihydroxy [1,25(OH)$_2$] vitamin D crosses the placenta from mother to fetus.

Mother	Placenta	Fetus
↑ Parathyroid hormone		Parathyroid hormone ↓
↓ Calcitonin		Calcitonin ↑
↓ PTH-rp		PTH-rp ↑
↑ Vitamin D ————		→ Vitamin D ↓
↑ 25-OH vitamin D ————		→ 25-OH vitamin D ↓
↑ 1,25(OH)$_2$ vitamin D	1,25(OH)$_2$ vitamin D	1,25(OH)$_2$ vitamin D ↓
↓ Calcium ————		→ Calcium ↑

The maternal-placental-fetal relationships of calciotropic hormones. Arrows represent comparative concentrations in mother and fetus. The placenta probably synthesizes its own supply of 1,25-dihydroxy vitamin D. (Adapted from Polin RA, Yoder MC, Burg FD (eds): Workbook in Practical Neonatology, 3rd ed. Philadelphia, W.B. Saunders, 2001.)

2. What perinatal factors are associated with hypocalcemia in the immediate newborn period?
- Prematurity
- Asphyxia (Apgar score < 6)
- Maternal diabetes
- Maternal hyperparathyroidism
- Transient congenital hypoparathyroidism
- Congenital absence or hypoplasia of the parathyroid glands (sporadic or as part of DiGeorge syndrome)

3. How is hypocalcemia diagnosed in premature infants in the first few days of life?

In newborn infants, there is a physiologic decline in serum total and ionized calcium during the first 48 hours of life. This decline is exaggerated in preterm infants compared with full-term infants, with a direct correlation between serum calcium and gestational age (see figure on following page). Because no symptoms are specific for early hypocalcemia in preterm infants, the diagnosis is made by demonstrating a serum calcium level < 7.0 mg/dl (1.75 mmol/L).

4. Describe the appropriate treatment for early hypocalcemia in premature infants.

This is a loaded question for the following reasons:
1. Hypocalcemia of prematurity is usually asymptomatic.
2. It resolves spontaneously.
3. Long-term follow-up studies have shown no benefit with treatment.
4. Total serum calcium is a poor predictor of ionized serum calcium in premature infants.

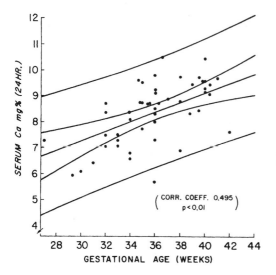

Serum calcium in relation to gestastional age at 24 hours of age. (From Tsang RC, et al: Possible pathogenetic factors in neonatal hypocalcemia of prematurity. J Pediatr 82: 423, 1973, with permission.)

5. Intravenous calcium is associated with complications such as cardiac arrhythmias and ulcerations due to soft tissue infiltration of the infusate. In addition, calcium therapy may block the normal physiologic adaptation to hypocalcemia in premature infants, which includes increasing serum levels of PTH and $1,25(OH)_2$ vitamin D in the first few days of life. Vitamin D therapy has no role at this early age, particularly in the absence of oral calcium intake.

In the absence of additional data, it is conventional to treat all serum calcium levels < 6.0 mg/dl, even in asymptomatic neonates. The addition of 200 mg/kg/day of 10% calcium gluconate to standard intravenous (IV) solutions provides 20 mg/kg/day of elemental calcium. If symptoms are present (especially cardiac arrhythmia or seizures), a bolus of 100 mg/kg of 10% calcium gluconate (10 mg/kg elemental calcium) may be given intravenously over 10 minutes with careful cardiac monitoring.

5. How much calcium do premature infants require for growth?

Calcium requirement is based on fetal intrauterine accretion rate (see figure on following page). Fetal calcium accrues exponentially throughout pregnancy (like most minerals). Of the 25–30 gm of total body calcium at 40 weeks' gestation, roughly two-thirds is accumulated during the last trimester of pregnancy. Thus, between 25 and 30 weeks' gestation, the estimated daily fetal calcium accretion rate is approximately 100 mg/kg/day of fetal body weight. After birth, the required calcium accretion rate does not change. However, the actual calcium requirement varies according to absorption and retention rates.

6. How can the calcium requirements for premature infants be met by oral feedings?

Recent studies in premature infants using stable isotopes of calcium showed a true calcium absorption rate of 50–90%. Thus, to meet an accretion rate of 100 mg/kg/day with an absorption rate of 75% and an assumed retention rate of 75% (which may be on the high side), oral intake of calcium for growing premature infants should be about 200 mg/kg/day. This large intake in infants with very low birth weight can be achieved only with special formulas for low-birth-weight infants or mineral fortifiers for breast milk-fed preterm infants.

7. How can the calcium requirements for premature infants be met by hyperalimentation solutions?

This problem is much more difficult to address, although intestinal absorption is not a factor. In the early weeks of life with fluid intakes of 150 mg/kg/day, it is difficult to exceed an IV calcium intake of 60 mg/kg/day in the smallest premature infants (weight < 1000 gm) with

CALCIUM. g/FOETUS

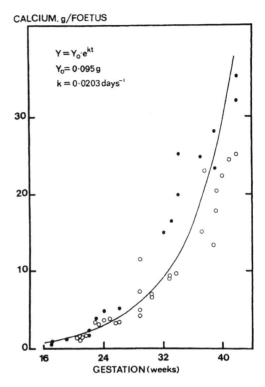

$$Y = Y_0 \cdot e^{kt}$$
$$Y_0 = 0.095 \, g$$
$$k = 0.0203 \, days^{-1}$$

Intrauterine calcium accretion rate in the human fetus from week 16 to week 40 of gestation. (From Shaw JCL: Evidence for the defective skeletal mineralization in low birth-weight infants: The absoprtion of calcium and fat. Pediatrics 57:16–25, 1976, with permission.)

GESTATION (weeks)

standard total parenteral nutrition (TPN) solutions. When the concentration of calcium exceeds 60 mg/dl (3 mEq/dl) in TPN solutions, precipitation with phosphate may occur, depending on variables such as temperature, pH, amino acid content, and even how the nutrients are added to the solution.

8. What is "breast milk rickets" in premature infants?

Clinical rickets develops in preterm infants with very low birth weight who are fed human milk not fortified with minerals and vitamins. Typically the disease presents after 8 weeks of life with severe hypophosphatemia, "relative hypercalcemia," and hypercalciuria. The x-ray findings mimic those of rickets due to vitamin D deficiency. The biochemical findings are due to low mineral intake. Because human milk is low in both calcium and phosphorus, the very low phosphorus intake (about 50% of calcium intake) severely limits deposition of calcium in bone. *Caution:* Because treatment with phosphorus alone can result in severe hypocalcemia, supplements of both minerals are imperative.

9. A 14-day-old, full-term infant presents with hypocalcemia and seizures responsive to IV calcium. What is the differential diagnosis? What acute dose of IV calcium is required to control the seizures?

Seizures secondary to hypocalcemia are very unlikely in a previously healthy, full-term infant at 2 weeks of age. The differential diagnosis includes congenital hypomagnesemia (rare), late infantile tetany associated with high phosphate load (e.g., feedings with cow milk), and acid–base disturbances secondary to diarrhea treated with alkali therapy.

Treatment of hypocalcemic seizures is the same for both premature and full-term infants. In general, 10% calcium gluconate containing 9.4 mg/ml of elemental calcium is the drug of choice. The usual dose of 2 ml/kg body weight (18 mg/kg of elemental calcium) should be given in a peripheral vein over 10 minutes with heart-rate monitoring.

HYPOGLYCEMIA

10. Define hypoglycemia.

In adults, hypoglycemia is defined as plasma glucose < 40 mg/dl. A plasma glucose concentraion of 70–100 mg/dl is considered normal, and the therapeutic target range for adults with hypoglycemia is > 60 mg/dl. The definition in neonates is controversial. Some physicians accept significantly lower plasma glucose concentrations as normal for neonates. However, in the absence of scientific evidence that neonates tolerate lower concentrations than adults, many clinicians now believe that values < 50 mg/dl are abnormal. This definition is supported by Koh et al., who demonstrated electrophysiologic changes in the brains of infants when glucose reaches 50 mg/dl.

11. Why is glucose important?

Glucose is the primary fuel for the brain and accounts for over 90% of total body oxygen consumption early in fasting. Because of their larger brain-to-body size ratio, infants have greater glucose requirements than adults. Hepatic glucose production rates in infants are approximately 6 mg/kg/min (3–6 times greater than in of adults).

12. List and explain the metabolic systems necessary for adaptation to fasting.

Hepatic glycogenolysis: mobilization of glucose from hepatic glycogen. This process is responsible for glucose production during the first 6–12 hours of a fast.

Hepatic gluconeogenesis: hepatic conversion of muscle-derived amino acids (particularly alanine) and triglyeride-derived glycerol to glucose. The rate of gluconeogenesis remains constant during fasting.

Lipolysis, fatty acid oxidation, and ketogenesis: generation of free fatty acids (a fuel that can be used by muscles but not by the brain) from adipose tissue and fatty acid-derived ketones (fuels that the brain can use) from the liver. The transition to fat oxidation and ketogenesis occurs 12–16 hours into a fast and spares excessive muscle breakdown.

13. List and explain the hormonal controls necessary for fasting adaptation.

Insulin: inhibits fasting metabolic systems.

Epinephrine: stimulates hepatic glycogenolysis, hepatic gluconeogenesis, and hepatic ketogenesis.

Glucagon: stimulates hepatic glycogenolysis.

Cortisol: stimulates hepatic gluconeogenesis.

Growth hormone: stimulates lipolysis.

14. What causes hypoglycemia in neonates?

Hypoglycemia results from either abnormal control of fasting adaptations or failure of a particular fasting metabolic system. In the first 12–24 hours of life, normal newborns are at increased risk for hypoglycemia because gluconeogenesis and especially ketogenesis are incompletely developed. Hypoglycemia occurring or persisting after the first 24 hours of life is abnormal and implies failure of one of the fasting systems.

15. Which hormonal abnormalitites may cause hypoglycemia in neonates?

• Hyperinsulinism (the most common cause of recurrent hypoglycemia in neonates)
• Hypopituitarism (combination of growth hormone, thyroid hormone, and cortisol deficiencies)

16. Which defects in fasting metabolic systems may cause hypoglycemia in neonates?

• Defects of glycogenolysis (glycogen storage diseases [GSDs]) are associated with hepatomegaly. Examples include deficiencies of debranching enzyme (GSD type 3), liver phosphorylase (GSD type 6), and phosphorylase kinase (GSD type 9).
• Defects of gluconeogenesis include deficiencies of glucose-6-phosphatase (GSD type 1) and fructose-1,6-diphosphastase. Defects of gluconeogenesis and glycogenolysis rarely

present in early infancy because neonates are not exposed to fasting for more than 4 hours at a time.

- Fatty acid oxidation disorders include medium-chain acyl dehydrogenase (MCAD) deficiency. Unless a neonate is breast-feeding poorly or experiences an illness that limits oral intake, a fatty acid oxidation disorder is unlikely to present in infancy.

17. What are "didja tubes"?

Didja tubes (as in "Did you obtain the critical blood samples at the time of hypoglycemia?") are of great help in identifying why fasting adapation has failed. Because bedside glucose meters are inaccurate at low blood glucose concentrations, documentation of hypoglycemia requires laboratory analysis of a serum specimen. Once hypoglycemia is confirmed (glucose = ≤ 50 mg/dl), blood is drawn before any intervention is initiated for analysis of the following:

- Insulin
- Free fatty acids
- Ketones
- Lactate/pyruvate
- Bicarbonate
- Ammonium
- Growth hormone
- Cortisol

18. Summarize the diagnostic work-up for neonates with hypoglycemia.

Blood glucose monitoring is essential. At the time of hypoglycemia, the critical laboratory samples and the glucagon stimulation test (to assess for hyperinsulinism) are performed. While you wait for the laboratory results, growth hormone and thyroxine (T4) can be assessed. Because growth hormone is tonically elevated in the newborn period, low concentrations of growth hormone and thyroid hormone suggest hypopituitarism. If hypopituitarism is suspected, provocative studies of growth hormone secretion, the hypothalamic-pituitary-adrenal axis, and the thyroid axis should be performed. If a fatty acid oxidation disorder is suspected, a serum acylcarnitine profile, serum carnitine levels, and urinary organic acids should be obtained.

19. How is a glucagon stimulation test done?

A glucagon stimulation test identifies accessible hepatic glucose stores. After the critical lab draw, glucagon (1.0 mg IV or intramuscularly) is administerd, and blood glucose is checked every 10 minutes for 40 minutes.

20. How are the results interpreted?

A positive glycemic response to glucagon is defined as an increase in blood glucose of ≥ 30 mg/dl. A positive glucagon result indicates inappropriate preservation of liver glycogen and is sensitive for hyperinsulinemic suppression of glycogenolysis. The only exceptions to this rule are neonates with hypopituitarism, who may have a positive glycemic response to glucagon.

21. What are the two types of hyperinsulinism in neonates?

Transient and congenital.

22. What causes transient hyperinsulinism?

Transient hyperinsulinism occurs in infants of diabetic mothers whose upregulated insulin secretion in response to a hyperglycemic fetal environment persists in the immediate postnatal period. In perinatally stressed neonates (e.g., infants who are small for gestational age or have birth asphyxia or toxemia), hyperinsulinism due to dysregulated insulin secretion may persist for up to several months after birth.

23. What causes congenital hyperinsulinism?

Genetic defects of insulin secretion include recessive mutations of the beta-cell sulfonylurea receptor/potassium channel genes and dominant gain of functional mutations of glucokinase and glutamate dehydrogenase. Dominant functional mutations are milder and usually present later in infancy.

24. What physical features suggest the cause of hypoglycemia in neonates?

Macrosomia. Because insulin is a growth factor, hyperinsulinism leads to macrosomia. Infants of diabetic mothers and infants with severe forms of congenital hyperinsulinism typically are large for gestational age. In addition, neonates with Beckwith-Wiedemann syndrome are macrosomic and may have hyperinsulinism.

Midline defects. Congenital pituitary deficiency may be associated with midline defects such as cleft lip, cleft palate, single central incisor, and micro-ophthalmia.

Micropenis. Congenital gonadotropin deficiency can cause micropenis.

Hepatomegaly. Glycogen storage diseases and fatty acid oxidation disorders may be associated with hepatomegaly.

25. How is hypoglycemia treated acutely?

Hypoglycemia can be treated emergently with oral or nasogastric tube feeding of dextrose or formula. If symptoms are severe, 200 mg/kg of dextrose (2 ml/kg of 10% dextrose) can be administered intravenously. Blood glucose should be checked within 15 minutes of intervention and subsequently monitored to ensure adequate treatment (plasma glucose > 60 mg/dl) and to prevent hypoglyemic episodes. If necessary, continuous IV dextrose is initiated (6 mg/kg/min).

26. What are the goals of long-term treatment?

To prevent brain damage with a manageable home regimen. The specific treatment depends on the cause of hypoglycemia.

27. What is the specific treatment for hypoglycemia due to hypopituitarism?

Appropriate hormone replacement.

28. How is transient hyperinsulinism treated?

Initial management consists of IV dextrose and frequent or continuous feeds. In persistent cases, diazoxide (5–15 mg/kg/day) may be effective in controlling insulin secretion.

29. Describe the treatment of congenital hyperinsulinism.

Congenital hyperinsulinism due to severe sulfonylurea receptor/potassium channel mutation is often resistant to diazoxide. Octreotide (a somatosatin analog) tempers excessive insulin secretion but rarely prevents hypoglycemia completely or normalizes fasting tolerance. Continuous glucagon infusion can stabilize blood glucose until surgery is performed, but experience with long-term use is limited. If the combination of octreotide and frequent feeds fails, pancreatectomy is necessary. Surgery may be curative if a focal lesion is present and completely resected.

30. What is the cornerstone of treatment for defects of glycogenolysis and gluconeogenesis?

Frequent feedings.

31. How are fatty acid oxidation disorders treated?

By instituting a high-carbohydrate diet and ensuring that fasting is limited to 12 hours. If an affected infant is feeding poorly or experiences vomiting, IV dextrose must be initiated emergently. The finding of euglycemia in the setting of a concurrent illness should not deter the clinician from initiating IV dextrose. By the time hypoglycemia is detected in fatty oxidation disorders, liver failure, cerebral edema, and cardiac toxicity are already present or developing. The mortality rate of > 25% during a first episode dramatizes the need for prompt intervention.

HYPERCALCEMIA

32. How many fractions of calcium are found in the serum? Which can be measured in the clinical laboratory?

There are three fractions of calcium in serum: ionized calcium (50%), calcium bound to serum proteins (40%), and calcium complexed to serum anions (10%). Ionized calcium and total calcium can be measured in most hospital laboratories.

33. What are the normal serum calcium values in full-term infants?

Normal values (in mg/dl, expressed as mean and range) depend on chronologic age:

Cord: 9.34 (8.2–11.1)
5 hours: 8.38 (7.3–9.2)
11 hours: 8.22 (6.9–10.2)
24 hours: 7.7 (6.2–9.0)
48 hours: 7.94 (5.9–9.7)

34. What are the normal serum values in preterm infants?

As in full-term infants, normal values (in mg/dl, expressed as mean ± standard deviation and range) depend on chronologic age:

1 week: 9.2 ± 1.1 (6.1–11.6)
3 weeks: 9.6 ± 0.5 (8.1–11.0)
5 weeks: 9.4 ± 0.5 (8.6–10.5)
7 weeks: 9.5 ± 0.7 (8.6–10.8)

35. What values "define" hypercalcemia in newborn infants?

Total serum calcium > 10.8 mg/dl or ionized serum calcium > 5.4 mg/dl.

36. List the manifestations of hypercalcemia in neonates.

- Lethargy
- Irritability
- Polyuria
- Vomiting
- Constipation
- Failure to thrive

37. What causes hypercalcemia in neonates?

- Iatrogenic hypercalcemia
- Subcutaneous fat necrosis
- Idiopathic infantile hypercalcemia
- Williams syndrome
- Hyperparathyroidism (primary and secondary)
- Parathyroid hormone-related peptide tumor
- Hyperprostaglandin E syndrome
- Hypophosphatasia
- Familial hypercalciuric hypercalcemia
- Blue diaper syndrome
- Thyrotoxicosis
- Vitamin A intoxication
- Chronic thiazide therapy
- Excessive maternal intake of vitamin D

38. How is acute hypercalcemia managed in newborn infants?

1. Promote diuresis by administering IV fluids (normal saline).
2. Administer furosemide, and monitor serum electrolytes carefully.
3. Hydrocortisone (1 mg/kg every 6 hours) is of value only in chronic situations to reduce intestinal absorption of calcium.

Neither ethylenediamine tetraacetic acid (EDTA) nor calcitonin can be recommended because of insufficient data.

39–44. A 3-day-old infant has a total serum calcium level of 13.2 mg/dl. She is preterm (33 weeks) and on IV fluids because of respiratory distress (resolving) secondary to transient tachypnea of the newborn. She was delivered by emergency cesarean section because of fetal distress. Her physical examination is otherwise unremarkable.

39. How likely is the diagnosis of Williams syndrome?

Williams syndrome is an unlikely diagnosis. Hypercalcemia is an infrequent finding, and most affected infants are small for gestational age and have some features of the "elfin" facies and/or cardiovascular findings consistent with supravalvular aortic stenosis.

40. Why is subcutaneous fat necrosis an unlikely diagnosis?

Subcutaneous fat necrosis is associated with bluish-red, indurated skin lesions.

41. After a complete family history and physical exam, how should your evaluation proceed?

Order the following tests:
- Serum total and ionized calcium
- Serum phosphorus
- Urinary calcium:creatinine ratio

42. What diagnoses are suggested by a low serum phosphorus level?

Phosphate depletion (unlikely at 3 days of age), hyperparathyroidism, and familial hypocalciuric hypercalcemia.

43. What is the most likely diagnosis?

Iatrogenic hypercalcemia. The infant received excessive calcium in the IV fluids. The second most likely diagnosis is idiopathic infantile hypercalcemia, a diagnosis of exclusion.

44. What is the proper amount of IV calcium for a 3-day-old preterm infant? How much phosphorus should be added?

A 3-day-old preterm infant should receive 54–75 mg/kg/day of elemental calcium in IV fluids. If IV fluids are to be continued for the long term (as in TPN), the ratio of elemental calcium to elemental phosphorus should be between 1.7:1 and 2:1 to optimize retention of both minerals.

45. Why is the diaper blue in blue diaper syndrome?

A defect in the intestinal transport of tryptophan causes excretion of blue, water-insoluble tryptophan metabolites. Why calcium concentrations are high is not well understood.

HYPOMAGNESEMIA AND HYPERMAGNESEMIA

46. What two types of magnesium reactions are important in human physiology?

Intracellular and extracellular.

47. Describe the important intracellular reactions.

Magnesium is the second most abundant intracellular cation after potassium and helps to regulate cellular metabolism. As part of the magnesium-adenosine triphosphate complex, it is essential for all biosynthetic processes, including glycolysis, formation of cyclic adenosine monophosphate, and transmission of the genetic code. In addition, any reaction that uses or produces energy requires magnesium.

48. Describe the important extracellular reactions.

Only 1% of magnesium is contained in extracellular fluid. However, extracellular concentrations are critical for maintenance of electrical potentials of nerve and muscle membranes and for the transmission of impulses across the neuromuscular junction. Magnesium and calcium may act synergistically or antagonistically in many of these processes.

49. How are millimoles (mmol) of magnesium converted to milliequivalents (mEq) and milligrams (mg)?

1 mmol = 2 mEq = 24 mg. Therefore, 1 mEq of magnesium = 12 mg.

50. How is magnesium regulated in the body?

Approximately 50–70% of ingested magnesium is absorbed in the normal intestine. Serum levels are regulated by the kidney. Under normal circumstances, 95–97% of filtered magnesium is reabsorbed. Sixty-five percent of the body stores of magnesium are in bone. Parathyroid hormone (PTH) increases the serum concentration by releasing magnesium from bone and decreasing renal excretion.

51. Define hypomagnesemia in neonates.

Hypomagnesemia is defined as a serum level < 1.5 mg/dl, but clinical signs usually do not develop unless the serum level falls below 1.2 mg/dl.

52. What causes magnesium depletion in neonates?
- Maternal diabetes
- Maternal magnesium deficiency
- Renal losses of magnesium in acidotic states
- Use of nutrient solutions containing insufficient amounts of magnesium
- Renal tubular defects
- Intestinal wasting of magnesium (rare X-linked condition)
- Gastrointestinal losses (through emesis, nasogastric suctioning, and diarrhea)
- Prematurity, which increases the risk for magnesium deficiency
- Intrauterine growth retardation

53. Discuss the signs and symptoms of magnesium deficiency in neonates.

Most infants are asymptomatic. On rare occasions the following signs and symptoms may be seen:

Color: pallor, cyanosis, or duskiness

Affect: out of touch with surroundings, apathetic, irritable when disturbed, restless

Eyes: staring with infrequent blinking, oculogyric crises

Heart: tachycardia (bradycardia during apneic episodes)

Respiration: brief apnea, sometimes followd by tachypnea

Neuromuscular system: motor weakness, transient spasticity, abnormal reflexes. If hypocalcemia develops (see below), the infant may show signs associated with calcium deficiency, including seizures.

54. How should hypomagnesemia be treated parenterally?

1. Hypomagnesemia usually is treated intravenously or intramuscularly with a 50% solution of magnesium sulfate.

2. One milliliter of a 50% solution contains 4 mEq of elemental magnesium. The usual dose is 0.1–0.25 ml/kg/day.

3. Serum magnesium levels should be monitored every 12 hours.

55. Describe the effects of hypomagnesemia on calcium homeostasis.

Hypomagnesemia usually increases the secretion of PTH, thereby increasing calcium levels. In chronic magnesium-deficient states, however, secretion of PTH is reduced. In such circumstances, hypomagnesemia may induce hypocalcemia.

56. What causes hypermagnesemia in neonates?
- Maternal treatment with magnesium (for preeclampsia or tocolysis)
- Excessive magnesium administration to neonate (TPN, antacids, treatment of pulmonary hypertension)

57. List the signs of hypermagnesemia in neonates.

• Flaccidity	• Respiratory insufficiency	• Ileus
• Unresponsiveness	• Apnea	• Delayed passage of meconium

In extreme cases, cardiorespiratory function ceases and death ensues.

58. How is hypermagnesemia treated?

1. Stop the administration of magnesium.
2. Make sure that the infant is well hydrated.
3. Consider diuretic therapy.

4. In severe cases, exchange transfusion (with acid-citrate-dextrose solution) is effective.
5. The effects of calcium salts are equivocal.

NEONATAL SCREENING

59. Neonatal screening commonly tests for which diseases?

- Hypothyroidism
- Phenylketonuria (PKU)
- Galactosemia
- Maple syrup urine disease (MSUD)
- Biotinidase deficiency
- Homocystinuria
- Sickle cell disease (SCD)
- Glucose-6-phosphate dehydrogenase deficiency (G6PDD)
- Congenital adrenal hyperplasia (CAH)

60. Which of these diseases is likely to be life-threatening in the neonatal period: (1) all; (2) none; (3) galactosemia, MSUD, and CAH; or (4) SCD, G6PDD, and biotinidase deficiency?

The answer is (3). Galactosemia can cause acute liver failure promptly after institution of milk feedings. It also predisposes neonates to *Escherichia coli* septicemia. MSUD causes lethal depression of the function of the central nervous system (CNS) in the neonatal period. Salt-losing CAH, caused by 21-hydroxylase deficency, can cause addisonian crisis with hypovolemic/hyponatremic shock, hypoglycemia, and (most danerous of all) severe hyperkalemia.

61. In which of these diseases is delayed or impaired development of the CNS expected if effective treatment is begun at 3 months of age: (1) all; (2) none; (3) PKU, hypothyroidism, MSUD, and galactosemia; or (4) PKU, hypothyroidism, and homocystinuria?

The answer is (3). Effective treatment of PKU, hypothyroidism, and MSUD must begin within the first few weeks of life to avoid significant problems in development. In infants with galactosemia, learning disabilities are quite prominent even if treatment is begun expectantly. Developmental disabilities are found in 50% of untreated homocystinuric patients, but the age by which treatment must begin is not known.

62. In which of these diseases may physical signs be present at birth: (1) none; (2) SCD, G6PDD, and homocystinuria; (3) galactosemia and CAH; or (4) galactosemia, CAH, and PKU?

The answer is (3). Some infants affected by galactosemia have cataracts at birth. The female infant with CAH due to 21-hydroxylase deficiency often has ambiguous genitalia (enlarged clitoris, labial fusion) at birth.

63. What are the benefits of detecting SCD by neonatal screening?

SCD presents at various ages and in various ways, but the major threat to life for small infants is bacterial sepsis, with *Streptococcus pneumoniae* high on the list of causative organisms. Preclinical detection of SCD allows prophylaxis against pneumococcal infection.

64. Why is screening for cystic fibrosis controversial, given that it is the most common inherited disease in Caucasians and that effective neonatal screening methods are available?

1. The clinical benefit of neonatal diagnosis has not been established unequivocally.

2. Because the disease is disabling and incurable, the screening process produces psychological stress in families of affected infants.

65. A 5-day-old breast-fed infant has a strongly positive test for urinary reducing substance but a negative test for urinary glucose. Explain these findings. What action should be taken?

In breast-fed infants, the dietary carbohydrate is lactose, which is hydrolyzed during absorption to glucose and galactose, both reducing sugars. Therefore, a non-glucose reducing substance in the urine is almost certainly galactose, and its presence strongly suggests the diagnosis of galactosemia. Intake of lactose should be stopped immediately and not reinstituted until galactosemia has been ruled out by assay of red blood cell galactose-1-PO4 uridylyltransferase.

Because galactosemia can be rapidly lethal, do not delay this decision until the result of the screening test is known.

66. What is the incidence of congenital hypothyroidism?

1 in 4000 liveborn infants.

67. What are the genetic implications of screening for hypothyroidism?

The vast majority of affected infants have thyroid dysgenesis of unknown, nonhereditary origin. However, the possible hereditary causes of congenital disease must be considered in the evaluation of all newborn infants with hypothyroidism.

INBORN ERRORS OF METABOLISM

68. What clinical signs suggest metabolic disease in neonates?

- Lethargy and coma
- Recurrent vomiting
- Tachypnea unrelated to pulmonary disease
- Marked hypotonia
- Seizures
- Dysmorphism
- Ocular abnormalities
- Visceromegaly
- Unusual odors
- Abnormalities of skin or hair
- Unstable body temperature

Note: The signs of metabolic disease are nonspecific. More common diseases such as sepsis must be considered in the differential diagnosis.

69. If a neonate misses one or two feedings, is large ketonuria likely to develop?

No. Large ketones usually are not detectable in the urine of normal newborn infants with fasting, including those with fasting-induced hypoglycemia. Conversely, ketonuria often is present in neonates with defects in gluconeogenesis and amino acid or organic acid metabolism. The rate of utilization of ketones as a fuel is greater in infants compared with children. Experimental data suggest that some inborn errors of metabolism may be associated with a secondary defect in ketone body utilization. Severe acidemia also may perturb the utilization of ketones.

70. Which metabolic disorders are associated with a distinctive odor?

- PKU
- MSUD
- Isovaleric acidemia
- Type I tyrosinemia
- Multiple carboxylase deficiency
- β-Methylcrotonyl-CoA carboxylase deficiency
- Type II glutaric aciduria

71. Which metabolic disorders are commonly associated with acidosis?

- Methylmalonic acidemia
- Propionic acidemia
- Isovaleric acidemia
- MSUD
- Primary lactic acidosis due to mitochondrial pyruvate dehydrogenase (PDH) complex deficiency and respiratory chain deficiencies
- Holocarboxylase synthetase deficiency
- Fructose 1,6-diphosphatase deficiency
- Succinyl CoA acetoacetate CoA transferase deficiency
- Ketothiolase deficiency
- Type II glutaric aciduria

72. What are the first items that the neonatal transport team must address in an infant with a suspected inborn error of metabolism?

1. ABCs: airway, breathing, circulation
2. Hypoglycemia, metabolic acidosis

73. What complications may the transport team encounter in infants with an inborn error?

- Coma
- Seizures
- Brain swelling
- Intracranial hemorrhage
- *E. coli* sepsis in infants with galactosemia

74. What congenital abnormalities are more common in infants born to women with PKU?

Microencephaly (mental retardation) and congenital heart defects, which are thought to result from high levels of phenylalanine.

75. Which inborn errors of metabolism are commonly associated with neonatal seizures?
- Nonketotic hyperglycemia
- Pyridoxine-responsive seizure disorders
- Peroxisomal disorders (e.g., neonatal adrenoleukodystrophy)
- Sulfite oxidase deficiency
- Glucose transporter (GLUT 1) deficiency with hypoglycorrhachia
- Disorders of ammonia metabolism (e.g., ornithine transcarbamylase deficiency)

76. What common metabolic disseases can cause Fanconi syndrome?
- Hereditary tyrosinemia
- Galactosemia
- Glycogen storage disease type I
- Hereditary fructose intolerance
- Pyroglutamic aciduria
- Cytochrome C oxidase deficiency

77. Summarize the initial diagnostic assessment of infants with suspected metabolic disease.
- Serum electrolytes
- Blood pH and partial pressure of carbon dioxide
- Blood lactate and pyruvate
- Urine organic acid quantitation
- Blood ammonia (urine orotic acid if elevated)
- Blood amino acid quantitation
- Liver function tests
- Ophthalmologic examination
- Urine Clinitest reaction (while the infant is ingesting a lactose-containing formula)

78. How can the five major kinds of metabolic diseases be distinguished?

	ORGANIC ACIDURIAS	PRIMARY LACTIC ACIDOSES	UREA CYCLE DEFECTS	CLASSIC GALACTOSEMIA	NONKETOTIC HYPERGLYCEMIA
Metabolic acidosis	Frequent	Frequent	No	No	No
Ketoaciduria	Frequent	Variable	No	No	No
Urine organic acids	Abnormal	Increased lactate	Normal	Nondiagnostic	Normal
Lactic acidosis	No	Frequent	No	No	No
Hyperammonemia	Usually < 500 µmol/L	Usually < 500 µmol/L	Usually > 500 µmol/L	No	No
Blood aminogram	Nondiagnostic	Increased alanine	Very abnormal*	Nondiagnostic	Marked increase in glycine
CSF aminogram	Nondiagnostic	Increased alanine	Very abnormal*	Nondiagnostic	Marked increase in glycine
Urine orotic acid	Usually normal	Normal	Very high†	Normal	Normal
Neutropenia	Frequent	Variable	Unusual	No	No
Thrombocytopenia	Frequent	Variable	Unusual	No	No
Urine Clinitest	Negative	Negative	Negative	Positive	Negative
Hepatic failure	No	Uncommon	No	Frequent	No
Cataracts	No	No	No	Frequent‡	No

* Often diagnostic in urea cycle defects.
† Major exception: in carbamyl phosphate synthetase deficiency, orotic acid is normal or low.
‡ May require slit-lamp examination for visualization.

Adapted from Yudkoff M: Inborn errors of metabolism presenting as catastrophic disease. In Spitzer A (ed): Intensive Care of the Fetus and Neonate. St. Louis, Mosby, 1996, p 1015.

THYROID DISORDERS

79. Summarize the embryonic stages of development of the fetal hypothalamic-pituitary-thyroid axis.

1. Thyroid tissue is first identified at the base of the tongue 16–17 days after conception.

2. By 7 weeks' gestation, the gland has migrated to its final position in the anterior neck and has developed its characteristic bilobed structure.

3. By 10 weeks' gestation the fetal thyroid gland is trapping iodine and synthesizing thyroxine (T4).

4. By 10 weeks' gestation the fetal hypothalamus is synthesizing thyrotropin-releasing hormone (TRH). Most fetal TRH, however, is made in extrahypothalamic tissues (placenta, pancreas). Hypothalamic TRH production does not mature fully until the perinatal period.

5. By 10–12 weeks' gestation the fetal pituitary gland is synthesizing thyroid-stimulating hormone (TSH).

80. When does the fetal hypothalamic-pituitary-thyroid axis begin to function?

The hypothalamic-pituitary-thyroid axis is in place by the end of the first trimester. The thyroid and pituitary glands reach mature secretory capacity by 30–35 weeks of gestation. The feedback interrelationship among the units is fully established when hypothalamic TRH maturation is completed by 1–2 months after birth.

81. Describe the pattern of secretion of fetal T4 during gestation.

The amount of T4 secreted by the fetal thyroid gland increases slowly until mid-gestation (20–24 weeks) when, stimulated by increasing amounts of TSH from the fetal pituitary, T4 levels begin to increase more rapidly, reaching a normal adult level by about 30 weeks' gestation. Thereafter T4 increases slowly to high normal levels at term.

82. Describe the pattern of T4 conversion to triiodothyronine (T3) during gestation.

Most of the circulating T4 is deiodinated by fetal peripheral tissues to an inactive metabolite, reverse T3 (rT3). Only a small amount of T4 is converted peripherally to active T3. Serum rT3 peaks at about 250 μg/dl at 30 weeks' gestation, then declines to term levels of about 150 μg/dl. The amount of ciriculating T3 is very low (< 15 ng/dl) until about 30 weeks' gestation, then increases slowly to reach a level of approximately 50 ng/dl (about one-third of maternal levels) by parturition.

83. Describe the pattern of TSH secretion during gestation.

The amount of circulating TSH begins to increase in mid-gestation (20 weeks) and reaches a peak level of approximately 15 μU/ml by 30 weeks' gestation. The TSH level then declines gradually to about 10 μU/ml at term.

84. Do maternal TSH and maternal iodine cross the placenta?

Maternal TSH does not cross the placenta, but maternal iodine crosses the placenta freely and is essential for the synthesis of thyroid hormones by the fetus.

85. Do maternal T3 and T4 have any effect on the fetus?

The placenta is a barrier to the passages of thyroid hormones and contains enzymes that break down maternal T4 and T3 into inactive metabolites. Only a small percentage of circulating maternal T4 and very little (if any) T3 reach the fetus. However, the amount of maternal T4 that does cross the placenta is significant. During the first 10–12 weeks of gestation, all of the circulating T4 in the fetus is from maternal sources; thus early brain development depends on maternal hormone. Even after the fetus synthesizes its own T4 in the second and third trimesters, maternal T4 is essential for normal neurologic development, including neuronal proliferation and maturation, dendritic arborization, and synapse formation. It accounts for about 30% of fetal T4 levels at term.

86. What evidence supports the essential role of maternal T4 during gestation?

    1. Children with intact thyroids born to mothers who were hypothyroid during pregnancy have subtle neurologic damage. They show greater distractibility and poorer aptitude and visual-motor skills when tested in mid-childhood than children born to euthyroid mothers.

    2. Neonates with thyroid aplasia or hypoplasia, whose mothers were euthyroid, are born with few, if any, overt signs of cretinism.

    3. If both mother and fetus are hypothyroid, the neonate has marked developmental delay and overt signs of cretinism.

87. What happens to TSH levels at parturition?

    Within 15–20 minutes after birth, the fetal pituitary releases a surge of TSH, probably in response to cooling. TSH reaches a peak of about 80 μU/ml in about 30 minutes, decreases rapidly over the first 24 hours of life, and then drops more gradually to levels comparable to normal adult levels by the end of the first 1–2 weeks of life.

88. How does the TSH surge affect T4 levels?

    Serum T4 levels increase rapidly, reaching a peak level of about 17 μg/dl at 24 hours. T4 then gradually decreases to levels at the upper limit of normal adult values over the first 4–5 weeks of life. Free T4 levels follow the same pattern, reaching a peak of 3.5 ng/dl at 24–36 hours.

89. How are T3 levels affected by parturition?

    The elimination of placental degradation products and the increasing maturation of hepatic deiodinating enzymes favor the conversion of T4 to T3 rather than to rT3. After birth, the levels of T3 rise rapidly to a peak of 250 ng/dl at 24–36 hours, then gradually fall over the next few weeks to levels found in infancy. The levels of rT3 continue to decline, and by the sixteenth week after birth rT3 has disappeared.

90. How do levels of thyroid hormone differ in premature and full-term infants?

    The levels of TRH, TSH, T4, free T4, and T3 are lower in premature infants than in full-term infants, and the postnatal surges of TSH and T4, although qualitatively similar, are blunted. These differences are related directly to gestational age: the lower the gestational age, the lower the levels and responses of thyroid-related hormones.

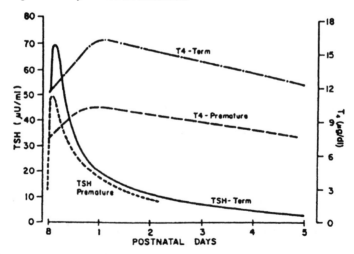

Changes in serum concentrations of thyroid-stimulating hormone (TSH) and thyroxine (T4) in full-term and premature infants during the first 5 days of life. (From Fisher DA, Klein AH: Thyroid development and disorders of thyroid function in the newborn. N Engl J Med 304:706, 1981, with permission.)

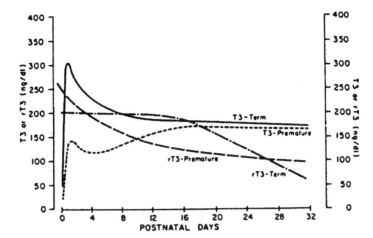

Changes in serum triiodothyronine (T3) and reverse T3 (rT3) concentrations in full-term and premature infants during the first month of life. (From Fisher DA, Klein AH: Thyroid development and disorders of thyroid function in the newborn. N Engl J Med 304:706, 1981, with permission.)

Serum Thryoxine (mg/dl) at Different Gestational Ages*

SAMPLE TIME	ESTIMATED GESTATIONAL AGE (WK)				
	30–31	31–33	34–35	36–37	TERM
Cord	6.5 (1.0)	7.5 (2.1)	6.7 (1.2)	7.5 (2.8)	8.2 (1.8)
3–10 days	7.7 (1.8)	8.5 (1.9)	10.0 (2.4)	12.7 (2.5)	15.9 (3.0)
11–20 days	7.5 (1.8)	8.3 (1.6)	10.5 (1.8)	11.2 (2.9)	12.2 (2.0)

* Mean (standard deviation).
Adapted from Cuestas RA: Thyroid function in healthy premature infants. J Pediatr 92:964, 1978, with permission.

91. Define hypothyroxinemia of prematurity.

The term refers to infants with low birth weight (30–35 weeks) or very low birth weight (< 30 weeks), who have an even more attenuated rise in T4, after which T4 levels drop below cord levels in the first week of life. Then they rise gradually over 3–6 weeks to approach levels of full-term infants.

Thyroid Function in Infants ≤ 28 Weeks Gestation*

POSTNATAL AGE	T4 (μg/dl)	T3 (ng/dl)	TSH (μU/ml)
Birth	3.8 (1.5)	58.6 (26)	16 (8)
24 hours	3.1 (1.6)	71.6 (26)	16 (8)
72 hours	2.7 (1.5)	65.1 (39.1)	11 (5)
1 week	2.3 (1.2)	58.6 (19.5)	12 (7)
3 weeks	3.9 (1.8)	71.6 (26)	11 (4)
4 weeks	4.0 (1.8)	71.6 (26)	11 (6)
6 weeks	4.7 (2.2)	78.1 (13)	12 (6)

T4 = thyroxine, T3 = triiodothyronine, TSH = thyroid-stimulating hormone.
• Mean (standard deviation).
Adapted from Mercado M, Yu VYH, Francis I, et al: Thyroid function in very preterm infants. Early Hum Devel 16:134, 1988, with permission.

92. What happens to thyroid tests in sick premature infants?

In the sick euthyroid or low T3 syndrome, the conversion of T4 to T3 is inhibited. Thus, illness exaggerates the normally hypothyroxinemic state in premature infants. T4 levels may be low or low normal for gestational age, whereas T3 levels are low and rT3 levels are high. However, free T4 is normal, and serum TSH levels are normal, an indication that the infant is not hypothyroid. In infants with very low birth weight and a poor TSH response, it may be difficult to distinguish the effects of illness from primary hypothyroidism. A high rT3 level suggests the former.

93. Should hypothyroxinemia of prematurity be treated?

The premature infant with low T4 and persistently elevated TSH has either transient or permanent hypothyroidism and should be treated with thyroxine until the nature of the condition becomes clear. However, whether premature infants with low T4 and normal TSH should be treated is controversial.

94. Summarize the arguments against treatment.

1. Hypothyroxinemia of prematurity is a physiologic phenomenon and resolves with age.

2. In sick premature infants, the physiologic hypothyroxinemia is exaggerated by the low levels of T3 and T4 associated with serious illness (sick euthyroid syndrome) and resolves when the child recovers.

3. Infants with low birth weight and gestational age > 30 weeks can increase serum TSH in response to true primary hypothyroidism. The TSH in the hypothyroxinemia of prematurity is normal.

4. Treatment with L-thyroxine has shown no benefit and carries a risk because thyroxine levels higher than normal for age may inhibit neural cell multiplication. In fact, the study by van Wassenaer et al. showed a loss of 10 points in mental development with treatment in infants of more than 27 weeks' gestation.

95. Summarize the arguments in favor of treatment.

1. Infants born prematurely are deprived of significant amounts of maternal T4 during a period critical for CNS development. They also are deprived of a significant source of iodine for thyroid hormone synthesis and storage.

2. Severe hypothyroxinemia (T4 > 2.6 standard deviations below the mean for the assay) is associated with risk of disabling cerebral palsy almost 11 times greater and a mean mental development score 15 points lower than in infants with hypothryoxinemia.

3. In the van Wassenaer study (see question 94, item 4) treatment with L-thyroxine was highly beneficial to infants of < 27 weeks' gestational age, resulting in an 18-point increase in mental development scores.

4. Because of their extreme immaturity, infants with very low birth weight and gestational age < 30 weeks cannot increase TSH in response to truly hypothyroid T4 levels. For the same reason, such infants cannot convert T4 to active T3.

96. Why do we screen for congenital hypothyroidism?

Signs and symptoms of hypothyroidism are subtle at birth, and the characteristic appearance of cretinism may not be apparent for 3–4 months. The brain requires thyroid hormone for normal development until about 2–3 years of age, and deficiency of thyroid hormone during this period causes irreversible brain damage to an extent related directly to the length of time of the hypothyroidism. Thus it is of vital importance to identify the hypothyroid infant as quickly as possible, even before clinical signs appear.

97. When and how is screening done?

A heel stick blood sample is taken at discharge or 3 days of life, whichever is earlier. In North America, thyroxine is measured first; then TSH is measured in samples with the lowest 10–29% of T4 results.

98. What is the overall incidence of congenital hypothyroidism?
1 in 4000 live births.

99. List the causes of congenital hypothyroidism and give the incidence of each.

CAUSE	INCIDENCE	PERCENT OF CASES
Thyroid dysgenesis (aplasia, hypoplasia, ectopy)	1:4000	75
Thyroid dyshormonogenesis	1:30,000	10
Hypothalamic-pituitary hypothyroidism	1:100,000	5
Transient hypothyroidism (secondary to drugs or maternal antibodies, idiopathic)	1:40,000	10

From Fisher FA: Disorders of the thyroid in the newborn and infant. In Sperling MA (ed): Pediatric Endocrinology. Philadelphia, W.B. Saunders, 1996, p 57, with permission.

100. Has neonatal screening been effective in preventing CNS damage?
Children identified as hypothyroid by screening usually are started on replacement therapy with L-thyroxine by 10 days to 3 weeks of life. If treatment is consistent and the dose of L-thyroxine is adequate, the results are quite good. Long-term follow-up studies show that IQ falls within the normal range. Even with optimal treatment, however, some children, especially those with no functioning thyroid tissue, show the irreversible effect of fetal hypothyroidism and have varying degrees of motor impairment and poor performance on IQ tests.

101. How does maternal Graves' disease affect the fetus and neonate?
The thyroid-stimulating immunoglobulins (TSIs) cross the placenta and may cause fetal thyrotoxicosis: goiter, tachycardia, rapid skeletal maturation, premature birth, and, occasionally, congestive heart failure. Long-term neurologic deficits may result because excessive thyroxine reduces the number of neurons that are formed.
Only about 1 in 70 neonates born to thyrotoxic mothers has clinical thyrotoxicosis. Such infants may show a phase of transient hypothyroidism due to antithyroid drugs (half-life = 2–3 days), then thyrotoxicosis secondary to maternal TSIs.

102. How may treatment of maternal Graves' disease affect the fetus and neonate?
1. Antithyroid drugs (propylthiouracil [PTU], methimazole) cross the placenta and may block the fetal thyroid, leading to fetal hypothyroidism.
2. Radioactive iodine crosses the placenta and ablates the fetal thyroid.
3. Beta-adrenergic agents (e.g., propranolol) cross the placenta and have been associated with intrauterine growth retardation, bradycardia, perinatal respiratory distress, and postnatal hypoglycemia.

103. What are the signs of neonatal thyrotoxicosis?
- Goiter
- Low birth weight with normal length
- Proptosis
- Periorbital edema
- Hyperactivity, hyperirritability
- Poor weight gain despite ravenous feeding
- Frequent stooling

104. Does neonatal thyrotoxicosis require treatment?
Neonatal thyrotoxicosis normally is a self-limited disease that subsides by about 3 months of age when maternal TSIs are metabolized. However, tachycardia, irritability, and poor weight gain require treatment with low-dose PTU with or without propranolol. The danger of treatment is oversuppression of the neonatal thyroid and consequent hypothyroidism.

105. What maternal drugs can adversely affect the fetal thyroid state?
- Iodide-containing medicines (e.g., saturated solution of potassium iodide, amiodarone)
- Antithyroid medications and beta-adrenergic blockers

Other drugs (e.g., dexamethasone) that cross the placenta and can affect the thyroid gland of an adult have not been shown to have any effect on the fetal thyroid gland.

106. How do iodide-containing medicines affect the fetal thyroid state?

The mature thyroid stops synthesis of T4 in the presence of excessive iodine (Wolff-Chaikoff effect) but escapes from this inhibition when intrathyroidal iodine pools are depleted. The fetal thyroid cannot "escape" and develops into a goiter that can be large enough to require emergency transection at birth. In addition, the continued blockade of T4 production by iodine leads to fetal hypothyroidism

Note: The premature infant is also unable to escape from the inhibitory effect of iodine and may become hypothyroid when subjected to multiple povidone-iodine washings or iodinated contrast agents.

107. Is breast-feeding contraindicated in mothers with Graves' disease?

Methimazole and carbamazole are excreted into breast milk in quantities that may affect the infant adversely. If breastfeeding cannot be avoided, the infant should undergo thyroid function tests at weekly intervals to avoid potential hypothyroidism. PTU is not a contraindication to breastfeeding because only about 0.1% is excreted in breast milk. The amounts of thyroxine and T3 in breast milk are too low to affect nursing infants.

108. Does breast feeding provide needed thyroxine to premature infants with an immature hypothalamic-pituitary-thyroid axis?

This question has not yet been answered.

ADRENAL DISORDERS

109. What enzyme abnormalities are associated with congenital adrenal hyperplasia?

Congenital adrenal hyperplasia is an autosomal recessive disorder that results from a deficiency of one of the five enzymes that convert cholesterol to cortisol:

1. 20,22-Desmolase   4. 21-Hydroxylase
2. 3-β-Hydroxysteroid dehydrogenase   5. 11-Hydroxylase
3. 17-α-Hydroxylase

110. List the major manifestations of each deficiency.

1. 20,22-Desmolase deficiency (congenital adrenal lipoid hyperplasia): salt wasting, ambiguous genitalia in males.

2. 3-β-Hydroxysteroid dehydrogenase deficiency: salt wasting, mild virilization in females, ambiguous genitalia in males.

3. 17-α-Hydroxylase deficiency: hypertension, ambiguous genitalia in males.

4. 21-Hydroxylase deficiency: manifestations depend on whether the deficiency is partial or complete. Partial deficiency results in virilization in females, and complete deficiency results in salt wasting and signs of cortisol deficiency (e.g., hypoglycemia, shock).

5. 11-Hydroxylase deficiency: salt retention and hypertension in 50–80% of cases, virilization in females.

111. In infants with CAH due to 21-hydroxylase deficiency, which of the following is abnormal: (1) genetic sex, (2) gonadal differentiation, (3) internal genital formation and structure, or (4) external genitalia in females?

The answer is (4). In females with congenital adrenal hyperplasia, the karyotype (genetic sex) is normal (46XX). The müllerian ducts develop normally into a uterus and fallopian tubes without secretion of antimüllerian hormone. No wolffian duct derivatives are formed because no fetal testis is present. The elevated adrenal androgen levels cause virilization of the external genitalia.

112. A female fetus is exposed to maternal androgenic substances at 10 weeks of gestation. What are the likely manifestations?

At 8–14 weeks of gestation, exposure to androgens may result in midline fusion of the labioscrotal folds, opening of the vagina and urethra into a common urogenital sinus, and (in severe cases) development of a penile urethra, prostate, and possibly seminal vesicles. Exposure after 12–14 weeks of gestation results only in clitoromegaly and hypertrophy of the labia majora.

113. List the sources of maternal androgens that cause masculinization.
- Androgen-secreting tumors
- Ingestion of synthetic progestins, androgens, or danazol (a derivative of testosterone)

114. A male fetus is exposed to maternal progestin at 10 weeks of gestation. What is the possible manifestation?

Exposure of male fetuses to progestin at 8–14 weeks of gestation may result in hypospadias.

115. What causes adrenal hemorrhage in neonates?

Adrenal hemorrhage occurs more frequently after breech delivery, with eventual calcification in some cases. Hypoxia, fetal distress, maternal diabetes and congenital syphilis also have been associated with adrenal hemorrhage.

116. What are the manifestations of adrenal hemorrhage?

Most infants with adrenal hemorrhage are asymptomtic.

117. Describe the evaluation of adrenal hemorrhage.

The evaluation should include a 60-minute adrenocorticotropic hormone stimulation test with measurement of baseline and 60-minute cortisols. The normal peak is > 20 µg/dl.

118. A pregnant woman has low urinary estriols. At delivery her male infant develops hyponatremia, hyperkalemia, and hypoglycemia. What diagnosis should you consider?

Congenital adrenal hypoplasia.

119. How common is congenital adrenal hypoplasia?

Congenital adrenal hypoplasia is an X-linked disorder affecting 1 in 12,500 live births.

120. With what other disorders may it be associated?
- Anencephaly
- Pituitary hypoplasia
- Gonadotropin deficiency

121. Why does the mother have low estriol levels?

Because the fetus contributes to the precursors for placental formation of maternal estriols.

122. What is steroidogenic acute regulatory (StAR) protein?

StAR protein is necessary for proper reduction of aldosterone, cortisone, and sex hormones. Its absence leads to feminization of males as part of congenital lipoid adrenal hyperplasia. In a subset of patients with congenital lipoid adrenal hyperplasia, mutations in StAR protein result in severe impairment of steroid biosynthesis in the adrenal glands and gonads.

123. What tests should be done after stopping dexamethasone therapy in neonates with adrenal insufficiency?

Adrenal suppression is a concern in pediatric patients who have received glucocorticoid therapy for more than 5 days. In neonates and premature infants, when and how the adrenal gland may respond after dexamethasone therapy are even more complex questions. Stimulation testing with a 250-µg dose of corticotropin uses a supraphysiologic stimulus and may give a false-positive cortisol response. The 1-µg corticotropin stimulation test is more sensitive for indicating whether adrenal cortical function is normal.

124. What is the best time to obtain a cortisol level in premature neonates?

Collect the blood specimen at any time. Circadian rhythms do not affect the level of cortisol in very premature infants. Infants with extremely low birth weight may have quite low cortisol levels (9.2 ± 9.8 µg/ml) and lack the typical early-morning rise in cortisol. Whether such low corticosteroid levels in premature infants with very low birth weight indicate adrenal insufficiency is not fully known.

125. A 3-day-old infant presents with salt wasting, vomiting, dehydration, hyperkalemia, hyponatremia, and acidosis. Which of the following are possible diagnoses: (1) congenital adrenal hyperplasia, (2) adrenal insufficiency, (3) pseudohypoaldosteronism, or (4) all of the above?

The answer is (4). The most common cause of such symptoms is congenital adrenal hyperplasia, followed by adrenal insufficiency. Pseudohypoaldosteronism is a rare cause of severe salt wasting in neonates.

126. What is pseudohypoaldosteronism?

Pseudohypoaldosteronism is an inherited disease (autosomal recessive or dominant pattern) characterized by renal tubular unresponsiveness to the kaliuretic and sodium and chloride reabsorptive effects of aldosterone. In contrast to congenital adrenal hyperplasia or adrenal insufficiency, it is accompanied by excessive levels of renin and aldosterone. Unresponsiveness to aldosterone may be generalized, in which case sodium excretion is increased in sweat, saliva, stool, and urine, or limited to the renal tubule, in which case sodium excretion is increased in urine only.

127. How is pseudohypoaldosteronism treated?

With salt supplementation and potassium-lowering agents such as kayexalate.

PITUITARY DISORDERS

128. When does growth hormone (GH) first appear in fetal plasma?

At 10 weeks' gestation. Levels increase in mid-gestation and decrease toward term.

129. Does placental GH contribute to fetal levels?

No. Placental GH is secreted only into the maternal circulation.

130. Describe the physiologic role of prolactin in neonates.

Fetal prolactin levels are first detectable at 10 weeks' gestation and increase progressively until delivery. Serum levels are 20-fold higher in fetuses than in adults. Levels decline rapidly over the first week after birth and may contribute to postnatal reduction in total body water. Cord blood prolactin levels are low in infants who develop respiratory distress syndrome.

131. When does the hypothalamic-pituitary-gonadal axis develop in the fetus?

Gonadotropin-releasing hormone (GnRH) is detectable in the hypothalamus at 8 weeks' gestation. Luteinizing hormone (LH) and follicle-stimulating hormone (FSH) are present in the pituitary gland by 11–12 weeks' gestation and at term are found in low levels in cord blood. The fetal testis responds to human chorionic gonadotropin (HCG), but the fetal ovary does not respond because it lacks HCG receptors.

132. List the common causes of elevated levels of antidiuretic hormone (ADH) in neonates.
- Birth asphyxia
- Infection with respiratory syncytial virus
- Acute blood loss
- Pain
- Periventricular hemorrhage

133. What manifestations of adrenocorticotropic hormone (ACTH) insufficiency are seen in neonates?
- Hypoglycemia   • Hyponatremia (without hyperkalemia)   • Direct hyperbilirubinemia

134. What disorders are associated with deficiencies of pituitary transcription factors?

Early evidence for the role of transcription factors in pituitary deficiencies was the discovery that *pit-1* gene mutation is the cause of the Snell dwarf mouse. In humans, Pit-1 deficiency results in pituitary gland hypoplasia and low levels of GH, TSH, and prolactin. Because Prop-1 (prophet of Pit-1) is needed for the expression of Pit-1, a deficiency of either factor results in the same defects. P-Lim is associated with deficiencies of all pituitary hormones except ACTH and with retinal colobomas.

135. What causes the transient surge of TSH in neonates?

The postnatal surge in TSH is believed to be mediated by TRH in response to the postdelivery cooling of the neonate exposed to the extrauterine environment.

136. Describe the secretory pattern of cortisol in full-term and premature neonates.

Both have a pulsatile pattern of cortisol secretion. Premature infants have a lower maximal secretory rate for cortisol. Both are capable of mounting a cortisol response to stress (e.g., surgery). The normal diurnal variation develops later in both.

137. What are the symptoms of GH deficiency in neonates?

The most common presenting symptom is hypoglycemia. Micropenis is also common in male neonates. Jaundice may be present for a prolonged period. Because GH is not necessary for intrauterine linear growth, intrauterine growth retardation is not a feature of GH deficiency.

138. Discuss the typical findings in neonates with hypogonadotropic hypogonadism (HHG).

In male neonates, HHG is associated with micropenis (stretched penile length < 2.5 cm). Undescended testes also may be present. In female neonates, there are no clinical findings of HHG.

139. What major malformations may be associated with disorders of the hypothalamic-pituitary axis in neonates?

Cleft lip and palate, optic nerve atrophy, septo-optic dysplasia, and holoprosencephaly.

140. What tumors may be associated with disorders of the hypothalamic-pituitary axis?

Hypothalamic hamartoblastoma (Pallister-Hall syndrome) and Rathke cleft pouch cyst.

141. What magnetic resonance findings have recently been recognized in infants with GH deficiency?

An ectopic pituitary "bright spot" and interrupted pituitary stalk.

INTERSEX DISORDERS

142. What is the major gene responsible for gonadal differentiation into testes?

The testes-determining factor (TDF), a relatively small segment on the short arm of the Y chromosome, has been linked to differentiation of primitive gonadal tissue into testes. In the absence of TDF, the undifferentiated gonadal tissue evolves into an ovary. The exact mechanisms by which the genes within the TDF locus lead to testicular differentiation are under investigation.

143. What two hormones, produced by the testes in utero, result in a phenotypic male?

Testosterone is produced by Leydig cells within the fetal testes by 6 weeks of gestation. In addition, the testes produce the peptide hormone, **müllerian inhibitory substance** (MIS), which eliminates all müllerian structures in the male. An isolated deficiency in MIS produces a normal external male phenotype, but the internal phenotype is characterized by a fallopian tube running parallel to the vas deferens.

144. What is the source of the major virilizing androgen?

Surprisingly, the testes are not the source of the major virilizing hormone. The testes produce testosterone, which has some virilizing properties. But the most potent virilizing hormone is dihydro-testosterone, which is produced in the peripheral genital tissues by the action of 5-alpha-reductase on testosterone. Dihydro-testosterone then diffuses locally to achieve its virilizing effects (a paracrine effect).

145. A male infant presents at delivery, but the family was told that amniocentesis showed a 46XX chromosomal pattern. What are the three possible explanations?

1. Congenital adrenal hyperplasia with secondary virilization of a gonadal female (the most common intersex diagnosis)
2. Sampling error during amniocentesis
3. XX male sex reversal syndrome (rare)

146. What finding on physical examination rules out congenital adrenal hyperplasia?
Documentation of normal testes within the scrotum.

147. How is the diagnosis of congenital adrenal hyperplasia confirmed?
The infant has intact ovaries, and no gonadal tissue is palpable in the inguinal or scrotal areas. Furthermore, normal uterine differentiation can be detected by ultrasound examination at the bedside.

148. How do sampling errors occur during amniocentesis?
The karyotype done during amniocentesis respresents a sampling of cells within the amnion. On rare occasions, some maternal cells are aspirated and used for the karyotype. This scenario can be confirmed or eliminated by repeating the karyotype in the neonatal period. In addition, ultrasound examination reveals no uterine structures if sampling error is the explantion.

149. What causes the XX male sex reversal syndrome?
The probable cause is translocation of some genetic material to the Y chromosome, which gives the appearance of two X chromosomes.

150. How is the diagnosis of XX male sex reversal syndrome confirmed?
Confirmation requires a fluorescence in situ hybridization (FISH) study with a series of cDNA probes for TDF in what appears to be an X chromosome. Ultrasound examination shows no uterine structures because MIS is produced by the testes.

151. Ultrasound and endocrine testing confirm a diagnosis of congenital adrenal hyperplasia in a female neonate with bilateral impalpable gonads and a complete phallus. What radiographic study is needed to complete the work-up?
A genitogram. A catheter is placed within the "penile urethra," which is actually a urogenital sinus. What appears to be a urethra is in fact a common channel into which the vagina and urethra are merged.

152. What is the purpose of the genitogram?
To determine where the vagina and urethra merge—just below the bladder neck (high insertion) or well below the bladder neck (low insertion). This anatomic information is crucial to planning genital reconstruction. Fortunately, most patients with congenital adrenal hyperplasia have a low insertion; thus, the vagina is quite close to the perineum, allowing a technically simpler vaginoplasty. Low insertions are more common even in virilized patients, such as the patient described in question 150. Twenty years ago, before ultrasound was sufficiently accurate, the genitogram was diagnostic. When contrast fills the vagina, it also outlines the cervical imprint.

153. Describe the sequelae of untreated congenital adrenal hyperplasia.
Congenital adrenal hyperplasia results from missing hydroxylase enzymes that modify steroid precursors and lead to the formation of cortisol and aldosterone. A major feature of the disorder is shunting of these mineralocorticoid precursors into the androgen biosynthetic pathways.

The result of this surge in androgens produces a wide spectrum of **genital ambiguity in female patients**. Without proper treatment the deficiency of cortisol and mineralocorticoids leaves patients **susceptible to stress**. Often a compensated, healthy patient deteriorates rapidly with only a minor medical condition. Deaths from fairly minor illnesses have been reported in patients with unrecognized congenital adrenal hyperplasia. Maintenance steroid supplements are life-saving. Many infants with severe loss of mineralocorticoids present in **hypovolemic shock** in the first week of life. In both boys and girls, the excessive androgens produce rapid growth in early life, accompanied by **premature closure of the epiphyses**. Such children are tall in childhood but short in adulthood. Another classic presentation in boys is **precocious puberty**, which can present as early as 5 years of age. Fortunately, all of these potential complications are avoidable if the diagnosis is established and the proper endocrine regimen is started.

154. You are asked to assess a neonate with nonpalpable gonads and genital ambiguity (severe hypospadias in a large phallus). What is the most likely diagnosis? Why?

The most likely diagnosis is congenital adrenal hyperplasia because it is the most common intersex diagnosis and because no genital tissue is palpable. Other diagnoses, such as mixed gonadal dysgenesis or hermaphroditism, generally present with one palpable gland.

155. Which *one* serum test has the greatest chance of confirming the correct diagnosis?

Several steps leading to cortisol synthesis may be affected and produce the virilized female phenotype. The most likely missing enzyme is 21-hydroxylase, and the result is a major accumulation of its immediate precursor, 17-hydroxy progesterone. A serum radioimmunoassay (RIA) for **17-hydroxy progesterone** should be diagnostic in 90% of cases. In the remaining 8–9%, a serum RIA for deoxycortisone establishes missing 21-hydroxylase activity. It is reasonable to send serum for both RIAs. If both assays are negative, further studies may be ordered.

156. What other factors should be considered in making the diagnosis?

The major clues to diagnosis in patients with genital ambiguity lie in a careful history of both patient and family and the physical examination. Other studies, such as ultrasound, genitogram, and especially serum or urine testing of metabolites, should be ordered in a highly organized manner to confirm clinical suspicion.

157. A neonate presents with severe penoscrotal hypospadias and a palpable gonad in the left hemiscrotum; the right hemiscrotum is empty. Amniocentesis showed a classic 46XX karyotype, and ultrasound shows a cystic structure behind the bladder but no uterus. The genitogram shows a vagina with low insertion and a tiny atretic uterine cavity. What is the differential diagnosis?

The two most likely diagnoses are mixed gonadal dysgenesis and true hermaphroditism. The combination of a descended gonad and virilization indicates the presence of some functional testicular tissue. An ovary never descends into the scrotum, and an ovotestis does so only in rare cases. In mixed gonadal dysgenesis, one gonad is a streak found within the abdomen, and one testis descends into an inguinal or scrotal position. True hermaphroditism is characterized by a combination of both ovarian and testicular tissue, which may be combined within one testis (ovotestis). The rudimentary vagina and uterus reflect inadequate production of MIS despite the presence of some testicular tissue. Because the action of MIS is also paracrine, the vaginal and uterine structures are lateralized primarily to the side opposite the testis.

158. How do you distinguish between the two possible diagnoses?

You must perform an exploratory laparotomy with direct visualization and biopsy of the gonads. Histologic assessment over 48 hours allows the pathologist to establish the most accurate diagnosis. Once the gonadal tissue is accurately assessed, a decision may be made about gender assignment. A second laparotomy at this point allows removal of the gonad that is inconsistent with gender assignment. In the patient described above, an ovary was found in the right pelvis along with an atretic fallopian tube and tiny atretic uterus. On the left side a testis was found within the scrotum.

159. Why should the karyotype be repeated?

In the patient described above, amniocentesis revealed a 46XX karyotype. A repeat study in the neonatal unit showed that 80 clones had a 46XX karyotype and that 20 clones had a 46X ring finding. The small ring of chromosomal material was a chromosomal loop that could not be identified until a FISH study was performed. The FISH study with TDF cDNA probes revealed hybridization to the ring chromosome, which provided evidence that TFD was present. This finding probably accounts for the development of a testis on one side.

160. A neonate presents with genital ambiguity, including significant clitoromegaly and a palpable gonad on the left side in a labioscrotal fold. The right gonad is palpable in the right inguinal canal. The family recently migrated from Dominica. What is the most likely diagnosis?

The most likely diagnosis is 5-alpha reductase deficiency, which was first characterized by its striking clinical presentation. Cases are clustered in Dominica, where the culture is extremely supportive.

161. Describe the typical clinical presentation and its underlying mechanism.

At puberty children raised as female develop a male phenotype and subsequently are assigned a male gender role. Such patients are genetic males with normal testes and normal testosterone levels. The missing element is the enzyme 5-alpha reductase, which converts testosterone to dihyrotestosterone (DHT). The process of male sexual differentiation is initiated in utero, but the major stimulus to phallic enlargement and scrotal fusion is DHT. At birth genital ambiguity is striking, but at puberty testosterone rises to such high levels that phallic enlargement occurs along with other secondary sexual characteristics.

162. How is the diagnosis established?

With cultured fibroblasts.

163. Why do men with 5-alpha reductase deficiency not develop benign prostatic hypertrophy (BPH) later in life?

DHT is a major molecular signal for prostatic enlargement. This observation, together with an understanding of basic steroid biochemistry, served as the basis for development of the drug finasteride (Proscar), which is used to prevent the onset of BPH. This historical footnote points out the importance of studying relatively rare disorders.

164. You are asked to evaluate a neonate in the delivery room. Amniocentesis during pregnancy revealed a 46XY karyotype, but the infant has a perfectly normal female phenotypic appearance. What is the most likely diagnosis?

Androgen insensitivity syndrome (AIS). Patients with AIS have a normal XY karyotype. The testes are fully developed but never descend, and the external genitalia are those of a normal female. Serum testosterone levels are markedly elevated, but no virilization takes place. Because of a mutation in the androgen receptor, androgen has no effect on its target tissues. AIS, in effect, is end-organ failure based on molecular mutation; it is a syndrome in the sense that several point mutations have been identified.

165. What are the likely findings on pelvic examination?

Absence of the uterus and upper two-thirds of the vagina. These structures originate from the müllerian ducts, which involute in response to secretion of MIS. The testes are normal and produce normal amounts of testosterone and MIS.

166. Describe the two presentations of AIS later in life.

1. Before the widespread use of amniocentesis, most patients presented with amenorrhea during puberty, which began normally with the development of pubic hair and breast enlargement. Thus, AIS must be considered in all female adolescents with primary amenorrhea.

2. Up to 30% of patients with AIS present with bilateral hernias at some point during their lifetime. However, only 1% of all female patients with inguinal hernias have AIS.

167. You are asked to evaluate a 6-week-old infant with hypospadias and one undescended, nonpalpable testis. Ultrasound demonstrates a small atretic uterine stripe behind the bladder, and the genitogram reveals a small vagina. The karyotype is 46XY. What is the next diagnostic procedure?

Exploratory laparotomy with gonadal biopsy.

168. At laparotomy a testis is found in the scrotal position, and a streak gonad is identified on the contralateral side. The streak is removed, and biopsy confirms that it is a normal testis. What is the diagnosis?

Mixed gonadal dysgenesis. If the streak had been an ovary, the diagnosis would be hermaphroditism. In many series, mixed gonadal dysgenesis is the second most common intersex state.

169. What is the likelihood of uncovering an intersex state in boys with hypospadias and an undescended testis?

An intersex state is found in 30% of such patients. In a recent review, an impalpable testis was associated with greater likelihood of an intersex state than a palpable testis. Severe penoscrotal hypospadias was more likely to be associated with an intersex state, but the incidence was also quite high in patients with midshaft hypospadias.

170. A male neonate in the intensive care unit has a right hernia and a left undescended testis. When the bulging hernia enlarges, intervention is recommended. The surgeon reports that a fallopian tube has been found in the hernia sac. What is the diagnosis?

Hernia uteri inguinalis.

171. What causes hernia uteri inguinalis?

Absence of MIS, which is produced by the testis and results in involution of müllerian ducts during the course of normal male sexual differentiation. A normal-appearing testis that produces testosterone may lack the capacity to synthesize or secrete MIS. The result is a normal external male phenotype with an accompanying fallopian tube and, in some instances, a uterus or prominent utricle.

172. How is hernia uteri inguinalis best managed?

The best management in a tiny neonate is to complete the hernia repair. The family must be given a detailed explanation of the findings as well as reassurances about the child's gender. When the neonate is stable, an ultrasound study and genitogram should be performed to search for vaginal and uterine structures. The fallopian tubes and vaginal and uterine segments can be managed later at the time of orchiopexy for the undescended testis. The surgeon must be careful in removing these structures and err on the side of leaving such tissues behind because of the risk of damaging the vas deferens and destroying whatever potential for fertility the patient may have.

173. Attempted circumcision at another institution results in complete amputation. An immediate attempt at replantation fails. Is gender reassignment the best option, or should a delayed phalloplasty be recommended?

This issue is controversial. Gender reassignment has been the treatment of choice for such rare but tragic cases, which arise from aphallia (normal scrotum, perineal urethra, and absent phallia), circumcision injury, or child abuse. Total phallic reconstruction is a multistage, Herculean task in adults, limited to a handful of centers around the world. In neonates or infants, it is even more surgically demanding and realistically cannot be done until the child is at least 6–8 years old. The boy must go through a critical period of development in an aphallic state before reconstruction can be performed.

174. What procedures are involved in gender reassignment surgery?

Bilateral orchiectomy and feminizing genitoplasty with creation of a labia and vagina from the scrotum.

175. How common is gender reassignment surgery?

There are no estimates of the incidence of pediatric gender reassignment surgery in the United States.

176. Discuss the major problems associated with gender reassignment surgery.

Unfortunately, gender reassignment treats the cosmetic aspects of sexuality. The long-term issue centers on the patient's ultimate gender identity. Surgeons may be able to fashion the external genitalia into a feminine appearance, but androgens already have imprinted a male pattern on the developing fetal brain. The concept of the brain as a sexual organ continues to gain acceptance not only in animal models but also in human studies.

177. Discuss the results of a recent follow-up study of a patient who underwent gender reassignment surgery.

In one case of gender reassignment surgery after circumcision injury, 8-year follow-up indicated that the procedure was successful. Thereafter the patient was lost to follow-up at the original institution. A recent case report identified the patient and reported long-term results. On reaching puberty the patient failed to gain a sense of female gender identity and at age 16 reverted to a male gender. This is not an isolated case report, and Diamond has called for an end to gender reassignment surgery in the neonatal period.

In light of this case report and a meeting convened by the National Institutes of Health on the topic of pediatric gender reassignment, the American Academy of Pediatrics/Section of Urology has convened a multidisciplinary panel to examine long-term outcomes in children with genital ambiguity. It is crucial to recognize how often such complex situations arise and to understand long-term outcomes not only in terms of cosmesis but also in terms of sexual function and, most importantly, gender identity.

BIBLIOGRAPHY

1. Allemand D, Grüters A, Beyer P, Weber B: Iodine in contrast agents and skin disinfectants is the major cause for hypothyroidism in premature infants during intensive care. Hormone Res 28:42–49, 1987.
2. Anand KJS, Aynsley-Green A: Measuring the severity of surgical stress in newborn infants. J Pediatr Surg 23:297–305, 1988.
3. American Academy of Pediatrics: Newborn screening for congenital hypothyroidism: Recommended guidelines. Pediatrics 91:1203–1209, 1993.
4. Behrman RE, Kliegman RM, Arvin AM: Hypomagnesemia. In Behrman RE, Kliegman RM, Arvin AM (eds): Nelson Textbook of Pediatrics, 15th ed. Philadelphia, W.B. Saunders, 1996, p 508.
5. Bose HS, Sugawara T, Strauss JF III, Miller WL: The pathophysiology and genetics of congenital lipoid adrenal hyperplasia. International Congenital Lipoid Adrenal Hyperplasia Consortium. N Engl J Med 335:1810–1818, 1996.
6. Burrow GH: Hypothyroidism during pregnancy. N Engl J Med 298:150–153, 1978.
7. Chowdhry P, Scanlon JW, Auerbach R, Abbassi V: Results of controlled double-blind study of thyroid replacement in very-low-birth-weight premature infants with hypothyroxinemia. Pediatrics 73:301–305, 1984.
8. Cuestas RA: Thyroid function in healthy premature infants. J Pediatr 92:964, 1978.
9. De Zegher F, Pernasetti F, Vanhole C, et al: A prismatic case: The prenatal role of thyroid hormone evidenced by fetomaternal Pit-1 deficiency. J Clin Endocrinol Metab 80:3127–3130, 1995.
10. Fisher FA: Disorders of the thyroid in the newborn and infant. In Sperling MA (ed): Pediatric Endocrinology. Philadelphia, W.B. Saunders, 1996, p 57.
11. Fisher DA: Fetal thyroid function: Diagnosis and management of fetal thyroid disorders. Clin Obstet Gynecol 40:16–31, 1997.
12. Fisher DA: The hypothyroxinemia of prematurity [editorial]. J Clin Endocrinol Metab 82:1701–1703, 1997.

13. Fisher DA: Thyroid function in premature infants. The hypothyroxinemia of prematurity. Emerg Concepts Perinat Med 25:999–1014, 1998.

14. Fisher DA, Dussault JH, Sack J, Chopra IJ: Ontogenesis of hypothalamic-pituitary-thyroid function and metabolism in man, sheep and rat. Rec Prog Hormone Res 33:59–116, 1977.

15. Fisher DA, Klein AH: Thyroid development and disorders of thyroid function in the newborn. N Engl J Med 304:706, 1981.

16. Fitzgerald JF: Cholestatic disorders of infancy. Pediatr Clin North Am 35:357, 1989.

17. Frank JE, Faix JE, Hermos RL, et al: Thyroid function in very low birth weight infants: Effects on neonatal hypothyroid screening. J Pediatr 128:548–554, 1996.

18. Franklin R, O'Grady C, Carpenter L: Neonatal thyroid function: Comparison between breast-fed and bottle-fed infants. J Pediatr 106:124–126, 1985.

19. Greer FR: Disorders of calicum homeostasis. In Spitzer AR: Intensive Care of the Fetus and Neonate. St. Louis, Mosby, 1996, pp 993–1012.

20. Habib A, McCarthy JS: Effects on the neonate of propranolol administered during pregnancy. J Pediatr 91:808–811, 1977.

21. Hanna CE, Jett PL, Laird MR, et al: Corticosteroid-binding globulin, total serum cortisol and stress in extremely low-birth-weight infants. Am J Perinatol 14:201–204, 1997.

22. Henzen C, Suter A, Lerch E, et al: Suppression and recovery of adrenal response after short-term, high-dose glucocorticoid treatment. Lancet 355:542–545, 2000.

23. Klein AH, Oddie TH, Parslow M, et al: Developmental changes in pituitary-thyroid function in the human fetus and newborn. Early Hum Devel 6:321–330, 1982.

24. Kooistra L, Laane C, Vulsma T, et al: Motor and cognitive development in children with congenital hypothyroidism: A long-term evaluation of the effects of neonatal treatment. J Pediatr 124:903–909, 1994.

25. LaFranchi S: Congenital hypothyroidism: Etiologies, diagnosis, and management. Thyroid 9:735–740, 1999.

26. Lamberg B-A, Ikonen E, Österlund K, et al: Antithyroid treatment of maternal hyperthyroidism during lactation. Clin Endocrinol 21:81–87, 1984.

27. Loughead JL, Tsang RC: Neonatal calcium and phosphorus metabolism. In Cowett RM (ed): Principles of Perinatal-Neonatal Medicine. New York, Springer-Verlag, 1998, pp 879–908.

28. Mercado M, Yu VYH, Francis I, et al: Thyroid function in very preterm infants. Early Hum Devel 16:134, 1988.

29. Metzger DL, Wright NM, Veldhuis JD, et al: Characterization of pulsatile secretion and clearance of plasma cortisol in premature and term neonates using deconvolution analysis. J Clin Endocrinol Metab 77:458–463, 1993.

30. Mischler EH, Wilfond BS, Fost N, et al: Cystic fibrosis newborn screening: Impact on reproductive behavior and implications for genetic counselling. Pediatrics 102:44–52, 1998.

31. Nakamura Y, Usui T, Mizuta H, et al: Characterization of prophet of *pit-1* gene expression in normal pituitary and pituitary adenomas in humans. J Clin Endocrinol Metab 84:1414–1419, 1999.

32. New England Congenital Hypothyroidism Collaborative: Elementary school performance of children with congenital hypothyroidism. J Pediatr 116:27–32, 1990.

33. Oberkotter LV, Periera GR, Paul MH, et al: Effect of breast-feeding vs. formula-feeding on circulating thyroxine levels in premature infants. J Pediatr 106:822–825, 1985.

34. Pacaud D, Huot C, Gattereau A, et al: Outcome in three siblings with antibody-mediated transient congenital hypothyroidism. J Pediatr 127:275–277, 1995.

35. Paxson CL Jr, Stoerner JW, Denson SE, et al: Syndrome of inappropriate antidiuretic hormone secretion in neonates with pneumothorax or atelectasis. J Pediatr 91:459–463, 1977.

36. Pfaffle R, Kim C, Otten B, et al: Pit-1: Clinical aspects. Hormone Res 45(Suppl):25, 1996.

37. Polin RA, Yoder MC, Burg FD (eds): Workbook in Practical Neonatology, 3rd ed. Philadelphia, W.B. Saunders, 2001.

38. Polin RA, Fox WW (eds): Fetal and Neonatal Physiology. Philadelphia, W.B. Saunders, 1998.

39. Porterfield SP, Hendrich CH: The role of thyroid hormones in prenatal and neonatal neurological development: Current perspectives. Endocr Rev 14:94–106, 1993.

40. Reuss ML, Paneth N, Pinto-Martin JA, et al: The relation of transient hypothyroxinemia in preterm infants to neurologic development at two years of age. N Engl J Med 334:821–827, 1996.

41. Roti E, Gnudi A, Braverman LE: The placental transport, synthesis and metabolism of hormones and drugs which affect thyroid function. Endocr Rev 4:131–147, 1983.

42. Roti E, Minelli R, Salvi M: Management of hyperthyroidism and hypothyroidism in the pregnant woman. J Clin Endocrinol Metab 81:1679–1682, 1996.

43. Rubin LP: Neonatal disorders of serum magnesium. In Taeusch HW, Ballard RA (eds): Avery's Diseases of the Newborn, 7th ed. Philadelphia, W.B. Saunders, 1998, pp 1189–1206.

44. Salerno M, Militerni R, DiMaio S, et al: Intellectual outcome at 12 years of age in congenital hypothyroidism. Eur J Endocrinol 141:105–110, 1999.

45. Shaw JCL: Evidence for the defective skeletal mineralization in low birthweight infants: The absoprtion of calcium and fat. Pediatrics 57:16–25, 1976.
46. Sornson MW, Wu W, Dasen JS, et al: Pituitary lineage determination by the Prophet of Pit-1 home-odomain factor defective in Ames mouse. Nature 384:327, 1996.
47. Thomas JL, et al: Premature infants: Analysis of serum during the first seven weeks. Clin Chem 14:272, 1968.
48. Thorpe-Beeston JG, Nicolaides KH, Felton CV, et al: Maturation of the secretion of thyroid hormone and thyroid-stimulating hormone in the fetus. N Engl J Med 324:532–536, 1991.
49. Tsang RC, et al: Possible pathogenetic factors in neonatal hypocalcemia of prematurity. J Pediatr 82:423, 1973.
50. Tsang RC, et al: Nutritional Needs of the Preterm Infant. Baltimore, Williams & Wilkins, 1993.
51. van Steensel-Moll HA, Hazelzet JA, van der Voort E, et al: Excessive secretion of antidiuretic hormone in infections with respiratory syncytial virus. Arch Dis Child 65:1237–1239, 1990.
52. van Wassenaer AG, Kok JH, de Vijlder JJM, et al: Effects of thryoxine supplementation on neurologic development in infants born at less than 30 weeks' gestation. N Engl J Med 336:21–26, 1997.
53. Yudkoff M: Inborn errors of metabolism presenting as catastrophic disease. In Spritzer A (ed): Intensive Care of the Fetus and Neonate. St. Louis, Mosby, 1996.

7. FLUID, ELECTROLYTES, AND RENAL DISORDERS

1. How does the principal function of the kidney differ in fetal and neonatal life?

The principal and unique function of the fetal kidney is the continuous provision of fluid and electrolytes into the amniotic cavity, which is essential for maintenance of amniotic fluid volume. In neonatal life, the kidney is responsible for maintenance of an appropriate fluid and electrolyte milieu.

2. Name the factors that contribute to the decline in renal vascular resistance postnatally.
- A fall in circulating catecholamine and renin levels
- A rise in vasodilating prostaglandins

3. What percentage of cardiac output do the kidneys receive in fetal life?

The kidneys receive 2–3% of cardiac output in fetal life (vs. 15–18% in adults).

4. When is nephrogenesis complete?

Nephrogenesis is complete at 36 weeks.

5. What are the changes in glomerular filtration rate that occur prenatally?

Before 36 weeks' gestation there is a gradual increase in glomerular filtration rate (GFR) through the period of nephrogenesis. Between 36 weeks and term gestation, the GFR remains stable and then increases dramatically at the time of birth. By 2 weeks of age, it has already doubled. In preterm infants born before the 34th week of gestation, the increase in GFR occurs more gradually.

6. Why is the fractional excretion of sodium higher in the newborn infant?
- Glomerular/tubular imbalance
- Intravascular volume expansion

7. How does sodium balance differ in the term and preterm infant?
- Term infants conserve sodium effectively after the first few hours of life (following intravascular volume contraction).
- Preterm infants conserve sodium less effectively because of the following:
  1. Decreased proximal tubular reabsorption
  2. Decreased response to aldosterone
  3. Different set point for glomerular-tubular balance

8. What are normal values for GFR in the newborn infant?

Glomerular Filtration Rate

NORMAL GFR	POSTNATAL AGE		
	1 WK	2–8 WK	> 8 WK
(ml/min/1.73 m^2)			
25–28 wk	11.0 ± 5.4	15.5 ± 6.2	47.4 ± 21.5
29–34 wk	15.3 ± 5.6	28.7 ± 13.9	51.4 ±
38–42 wk	40.6 ± 14.8	65.8 ± 24.8	95.7 ± 21.7

9. What are normal values for creatinine in the newborn infant?

Normal Creatinine Values

	POSTNATAL AGE		
	1 WK	2–8 WK	> 8 WK
Gestational age			
25–28 wk	1.4 ± 0.8	0.9 ± 0.5	0.4 ± 0.2
29–34 wk	0.9 ± 0.3	0.7 ± 0.3	0.3 ±
38–42 wk	0.5 ± 0.1	0.4 ± 0.1	0.4 ± 0.1

10. What are the developmental differences in acidification mechanisms in the newborn infant?
• H^+ excretion in the preterm infant is decreased.
• Both term and preterm infants exhibit an altered threshold for bicarbonate reabsorption at birth.
• In term infants the bicarbonate wastage disappears by 1–2 weeks of life; however, in preterm infants it may be persistent.

11. What are the developmental differences in water conservation and excretion in the newborn infant?
Although the capacity to dilute urine is normal, concentrating ability is limited in the immediate newborn period because of (1) diminished tonicity of the renal medullary interstitium and (2) diminished response to arginine vasopressin (AVP).

12. Why do preterm infants have difficulty in excreting a potassium load?
Preterm infants have difficulty excreting potassium for the following reasons:
• Distal immaturity of sodium-potassium-adenosine triphosphatase (Na^+-K^+-ATPase)
• Reduced permeability of peritubular cells
• Diminished tubular surface area
• Diminished GFR

13. When should the time of first voiding be considered delayed?
• Ninety-seven percent of infants pass urine in the first 24 hours of life and 100% by 48 hours.
• During the first 2 days of life, infants urinate from 2–6 times per day.

Time of First Void in 500 Infants

	395 FULL-TERM INFANTS		80 PRETERM INFANTS		25 POST-TERM INFANTS	
HOURS	NO. OF INFANTS	CUMULATIVE %	NO. OF INFANTS	CUMULATIVE %	NO. OF INFANTS	CUMULATIVE %
In delivery room	51	12.9	17	21.2	3	12
1–8	151	51.1	50	83.7	4	38
9–16	158	91.1	12	98.7	14	84
17–24	35	100	1	100	4	100
> 24	0	—	0	—	0	—

Adapted from Clark DA: Time of first void and first stool in 500 newborns. Pediatrics 60:457, 1977.

MAINTENANCE FLUID REQUIREMENTS

14. Why do premature infants lose weight after birth?
Premature infants excrete water and sodium shortly after birth, resulting in a decrease in extracellular water volume (see figure, next page). Although the cause of the decrease is unknown, it is generally accepted that the decrease in extracellular volume is physiologically appropriate because there is increased risk of a patent ductus arteriosus, necrotizing enterocolitis, and

bronchopulmonary dysplasia when one tries to prevent the change. The same phenomenon probably occurs in term infants, but this assumption has not been well documented.

Postnatal changes in body weight, extracellular fluid volume, and sodium balance. (From Shaffer SG, Weismann DN: Fluid requirements in the preterm infant. Clin Perinatol 19:233, 1992, with permission.)

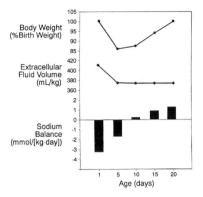

15. What are the main variables to consider when estimating insensible water loss?

The most important determinants of insensible water loss (IWL) are gestational age, postnatal age, and environment. IWL decreases with increasing gestational and postnatal age, and it increases with increasing air temperature, decreasing ambient humidity, and exposure to radiant energy (see figure). Therefore, IWL is lower in a humidified incubator than under a radiant warmer.

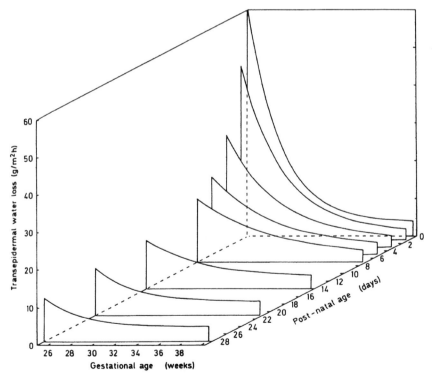

Transdermal water loss as a function of gestational and postnatal age in naked, appropriate-for-gestational-age infants in a neutral thermal environment in incubators with 50% ambient humidity. (From Hammarlund K, Sedin G, Strömberg B: Transepidermal water loss in newborn infants. Part VIII: Relation to gestational age and post-natal age in appropriate and small for gestational infants. Acta Paediatr Scand 72:721–728, 1983, with permission.)

16. What concentration of dextrose is ordered for infants who must avoid oral ingestion?

The relevant variable is the dextrose administration rate. Neonates normally produce 4–8 mg/kg/min of glucose endogenously. Administration at this rate usually maintains serum glucose concentration in the normal range and conserves glycogen stores. Once the rate of water administration is determined, a dextrose concentration is selected that provides somewhere between 4 and 8 mg/kg/min. In some infants, higher glucose infusion rates may be necessary.

17. How much sodium should be given on the first day of life?

In the absence of unusual sodium losses (i.e., loss of gastrointestinal or cerebrospinal fluid), no sodium should be given. During the first day of life, urine excretion is low (0.5–2 ml/kg/hr); and, in the absence of abnormal sodium losses, the kidney is the principal route of sodium loss. Thus, sodium loss is low so long as urinary output is low. Moreover, if IWL is unexpectedly high or with the onset of the postnatal diuresis (when water loss often exceeds sodium loss), serum sodium (Na^+) often rises. Therefore, it is usually best to withhold sodium initially, especially in the extremely premature infant who is particularly at risk for developing significant hypernatremia in the first few days of life.

18. When should maintenance potassium be started in an extremely premature infant?

The main route of potassium loss is in the urine. Urine losses are low initially because GFR and urine output are relatively low after birth. Moreover, plasma potassium (K^+) may rise in extremely premature infants even in the absence of exogenous potassium. Therefore, potassium should be withheld until it can be ascertained that renal function is normal and, in extremely premature babies, plasma K^+ is normal and not increasing.

19. What are the maintenance fluid and electrolyte (Na+, K+, Cl–) requirements for the preterm infant in the first month of life?

Fluid Recommendations for Preterm Infants

TRANSITIONAL PHASE (FIRST 3–5 DAYS)					
WEIGHT (gm)	WEIGHT LOSS (%)	WATER* (ml/kg/day)	NA+ (mEq/kg/day)	CL– (mEq/kg/day)	K+ (mEq/Kg/day)
< 1000	15–20	90–140	0–1	0–1	0
1001–1500	10–15	80–120	0–1	0–1	0–1
1501–2000	5–10	70–100	0–1	0–1	0–1
< 2000	5–10	60–80	0–1	0–1	0–1

STABILIZATION PHASE (< 14 DAYS)					
WEIGHT (gm)	WEIGHT LOSS (%)	WATER (ml/kg/day)	NA+ (mEq/kg/day)	CL– (mEq/kg/day)	K+ (mEq/Kg/day)
< 1000	0	80–120	2–3	2–3	1–2
1001–1500	0	80–120	2–3	2–3	1–2
1501–2000	0	80–120	2–3	2–3	1–2
< 2000	0	80–120	2–3	2–3	1–2

GROWTH PHASE (> 14 DAYS)					
WEIGHT (gm)	WEIGHT GAIN (gm/day)	FEEDINGS (ml/kg/day)	NA+ (mEq/kg/day)	CL– (mEq/kg/day)	K+ (mEq/Kg/day)
< 1000	15–20	150–200	3–5	3–5	2–3
1001–1500	15–20	150–200	3–5	3–5	2–3

* Requirements are 10–20% less with a humidified isolette or plastic shield

20. Baby R is a 22-hour-old, 25-weeks' gestation male in a humidified incubator who has received 150 ml/kg/day of fluid during the first day of life. Serum sodium is 128 mmol/L. Should sodium intake be increased?

Not necessarily. Serum Na^+ is the concentration, not the amount, of sodium in the extracellular fluid (ECF) space. If it is abnormal, the amount of sodium in the ECF space is abnormal **for the amount of water** in the ECF space. Thus, serum Na^+ may be low because there is too little extracellular sodium and/or too much extracellular water. Furthermore, the ECF space may be contracted, normal, or expanded in either of these cases. The most common cause of hyponatremia in the neonate is excess fluid administration. In such situations, the serum Na^+ will rise with fluid restriction.

21. Which should be used, birth weight or daily weight, to calculate water and sodium requirements during the first week of life?

You should use what the attending tells you to use! After the first day of life, however, it is the absolute fluid and electrolyte intake (ml or mmol/day) **relative to the previous 12–24 hours** that one should be thinking about. In other words, should the absolute fluid or electrolyte intake be more or less than it was previously? The answer depends on what fluid and electrolyte balances resulted from the previous intakes and on what water and electrolyte losses are anticipated. There is no magic amount of water/kg/day that is appropriate for all infants, even at the same weight, gestational age, and postnatal age, and in the same environment. If the infant loses more water (and therefore weight) than you judge to be appropriate and you anticipate that water losses will remain approximately the same, the absolute amount of water (ml/day) given should be increased. However, if the current weight is used to calculate fluid requirements, the absolute amount of water administered may be only slightly more or even less than the amount given the day before. For example, an 860-gm infant loses 110 gm (~13% of birth weight) in the first day of life after receiving 100 ml/kg/day (86/ml/day). You decide this rate of weight loss is too great and increase water intake by 25% to 125 ml/kg/day. Based on the current weight of 750 gm, however, this is only 94 ml/day, which is less than that given the previous day. If water losses remain the same, weight loss will be even greater over the next 24 hours despite an increase in water intake.

ACID–BASE BALANCE

22. How are acid–base measurements made?

Arterial oxygen activity is measured amperometrically by the Clark electrode. The reduction reaction of interest is as follows: $4e^- + O_2 + 2H_2O = 4OH^-$. Current flows in linear proportion to the activity of dissolved oxygen.

Hydrogen ion concentration (pH) is measured potentiometrically using a complicated system that employs two electrodes (usually Ag/AgCl) designed such that the potential between them is sensitive to the concentration of H^+ ions in the intervening medium.

Carbon dioxide (CO_2) activity is measured using an electrode with a semipermeable membrane that allows only CO_2 to diffuse into the electrode compartment, where it is converted to carbonic acid. The hydrogen ions produced by this reaction are then measured as above. The semipermeable membrane ensures that this measurement is completely independent of blood pH.

Bicarbonate is not measured, but is calculated from the Henderson-Hasselbalch equation:

$$pH = \frac{pK' + \log(HCO_3^-)}{(0.0307 \times pCO_2)}, \text{ where } 0.0307 = \text{solubility coefficient of } CO_2 \text{ at } 37°C$$

The equation uses pK', not just pK, because the pK is a composite of two reaction constants and only an "apparent" pK for H_2CO_3 dissociation.

23. What is base excess? How is it measured?

The total blood buffers of human adults are comprised of the buffers listed at the end of the paragraph. Values for infants are 3–4 mEq/L blood lower, so infants tend to have a persistent base deficit of that amount. The effect of these buffers is to establish and stabilize a pH of roughly 7.40 in the blood.

Plasma HCO_3^-	24 mEq/L blood
Plasma protein	13 mEq/L blood
Red cell HCO_3^-	14 mEq/L blood
Red cell hemoglobin	6 mEq/L blood

Base deficit or excess is the difference between the sum of these values and what actually is measured (or calculated) in the test sample.

Thus, base excess is defined as the number of millimoles of strong base or strong acid needed to titrate 1 L of blood (Hgb = 15.0 gm/dl) to pH = 7.40 at 37°C while pCO_2 is held at 40 mmHg (at which point the buffers have been restored to normal values).

It may be calculated from the following equation:

$$BE = [1 - 0.014(Hgb)] \{[HCO_3^-] - 24 + [1.43(Hgb) + 7.7](pH - 7.4)\}$$

24. In acid–base disorders in human biology, in which body compartment is the measurement made?

Acid–base measurements are made of the ECF, which includes the intravascular and the interstitial fluid compartments. Intracellular acid–base status, which likely influences cell function significantly, is different and not routinely measured. Because CO_2 exchanges with the intracellular fluids much more rapidly than HCO_3^-, it is possible for rapid changes in pCO_2 to change the acid–base profile of the two compartments in different directions and at different rates. When attempting to treat acid–base disorders, pediatricians must consider the possible consequences: worsening intracellular acidosis in the face of alkalinization of the ECF with infusions of bicarbonate.

25. What are the principal mechanisms whereby infants compensate for abnormal acid–base profiles?

Metabolic alkalosis	Compensation: hypoventilation
Metabolic acidosis	Compensation: hyperventilation
Respiratory acidosis	Compensation: increased renal absorption of bicarbonate
Respiratory alkalosis	Compensation: diminished renal retention of bicarbonate

26. Explain the importance of the volume of distribution in correcting acid–base derangements.

After a known amount of solute is introduced into a solution, the concentration is measured, and the apparent volume in which the solute is distributed is calculated. This volume is called the volume of distribution, which is used to estimate how much solute is needed to change the measured concentration of that solute. For simple, single compartments and inert solutes, the calculation measures the true volume. For multicompartment systems and unstable solutes, the solute may be distributed unevenly (i.e., either concentrated in or excluded from various compartments), metabolized, or otherwise eliminated. In these systems, the calculated volume is different from the true volume in which the solute is distributed. Because of its interaction with a number of buffer systems, both intracellular and extracellular, and elimination as CO_2 through the lungs, the volume of distribution of bicarbonate is variable and difficult to predict. A good guess for use in dosing is 30% of body weight.

27. What do we know for sure about the indications for the therapeutic use of sodium bicarbonate in pediatrics?

Much less than you think. As a general rule, replacement of bicarbonate when body losses of bicarbonate are excessive (e.g., through the stool or urine) is appropriate. On the other hand, evidence documenting the value of sodium bicarbonate infusions to correct acidosis from many, if not most, other causes is very sketchy; therefore, sodium bicarbonate–replacement treatment should be used cautiously, if at all. Although it is relatively easy to make the numbers in the ECF change in the desired direction, it is much more difficult to be certain that the patient will improve. Review the literature thoroughly before reaching for the alkali.

28. Is an infant able to make more or less acid when the pH is out of the normal range and thereby help in the correction of systemic acidosis?

The answer is yes. According to Hood and Tannen, "There is convincing evidence that small changes in systemic pH modify the rate of endogenous acid production in a direction and amount that can attenuate the effect of an acid challenge in a variety of physiologic and pathologic situation."

29. What mechanism underlies dilution acidosis and contraction alkalosis?

When the concentration of HCO_3^- is changed by increasing or decreasing the volume in which it is distributed and the pCO_2 remains constant, the pH changes in the direction dictated by the Henderson-Hasselbalch equation.

30. What is the difference between the units torr and mmHg?

There is no difference.

DIURETICS

31. Furosemide and bumetanide are loop diuretics that clinicians commonly prescribe for infants who have one of various diseases including respiratory distress syndrome, bronchopulmonary dysplasia, posthemorrhagic hydrocephalus, and congenital heart disease. What damage can chronic administrative loop diuretics inflict on the kidney and/or urinary tract?

Loop diuretics induce hypercalciuria by inhibiting renal tubular calcium reabsorption. Therefore, chronic administration of these agents can cause **nephrocalcinosis** and/or calcium **nephrolithiasis**.

32. How does one know if a patient is at risk for developing furosemide-induced renal and/or genitourinary disease?

Hypercalciuria induced by loop diuretics is a risk factor for nephrolithiasis and/or nephrocalcinosis. Urinary calcium excretion can be evaluated by calculating the urinary calcium concentration/urinary creatinine (Uca/Ucreat) concentration ratio from a random urine specimen or in an aliquot of a timed urine collection. Hypercalciuria in the newborn is identified when the Uca/Ucreat concentration ratio is significantly greater than 0.8.

33. Explain the means by which furosemide-induced hypercalciuria and the consequent risk of nephrocalcinosis/nephrolithiasis can be reversed.

Obviously, the best way to treat hypercalciuria that is induced by loop diuretics is to discontinue treatment. However, discontinuation is not always possible. Thiazide diuretics have an anticalciuretic effect. Thus, changing an infant's diuretic regimen from furosemide/bumetanide to a thiazide should reduce urinary calcium excretion. If it is not feasible to discontinue treatment with a loop diuretic, adding a thiazide may effectively reverse hypercalciuria, thereby reducing the risk of nephrocalcinosis and/or nephrolithiasis.

34. What is the most rational treatment for the hypokalemic, hypochloremic metabolic alkalosis that may occur in newborns who receive intensive diuretic therapy?

The rational treatment is spironolactone and potassium chloride supplementation. Diuretic therapy induces a reduction in effective intra-arterial volume and thereby activates the renin-angiotensin-aldosterone system, which, in turn, stimulates secretion of potassium in the distal tubule. Blocking the effect of aldosterone on the distal tubule, therefore, should counteract the metabolic consequences of pharmacologic diuresis. Accordingly, adding **spironolactone**, a competitive inhibitor of aldosterone, to the diuretic regimen improves the derangements in serum bicarbonate and potassium concentrations. Recent data also suggest that spironolactone therapy may improve cardiac function by a mechanism that is independent of its effect on the kidney.

35. How can the addition of acetazolamide be detrimental to infants who are being treated with other diuretics?

Some neonatologists and cardiologists prescribe acetazolamide, an inhibitor of carbonic anhydrase, to treat the alkalosis that is caused by diuretic therapy. Although acetazolamide may lower the blood bicarbonate concentration by virtue of its ability to block reabsorption of bicarbonate in the proximal tubule, it also increases renal potassium excretion. Therefore, treatment with acetazolamide may cause an undesirable decrease of the patient's already low serum potassium concentration.

DIFFERENTIAL DIAGNOSIS AND EVALUATION OF OLIGURIA

36. Does the fetus make urine? If so, where does it go?

Urine is made by the fetus in increasing amounts as gestation advances. Fetal urine, along with tracheobronchial secretions, is an important contributor to amniotic fluid. The process is dynamic, with amniotic fluid being secreted continuously, then swallowed and reabsorbed from the gastrointestinal tract. Fetal oliguria may produce oligohydramnios, and swallowing difficulty or obstruction in the gastrointestinal tract may produce produce polyhydramnios.

37. What determines urine output in the postnatal period?

The volume of urine in the postnatal period is determined by water intake, glomerular filtration rate, the concentration gradient in the renal medullary interstitium, and the presence or absence of antidiuretic hormone (ADH).

38. Is the urinary concentrating ability of an infant the same as that for older children? If not, why is it different?

Children and adults can concentrate the urine maximally to 1200 mOsm/L. Infants can concentrate only to 700 mOsm/L or less. Concentration ability is limited in infants for several reasons. Protein intake by the infant is used to make new cells during this period of rapid growth, and relatively little nitrogen is diverted to urea. Urea is an important component of the tonicity of the medullary interstitium and the osmolality of urine. Additional factors are the relatively short loops of Henle in the neonatal nephrons that limit the surface area available for equilibration with the interstitium and a high level of prostaglandins that could increase medullary blood flow and "wash out" the medullary concentration gradient and also blunt the ability of ADH to increase water reabsorption. There may as well be decreased production of cyclic adenosine monophosphate (cAMP) in response to ADH, decreasing the insertion of water channels into the collecting duct.

39. The nurse says a 3-day-old infant is oliguric. You say, "How do you know?" What qualifies as oliguria?

Your question is not so naive, given the wide range of urine volumes from the most dilute to the most concentrated. The nurse likely responds on the basis of physical evidence; e.g., she may say that the infant had only three wet diapers over the past 24 hours. If the baby is in an intensive care unit and the urine volume is being quantified, a rate of urine flow can be calculated. Within the first 48 hours after delivery the volume may be as low as 0.5–0.7 ml/kg/hr, but beyond this period it is greater than 1 ml/kg/hr. Values less than 1 ml, if persistent, qualify for oliguria.

40. If an infant is found to be oliguric, what are the possible causes?

It is most useful to approach the differential diagnosis in terms of the factors that determine urine output (see question 37). First, one should evaluate the intake, look for signs of dehydration, and reexamine fluid requirements, taking into account gestational age and the use of lights and warmers, which increase fluid requirements. A decrease in GFR is manifested by a rising serum creatinine concentration. This acute renal failure should be analyzed for prerenal causes (e.g., congestive heart failure, increased insensible water loss), intrarenal causes (e.g., acute tubular necrosis following perinatal asphyxia, renal malformations), and postrenal causes (e.g., obstruction, often posterior urethral valves). An increase in ADH leading to increased water reabsorption and oliguria occurs in heart failure. The syndrome of inappropriate secretion of ADH (SIADH) occurs only rarely in the neonatal period.

41. An oliguric infant had a serum creatinine of 0.7 mg/dl at birth and 1.0 mg/dl at 48 hours of life? How do you interpret these levels?

The serum creatinine of the infant at birth reflects that of his or her mother. Thereafter, the level in a term infant should decline to the normal value of 0.3–0.4 mg/dl. The rate of decline varies depending on the initial GFR, rate of increase in GFR, and gestational age. The important point is that the serum creatinine should decline. In this case, it is rising and therefore is abnormal.

42. How can the urine sodium concentration be helpful in evaluating oliguria?

Urinary indices to separate prerenal acute renal failure (ARF) from intrarenal ARF are not as useful in neonates as in older children and adults. The best index is the fractional excretion of sodium (FE_{Na}), which is calculated as follows:

$$\frac{(U_{Na})(Screat)}{(S_{Na})(Ucreat)} \times 100$$

Prerenal failure is associated with $FE_{Na} \leq 2.5\%$, whereas intrarenal ARF is associated with $FE_{Na} \geq 3\%$. However, because of overlap between the two groups, specificity is limited. Premature infants with gestations < 32 weeks have a high rate of sodium excretion; therefore, a high FE_{Na} is not useful as an index. However, if FE_{Na} is low, prerenal ARF is suggested.

43. The nurse says a 2-day-old infant is oliguric. He has respiratory distress and is on a respirator. In reviewing his chart, you note that his mother had oligohydramnios. Several people have noted that the baby looks "funny." Can you hazard an armchair differential diagnosis before going to see the baby?

Oligohydramnios may be associated with severe renal anomalies that produce fetal oliguria. The lack of amniotic fluid can produce a fetal compression syndrome characterized by positional abnormalities of the extremities, a characteristic facial appearance, and pulmonary hypoplasia. The classic renal anomaly is renal agenesis, and the facial appearance in this condition is known as Potter's facies. A similar syndrome can be produced by autosomal recessive (infantile) polycystic kidney disease (ARPKD) or severe obstructive uropathy involving both kidneys, the bladder neck, or urethra. If the nurse adds that the baby's abdomen is very distended, the most likely suspicion is ARPKD and the less likely is severe obstruction.

44. In the case of this 2-day-old infant, what diagnostic findings might the physical examination show?

The physical examination might show large abdominal masses in ARPKD or in obstruction that produce hydronephrosis, but no masses in renal agenesis.

45. Which initial test would help in the evaluation?

The most helpful initial test would be abdominal sonography, concentrating on the kidneys, ureters, and bladder.

DIFFERENTIAL DIAGNOSIS AND EVALUATION OF POLYURIA

46. A newborn male infant is found to have renal failure due to obstructive uropathy from posterior urethral valves. A catheter is inserted into the bladder through the urethra. There is a large diuresis, and the acute renal failure gradually subsides with normalization of the serum creatinine. Months later the mother complains that her infant requires many more changes of diapers than did her other children. What is the explanation?

Severe obstruction of the urinary tract during nephrogenesis may lead to renal maldevelopment resulting in renal dysplasia. An early sign of dysplasia is a renal concentrating defect that manifests as polyuria and polydipsia. Some affected children maintain a normal glomerular filtration rate throughout life, but others have a slowly progressive decline in renal function resulting in endstage renal disease, often during the teenage years.

47. What constitutes polyuria in the newborn period?
Infants with polyuria have a rate of excretion of urine that is 4 to 5 ml/kg/hr or greater.

48. The mother of a 2-month-old infant complains about a large urine output, which she believes is due to his drinking too much water, and she is trying to control it by limiting fluid intake. What is wrong with her reasoning?
Psychogenic water drinking does not occur in infants. The infant may be drinking excessive amounts of water to compensate for a urinary concentrating defect and to maintain water balance. In such cases, limiting oral intake results in dehydration.

49. If this infant is fluid-restricted, what would you expect his serum electrolytes to show?
The serum electrolytes most likely would show hypernatremia because of a negative water balance. The sodium balance probably is normal.

50. An infant born prematurely to a mother who had polyhydramnios required mechanical ventilation for 1 week. At 6 days of life he had a rising serum creatinine, hypotension with cool extremities, hyponatremia, and mild hypokalemia. Despite the appearance of acute renal failure and hypovolemia, the infant had a large urine output with a high urinary concentration of sodium. What might be the cause? Is treatment available?
Neither central nor nephrogenic diabetes insipidus commonly presents with polyuria in the newborn period, but the neonatal form of Bartter syndrome, also known as hyperprostaglandin syndrome, may present this way. In such cases, the mothers have polyhydramnios due to increased fetal urine excretion, and the infants are often born prematurely. Postnatally, polyuria and renal sodium wasting continue, resulting in hypovolemia and prerenal acute renal failure. Infants with Bartter syndrome also have hypercalciuria and increased excretion of prostaglandin E_2. Findings may include hypokalemia and elevated serum bicarbonate, but not as frequently in infants as in older children with Bartter syndrome.

The defect appears to be in the ascending limb of the loop of Henle involving the Na-K-2Cl transporter and the potassium channel. Treatment with a prostaglandin inhibitor reverses many of the abnormalities. Salt-losing adrenal insufficiency must be excluded, but is usually associated with hyperkalemia and acidosis.

POTTER SYNDROME AND OLIGOHYDRAMNIOS SEQUENCE

51. What are the features of the oligohydramnios sequence (Potter syndrome)?
Typical signs of the oligohydramnios sequence include deformation of the limbs, pulmonary hypoplasia, and the physical features of flat face, beaked nose, and low-set ears. The ears appear big because they are simple. There may also be heterotopic brain malformations.

52. What are the causes of the oligohydramnios sequence?

Obstructive uropathy	Posterior urethral valves
	Prune belly syndrome
Renal anomalies	Bilateral renal agenesis
	Bilateral renal cystic dysplasia
	Renal tubular dysgenesis
	Autosomal recessive polycystic kidneys
	Autosomal dominant polycystic kidneys
Chronic leakage of amniotic fluid	

53. What are the inheritance patterns for conditions causing oligohydramnios sequence?

Posterior urethral valves	Sporadic
Prune belly syndrome	Sporadic
Bilateral renal agenesis	Sporadic, recessive, or dominant
Bilateral renal cystic dysplasia	Sporadic, recessive, or dominant
Renal tubular dysgenesis	Sporadic or recessive
Autosomal recessive polycystic kidneys	Recessive: chromosome 6p21
Autosomal dominant polycystic kidneys	Dominant: chromosome 16p

54. What are the causes of small kidneys in neonates?

Inherited or congenital	Renal hypoplasia
	Renal dysplasia
	Oligomeganephronic hypoplasia
Acquired	Renal venous thrombosis (kidneys are initially large)
	Renovascular accidents

55. How are small kidneys diagnosed? How do they present clinically?

Diagnosis of small kidneys:

In utero	Oligohydramnios
	Fetal ultrasound
At birth	As part of a syndrome
	Oligohydramnios sequence
	Polydipsia, polyuria
Infancy	Failure to thrive
	Urinary tract infection

HYPERKALEMIA IN PREMATURE INFANTS

56. What is the definition of hyperkalemia?

Hyperkalemia is a high serum potassium concentration in the blood of ≥ 6.7 mEq/L.

57. What are the two ways that hyperkalemia develops in premature infants?

Hyperkalemia develops in the premature infant either from a positive potassium balance arising from increased intake or reduced excretion of potassium, or it develops from a shift of potassium from the intracellular fluid space (ICF) to the extracellular fluid space (ECF).

58. What is the incidence of hyperkalemia in premature infants?

In infants weighing ≤ 1000 gm, the incidence ranges from 15–50%. However, some studies may have overstated the problem because a hemolytic specimen can artificially elevate the value of serum potassium reported by the laboratory.

59. What is nonoliguric hyperkalemia?

Nonoliguric hyperkalemia is a rise in the serum potassium concentration (≥ 6.7 mEq/L) in the absence of a falling or low urine output. In contrast with older children, infants with nonoliguric hyperkalemia do not demonstrate a lower rate of urine production than age- and weight-matched controls.

60. What is the pathophysiology of nonoliguric hyperkalemia?

In the premature infant hyperkalemia can develop from a state of positive potassium balance or an internal shift of potassium. Although premature infants have some difficulty in excreting a potassium load, nonoliguric hyperkalemia develops in the first 72–96 hours of life when potassium intake is minimal. Therefore, excess administration of potassium is not an important variable. Most infants who develop nonoliguric hyperkalemia are in a state of **negative potassium balance.** In affected infants, the ratio of intracellular to extracellular potassium is significantly lower than in controls. In addition, infants with nonoliguric hyperkalemia are in a state of volume contraction and their levels of Na+,K+-ATPase are lower. Therefore, nonoliguric hyperkalemia is likely due to a shift of potassium from the intracellular fluid space to the extracellular fluid space.

61. What are the consequences of hyperkalemia in the premature infant?

Most of the time, there are minimal untoward effects, but an occasional infant may develop tachyarrhythmias.

62. What are the available treatments for nonoliguric hyperkalemia?
• Continuous infusion of insulin
• Treatment with sodium bicarbonate
• Na+,K+ exchange resins
• Calcium infusions
Note: None of the strategies have been studied rigorously or proved to be efficacious.

63. What is the role of insulin and glucose in reducing serum potassium levels?

The reported mechanisms of action are complicated and not well understood.
• Although insulin transports glucose into the cell, it is not the primary mechanism for shifting potassium.
• Insulin induces the enzyme Na+,K+-ATPase, which is independent of glucose.
• Glucose is needed to prevent hypoglycemia and not to transport potassium.
• The efficacy of glucose and insulin in affected infants has not been proved.

64. What is the role of hydration in infants with nonoliguric hyperkalemia?

Hyperkalemic infants have urinary indices that indicate a state of prerenal volume contraction. When serum potassium values rise above 6 mEq/L and serum creatinine and BUN increase in a proportionate fashion, fluid intake should be increased by 25–30%. By improving the intravascular volume status, a greater potassium load is delivered at the glomerular level, resulting in higher potassium excretion.

RENAL TUBULAR ACIDOSIS

65. What is the normal serum bicarbonate level for gestational age?

During the first year of life, the plasma concentration of bicarbonate is approximately 22 mEq/L ± 1.9 mEq/L, compared with 26 mEq/L ± 1.0 mEq/L in adults. The bicarbonate concentration is lower in term infants (20 mEq/L ± 2.8 mEq/L) and even lower in preterm infants (17 mEq/L ± 1.2 mEq/L), with two standard deviations including values as low as 14.5 mEq/L. Children generally have a bicarbonate level of 23 mEq/L ± 1.0 mEq/L.

66. How well do premature infants reabsorb bicarbonate?

Preterm infants have a depressed renal threshold for bicarbonate. A close negative correlation has been found between bicarbonate threshold and urinary sodium excretion, suggesting that the limited renal capacity to reabsorb sodium may account for the low bicarbonate threshold in premature infants. However, the reabsorption of bicarbonate in the proximal tubule is generally complete in preterm infants, with maximal reabsorptive rates comparable to adult tubules (2.5–2.6 mEq/dL glomerular filtrate). Thus, in early life, the intrinsic capacity of the proximal tubule to reabsorb bicarbonate appears adequate to handle the filtered load of bicarbonate. Bicarbonate reabsorption will improve if the extracellular volume is allowed to contract.

67. Do infants excrete more or less titratable acid and ammonia per kg body weight compared with older children?

The titratable acid excretion rate in term infants < 1 month old is about one-half and the ammonium excretion rate about two-thirds of that of older children and adults. Preterm infants have even lower rates. Net acid excretion rates (titratable acid plus ammonium) are lower than in infants older than 1 months. After 1 month of age, the net acid excretion rate in full-term infants is similar to that in older children and adults when expressed per 1.73 m². Preterm infants also increase their rates of titratable acid and ammonium excretion with maturation, but these rates still remain lower than in full-term infants even up to the age of 4 months.

68. What are the signs and symptoms of renal tubular acidosis?

Rental tubular acidosis (RTA) usually presents with nonspecific symptoms such as failure to thrive, lethargy, vomiting, and tachypnea. The hallmark is the presence of hyperchloremic metabolic acidosis. The most common cause of hyperchloremic metabolic acidosis is not related to the kidney, but is caused by diarrhea with loss of base in the stool. This is also a form of RTA—rectal tubular acidosis.

69. What are the types of RTA?

Type 1—impairment of distal acidification
Type 2—impairment of bicarbonate reclamation
Type 3—combination of types 1 and 2
Type 4—secondary to a lack, or insensitivity to, aldosterone
All four types are associated with a hyperchloremic, normal anion gap acidosis.

70. How does one make the diagnosis of the different types of RTA?

Because **proximal RTA** (classic type II) results from a defect in reabsorption of filtered bicarbonate by the proximal renal tubule, the diagnosis is made by showing reduced bicarbonate reabsorption when the serum bicarbonate level is normal.

Distal RTA (classic type I) is characterized by the inability to acidify the urine adequately. Thus, the diagnosis is made by demonstrating an inability to lower the urine pH below 5.5 in the setting of metabolic acidemia.

Type IV RTA results from a deficiency of aldosterone or tubular unresponsiveness to its effects. As a result of the aldosterone deficiency or an insensitivity to its effects, hyperkalemia ensues because of decreased excretion and impairs ammonium generation. Titratable acid excretion is less impaired, and patients with type IV RTA can acidify the urine to 5.5 in acidotic situations. Thus, if metabolic acidosis is present and the serum potassium is high (> 5 mEq/L) with a urinary pH < 5.5, one should consider the possibility of type IV RTA. Plasma renin and aldosterone should be measured after salt restriction or furosemide administration to determine whether there is a deficiency or resistance to aldosterone.

71. What is late metabolic acidosis?

The term *late metabolic acidosis* is used to describe premature infants who have poor weight gain and hyperchloremic metabolic acidosis that appeared in the 2nd–3rd weeks of life. The acidosis is the result of formula that contains excessive metabolic acid precursors that overload the immature kidney's ability to excrete them. With the current formulas for premature infants, late metabolic acidosis has largely disappeared.

72. What type of RTA is seen in Fanconi syndrome?

Fanconi syndrome is a global disorder of proximal tubular function, including bicarbonate reabsorption. Type II RTA is the kind of RTA in Fanconi syndrome.

73. What type of RTA is seen in congenital adrenal hyperplasia?

Type IV RTA

74. What type of RTA is associated with pseudohypoaldosteronism?

Pseudohypoaldosteronism is an inherited unresponsiveness to aldosterone due to to a receptor defect. Type I pseudohypoaldosteronism is an autosomal recessive trait that presents in infancy with volume contraction, hyponatremia, hyperkalemia, metabolic acidosis, and severe salt wasting. Patients with this trait have type IV RTA.

75. Describe the usual causes of type IV RTA in neonates.

Obstructive uropathy	21-hydroxylase deficiency (CAH)
Adrenal insufficiency	Type I pseudohypoaldosteronism

76. How low can the premature infant reduce the urine pH?

During the first three weeks of life, a premature infant can reduce the urine pH only to 6.0 ± 0.1. After 1 month, the urine pH can be reduced to 5.2 ± 0.4.

OBSTRUCTIVE UROPATHY

77. What is the differential diagnosis of antenatal hydronephrosis?

Anomalous ureteropelvic junction/ureter opelvic junction obstruction	Ectopic ureter
Multicystic kidney	Posterior urethral valves
Retrocaval ureter	Prune belly syndrome
Primary obstructive megaureter	Urethral atresia
Nonrefluxing, nonobstructed megaureter	Hydrocolpos
Vesicoureteral reflux	Pelvic tumor
Midureteral stricture	Cloacal abnormality
Ectopic ureterocele	Idiopathic

From Elder JS: Antenatal hydronephrosis: Fetal and neonatal management. Pediatr Clin North Am 44:1301, 1997, with permission.

78. What does the postnatal evaluation of a neonate with an abnormal prenatal ultrasound include?

A renal and bladder ultrasound should be performed to evaluate renal length, degree of caliectasis, parenchymal thickness, the presence or absence of ureteral dilation, and bladder wall thickening, and to determine if a dilated posterior urethra or a ureterocele is present. If hydronephrosis is present, a voiding cystourethrogram (VCUG) and a renal scan (DTPA or MAG-3) are recommended to exclude vesicoureteral reflux and obstruction, respectively. The latter two studies may be postponed for 4–6 weeks so long as there is no significant bilateral disease or pathology affecting a solitary kidney. Prophylactic antibiotic therapy with amoxicillin, 50 mg daily, is recommended until studies are complete.

79. What if the initial renal ultrasound is normal?

Relative oliguria in the first 48 hours of life can cause transient normalization of the renal ultrasound at the time of discharge. Because studies have shown significant pathology even with normal neonatal ultrasound, antibiotic prophylaxis and repeat ultrasound are recommended.

80. What is ureteropelvic junction obstruction? How is it diagnosed and managed?

Ureteropelvic junction (UPJ) obstruction is the most common cause of hydronephrosis in children. Diagnosis requires the presence of hydronephrosis (ultrasound with dilated renal pelvis in the absence of a dilated ureter) and determination of significance by the use of diuretic renography. Many cases are managed expectantly. Pyeloplasty, excision of the stenotic segment, is usually necessary in cases in which neonates have an abdominal mass, bilateral hydronephrosis, or a solitary kidney.

81. What is a ureterocele? How does it cause obstruction?

A ureterocele is a cystic dilatation of the distal end of the ureter. It is obstructive because it may extend through the bladder neck (ectopic) but may remain entirely within the bladder (intravesical). Ureteroceles affect girls more than boys and are usually associated with the upper pole of a completely duplicated collecting system, although in some cases the ureter may drain a single collecting system. Ultrasound shows hydronephrosis in the upper pole, dilated ureter, and the ureterocele in the bladder.

POSTERIOR URETHRAL VALVES

82. What are posterior urethral valves?

Posterior urethral valves (PUVs) are classified as type 1 or type 3, based on the cause of obstruction. A type 1 PUV is the most common (95%) and represents an obstructing membrane extending from the verumontanum at the base of the prostatic urethra to the more distal anterior portion of the membranous urethra. This membrane contains only a small opening through which urine can pass; as the urine flows, the membrane billows out in a windsock fashion as a one-way flap valve causing obstruction. The degree of obstruction varies, depending on the size of the opening of the membrane. A type 3 valve is less common (5%) and is caused by a thin transverse membrane across the urethra, which develops from incomplete dissolution of the urogenital diaphragm, causing urinary obstruction.

83. Describe the most common presentation of a PUV.

Currently, antenatal ultrasound demonstrating bilateral hydroureteronephrosis, a dilated, thick-walled bladder with poor emptying, and occasionally oligohydramnios are the most common presentations. If not detected antenatally, a PUV presents variably, based on the degree of urinary obstruction. Palpable abdominal masses, including a distended bladder, ureter, or renal pelvis, suggest urinary tract obstruction and PUV. Respiratory distress or pulmonary hypoplasia, renal insufficiency or failure, or urosepsis may all be presenting signs of PUVs in newborns. If missed in the neonatal period, urinary obstruction from valves can present later in life as diurnal enuresis due to bladder dysfunction.

84. Name some consequences of PUVs.

- Glomerular and renal tubular dysfunction causing renal insufficiency, poor urinary concentrating ability, and polyuria
- Urinary tract dilatation, including hydroureteronephrosis and bladder dilatation, and secondary to obstruction, polyuria, bladder dysfunction, and vesicoureteral reflux
- Vesicoureteral reflux, which is found in one-third to one-half of boys with valves
- Bladder dysfunction, including a wide spectrum from bladder atony (poor contractility), bladder instability (hyperactive bladder with frequent bladder contractions), poor bladder compliance due to thickening of the bladder wall, to inability to store normal urine volumes
- Valve bladder syndrome, which is a constellation of findings including renal tubular dysfunction, polyuria, ureteral obstruction, bladder dysfunction, and incontinence

85. Does intervention after fetal diagnosis ultimately improve renal function?

There is no evidence that intervention ultimately improves renal function. Fetal intervention, including vesicoamniotic shunt placement, is performed when progressive oligohydramnios is noted on serial fetal ultrasounds in order to improve amniotic fluid levels. Oligohydramnios is detrimental to pulmonary development and may cause pulmonary hypoplasia. Correcting oligohydramnios is thought to allow better expansion of the chest wall and lung development, lessening the chance of pulmonary hypoplasia, but it has not been shown to affect overall renal function.

86. Which conditions can be confused with PUVs on fetal ultrasound?

- Prune belly syndrome
- Severe bilateral vesicoureteral reflux with distended bladder

87. Which conditions are associated with improved prognosis?

Conditions that allow decompression of the urinary tract ("pop-off" mechanism) have a better prognosis. Such conditions include bladder diverticular formation; bladder ascites; and valves, unilateral reflux, and dysplasia (VURD) syndrome. Urinary ascites is caused by transudation of urine across a renal calyceal fornix into the peritoneal cavity and relief of obstruction. VURD syndrome is noted when one kidney refluxes with subsequent renal dysplasia on that side, offering protection for the contralateral kidney.

88. What fetal parameters are associated with good postnatal renal function?
- Normal/moderately decreased level of amniotic fluid
- Normal/slightly increased renal parenchymal echogenicity by fetal sonography
- Fetal urinary chemistries:
  - Sodium, < 100 mEq/L
  - Chloride, < 90 mEq/L
  - Osmolarity, < 210 mOsm
  - Urinary output, > 2 ml/hr

HEMATURIA

89. Is hematuria ever a normal finding in the newborn infant?
No! Hematuria is never physiologic, but it can be a common finding in sick premature infants.

90. How is hematuria defined?
$\geq$ 5 red blood cells/high power field

91. What are the causes of hematuria in the newborn infant?
- Perinatal asphyxia
- Renovascular accident (renal vein or renal artery thrombosis)
- Neoplasia
- Obstructive uropathy
- Coagulopathies
- Urinary tract infection
- Trauma (most often suprapubic aspiration)
- Congenital malformation including polycystic disease

92. How should infants with hematuria be evaluated?
- Exclude other causes of red urine, such as urates, porphyrins, bile pigments, myoglobin and hemoglobin.
- Obtain a microscopic evaluation on a fresh specimen (when examination is delayed, red blood cells can hemolyse).
- Decide whether the blood comes from upper or lower tracts (the presence of dysmorphic red cells or casts indicates parenchymal renal disease).
- Exclude extraurinary sources of blood, such as vaginal, rectal, or perineal sources.
- Obtain a urine culture if infection is suspected.
- Obtain a renal ultrasound study if hematuria is persistent.
- Exclude a coagulopathy.
- Determine blood urea nitrogen (BUN) and creatinine levels

CONGENITAL NEPHROTIC SYNDROME

93. What is the definition of congenital nephrotic syndrome?
The term *congenital nephrotic syndrome* is used to describe a patient who develops the nephrotic syndrome during the first 3 months of life. Nephrotic syndrome is a constellation of abnormalities that includes (1) nephrotic-range proteinuria, defined as a urinary protein excretion > 100 mg/m^2 body surface area/24 hr, calculated from a timed urine collection, or a ratio of urine protein concentration (mg/dl)/urine creatinine concentration (mg/dl) > 2.0–2.5, calculated from a single spot urine; (2) nephrotic range hypoalbuminemia with serum albumin concentrations < 2.5 gm/dl; (3) hyperlipemia, determined from the results of measurements of serum cholesterol and/or triglyceride concentrations; and (4) peripheral edema that may be present in many patients.

94. Newborns may have proteinuria that occurs without complete nephrotic syndrome. How does one interpret isolated proteinuria?

Abnormal proteinuria is defined as urine protein excretion > 100 mg/m^2 body surface area/24 hr, calculated from a timed urine collection, or a ratio of urine protein (mg/dl)/urine creatinine (mg/dl) > 0.2, calculated from a spot urine specimen. Normal preterm infants are more likely to have proteinuria than are term infants. Abnormal proteinuria can occur in newborns as a result of various pathologic processes, including chronic volume depletion, congestive heart failure, and interstitial nephritis due to antibiotic administration. However, nephrotic-range proteinuria, as defined above, suggests significant damage to glomerular epithelial cells caused by some pathologic process. Therefore, discovery of nephrotic-range proteinuria, even in the absence of the full nephrotic syndrome, should prompt an aggressive evaluation.

95. Describe the disease that can cause congenital nephrotic syndrome in the first 3 months of life.

By contrast with older children with nephrotic syndrome whose underlying renal pathology is most often minimal change disease, newborns and infants who develop nephrotic syndrome are likely to suffer from a genetically determined disease. The most common cause is congenital nephrotic syndrome (CNS) of the Finnish type, an autosomal recessive disease that is most common among Finns, although cases have been reported from all over the world. A less common cause of CNS is diffuse mesangial sclerosis (DMS). DMS seems to have a genetic basis, but the exact mode of inheritance is unknown. Patients with DMS tend to develop nephrotic syndrome at an older age than do patients with the Finnish type.

Other renal lesions that can cause neonatal nephrotic syndrome may be associated with malformations that are not inherited in a known Mendelian fashion. An example is Drash syndrome, a combination of ambiguous or female external genitalia with gonadal dysgenesis, a 46XY genotype, and a predilection for the development of nephroblastoma.

Congenital infections may also cause nephrotic syndrome in the neonate. Congenital syphilis is the most common infectious association, but hepatitis B, HIV, and CMV infections have also caused CNS. Many patients with CNS due to a congenital infection demonstrate depressed serum concentrations of one or more components of the complement system.

96. What pre- or perinatal abnormalities should alert the perinatologist to the possibility that a newborn may have or may develop congenital nephrotic syndrome?

Most patients with congenital nephrotic syndrome of the Finnish type (CNF) had a large placenta (mean placental/fetal weight $= 0.4$) and were born preterm and small for gestational age. Prenatal evaluation of the mother of a patient with CNF will have demonstrated elevated concentrations of alpha-fetoprotein in both the amniotic fluid and the mother's blood. These abnormalities are not observed in mother–infant pairs afflicted with other forms of CNS. Infants with nephrotic syndrome due to congenital syphilis exhibit the stigmata of congenital lues.

97. Which evaluation is appropriate for the newborn with the nephrotic syndrome?

The evaluation should be, as usual, driven by the differential diagnosis. Although the most likely underlying diagnosis is congenital primary glomerular disease, causes of secondary nephrotic syndrome should be pursued. A careful physical examination and renal/pelvic imaging (ultrasonogram) will identify any abnormalities of the external genitalia, the internal reproductive organs, or the kidneys, such as nephroblastomatosis or Wilms tumor, that may suggest Drash syndrome or other malformation syndromes associated with congenital nephrotic syndrome. A family history of consanguinity, of fetal or neonatal demise, or of renal failure may be useful in suggesting a genetic cause for the nephrotic syndrome. Blood should be drawn to measure the levels of serum complement and complement components and to uncover evidence of prenatal infection with syphilis, hepatitis B or C, HIV, CMV, *Toxoplasma gondii*, or malaria. If the imaging and serologic evaluations are unrevealing, a renal biopsy should be performed to make a diagnosis and, thereby, to guide future management.

98. What is the prognosis for children who develop nephrotic syndrome in the newborn period?

As a group, patients who develop nephrotic syndrome in the newborn period have a grim prognosis. The majority will die before reaching the age of 3 years. The complications of CNS that are responsible for the morbidity and mortality include bacterial infections and developmental delay, which are especially common among patients with CBS; growth failure; thrombotic events; acute or chronic renal failure; complications of renal transplantation; and Wilms tumor among patients with Drash syndrome.

NEPHROCALCINOSIS

99. How is the diagnosis of nephrocalcinosis usually made in an infant?

Nephrocalcinosis is usually suggested by the findings on a renal ultrasound of a hyperechoic renal medulla, commonly in a very-low-birth-weight (VLBW) infant. Nephrocalcinosis results from microscopic calcification in the medullary portion of the kidney but often is accompanied by hyperechoic foci in the calyces, which represent renal calculi as well. Nephrocalcinosis can present with hematuria or urinary tract infection, but it is usually an incidental finding.

100. A 6-week-old premature infant, 28 weeks' gestation, with bronchopulmonary dysplasia (BPD) is found to have nephrocalcinosis. The infant has been treated for several weeks with Lasix. Is long-term furosemide therapy the only known cause of nephrocalcinosis in infancy?

The association of long-term Lasix therapy and nephrocalcinosis has been well recognized since the original description by Hufnagle et al. in 1982. There are, however, other diagnostic considerations for the infant with nephrocalcinosis, which are outlined in the table below.

NORMOCALCEMIC HYPERCALCIURIA	HYPERCALCEMIC HYPERCALCIURIA	NORMOCALCIURIC NEPHROCALCINOSIS
Furosemide therapy	Hyperparathyroidism	Primary hyperoxaluria
Bartter syndrome	Hypophosphatasia	Enteric hyperoxaluria
Distal renal tubular acidosis	Williams syndrome	Renal candidiasis
Hyperprostaglandin E	Idiopathic infantile hypercalcemia	Long-term acetazolamide therapy
	Subcutaneous fat necrosis	Dystrophic calcifications

Adapted from Karlowicz MG, Adelman RD: Renal calcification in the first year of life. Pediatr Clin North Am 42:1397–1413, 1995.

101. Hypercalciuria is an important diagnostic consideration in an infant with nephrocalcinosis. What is the normal range for calcium excretion in infants?

The value for hypercalciuria, if defined as calcium excretion of greater than the 95th percentile for an age-matched cohort, is different in infants compared with older children. In infants < 7 months old, the 95th percentile for urinary calcium/creatinine (mg/mg) was reported by Sargent et al. to be 0.86, and in children 7–18 months old the value was 0.60. In another study, VLBW infants with nephrocalcinosis had a mean urinary calcium/creatinine of 0.49 compared with 0.11 in controls. The relatively low calcium excretion in the controls of this study conflicted with the mich higher levels in the first study and are in the range described for older children. This discrepancy has resulted in confusion in the evaluation of infants with nephrocalcinosis.

102. What is the suggested therapy for an infant with nephrocalcinosis?

Treatment of the primary cause can be important in cases not caused by long-term furosemide therapy. In infants taking furosemide, substitution of a thiazide diuretic for furosemide can decrease the calcium excretion and result in shrinkage of calculi and improvement of the medullary nephrocalcinosis. The long-term prognosis has been correlated to the course of the urinary calcium excretion.

103. What is the long-term prognosis in infants with nephrocalcinosis?

Long-term studies of premature infants with nephrocalcinosis have suggested that 30–50% of the children continue to have evidence of renal calcification up to 5 years after diagnosis. There is some evidence of a slightly decreased glomerular filtration rate and tubular function, but some of these findings may be the result of a premature birth and not specific for the history of nephrocalcinosis.

HYPERTENSION

104. Discuss the environmental and technical factors that can affect blood pressure measurements in the newborn.

Various factors alter the relationship between blood pressure (BP) as recorded on the neonatal intensive care unit (NICU) flow sheet and the patient's true average baseline BP. For example, BP readings are affected by the patient's position (pressures measured when the patient is supine are slightly higher than those obtained when the patient is prone), by recent medical manipulations, or by recent feeding. Cuff inflation, by itself, can stimulate the startle response that can cause a transient increase in BP. In addition, body geography has an impact on BP measurements: pressures measured in the legs are normally somewhat higher than those measured in the arms.

105. Which newborn has hypertension?

This question is often difficult to answer. There are published data about the normal ranges of systolic and diastolic blood pressures for term newborns and premature infants at various gestational ages. These data, however, were derived from BP measurements that were obtained randomly, without respect to the patient's sate of alertness or agitation.

A single random recording of elevated BP may not have clinical significance because it may not exemplify the patient's average BP. A more representative BP measurement is recorded when the infant has not been fed or manipulated for 90 minutes before the evaluation; further refinement is achieved when several BP measurements are made over a period of 5–10 minutes.

The diagnosis of hypertension should be made only if the systolic and diastolic BPs are above the 95th percentile on at least three separate BP measurements recorded at 2-minute intervals during a time when the infant is quiet and otherwise undisturbed.

106. What is the most common cause of hypertension among patients in the neonatal intensive care unit?

The most common cause of hypertension among patients in the NICU is renal artery thrombosis due to thrombotic emboli that are released from an umbilical artery catheter (UAC). The thrombotic lesions usually occur in the peripheral circulation of one kidney, although there may be bilateral lesions. In the most serious situation, segmental thrombosis may propagate backward and occlude one or both main renal arteries.

107. What is the blood pressure profile of a patient whose hypertension is due to a complication related to an umbilical artery catheter?

Most patients who develop hypertension as a result of complications from a UAC are normotensive until the UAC is pulled. When the UAC is removed, hypertension often develops abruptly. The onset of hypertension in this situation coincides with the embolization of renal vessels by clots that are sheared from the tip of the catheter during its withdrawal.

108. What is the treatment of choice for newborns with hypertension related to a complication from the umbilical artery catheter?

UAC-related hypertension is generated by high circulating concentrations of angiotensin II. Angiotensin II production can be blocked by use of drugs that inhibit angiotensin-converting enzyme (ACE inhibitors). Captopril, 0.5 mg/kg/day divided into three or four daily doses, is often able to normalize BP. The daily dose may be increased to 2–4 mg/kg, if needed. Other ACE inhibitors such as enalapril or lisinopril may be used with equally beneficial effects, but dosing of these drugs for very small patients may be problematic for the pharmacist.

109. What role do endocrine hormones play in neonatal hypertension?

Most cases of hypertension in the newborn are due to excessive circulating concentrations of hormones that cause hypertension as a result of their ability to increase peripheral vascular resistance and/or by virtue of their ability to cause salt and water retention.

Renin produced by the kidney in response to either UAC-related renal artery thrombosis or to congenital renal artery stenosis generates angiotensin I. Angiotensin I is converted to angiotensin II (AII) by action of angiotensin-converting enzyme that is present in the kidney, lung, placenta, brain, and other organs. AII has multiple effects when it circulates in the blood, including increased peripheral vascular resistance, augmented production and release of aldosterone by the adrenal glands, and stimulation of thirst and salt craving. All of these AII actions cause an increase in blood pressure.

Rare endocrine disorders such as virilizing adrenal hyperplasia due to 11β-hydroxylase deficiency and primary hyperaldosteronism may cause neonatal hypertension due to overproduction of mineralocorticoid (desoxycorticosterone in the case of 11β-hydroxylase deficiency; aldosterone in the patient with hyperaldosteronism). The overproduction of mineralocorticoid in these diseases causes hypertension via inappropriate renal salt and water retention. There may also be a mineralocorticoid-mediated hypokalemic metabolic alkalosis.

Prenatal or postnatal exposure to exogenous steroids (e.g., betamethasone, prednisone, or methylprednisolone) can, likewise, cause hypertension in the newborn.

110. What abnormality of the physical examination of a hypertensive infant suggests that coarctation of the aorta may be the cause of the elevated blood pressure?

Despite the conventional wisdom that coarctation of the aorta is associated with a cardiac murmur and absent femoral pulses, many newborns with aortic coarctation do not fit the mold. In hypertensive infants, it is crucial to measure BP in both upper and lower extremities. Coarctation of the aorta should be suspected if the systolic pressure in the leg is more than 10 mmHg lower than the systolic pressure in the arms.

RENAL VEIN THROMBOSIS

111. Renal venous thrombosis occurs rarely among newborn infants. Most cases are idiopathic. What are some maternal and infant factors that increase the risk of renal venous thrombosis?

Maternal factors known to increase the risk of renal venous thrombosis (RVT) in the newborn include diabetes mellitus, elevated levels of IgG anticardiolipin antibody, and activated protein C resistance.

Infants with hemoglobin SS or inherited thrombophilic disorders, such as a deficiency of protein S, protein C, or antithrombin III, have an increased risk of RVT. Newborns who are otherwise normal may develop RVT if they have experienced perinatal asphyxia, an episode of sepsis, or hyperosmolarity and dehydration due to, for example, administration of IV radio-contrast or fluid losses as a result of vomiting or diarrhea.

112. What signs and symptoms suggest the occurrence of renal venous thrombosis in the newborn?

The clinician should suspect the diagnosis of RVT if a newborn develops hematuria, often gross hematuria, in association with a swollen kidney, palpable as a flank mass, and abrupt or progressive elevation of the plasma creatinine concentration, especially if these abnormalities are accompanied by thrombocytopenia. RVT may not, however, always induce dramatic clinical or laboratory changes. For example, a newborn with RVT may produce urine that is clear yellow;

microscopic hematuria with or without proteinuria may be the only urinary abnormality. Even when the RVT does not cause major changes in the urinalysis, however, there is usually a measurable deterioration of renal function, thrombocytopenia, and perhaps a transient elevation of blood pressure.

113. Which imaging studies are helpful and which may be harmful when one is trying to diagnose renal venous thrombosis?

Renal ultrasonography is a useful tool. It is noninvasive and usually identifies areas of the kidney that are affected by RVT. Renal parenchyma that experiences obstruction to venous drainage appears swollen and hyperechoic.

Renal scans, using intravenous injections of technetium diethylenetriaminepentaacetic acid (DTPA) or technetium dimercaptosuccinic acid (DMSA), demonstrate perfusion defects in the areas that are drained by the thrombosed renal vessels. These scans, however, do not provide anatomic detail, nor are they able to differentiate between arterial and venous renovascular disease. Furthermore, the utility of renal scans is limited by the fact that they generally require the sick infant to be transported from the neonatal unit to the nuclear medicine department.

Because RVT may be caused by serum hyperosmolarity, intravenous administration of hypertonic radiocontrast agents may be ill-advised. Therefore, the clinician should avoid ordering studies such as intravenous pyelography (IVP) or computed tomography (CT) that may require administration of intravenous contrast agents.

114. Which fluid and electrolyte abnormalities may occur in an infant with renal venous thrombosis?

Infants with renal venous thrombosis commonly experience a period of renal insufficiency that results in the following fluid and electrolyte abnormalities:

1. Oliguria, fluid retention, and hyponatremia
2. Metabolic acidosis
3. Hyperphosphatemia
4. Hypocalcemia

115. Is there a role for thrombectomy or nephrectomy of kidneys with renal venous thrombosis?

Neither thrombectomy nor nephrectomy has a role. Thrombectomy is unlikely to provide benefit because most cases of RVT begin in the peripheral renal venous circulation; therefore, removal of any clot that may be present in the main renal vein is not likely to restore venous drainage to the bulk of the affected renal parenchyma. Some advocate attempting thrombectomy when bilateral RVT also involves the inferior vena cava; however, there is little evidence to support the notion that the procedure, even in the most dire circumstances, improves either long-term patient survival or ultimate renal function.

Because many, if not most, kidneys with RVT ultimately recover some function as a result of recanalization of thrombosed vessels, nephrectomy of the affected kidney in the acute or subacute phase of RVT should be discouraged. Evidence is insubstantive that nephrectomy improves patient survival, and it certainly leads to a decrease in functional nephron mass.

116. Is thrombolytic (e.g., urokinase, tissue plasminogen activator [TPA]) or anticoagulant therapy useful in neonates with renal venous thrombosis?

The usefulness of thrombolytic or anticoagulant therapy must be qualified by such terms as *maybe* or *sometimes*.

Infusion of thrombocytic agents, either locally or systemically, has been employed with some success in patients with RVT or with renal arterial thrombosis. The risk of hemorrhagic complications, however, is significant. Because thrombolysis and venous recanalization occur as part of the normal resolution of RVT, it is not clear that pharmacologic thrombolytic therapy carries a favorable risk/benefit ratio.

Anticoagulant intervention aimed at prevention of extension of RVT into previously uninvolved venous structures may be appropriate for some patients, particularly those who have congenital thrombophilic disorders. The prothrombotic factors that lead to RVT formation and propagation in most newborns can be eliminated without anticoagulant therapy (e.g., hyperosmolarity, dehydration). However, anticoagulants may protect infants with intrinsic abnormalities of the coagulation cascade from experiencing secondary thrombotic events.

PRUNE BELLY SYNDROME

117. What is prune belly syndrome?

Prune belly syndrome (PBS) consists of (1) absent or decreased abdominal musculature, causing the abdomen of the recumbent newborn to appear wrinkled or prune-like; (2) undescended testes; and (3) abnormalities of the kidneys and urinary tract.

118. What are the most common urinary tract anomalies that occur in patients with prune belly syndrome?

From bottom to top, the most common urinary tract anomalies are the following:

1. The bladder neck is patulous.

2. The bladder is capacious. The bladder wall may be thickened, but the internal contour of the bladder is smooth, without trabeculations or diverticuli. Often the bladder communicates with a patent urachus.

3. Ureteral abnormalities commonly consist of irregular dilatations and narrowings, usually most dramatic in the lower ureteral segments.

4. The kidneys are often small, with or without dilatation of the collecting system.

Of importance, the anatomic abnormalities of the urinary tract in patients with PBS may be due to **primary, intrinsic, and diffuse defects of embryologic development** of the structures involved, which are different from the **discrete lesions** of obstruction or reflux that may occur in the urinary tract of otherwise normal newborns, although they may appear similar to those that occur in PBS. For example, the large, thick-walled bladder of patients with PBS may occur in the absence of bladder outlet obstruction, although the bladder may bear a resemblance to that of a patient with posterior urethral valves. Likewise, while ureteral dilatation in otherwise normal infants is commonly associated with vesicoureteral reflux (VUR) or obstruction, a similar ureteral lesion in a patient with PBS may occur in the absence of reflux or obstruction.

119. What important anomalies outside the genitourinary system occur more commonly among patients with prune belly syndrome than among otherwise normal neonates? What are their causes?

Patients with PBS often have problems that are related to pulmonary hypoplasia; hip dislocation or subluxation; talipes equinovarus; congenital cardiac disease, especially atrial septal defect, ventricular septal defect, and tetralogy of Fallot; and gastrointestinal anomalies.

The urologic/renal dysfunction in patients with PBS is almost certainly responsible for some of the nonurologic complications. For example, oligohydramnios, a common complication of PBS pregnancies, accounts for the pulmonary hypoplasia, the hip dislocation or subluxation, and the talipes equinovarus that may be seen in these newborns. It is uncertain how the components of PBS cause the excess prevalence of other anomalies that occur in the heart and in the gastrointestinal tract.

120. Which diagnostic studies assist the neonatologist in evaluating a child with prune belly syndrome?

A newborn with PBS requires an exhaustive evaluation of the urinary tract anatomy. The aim of the evaluation is to identify the extent of anatomical abnormalities and, more importantly, to diagnose lesions that may require urgent intervention. Therefore, the initial workup should include (1) **abdominal and pelvic ultrasonography** to provide a basic *road map* of the genitourinary (GU) anomalies and (2) **voiding cystourethrography** to diagnose VUR and reflux into a patent urachus. Either diagnosis, VUR or patent urachus, mandates initiation of antibiotic prophylaxis. If the infant is stable enough to be transported, other imaging studies significantly enhance understanding of the GU pathology. Computerized axial tomograms (CAT scan) of the abdomen, performed before and after intravenous administration of radiocontrast material, likely reveals more anatomic detail than ultrasound and, in addition, provides a qualitative assessment of comparative renal function (i.e., right vs. left kidney). **Renal scan using DTPA** localizes any points of obstruction between the kidneys and the bladder and provides a quantitative estimate of the comparative function of the two kidneys.

Because the infant with PBS may also harbor gastrointestinal (GI) and cardiac anomalies, the wise neonatologist will oder an **upper GI series with small bowel follow-through**, a **barium enema**, an **electrocardiogram (EKG)**, and an **echocardiogram.**

121. What is the role for surgical intervention in patients with prune belly syndrome?

Every newborn with PBS should be evaluated by a pediatric urologist. However, intervention in the newborn period should be limited to the least invasive procedures that are available and be used only when necessary to relieve high-grade obstruction in the urinary tract. More extensive genitourinary reconstructive procedures should be postponed to a later date and, in fact, may not be necessary at all. There is considerable controversy about whether surgical intervention is appropriate in boys with PBS when their GU anomalies are not associated with obstruction or VUR.

At some point, the surgeon must deal with the intra-abdominal cryptorchidism. Orchidectomy, as a means to prevent testicular neoplasia, is an option because the reproductive potential of boys with PBS is probably low. An alternate approach is to relocate the abdominal testes into the scrotum by one of a variety of complex surgeries. In any case, these surgical interventions can wait until the infant is several months old.

Surgical plication of the lax abdominal musculature is important for the psychological well-being of patients with PBS, but this cosmetic reconstruction should probably not be performed in the newborn.

122. What are other names for prune belly syndrome?

Prune belly syndrome is also known as the Eagle-Barrett syndrome and as triad syndrome. Eagle and Barrett should not be awarded historic primacy because their 1950 report of nine cases of PBS reiterated a description of the syndrome that had been published by R. W. Parker some 55 years earlier. The term *triad syndrome* may be appropriate, although it is neither specific nor descriptive.

123. Parents almost always smile when they see that their infant has dimples. Some dimples, however, can constantly remind parents that their child has prune belly syndrome. Where are these dimples?

Many patients with PBS have dimples on the lateral aspect of the knees and/or elbows.

CYSTIC KIDNEY DISEASE

124. What is the definition of multicystic renal disease?

A multicystic kidney is the result of abnormal metanephric differentiation. There is no continuity between glomeruli and calyces, and the kidney does not function. The contralateral kidney may be normal, absent, hydronephrotic, ectopic, or dysplastic.

125. What is the definition of renal cystic dysplasia?

Renal cystic dysplasia involves unilateral or bilateral, usually cystic kidneys with disorganized architecture. It often contains ectopic tissues (cartilage, muscle) and results in reduced renal function.

126. What is the definition of polycystic renal disease?

With polycystic renal disease, there are many cysts in both kidneys, no dysplasia, and continuity between glomeruli and calyces. The kidneys are often large.

127. Describe the management of autosomal recessive polycystic kidney disease in the neonate.

- Offer parents the option of withdrawal of life support.
- Treat the hyponatremia with furosemide.
- Treat the hypertension with an ACE-inhibitor.
- Ventilate; drain pneumothoraces.
- Perform uninephrectomy, if massive nephromegaly, for adequate enteral feeding.
- Perform bilateral nephrectomy, if massive nephromegaly, for better ventilation.
- Order peritoneal dialysis for chronic renal failure.

128. What is the prognosis of autosomal recessive polycystic kidney disease?

Life-table survival rates calculated from birth:

	86% alive at 3 months
	79% alive at 1 year
	51% alive at 10 years
	46% alive at 15 years
Patients who survive to age 1 year:	82% alive at 10 years

129. What is the probability of requiring antihypertensive treatment?

The probability of requiring antihypertensive treatment is 39% at 1 year and 60% at 15 years of age.

130. Name some additional complications that can occur in infants with autosomal recessive polycystic disease.

- Bleeding from gastroesophageal varices
- Hypersplenism with combinations of anemia, leukopenia, and thrombocytopenia
- Urinary tract infections in 30%
- Growth retardation in 25%
- Rare cases of cholangiocarcinoma

131. Can autosomal dominant polycystic kidney disease present in the neonate?

Patients with polycystic kidney disease (ADPKD) and patients with a maternal history of tuberous sclerosis may have polycystic kidneys in the neonatal period.

132. What are the indications for liver and renal biopsies in neonates with polycystic kidneys?

There are no indications for biopsies in these patients. Careful evaluation with ultrasonography is sufficient for diagnostic and treatment purposes.

133. In which conditions may there be an association between abnormal kidneys and congenital hepatic fibrosis?

Congenital hepatic fibrosis (CHF) and polycystic kidneys
- Autosomal recessive polycystic kidneys
- Autosomal dominant polycystic kidneys

CHF and hereditary tubulointerstitial nephritis
- Juvenile nephronophthisis
- Biedl-Bardet syndrome
- Jeune syndrome (asphyxiating thoracic chondrodystrophy)

CHF and hereditary renal dysplasia
- Meckel syndrome
- Chondrodysplasia syndromes
- Renal-hepatic-pancreatic cystic dysplasia (Ivermark syndrome)
- Zellweger syndrome

EXTROPHY

134. What are the correct terms for the developmental defect shown in the figure?
The correct terms for the developmental defect shown (*right*) are bladder extrophy and epispadias.

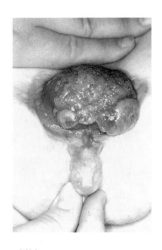

135. When does this developmental defect occur?
Bladder closure takes place between the 6th and 8th weeks of fetal life.

136. When should the extrophy-epispadias complex be repaired?
Bladder extrophy should be closed in the first 48 hours of life to ensure the best possible technical results for achieving long-term continence.

137. Should one be concerned with upper tract anomalies in children with bladder extrophy?
No. The upper urinary tract is almost always normal in these children.

138. What is the risk of recurrence in subsequent pregnancies?
The risk is no greater than that for the general population, which is 1:50,000 live births.

139. True or false: The extrophy-epispadias complex is decreasing in incidence nationwide.
True. The reasons are not entirely clear; however, it appears that the widespread use of prenatal ultrasonography and elective termination have had a significant impact on the incidence of bladder extrophy worldwide.

HYPOSPADIAS

140. What is the developmental defect shown in the figure?
The developmental defect pictured to the right is called hypospadias.

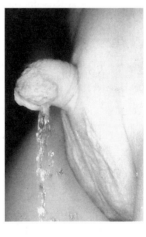

141. Does the child shown in the figure need immediate surgical attention?
No. Surgical correction is best done somewhere between 6 and 12 months of life, assuming there are no additional medical issues.

142. When during development did this lesion occur?
Penile development takes place between 12 and 15 weeks of gestation.

143. Hypospadias in association with bilateral nonpalpable gonads demands what kind of evaluation?
Chromosomal evaluation is mandatory in infants with hypospadias and nonpalpable gonads. One must rule out virilizing congenital adrenal hyperplasia in order to prevent errors in gender assignment and avoid a risk of a salt-losing crisis in the infant.

144. How common are other genitourinary abnormalities in infants with distal hypospadias?
Rare. There is no greater incidence of other genital urinary anomalies in infants with distal hypospadias.

145. What is happening to the incidence of hypospadias nationwide?

The incidence of hypospadias is increasing nationwide. The reason is not entirely clear, but it may have to do with increasing maternal age and increasing incidence of in vitro fertilization.

BIBLIOGRAPHY

1. Cendron M, Elder JS, Duckett JW: Perinatal urology. In Gilenwater JY, Grayhack JT, Howards SS, Duckett JW (eds): Adult and Pediatric Urology, 3rd ed. St. Louis, Mosby, 1996, pp 2075–2169.
2. Clark DA: Time of first void and first stool in 500 newborns. Pediatrics 60:457–459, 1977.
3. Dell RB: Normal acid-base regulation. In Winters RW (ed): The Body Fluids in Pediatrics, 1st ed. Boston, Little, Brown, 1973.
4. Duncan BW, Adzick NS, Longaker MT, et al: In utero arterial embolism from renal vein thrombosis with successful postnatal thrombolytic therapy. J Pediatr Surg 26:741–743, 1991.
5. Edelmann CM Jr, Rodriguez-Soriano J, Boichis H, et al: Renal bicarbonate reabsorption and hydrogen ion excretion in normal infants. J Clin Invest 46:1309–1317, 1967.
6. Elder JS: Antenatal hydronephrosis: Fetal and neonatal management. Pediatr Clin North Am 44:1299–1321, 1997.
7. Ellis EN, Arnold WC: Use of urinary indexes in renal failure in the newborn. Am J Dis Child 136:615–617, 1982.
8. Fick GM, Gabow PA: Hereditary and acquired cystic disease of the kidney. Kidney Int 46:961–964, 1994.
9. Fukuda Y, Kojima T, Ono A, et al: Factors causing hyperkalemia in premature infants. Am J Perinatol 6(1):76–79, 1989.
10. Gasser B, Mauss Y, Ghnassia JP, et al: A quantitative study of normal nephrogenesis in the human fetus: Its implications in the natural history of kidney changes due to low obstructive uropathies. Fetal Diagn Ther 8:8:371–384, 1993.
11. Gaudio KM, Siegel NJ: Pathogenesis and treatment of acute renal failure. Pediatr Clin North Am 34:771–787, 1987.
12. Glick PL, Harrison MR, Golbus MS, et al: Management of the fetus with congenital hydronephrosis II: Prognostic criteria and selection for treatment. J Pediatr Surg 20:376–387, 1985.
13. Goble MM: Hypertension in infancy. Pediatr Clin North Am 40:105–114, 1993.
14. Gonzalez ET: Posterior urethral valves and other urethral anomalies. In Campbell MF, et al (eds): Campbell's Urology, 7th ed. Philadelphia, W.B. Saunders, 1998, pp 2069–2091.
15. Gruskay J, Costarino AT, Polin RA, et al: Nonoliguric hyperkalemia in the premature infant weighing less than 1000 grams. J Pediatr 113:381–386, 1988.
16. Hammarlund K, Sedin G, Strömberg B: Transepidermal water loss in newborn infants. Part VIII: Relation to gestational age and post-natal age in appropriate and small for gestational infants. Acta Paediatr Scand 72:721–728, 1983.
17. Hawdon JM, Ward Platt MP, Aynsley-Green A: Prevention and management of neonatal hypoglycemia. Arch Dis Child 70:F54–F65, 1994.
18. Hood VL, Tannen RL: Protection of acid-base balance by pH regulation of acid production. N Engl J Med 339:819–826, 1998.
19. Hoover DL, Duckett JW: Posterior urethral valves, unilateral reflux and renal dysplasia: A syndrome. J Urol 128:994–997, 1982.
20. Ing FF, Starc TJ, Griffits SP, Gersony WM: Early diagnosis of coarctation of the aorta in children: A continuing dilemma. Pediatrics 98:378–382, 1996.
21. Jee LD, Rickwood AM, Turnock RR: Posterior urethral valves: Does prenatal diagnosis influence prognosis? Br J Urol 72:830–833, 1993.
22. Kaplan BS, Fay J, Shah V, et al: TM autosomal recessive polycystic kidney disease. Pediatr Nephrol 3:43–49, 1989.
23. Karlowicz MG, Adelman RD: Renal calcification in the first year of life. Pediatr Clin North Am 42:1397–1413, 1995.
24. Libenson MH, Kaye EM, Rosman NP, Gilmore HE: Acetazolamide and furosemide for posthemorrhagic hydrocephalus of the newborn. Pediatric Neurology 20:185–191, 1999.
25. Lorenz JM: Fluid and electrolyte management during the first week of life. In Fletcher J, Polin RA (eds): Workbook in Practical Neonatology, 3rd ed. Philadelphia, W.B. Saunders, 2000.
26. Lorenz JM, Kleinman LI, Disney TA: Renal response of newborn dogs to potassium loading. Am J Physiol 251:F513–F519, 1986.
27. Machin GA: Diseases causing fetal and neonatal ascites. Pediatr Pathol 4:195–211, 1985.
28. Malone TA: Glucose and insulin versus cation-exchange resin for the treatment of hyperkalemia in very low birth weight infants. J Pediatr 118:121–123, 1991.
29. Moore RD: Effects of insulin upon ion transport. Biochim Biophys Acta 737:1–49, 1983.

30. Nawankwo MU, Torenz JM, Gardiner JC: A standard protocol for blood pressure measurement in the newborn. Pediatrics 99(6):E10, 1997.

31. Ogborn MR: Polycystic kidney disease—a truly pediatric problem. Pediatr Nephrol 8:762–767, 1994.

32. Peters CA: Obstruction of the fetal urinary tract. J Am Soc Nephrol 8:653–663, 1997.

33. Rodriguez-Soriano J: Bartter and related syndromes: The puzzle is almost solved. Pediatr Nephrol 12:315–327, 1998.

34. Rosendaal FR: Thrombosis in the young: Epidemiology and risk factors. A focus on venous thrombosis. Thromb Haemost 78:1–6, 1997.

35. Roy S, Dillon MJ, Trompeter RS, Barratt TM: Autosomal recessive polycystic kidney disease: Long-term outcome of neonatal survivors. Pediatr Nephrol 11:302–306, 1997.

36. Sargent JD, Stukel TA, Kresel J, Klein RZ: Normal values for random urinary calcium to creatinine ratios in infancy. J Pediatr 123:393–397, 1993.

37. Schwartz GJ, Haycock GB, Edelmann CM Jr, Spitzer A: Late metabolic acidosis: A reassessment of the definition. J Pediatr 95:102–107, 1979.

38. Shaffer SG, Weismann DN: Fluid requirements in the preterm infant. Clin Perinatol 19:233–250, 1992.

39. Shaffer SG, Kilbride HW, Hayen LK, et al: Hyperkalemia in very low birth weight infants. J Pediatr 121:275–279, 1992.

40. Simon DB, Lifton RP: The molecular basis of inherited hypokalemic alkalosis: Bartter's and Gitelman's syndrome. Am J Physiol 271:F961–F966, 1996.

41. Stefano JL, Norman ME: Insulin therapy for nonoliguric hyperkalemia in the extremely low birth weight infant: Is it effective? [abstract]. Pediatr Res 31:66A, 1992.

42. Stefano JL, Norman ME: Nitrogen balance in extremely low birth weight infants with nonoliguric hyperkalemia J Pediatr 123:632–635, 1993.

43. Stefano JL, Norman ME, Morales MC, et al: Decreased erythrocyte Na^+,K^+-ATPase activity associated with cellular potassium loss in extremely low birth weight infants with nonoliguric hyperkalemia. J Pediatr 122:276–284, 1993.

44. Svenningsen NW: Renal acid-base titration studies in infants with and without metabolic acidosis. Pediatr Res 8:659–672, 1974.

45. Tan KL: Blood pressure in very low birth weight infants in the first 70 days of life. J Pediatr 112:266–270, 1988.

8. GASTROENTEROLOGY AND NUTRITION

ANATOMIC AND FUNCTIONAL DEVELOPMENT OF THE GASTROINTESTINAL TRACT

1. At what gestational age is the anatomic development of the gastrointestinal tract (including the liver) complete?

By 12 weeks. Starting as a straight tube, the gastrointestinal (GI) tract undergoes a process of elongation and organ development from primitive buds (anlages) responsible for liver and pancreas organogenesis. The rapid elongation brings the bowel outside of the abdominal cavity until week 11, when counterclockwise rotation around the axis of the superior mesenteric artery brings the cecum to the right lower quadrant and the duodenum to its final location.

2. When is villus morphology and function fully developed?

Fetal small intestine is morphologically recognizable by week 8 of gestation. Between weeks 10 and 14, the typical finger-like projections develop, and the microvilli become denser at the apical surface of the enterocyte. Maturation of the villi progresses in a caudal direction. By 14 weeks, most fetal intestinal enzymes activities, including sucrase, maltase, and alkaline phosphatase, are at near adult levels. Lactase activity, however, remains low until the end of gestation.

3. What are the most common anomalies resulting from abnormal separation of the respiratory and GI tracts during embryogenesis?

Tracheoesophageal fistula and esophageal atresia in various combinations are the result of failure to separate of the once-joined esophagus and trachea, both growing from the primitive foregut and elongating during development. A laryngotracheoesophageal cleft can also occur when the defect is more proximal. It is estimated that these anomalies occur in 2–3 cases per 10,000 live births.

4. What is the Meckel's diverticulum?

The Meckel's diverticulum is the remnant of the omphalomesenteric (vitelline) duct, which connected the intestine to the yolk sac. This conduit usually involutes by week 9 of gestation. In one-third of cases, the diverticulum contains ectopic gastric acid–producing cells, which are responsible for the bleeding complications of this anomaly. Intussusception, internal herniation around a fibrotic band connecting the intestine to the abdominal wall, or diverticulitis can also occur. Two percent to 10% of patients with Meckel's diverticulum also have umbilical abnormalities (cysts, mucosal "polyps," vitelline duct cysts, sinuses).

5. What are Ladd's bands? Why are they important?

Ladd's bands are abnormal mesenteric ligaments crossing from the abnormally located cecum to the duodenum, causing obstruction of the second portion of the duodenum in cases of malrotation. As a result of incomplete rotation, the duodenal-jejunal loop ends up to the right of the spine, and the intestine is narrowly fixated on a vascular pedicle, which includes the superior mesenteric artery and vein. Volvulus around this pedicle is a serious complication with potential catastrophic results: infarction of the midgut and resulting short bowel syndrome.

6. Why is loss of intestinal length as a result of necrotizing enterocolitis or other complications more serious in a full-term infant than a premature infant?

Intestinal lengthening occurs more rapidly in the last trimester of gestation, but it slows down considerably thereafter. As a result, a full-term infant has less potential for compensatory growth. The small intestine elongates an estimated 1000-fold from the fourth to the fortieth week. The full length of small bowel in a full-term infant is approximately 300 cm.

7. What is the rationale for the maxim: "it takes a heart to make a liver"?

Formation of the primitive liver is a result of signaling from the closely apposed cardiac mesoderm against the foregut endoderm. Extracellular matrix proteins, such as fibroblast growth factors, diffusing from the cardiac tissue probably mediate this induction. Differentiation of hepatocytes are temporally closely related to the development of biliary and pancreatic ductal structures arising from duodenal buds.

8. What is the ductal plate?

The ductal plate is the one-cell layer of hepatocyte precursors that surrounds the portal vein and its branches. A remodeling of this ductal plate, starting after 12 weeks' gestation, results in formation of the intrahepatic bile ducts. Embryonic-type biliary atresia, congenital hepatic fibrosis, and cystic dilatation of the intrahepatic bile ducts can result from anomalies of ductal plate remodeling.

9. What is pancreas divisum?

Failure of fusion of the ventral and dorsal pancreatic ducts around 7 weeks' gestation results in a divisum anatomy. Normally, the head of the pancreas is derived from the ventral pancreatic bud, whereas the body and tail stem from the dorsal anlage. Each bud carries its duct, but eventually they fuse and drain into the main duct of Wirsung. The dorsal bud duct can remain as the accessory duct of Santorini. Pancreatic duct anomalies can result in recurrent pancreatitis, especially when associated with a common channel draining biliary secretions.

10. What is the origin of the cells in the ganglia of the enteric nervous system (ENS)?

Neural cells from the embryonic neural plate migrate along the developing intestinal tube and eventually reach all areas of the bowel brought there by signaling molecules found in the extracellular matrix. These cells reach the stomach at around 7 weeks and the end of the colon by 12 weeks. The sympathetic and parasympathetic nerves will innervate various regions of the gut, providing important modulatory afferent and efferent pathways.

MECONIUM

11. What is the composition of meconium?

Meconium is composed of substances either swallowed by the fetus or secreted into the fetal GI tract during gestation. Its composition includes squamous epithelial cells (squames), lanugo hair, vernix, sloughed mucosal cells, bile salts and pigments, and pancreatic enzymes.

12. What stimulates the passage of meconium?

The multiple stimuli for meconium passage involve the interactions of quantity of meconium, gestational age, motilin and other GI hormones, and catecholamines. The "distressed" fetus may pass meconium during episodes of hypoxia.

13. When is meconium passed in the term infant?

Approximately 15% of deliveries at term have meconium in the amniotic fluid, suggesting that those fetuses have passed meconium in utero. Most term neonates pass meconium by 24 hours of postnatal age; 99% of term neonates stool by 36 hours of age.

14. When is meconium passed in the preterm infant?

The data are quite different for preterm neonates than term infants. For babies of birth weights less than 1000 g, the median postnatal age at passage of the first stool is 3 days, with 85% of babies passing stool by approximately 10 days. Almost 80% of babies within this weight range pass stool prior to initiation of enteral feedings. In preterm infants, the time of passage of the first stool does not correlate with gestational age, birth weight, or appropriateness of intrauterine growth.

FETAL GROWTH ASSESSMENT

15. Why is it important to routinely monitor fetal growth during the pregnancy?
Intrauterine growth is one of the most important signs of fetal well being and one of the most reliable indicators of pathologic conditions that affect the mother and the fetus during pregnancy. In addition, alterations in fetal growth have great implications in the acute and long-term management of the fetus and the newborn infant.

16. What do the terms low birth weight (LBW), very low birth weight (VLBW), and extremely low birth weight (ELBW) indicate?
LBW: < 2500 g
VLBW: < 1500 g
ELBW: < 1000 g
This classification is clinically relevant because neonatal morbidity and mortality are strongly correlated with the infants' gestational age and birth weight.

17. What is the difference between an intrauterine-growth-retarded (IUGR) and a small-for-gestational-age (SGA) infant?
The two terms are used to refer to infants born with a birth weight for gestational age that falls below the 10th percentile on the intrauterine growth chart. However, IUGR denotes the presence of a pathologic process during the pregnancy that results in fetal growth restriction whereas SGA denotes all infants whose weight fall below the 10th percentile from growth retardation, biologic diversity, or unidentifiable causes.

18. What are the most common causes of intrauterine growth retardation?

Intrinsic (fetal) causes:	*Extrinsic (maternal/placental) causes:*
Constitutional (parents of small stature)	Maternal age < 16 years and > 35 years
Genetic (congenital/chromosomal anomalies)	Maternal illness (cardiac, anemia, malnutrition)
Toxic (alcohol, nicotine, virus, hydantoin, coumarin)	Placental dysfunction (hypertension, infection, vascular accident, diabetes)
Infection (TORCH, syphilis, malaria)	Multiple gestation
Teratogenic (radiation, drugs)	Demographic (low socioeconomic status, race)
	Behavioral (low educational status, stress, teenage pregnancy)
	In-utero constraint (extrinsic mass, tumor)

Adeniyi-Jones S: Intrauterine growth retardation. In Spitzer AR (ed): Intensive Care of the Fetus and Neonate. Philadelphia, W.B. Saunders, 1996, p 137.

19. What are the clinical complications associated with intrauterine growth retardation? Why do they occur?

TYPES OF COMPLICATIONS	ETIOLOGY
Perinatal asphyxia	Acute hypoxia during labor in fetus with compromised placental blood flow
Hypothermia	Increased surface area for body-mass ratio and decreased subcutaneous fat
Hypoglycemia	Increased glucose utilization Impaired free fatty acid oxidation

(Table continued on next page.)

TYPES OF COMPLICATIONS	ETIOLOGY
Hypoglycemia *(cont.)*	Attenuation of adrenergic hormones
	Decreased glucose production
Hyperviscosity	Chronic fetal hypoxia
	Increased red blood cell (RBC) mass
	Sludging of RBC in microcirculation
Altered immunity	Analogous to malnourished children
	Reduction in serum IgG levels
	Decreased thymic weight
	Decreased T-lymphocyte counts
	Decreased qualitative T-cell function

20. What causes neonates to be large for gestational age (LGA)?

Infants with birth weight above the 90th percentile of the intrauterine growth chart are classified as LGA. Maternal diabetes is the most common cause of fetal growth acceleration due to the induction of fetal hyperinsulinism during the gestation. Other causes include fetal hydrops (edema), Beckwith-Wiedemann syndrome, transposition of the great vessels, and maternal obesity.

Lubchenco LO: The infant who is large for gestational age. In The High Risk Infant. Philadelphia, W.B. Saunders, 1976, p 165.

21. Is assessment of Doppler flow velocity useful in the evaluation of growth-retarded infants?

Utero-placental and fetal-placental blood flow velocities have been assessed during the pregnancy, and normal standard curves have been developed. Blood-flow velocities may be altered in pregnancies complicated by hypertension, proteinuria, and fetal growth retardation. Doppler studies demonstrating raised pulsatility indices with absent end-diastolic flow are associated with poor perinatal outcomes (i.e., death, hemorrhage, and necrotizing enterocolitis).

Hackett GA, et al: Doppler studies in growth retarded fetus and prediction of neonatal necrotizing enterocolitis, hemorrhage, and neonatal morbidity. BMJ 294:13, 1987.

22. Is it clinically useful to classify SGA infants as symmetric and asymmetric?

Infants who are symmetrically growth retarded have proportionally reduced size in weight, length, and head circumference. This type of growth retardation starts early in pregnancy, and it is often secondary to congenital infection, chromosomal abnormalities, and dysmorphic syndromes. Most IUGR babies are, however, asymmetrically growth retarded with the most severe growth reduction in weight, less severe length reduction, and relative head sparing. Asymmetric IUGR is caused by extrinsic factors that occur late in gestation such as pregnancy-induced hypertension syndromes. Asymmetric IUGR infants have a better long-term growth and developmental outcome than symmetric IUGR infants.

Walther FJ: Growth and development of term-disproportionate small-for-gestational-age infants at age of 7 years. Early Hum Dev 18:1, 1988.

MEDICAL PROBLEMS OF THE GROWTH-RETARDED INFANT

23. What are the long-term consequences of IUGR?

Development. Because the group is heterogeneous, the outcome is dependent on perinatal events, the etiology of growth retardation, and the postnatal socioeconomic environment. In general, the asymmetric growth-retarded baby does not show significant differences in intelligence or neurologic sequelae, but does demonstrate differences in school performance related to abnormalities in behavior and learning.

Health effects. An increased risk of hypertension is found in adolescents and young adults. Growth-retarded infants with a low ponderal index are at increased risk from syndrome X

(non–insulin dependent diabetes mellitus, hypertension, and hyperlipidemia) and death from cardiovascular disease by the age of 65 years (Barker hypothesis).

Growth. Fetuses that experienced growth failure after 26 weeks gestation (asymmetric
growth retardation) exhibit a period of catch-up growth during the first 6 months of life. However,
their ultimate stature is frequently less than an appropriate-for-gestational-age (AGA) baby.

CALORIC REQUIREMENTS

24. What is the significance of energy balance?

Energy, being neither created nor destroyed, conforms to classic balance relationships.
Energy balance is a state of equilibrium when energy intake equals expenditure plus losses. If
energy intake exceeds expenditure plus losses, the infant is in positive balance, and excess calories are stored. If energy intake is less than expenditure plus losses, the infant is in negative balance, and calories are mobilized from body stores. Maintenance or basal energy requirements are
the energy needs required to cover basal metabolic rate or resting energy expenditure; total
energy expenditure in infants is the sum of the energy required for basal metabolic rate, activity,
thermoregulation, diet-induced thermogenesis, and growth. The energy balance equation may be
stated as follows:

$$\text{Gross energy intake} = \text{energy excreted} + \text{energy expended} + \text{energy stored}$$
or
$$\text{Metabolizable energy} = \text{energy expended} + \text{energy stored}$$

ENERGY INTAKE	METABOLIZABLE ENERGY	ENERGY EXPENDED	• *BASAL METABOLIC RATE* • *ACTIVITY* • *SYNTHESIS* • *THERMOREGULATION*
		ENERGY STORED	*FAT & PROTEIN*
	LOSSES		

Putet G, Senterre J, Rigo J, Salle B: Energy balance and composition of body weight. Energy metabolism, nutrition and growth in premature infants. Biol Neonate 52(suppl 1):17–24, 1987.

25. What are the caloric requirements of LBW infants?

LBW infants require at least 120 cal/kg/day, partitioned to approximately 75 cal/kg/day for
resting expenditure and the remainder for specific dynamic action (SDA 10 cal/kg/day), replacement of inevitable stool losses (10 cal/kg/day) and growth (25 cal/kg/day)

Caloric Requirements of Low Birth Weight Infants (in cal/kg/day)

Resting*	50–75
SDA	5–8% of total intake
Stool losses	10% of total intake
Growth	25–45
Total†	85–142

* Estimate includes caloric expenditure for maintenance of basal metabolism plus activity and response to
  cold stress
† Includes sum of resting and growth requirements for specific dynamic action [SDA] and replacement of
  stool losses plus an increment of 15–18%.

26. What is respiratory quotient and what is its significance?

Respiratory quotient (RQ) is the ratio of the volume of CO_2 produced to the volume of O_2
consumed per unit of time (Vco_2/Vo_2). The proportion of the amount of CO_2 produced to the

amount of O_2 consumed varies with the type of nutrient oxidized. In addition, the energy produced varies with the type of substrate burned. Thus, various substrates will differ in RQs, and varying proportions of different nutrients will result in different energy production per liter of O_2 consumption or CO_2 production. The RQs and caloric equivalents of O_2 and CO_2 for carbohydrate, fat, and protein are shown in the table.

	RQ	ENERGY PRODUCED/L OF O_2 (kcal)	ENERGY PRODUCED/L OF CO_2 (kcal)
Carbohydrate	1.00	5.0	5.0
Fat	0.71	4.7	6.6
Protein	0.80	4.5	5.6

Lehninger AL: Biochemistry: The Molecular Basis of Cell Structure and Function. New York, Worth Publishers, 1975, p 825.

27. What factors affect energy expenditure during the neonatal period?

Multiple factors may affect energy expenditure during the neonatal period. Briefly, some of the most significant factors are:

Age. Neonates have twice the rate of energy expenditure as adults (50 versus 25 kcal/kg/day). The resting energy expenditure increases steadily from birth, peaks between 3 and 6 months of age, and then steadily declines.

Dietary intake. Two effects of dietary intake have been described. The first is the immediate effect of a meal on energy expenditure, referred to as **diet-induced thermogenesis** (also known as specific dynamic action, thermic effect of food, or postprandial thermogenesis). This is thought to represent the energy necessary for absorption and assimilation of nutrients. The second is the **long-term effect of diet**, with higher levels of dietary intake leading to increased rates of energy expenditure.

Ambient temperature. Energy expenditure may be nearly doubled under extreme environmental conditions.

Activity. Activity contributes approximately 10% to total energy expenditure in the neonatal period. Differences in energy expenditure have been demonstrated in various activity states (e.g., active and quiet sleep) in both term and preterm infants.

Biologic variability. Biologic variation has been observed in respiratory calorimetry measurements made in relatively homogenous groups of infants studied under neutral thermal environment over prolonged periods after a feeding. Most likely, both interindividual and intraindividual variability are significant.

28. What is the energy cost of growth?

The energy cost of growth includes the energy used for synthesis of new tissues (absorption, metabolism, and assimilation of fat and protein) and the energy stored in these new tissues. The energy cost of growth varies with the type of tissue added during growth. The precise caloric requirements for growth are unknown. A wide range of values for energy cost of growth in neonates has been determined (1.2–6 kcal/g of weight gain). Separate evaluations of energy expenditure requirement for fat and protein deposition in premature newborns estimate that 1 g of protein deposition requires 7.8 kcal, and 1 g of fat requires 1.6 kcal.

CARBOHYDRATE REQUIREMENTS

29. How are carbohydrate requirements estimated in newborn infants?

Strict carbohydrate requirements are difficult to estimate because glucose, a preferred metabolic fuel for many organs including the brain, is synthesized endogenously from other compounds. Several methods have been used to assess carbohydrate requirements in neonates:

1. Breast milk intake of lactose (assuming breast milk provides optimal intakes of all nutrients)

2. Constant infusion of labeled glucose to determine the rates of glucose production and oxidation (as a reflection of overall carbohydrate metabolism)

3. Altering the amount of the carbohydrate intake in the diet and determining its effect on energy metabolism and nitrogen retention.

Results from these different methods indicate that carbohydrates should contribute approximately 40% to the total calories of the diet in newborn infants.

30. The rate of endogenous glucose production in neonates has been estimated to range from 4 to 6 mg/kg/min. Do these values represent the ideal carbohydrate intake for neonates?

No. The rates of glucose endogenous production should be regarded only as the *minimal* carbohydrate requirement because of the methods and conditions in which these measurements were performed. These studies were done in neonates under basal or resting metabolic conditions and during fasting periods. In addition, they did not take into account the energy cost of physical activity, growth, and thermic effect of feeding. Higher values ranging from 5.8 to 6.8 mg/kg/min have been used as guidelines for the initiation of glucose infusion in neonates receiving parenteral nutrition.

Denne SC: Carbohydrate requirements. In Polin RA, Fox WW (eds): Fetal and Neonatal Physiology, 2nd ed. Philadelphia, W.B. Saunders, 1998, pp 325–327.

31. Can an excessive intake of carbohydrate be toxic for the neonate?

Yes. Excessive intake of carbohydrate in infant feedings may lead to delayed gastric emptying, emesis, diarrhea, and abdominal distention due to excessive gas formation. The excessive administration of intravenous glucose, at rates exceeding 13.8 mg/kg/min, may be associated with metabolic complications such as hyperglycemia, glycosuria, and osmotic diuresis. In addition, the excessive glucose metabolized is stored mainly as fat.

Sauer PJJ, et al: Glucose oxidation rates in newborn infants measured with indirect calorimetry and U-13C glucose. Clin Sci (Colch) 70:587, 1986.

32. Why do premature infant formulas contain a comparable amount of lactose and glucose polymers?

- Premature infants have a limited ability to digest lactose because intestinal lactase does not reach maximal activity until near term.
- Glucose polymers are well digested and absorbed by premature infants.
- The use of glucose polymers allows the osmolality of the formula to remain low, even at at high-caloric density of 24 kcal/30 ml (< 300 mOsm/L).

33. What is the metabolic fate of the lactose malabsorbed by the small intestine?

The malabsorbed lactose is fermented in the colon, forming various gases such as carbon dioxide, methane, and hydrogen and short chain fatty acids such as acetate, propionate, and butyrate. These short chain fatty acids are absorbed in the colon, reducing energy losses in the stools and maintaining the nutriture and function of the colon. Despite these putative benefits of lactose fermentation, there are metabolic concerns that result from the reduced digestion and absorption of lactose in the small intestine such as:

1. Decreased insulin secretion and a reduced effect on protein synthesis

2. Lower adenosine triphosphate (ATP) formation when lactose is fermented to acetate instead of following the glucose metabolic pathways

3. Possible increased risk of necrotizing enterocolitis

PROTEIN REQUIREMENTS

34. What are essential amino acids?

The amino acids that cannot be synthesized in the body are regarded as essential amino acids:

Leucine	Threonine	Phenylalanine
Isoleucine	Methionine	Tryptophan
Valine	Lysine	Histidine

35. Which amino acids are considered conditionally essential for the preterm infants?
Cysteine, tyrosine, and taurine, because of immaturity of the enzymes (decreased activity) involved in their synthesis.

36. What is the whey-to-casein ratio of cow's milk and human milk protein?
The whey-to-casein ratio of cow's milk protein is 18:82 and that of human milk protein is 60:40.

37. How does the whey-to-casein ratio change during lactation?
The ratio of whey to casein is about 90:10 at the beginning of lactation and rapidly decreases to 60:40 (or even 50:50) in mature milk.

38. What is the predominant whey protein in human milk and cow's milk?
The predominant whey protein in cow's milk is β lactoglobulin, and the predominant whey protein in human milk is α lactalbumin.

39. What are the non-nutritive roles of protein in human milk?
- Whey proteins are known to be involved in the immune response (immunoglobulins), lactose synthesis (α-lactalbumin), and other host defenses (lactoferrin).
- Casein phosphopeptides are believed to enhance the absorption of minerals.
- Casein fragments are thought to increase intestinal motility.
- Glycoproteins (e.g., κ-casein) may promote the growth of certain beneficial bacteria. (Early premature milk may lack κ-casein.)

40. Name the methods used for determining protein requirements.
- Factorial method (based on reference data of infant body composition)
- Balance method (protein intake = protein retention + inevitable protein losses)
- Indices of protein nutritional status (e.g., plasma albumin and transthyretin concentrations; protein intake required to maintain these indices within an acceptable range)
- Stable isotope tracer techniques (insight into how metabolism changes with clinical state or nutritional status and thus an assessment of protein requirement)

41. What is a lactobezoar?
Lactobezoars are intragastric masses composed of partially digested milk curd (casein, fat, and calcium). Rarely seen now, lactobezoars were reported in LBW infants (< 2000 g) fed casein-predominant formulas.

42. What is the protein requirement of full-term and of preterm infants?
The recommended protein intake for full-term infants is 2–2.5 g/kg/day and for preterm infants is 3–4 g/kg/day.

43. What factors may affect protein utilization in the neonate?

Energy intake	Intake of other nutrients
Quality of protein intake	Infections and stress

44. What is the protein content of currently available formulas?
- Term formulas (e.g., Similac, Enfamil)—2.1 g/100 kcal
- Preterm formulas (e.g., Similac Special Care, Enfamil Premature)—2.7–3 g/100 kcal
- Follow-up formulas for LBW weight infants (e.g., Similac NeoSure, EnfaCare)—2.6–2.8 g/100 kcal

45. What is the rate of protein loss in premature infants who receive only 10% dextrose and water in the immediate newborn period?

ELBW infants (< 1000 g) who receive only glucose lose 1.2 g/kg/day. More mature infants lose protein at a slower rate (0.9 g/kg/day at 28 weeks and 0.7 g/kg/day at 31 weeks). Any protein deficits that are accrued must be replaced.

46. How can the protein losses be minimized?

Early provision of protein (1.0–1.5 g/kg/day) along with minimal calories (30 cal/kg/day) can stem the protein losses in ELBW infants.

47. How do protein requirements differ when protein is delivered parenterally versus enterally?

Protein requirements are higher parenterally because preterm infants retain only 50% of amino acids administered intravenously but 70–75% of formula or human milk protein.

48. What is the ideal calorie-to-protein ratio to ensure complete assimilation of protein?

Enteral feedings: ~ 30 cal/g of protein
Parenteral feedings: 20–30 cal/g of protein (based on limited data)

LIPID REQUIREMENTS

49. What are the beneficial effects of lipid emulsions in the premature infant?
- Provision of calories (in a calorically dense form)
- Prevention of essential fatty acid deficiency

50. In human milk, what is the percentage of calories provided by fat?
40–55%.

51. What is the source of fat in breast milk?

Most of the fat in breast milk is formed from circulating lipids derived from the mother's diet. A small amount of fat is synthesized by the breast itself; that percentage increases in women receiving a low-fat–high-carbohydrate diet.

52. What structural features of fatty acids improve enteral absorption?
- Shorter chain length—medium chain triglycerides are absorbed more efficiently than long chain triglycerides.
- Fatty acids with double bonds are absorbed more efficiently.

53. What are the energy contents of long and medium chain triglycerides?

Long chain triglycerides: 9 cal/g
Medium chain triglycerides: ~ 7.5 cal/g

54. What is the energy cost of synthesizing fat from carbohydrate?

Synthesis of fat from glucose requires about 25% of the glucose energy invested in synthesis. In comparison, synthesis of fat from fat requires only 1–4% of the energy invested.

55. What fatty acids are essential for the fetus and premature infant?

All human beings have a requirement for linoleic and linolenic acid. These are 18-carbon omega-6 and omega-3 fatty acids, respectively. Linoleic and linolenic acid serve as precursors for long chain polyunsaturated fatty acids (LCPUFAs) such as arachidonic (a 20-carbon omega-6 fatty acid), eicosapentaenoic (a 20-carbon omega-3 fatty acid), and docosahexaenoic acid (a 22-carbon omega-3 fatty acid). LCPUFAs are essential components of membranes and are particularly important in membrane-rich tissues such as the brain. In addition, eicosapentaenoic and arachidonic acids are precursors for prostaglandins, leukotrienes, and other lipid mediators. The fetus receives essential fatty acids (including LCPUFAs) transplacentally, and breast-fed babies receive them in breast milk. Vegetable oil–based formulas do not contain LCPUFAs, and the ability of preterm infants to synthesize LCPUFAs from linoleic and linolenic acid may be limited.

56. What are the current recommendations for LCPUFA supplementation?
In Europe, the recommendation is that formulas designed for preterm infants contain LCPUFAs in addition to linoleic and linolenic acid. Because of a concern about the effect of LCPUFA supplementation on postnatal growth, a similar recommendation has not been made in the United States.

57. What are the side effects of LCPUFA depletion?
- Omega-6 LCPUFA-reduced growth
- Omega-3 LCPUFA alterations in electroretinogram responses, reduced visual acuity, and possible cognitive abnormalities

58. What is the advantage of supplying calories as lipid rather than carbohydrate in infants with chronic lung disease?
The respiratory quotient of lipids is lower than that of carbohydrate. Therefore, the use of lipid infusions should theoretically decrease CO_2 production in infants with bronchopulmonary dysplasia.

59. What is the advantage of using a 20% lipid emulsion versus a 10% lipid emulsion in newborn infants?
Twenty-percent lipid emulsions are cleared from the circulation more rapidly than 10% emulsions. Ten-percent lipid emulsions contain proportionately more emulsifier (egg yolk phospholipid). In 10% emulsions, the phospholipid-to-triglyceride ratio is 0.12, and in 20% emulsions the ratio is 0.06. The excess phospholipid forms bilayer vesicles that extract free cholesterol from peripheral cell membranes to form lipoprotein X. Lipoprotein X is cleared very slowly from the circulation (half-life = 2 days).

60. What is the maximum acceptable triglyceride level in infants receiving lipid emulsions and how often should they be checked?
150 mg/dl. routine monitoring of serum triglycerides is necessary as they are being advanced.

TOTAL PARENTERAL NUTRITION: MONITORING AND COMPLICATIONS

61. Total parenteral nutrition (TPN) regimens for neonates are commonly prescribed with a calorie distribution of 8–10% from amino acids, 30–40% from lipid emulsions, and 50–60% from dextrose. What are the metabolic advantages of using different regimens containing high carbohydrate (67%) and low fat (5%) or low carbohydrate (34%) and high fat (58%)?
There are none. The administration of TPN solutions containing a moderate carbohydrate (60%) to fat (32%) ratio has been shown to result in a higher nitrogen retention rate than that of the unbalanced regimens.
Nose O, Tipton JR, Ament ME, Yabuuchi H: Effect of energy source on changes in energy expenditure, respiratory quotient and nitrogen balance during total parenteral nutrition in children. Pediatr Res 21:438–541, 1987.

62. Hyperglycemia is a common complication observed in ELBW infants receiving parenteral nutrition. Should insulin infusions be provided routinely to these infants?
No. Insulin infusions are recommended for infants < 1000 g who develop hyperglycemia with serum glucose in excess of 150 mg/dl and glycosuria during the course of parenteral nutrition providing low glucose infusion rates (< 12 mg/kg/min). In these infants, insulin infusions at

rates of 0.04–0.1 U/kg/hr have been shown to improve glucose tolerance and to promote weight gain, as compared to control infants.

Collin JW, Hoppe M: A controlled trial of insulin infusion and parenteral nutrition in extremely low birth weight infants with glucose intolerance. J Pediatr 118:921–927, 1991.

63. The clearance of intravenous fat emulsions in neonates is improved by all of the following measures except:
   A. Increasing the period of infusion from 8 to 24 hours
   B. Adding a low dose of heparin to the TPN solutions (1 U/ml)
   C. Exposing the fat emulsions to ambient light or to phototherapy lights
   D. Using 20% instead of 10% lipid emulsions
   C. Exposure of lipid emulsions to ambient or to phototherapy lights increases the formation of triglyceride hydroperoxide radicals but does not enhance lipid clearance. Lipid clearance in neonates is improved by prolonging the infusion period, by adding heparin to TPN solutions (which releases the lipoprotein lipase from capillary endothelial cells) and by using 20% lipid emulsions, which contain a lower phospholipid content than 10% lipid emulsions.

64. Why do premature infants who receive prolonged courses of parenteral nutrition develop osteopenia resulting in pathologic bone fractures?
   The development of osteopenia during the course of TPN in premature infants is believed to result from the inability to provide the calcium and phosphorus required for proper bone mineralization. The solubility of calcium and phosphorus in TPN solutions can be improved by providing a high amino acid intake and by the supplementation of cysteine hydrochloride. These measures allow for a greater but still inadequate intake of calcium and phosphorus. The administration of calciuric diuretics such as furosemide, the use of postnatal steroids, and the development of cholestatic liver disease further aggravate calcium homeostasis in these patients. The IV administration of vitamin D does not prevent the occurrence of TPN-induced osteopenia.

Koo WWK, Tsang RC, Steichen JJ, et al: Parenteral nutrition in infants: The effect of high versus low calcium and phosphorus content. J Pediatr Gastroent Nutr 6:96–104, 1980.

65. Which of the trace elements in TPN solutions can be potentially toxic for patients with cholestatic liver disease?
   Copper and manganese. Both of these trace elements are metabolized in the liver and primarily excreted in bile. Therefore, the chronic administration of trace elements in patients with cholestasis can potentially result in toxic states. Manganese and copper supplements should be withheld from TPN solutions when hepatic cholestasis is present. Monitoring of serum levels of copper and manganese levels is indicated in patients with cholestasis who require prolonged course of TPN.

66. What is the most common complication of TPN administered by peripheral vein catheters?
   The accidental infiltration of TPN solution into the subcutaneous fat tissue resulting in skin necrosis. This complication can be minimized by lowering the osmolality of TPN solution through the administration of dextrose concentrations not exceeding 10% and by the concomitant administration of lipid emulsions.

67. What is the most common cause of bacterial infection in neonates receiving TPN by central vein catheter?
   Staphylococcus epidermidis remains the most common cause of bacterial sepsis during the course of TPN. Other organisms include *S. aureus, Escherichia coli, Pseudomonas* species, *Klebsiella* species, and *Candida albicans*. TPN-related infections are more common in the smallest and sickest infants receiving prolonged courses of TPN via a central catheter. The rate of these infections can be reduced by aseptic preparation of TPN solutions and by avoiding the use of the TPN catheter for blood transfusions, administration of medications, and blood sampling.

ENTERAL NUTRITION

68. What is the carbohydrate source in human milk and in term and preterm formulas?

Lactose is the major source of carbohydrate in human milk and in formulas for term infants. The preterm formulas contain a mixture of lactose and glucose polymers to compensate for the developmental lag in the intestinal mucosal lactase activity. Glycosidase enzymes involved in the digestion of glucose polymers are active in preterm infants.

69. Why is the fat absorption of preterm infants lower than that of term infants?

The lower fat absorption reported in preterm infants is attributed to their relative deficiency of pancreatic lipase and bile salts.

70. Why is the fat of human milk well absorbed by preterm infants?

The human milk triglyceride molecule has palmitic acid in the β position and is more easily absorbed compared to triglyceride molecules of cow's milk, vegetable fats, and animal fat that have palmitic acid in the α position. Presence of human milk lipase also improves fat absorption.

71. When should soy protein-based formulas be used for feeding infants?

Soy formulas are recommended for:
• Infants with lactase deficiency and galactosemia (soy formulas are lactose free)
• Infants with IgE-mediated allergy to cow's milk protein
• Infants of parents requesting vegetarian-based diet

72. What essential amino acid is added to soy-based infant formulas?

Because soy protein has low concentrations of methionine, this amino acid is added to all soy-based formulas.

73. When can preterm infants be nippled successfully?

The success of feeding a preterm infant by nipple is dependent on the ability of the infant to coordinate sucking and swallowing, which develops at about 33–34 weeks of gestational age.

74. Why may transpyloric feedings result in fat malabsorption?

Transpyloric feeds may result in fat malabsorption as a result of bypassing the lipolytic effect of gastric lipase.

75. Why are early minimal enteral feedings recommended for preterm infants receiving parenteral nutrition?

Gastrointestinal hormones, gastrin, enteroglucagon, and pancreatic polypeptide may have a trophic effect on the gut. Postnatal surges of these hormones are reported in enterally fed preterm infants. Small enteral feeding has also been reported to produce more mature small intestinal motor activity patterns in preterm infants. Thus, early minimal enteral feedings given along with parenteral nutrition may improve subsequent enteral feeding tolerance and shorten the time to achieve full enteral intake.

76. What are the reported advantages of feeding human milk to preterm infants over the commercially available infant formulas?

• Data suggesting lower incidence of necrotizing enterocolitis in preterm infants fed human milk have been reported and are believed to be due to the immunologic properties of human milk (cellular components, immunoglobulins, lactoferrin, lysozyme).
• Faster gastric emptying in preterm infants fed human milk compared to hose fed bovine milk–derived formulas has been reported.
• Improved long-term cognitive development has been correlated with human milk feedings in the preterm infant.

77. Does human milk meet the nutritional requirement of preterm infants (birth weight < 1500 g)?

Growth rates of preterm infants fed banked human milk or their own mother's milk are lower than that of infants fed preterm formulas. In addition, the calcium and phosphorus content of human milk is insufficient to support adequate skeletal mineralization. Supplementation of human milk with available human milk fortifiers that provide protein, calcium, phosphorus, sodium, zinc, and vitamins helps overcome the nutritional inadequacies.

BREAST-FEEDING

78. What are the determinants of milk volume (milk production)?

Initially, hormonal factors (prolactin and oxytocin) affect the synthesis and secretion of milk. Once milk "comes in," tight junctions close and lactation shifts from endocrine control to autocrine control, or control driven by milk removal. The frequency of breast-feeding then becomes the most important factor affecting the continuation of adequate milk production. The term infant should receive at least 8–12 feedings per day in the first week and more than 6 per day thereafter. So that the volume of residual milk is minimized, mothers should alternate the breast they start on the next feeding. Maternal diet and fluid intake rarely affect milk volume. In severe malnutrition, there *may* be diminished milk production.

There are no magic potions or medication that increase milk production. If mothers are producing a low milk volume, the administration of metoclopramide will occasionally increase serum prolactin and increase milk production. Unfortunately, there are side effects of this medication, including sedation and extrapyramidal neurologic signs. Oxytocin will not increase milk production, but it may help milk ejection (once milk already has been synthesized). Herbal remedies have been advocated, but no data are available that determine their efficacy or risk.

Fatigue and stress also affect milk production adversely. A small percentage of women (2–5%) have lactation insufficiency and cannot produce adequate quantities of milk.

79. What are the contraindications for breast-feeding?

- Galactosemia
- Substance abuse/use: cocaine, narcotics, stimulants
- Miliary tuberculosis (avoid breastfeeding until adequate therapy for about 2 weeks)
- Human immunodeficiency virus (HIV). This contraindication has far-reaching global concerns. In the U.S., women who test positive for HIV should not breast feed. The risk/benefit ratios must be determined for particular populations. Efforts are underway to determine the risk/benefit ratio and cost/benefit ratio for the use of antiretroviral therapy along with breast-feeding or the use of infant formula in high-risk populations.
- Medications. Only a few medications are incompatible with breast-feeding:

Bromocriptine (suppresses lactation)	Amiodarone
Ergotamine	Thiouracils
Chemotherapeutic agents	Metronidazole
Radiopharmaceuticals	Clonapin
Phenindione	Salts containing bromide and gold
Amantidine	

80. For how many months should mothers breast-feed their infants?

The American Academy of Pediatrics recommends 1 year but does not discourage continued breast-feeding thereafter.

American Academy of Pediatrics, Work Group on Breastfeeding: Breastfeeding and the use of human milk. Pediatrics 100:1035–1039, 1997.

81. What are the major public policy issues regarding breast-feeding?

1. **"Right-to-Breast Feed" legislation.** In September 1999, President Clinton signed legislation stating that breast-feeding could not be banned on federal property. The right-to-breast

feed provision was included in the annual spending bill for the Department of Treasury and the Postal Service. The law prohibits the use of federal funds to "implement, administer, or enforce any prohibition on women breastfeeding their children in Federal buildings or on Federal property." It was added to the measure at the urging of Rep. Carolyn Maloney (D-NY), who introduced the "right to Breast Feed Act."

2. **Baby Friendly Hospital Initiative.** The World Health Organization (WHO) and United Nations International Children's Emergency Fund (UNICEF) global ten-step program to increase the success of breast-feeding has a parallel program in the United States, The Baby Friendly Hospital Initiative (BFHI). The BFHI is a program where hospitals can be credentialed as "baby friendly." The ten-step program that should be adopted by hospitals is as follows:

1. A written breast-feeding policy should be available.
2. The health care staff should be trained to implement the policy.
3. All pregnant women should be educated in prenatal classes and visits.
4. Breast-feeding should be initiated within 1 hour of birth.
5. Caregivers should be able to demonstrate how to breast feed and maintain lactation.
6. Only breast milk should be used, unless medically not indicated.
7. Rooming-in should be practiced 24 hours/day.
8. Caregivers should encourage breast-feeding on demand.
9. No artificial nipples or pacifiers should be provided until breast-feeding is established.
10. Caregivers should facilitate the development of breast-feeding support groups.

World Health Organization and UNICEF: Protecting, Promoting, and Supporting Breastfeeding: The Special Role of Maternity Services. Geneva, Switzerland, World Health Organization, 1989.

UNICEF: Take the Baby-Friendly Hospital Initiative! A Global Effort with Hospitals, Health Services, and Parents to Breastfeed Babies for the Best Start in Life. New York, UNICEF, 1991.

82. *Case.* A mother has breastfed her 5-week-old infant exclusively. She now calls with a concern that she has recently noticed a burning pain in her nipple during breast-feeding. You examine the mother and note some erythema of her areola. You diagnose a fissure and advise her to use dry heat and a few drops of milk on her areola after breast-feeding. She calls back in a few days saying that the pain is increasing. What other diagnosis should you consider?

This is not an uncommon presentation for a *Candida* infection of the nipple. You should have the mother bring her infant to your office and examine the infant for evidence of perioral thrush. If present, the baby should be treated with an oral medication and the mother with an antifungal.

83. A mother calls you and explains that she is worried because her 4-day-old baby is not receiving enough breast milk. How do you assess whether a newborn is receiving sufficient amounts of breast milk in the first week after birth?

Understand why the mother is concerned. Some of the following factors should influence your decision either to see the mother and baby or to reassure the mother over the phone: frequency of feeding (8–12 times in 24 hours, no interval longer than 4 hours), urine output (light yellow stained diapers), and stool output (no more meconium stools after day 3). Some practitioners use the following rough guide for urine and stool output in the first week: minimum of 1 urine output in the first 24 hours, 2–3 in the next 24 hours, about 4–6 on day 3, and 6–8 on day 5; stools should be 1 per day on day 1 and 2, 2 per day on day 3, and 4 or more afterward. The mother should sense that her milk has "come in" between the second and fourth days postpartum. The baby should have established feeding activities, such as lip smacking and rooting; you should hear swallows; and the baby should be satisfied after a feeding. Feeding activities, however, vary widely. Some adequately hydrated infants are sleepy and need coaching with feedings. If a mother experiences leaking from one breast while the child is nursing at the other, her milk supply is usually quite adequate.

84. *Case.* You see a 5-day-old male infant in the office for a routine check after early hospital discharge. The mother reports no particular problems; he is much easier to manage than she thought a newborn would be. She is breast-feeding every 3 hours but lets him sleep at night (last night he slept for 6 hours). About once a day she notes that he has dark yellow

urine in his diaper. He had a dark green, tarry stool yesterday. The mother thinks her milk has "come in," but she acknowledges no signs of engorgement. You examine the infant and note jaundice to the level of the umbilicus and dry skin, but moist mucous membranes. He is responsive and alert. You examine the mother and note that her breasts are moderately engorged. The infant's body weight is 11 ounces below his birth weight of 7 pounds, 8 ounces. You check his serum bilirubin concentration, which is 11 mg/dl. There is no blood group incompatibility. How would you manage this case and what would you advise the mother?

You should observe a breast-feeding to ensure that the baby has a good latch-on to the breast and is able to suck and swallow. You advise the mother to breast feed every 2 hours and to supplement the baby with formula. As the baby takes more milk from the breast, he will take less formula and will wean himself. You do not advise water supplements. The baby needs calories. His bilirubin level should decline. If the mother had not been making milk, you might suggest that she mechanically express her milk after every feeding to increase stimulation. You must schedule a return visit in 24–48 hours to assess the infant.

85. What is the most variable nutrient in human milk?

Fat is the most variable content of all nutrients in human milk. The fat content rises slightly during lactation, increases from the beginning (foremilk) to the end (hindmilk) of the feeding, varies among women (probably a direct effect of body fat stores), and varies over the course of the day. If mother does not completely empty her breast after feeding, the baby will not receive all the calories (fat). Mothers using mechanical methods to express their milk may not completely empty the breast.

86. Breast-feeding the premature infant can be a challenge. How do you advance from tube-feeding to breast-feeding in the premature infant?

Note the sucking and swallowing ability of infant. Parental skills, infant feeding cues, and timing of feedings should also be considered. Begin one breast-feeding in place of or in addition to the tube-feeding. If the latch-on is good and clinical signs of sucking, swallowing, and some drooling of milk are noted, then continue the process each day. It is not accurate to withdraw milk from an indwelling feeding tube to assess milk intake from breast-feeding. Gastric emptying from the stomach after a human milk feeding is rapid. Clinical signs of feeding activity and maternal assessment of breast emptying are inexact measures of milk intake and may not reflect small amounts consumed. The test-weighing technique has gained widespread use to better assess milk intake from breast-feeding. The infant is weighed before and immediately after a breast-feeding session. The technique requires an electronic scale and strict attention to details such as not unwrapping the infant or changing diapers before the reweighing is done. The replacement of tube-feeding with oral feeding also can be monitored by daily weight gain.

Meier P, Lysakowski TY, Engstrom JL: The accuracy of test weighing for preterm infants. J Pediatr Gastroenterol Nutr 10:62–65, 1990.

87. Do mothers benefit from breast-feeding?

Postpartum weight loss and uterine involution may be more rapid with breast-feeding. The postpartum amenorrhea during lactation is an acknowledged method of child spacing, especially for 4–6 months. This technique is most reliable if breast-feeding is practiced around the clock. Several reports now suggest that women who breast fed their infants had a decreased incidence of premenopausal breast cancer and ovarian cancer. Women who breast fed their infants also may have a decreased incidence of osteoporosis.

Labbok MH: Health sequelae of breastfeeding for the mother. Clin Perinatol 26:491–503, 1999.

88. What are "tandrieres" and how are they prevented?

"Tandrieres" are little fissures in the breast. In the 1500s, Laurent Joubert of Montpellier (1529–1582) theorized that tandrieres resulted from cracking and splitting of the nipples from the first milk. He recommended that the nipples and breasts be softened with cool bacon fat before the first milk arrived. Joubert wrote a number of medical books and was most famous for his textbook *Popular Errors*. Joubert was a controversial figure because he wrote about sexual matters that were considered taboo. At the age of 53, he disappeared on a stormy night on the way to a home visit in a neighboring village.

Joubert L: Popular Errors. Translated by GD de Rocher. Tuscaloosa, University of Alabama Press, 1989.

VITAMINS AND TRACE MINERALS

89. A 2-month-old preterm infant (with an estimated gestational age of 26 weeks) develops osteopenia of prematurity and fractures of both humeri. The infant is receiving 400 units of vitamin D/day. Should the dose of vitamin D be increased?

No! Contrary to earlier theory, osteopenia of prematurity results primarily from inadequate intake of mineral substrate (calcium and phosphorus) and not vitamin D. High doses of vitamin D do not appear to aid in the prevention or treatment of osteopenia of prematurity. Infants born prematurely are at risk for developing osteopenia because of limited accretion of bone mass in utero (fetal accretion rates from 25 to 40 weeks gestation: 92–119 mg calcium/kg/day and 59–74 mg phosphorus/kg/day) and greater need for bone nutrients compared to term infants. Preterm infants often receive limited intravenous and enteral calcium until full enteral feedings are established. Diuretics and steroids, as well as physical inactivity, have a negative effect on bone mineralization. In order to mimic fetal accretion, an enteral intake of 120–230 mg/kg/day of calcium and 60–140 mg/kg/day of phosphorus is recommended for preterm infants. This amount is provided by 150 cc/kg/day of premature infant formula or fortified breastmilk.

90. A 6-week-old infant is recovering from necrotizing enterocolitis that necessitated resection of two-thirds of the jejunum and placement of an ileostomy. When enteral feedings are restarted, the drainage from the ileostomy becomes excessive. The infant is growing poorly (despite an adequate caloric intake) and develops vesiculobullous and eczematous lesions around the eyes, mouth, and genitals. What mineral deficiency should be considered?

Infants with abnormal gastrointestinal losses (persistent diarrhea, excessive ileostomy drainage) may be at risk for zinc deficiency because fecal loss is the major excretory route. Signs of zinc deficiency include poor wound healing, poor linear growth, decreased appetite, hair loss, depressed immune function, and skin lesions.

Causes of Zinc Deficiency in Low Birth Weight Infants

- Poor zinc sores
- Increased requirement for growth
- Prolonged intravenous nutrition containing inadequate zinc
- Abnormally low zinc content of mother's milk
- Supplements of iron or copper which compete with zinc for absorption

---

Adapted from Atkinson SA, Zlotkin S: Recognizing deficiencies and excesses of zinc, copper, and other trace elements. In Tsang RC, et al (eds): Nutrition during Infancy. Cincinnati, Digital Educational Publishing, 1997.

91. The requirements for what nutrient are increased under phototherapy?

Riboflavin is a photosensitive vitamin, and requirements may be increased in infants being treated with phototherapy.

92. Is fluoride an essential nutrient for the newborn infant?

Although fluoride has been considered "beneficial for humans," its essentialness has not been confirmed. Fluoride supplementation is not recommended from birth because of questions concerning whether the benefit of fluoride warrants the risk of dental fluorosis. Commercial infant formulas do not contain fluoride.

93. What is the scientific rationale for administering vitamin A to prevent bronchopulmonary dysplasia (BPD)?
- Lung differentiation is affected by vitamin A.
- Vitamin A deficiency causes replacement of mucus-secreting epithelium by stratified squamous keratinizing epithelium in the trachea and bronchi.
- BPD has been associated with vitamin A deficiency in VLBW preterm infants.
- Premature birth deprives the newborn infant of the supply of retinol (vitamin A).
- The histopathology of BPD includes findings commonly seen with vitamin A deficiency (loss of ciliated cells and keratinizing metaplasia).

94. Does supplementation with vitamin A decrease the likelihood a preterm infant will develop BPD?

Tyson et al. recently published a blinded, randomized study investigating whether vitamin A (5000 U IM × 4 wk) decreased the incidence of BPD or death at 36 weeks gestation (N = 807 infants with RDS; mean BW 770 g). Death or chronic lung disease occurred in significantly fewer infants in the treatment group (55 v. 62%). Relative risk was 0.89 (CI 0.80–0.99). Overall, 1 additional infant survived without chronic lung disease for every 14–15 who were treated with vitamin A.

95. What are the concentrations of water-soluble vitamins in mature human milk and how do they compare with the recommended dietary allowances for healthy full-term infants?

	HUMAN MILK	AAP, CON* (units/100 kcal)
Thiamin (μg)	31 (21–36)	40
Riboflavin (μg)	56 (42–85)	60
Niacin (mg)	0.29 (0.27–0.34)	0.25 (0.8)
Vitamin B_6 (μg)	20 (15–30)	35
Pantothenic acid (mg)	0.6 (0.3–1.0)	0.3
Biotin (μg)	0.7 (0.6–1.1)	1.5
Folate (μg)	7 (6–12)	4
Vitamin B_{12} (μg)	0.10 (0.07–0.16)	0.15
Vitamin C (mg)	8 (5–13)	8

* Committee on Nutrition of the American Academy of Pediatrics
Adapted from Schlaner RJ. Who needs water soluble vitamins? In Tsang RC, et al (eds): Nutrition during Infancy. Cincinnati, Digital Educational Publishing, 1997.

IRON REQUIREMENTS

96. How long can iron stores meet the needs of full-term, LBW, and preterm infants before supplementation is necessary?

The quantity of iron stored is proportional to the birth weight of the infant. On average, the iron stores in a full-term infant can meet the infant's iron requirement until 4–6 months of age and that of LBW and preterm infants until 2–3 months of age. Transfused infants, however, may have greater iron stores.

97. What are the daily dietary iron requirements for term, LBW, and preterm infants?

The estimated daily requirement is 1 mg/kg/day for term infants and 2–4 mg/kg/day for LBW and preterm infants.

98. Do breast-fed infants require iron supplementation?

Although the bioavailability of iron in breast milk is high (because of the presence of lactoferrin, which enhances iron absorption), the content is relatively low. Additional sources of iron are recommended for breast-fed infants after 4–6 months of age.

99. What is the iron content of hemoglobin?

Each gram of hemoglobin contains 3.4 mg of iron.

100. Where is iron absorbed and what factors can influence iron absorption?

Dietary iron is absorbed in the duodenum and the proximal jejunum. Absorption is influenced by iron need and also by the dietary source. The majority of the dietary iron (in plant foods and fortified food products) is non-heme iron. Ascorbic acid enhances the absorption of non-heme iron, and calcium, phytates, manganese, and polyphenols decrease it.

101. Do premature infants need more or less iron than term infants?

Overall, premature infants will need more iron than term infants during their first postnatal year. The reason for this increased need stems from two factors. First, iron is accreted primarily during the last trimester. The fetus maintains a fairly steady 75 mg of elemental iron per kilogram body weight during this time period. At 24 weeks gestation, the fetus has 37.5 mg of total body iron, whereas at term the newborn has 225 mg. Therefore, premature birth results in significantly reduced total body iron. Second, the premature infant has a more rapid rate of growth per kilogram of body weight than the term infant. The blood volume must increase in proportion to that elevated growth rate. Iron intake must increase to support the increase in hemoglobin mass. Thus, whereas the term newborn needs approximately 1 mg/kg of iron per day, the preterm infant needs between 2 and 4 mg/kg/day. The more premature the infant, the greater the need.

102. What groups of term neonates are at increased risk of low iron stores at birth?

Growth-retarded infants and infants of diabetic mothers (IDMs) are two groups of infants at risk for reduced iron stores. Fifty percent of IUGR infants and 65% of infants of diabetics have cord serum ferritin concentrations below the fifth percentile (60 µg/L). In the case of IUGR infants, the etiology is probably related to impaired placental nutrient transport (they have protein-energy malnutrition as well, as defined by their IUGR). The pathophysiology of low iron stores in IDMs is more complex. Chronic maternal hyperglycemia results in chronic fetal hyperglycemia and hyperinsulinemia, both of which increase the oxygen consumption of the fetus by approximately 30%. Chronic fetal hypoxia leads to increased erythropoietin secretion and secondary polycythemia, which in turn requires increased iron delivery. Each extra gram of hemoglobin synthesized by the fetus requires an additional 3.49 mg of elemental iron delivered by the placenta. The human placenta is apparently not capable of upregulating placental transport to that extent, leaving the fetus dependent on its accreted iron stores to support the expanding fetal blood volume. The end result is that the IDM's iron is redistributed away from storage and nonstorage tissues and into the red cell mass. It does not appear that either group needs additional dietary iron postnatally, suggesting that the neonatal intestine avidly absorbs iron.

Chockalingam UM, Murphy E, Ophoven JC, et al: Cord transferrin and ferritin values in newborn infants at risk for prenatal uteroplacental insufficiency and chronic hypoxia. J Pediatr 111:283–286, 1987.

Stonestreet BS, Goldstein M, Oh W, Widness JA: Effect of prolonged hyperinsulinemia on erythropoiesis in fetal sheep. Am J Physiol 257:R1199–R1204, 1989.

Widness JA, Susa JB, Garcia JF, et al: Increased erythropoiesis and elevated erythropoietin in infants born to diabetic mothers and in hyperinsulinemic rhesus fetuses. J Clin Invest 67:637–642, 1981.

103. What is the effect of recombinant human erythropoietin (rhEpo) on the iron needs of the premature infant?

Erythropoietin increases the need for iron by up to threefold to 6 mg/kg/day. In the national collaborative trial of rhEpo for preterm infants, 6 mg/kg/day maintained steady ferritin concentrations over the duration of the study. Premature infants traditionally have depended on two sources of iron: dietary and blood transfusion. In the past when blood transfusion was more liberally prescribed, preterm infants received a large amount of iron by this route. The practice of administering erythropoietin to decrease donor exposure in preterm infants (along with the more stringent criteria for transfusions) has resulted in the infants being dependent on their own iron stores and any dietary iron they are receiving to fuel the hemoglobin response. Studies of erythropoietin given to sheep of varying degrees of iron sufficiency clearly demonstrate that the degree of he-moglobin response is directly related to the iron sufficiency of the animal. Knowing that preterm infants have much lower iron reserves (and thus a greater chance of not responding to rhEpo) prompted the investigators in the national collaborative trial to administer 6 mg/kg of iron to the infants.

Shannon KM, Keith JF 3rd, Mentzer WC, et al: Recombinant human erythropoietin stimulates erythro-poiesis and reduces erythrocyte transfusions in very low birth weight preterm infants. Pediatrics 85:1–8, 1995.

104. True or false: The premature infant is iron overloaded at hospital discharge?

This is a trick question. In fact, the preterm infant could be iron deficient, iron neutral, or iron overloaded. As noted above, preterm AGA infants start with approximately 75 mg of iron per kg of body weight. This amount of iron is considered sufficient for the neonatal period, and iron supplementation probably should not begin until the preterm infant is at least 2 weeks of age. Preterm infants are born with very immature antioxidant systems, and there is concern that large doses of iron could overwhelm the system and lead to disease that is related to oxidant stress (e.g., retinopathy of prematurity, bronchopulmonary dysplasia). On the other hand, the rapid growth rate of the preterm infants results in a rapid expansion of the blood volume, and iron is required to support this growth. By the end of the hospital period, the preterm infant may have been exposed to a wide range of iron intake and iron loss. Those who are born at low gestational ages, who have a benign neonatal course, and who are fed a low iron diet (e.g., breast milk with-out iron supplementation) are at high risk of utilizing all the available stores soon after discharge. These infants need to have their iron and hemoglobin status checked earlier than the usual 9 months of age recommended for term infants. In contrast, the sick preterm infant who requires multiple transfusions to maintain cardiovascular stability may be at high risk for iron overload. Preterm infants can have ferritin concentrations of 500 µg/dl at discharge, suggesting significant iron loading of the liver.

105. Is placental iron transport dependent on maternal iron status, fetal iron status, or both?

Both. Early studies clearly establish a relationship between maternal iron stores as indexed by her ferritin concentration and the infant's cord serum ferritin concentration. This relationship appeared to be particularly strong when the mother was suffering from profound iron deficiency. However, lesser degrees of iron deficiency did not seem to influence fetal iron status. In fact, the fetus manages to maintain iron sufficiency in the face of maternal iron deficiency. Conversely, certain fetuses can become iron deficient in spite of maternal iron sufficiency. This occurs when placental iron transport is disturbed by utero-placental vascular insufficiency resulting in in-trauterine growth retardation and when fetal iron demand exceeds placental iron transport ability. The latter is seen in pregnancies complicated by diabetes mellitus and chronic fetal hypoxia with augmented secondary fetal erythropoiesis. In pregnancies complicated by fetal iron deficiency as indexed by a low cord serum ferritin concentration or decreased placental iron content, the ex-pression of iron transport proteins such as the transferrin receptor is increased on the apical (ma-ternal-facing) membrane of the syncytiotrophoblast. Studies have shown that this upregulation is most likely in response to the iron status of the syncytiotrophoblast, which besides being a ge-nomically fetal cell also closely reflects the fetal iron status. This upregulation is achieved by in-tracellular iron regulatory proteins that bind transferrin receptor mRNA, stabilizing it to produce more copies of the receptor and leading to greater iron transport. Thus, the fetus appears to regu-late its own iron accretion! A similar system has been described for the transport of certain amino acids by the placenta.

Bergamaschi G, Bergamaschi P, Carlevati S, Cazzola M: Transferrin receptor expression in the human placenta. Haematologica 754:220–223, 1990.

Petry CD, Wobken JD, McKay H, et al: Placental transferrin receptor in diabetic pregnancies with in-creased fetal iron demand. Am J Physiol 267:E507–E514, 1994.

Georgieff MK, Berry SA, Wobken JA, Leibold EA: Increased placental iron regulatory protein-1 ex-pression in diabetic pregnancies complicated by fetal iron deficiency. Placenta 20:87–93, 1999.

GASTROESOPHAGEAL REFLUX

106. How many infants have reflux?

Up to 50% of normal infants will regurgitate two or more times a day. By 12 months of age, the incidence decreases to 1%. In the first year of life, 6–7% of all infants come to medical attention for gastroesophageal reflux (GER) symptoms. Up to 10% of VLBW babies will have symptomatic GER associated with apnea, bradycardia, or bronchopulmonary dysplasia.

Hyman PE: Gastroesophageal reflux: One reason why baby won't eat. J Pediatr 125:S103–S109, 1994.
Orenstein SR: Infantile reflux: Different from adult reflux. Am J Med 103:114S–119S, 1997.

107. What findings differentiate physiologic GER of infancy from pathologic reflux?
- Weight loss
- Failure to thrive
- Excessive irritability
- Feeding aversion
- Respiratory symptoms (persistent cough, choking, wheezing, pneumonia)
- Apnea
- Esophagitis
- Hemoccult positive stools

108. When should an infant with GER be referred to a specialist?

Referral is appropriate when symptoms fail to resolve with nonpharmacologic management or a brief course of pharmacotherapy. Other indications for referral are diagnostic testing beyond radiographic studies, persistence of symptoms beyond 1 year of age, the presence of severe symptoms, and when surgical intervention is being considered.

109. What factors predispose premature infants to symptomatic GER?
- Gastric compliance is lower, promoting transient lower esophageal sphincter (LES) relaxation of lower gastric volumes.
- Esophageal motor activity is less frequently peristaltic in premature infants, which can impair the return of refluxed material to the stomach.
- The oropharyngeal function of premature infants is immature. Material refluxed to the oropharynx is cleared less readily.
- Hypotonia may predispose to postures that promote reflux or delay its clearance.
- Nasogastric orogastric tubes may stent open the LES.
- Caffeine causes LES relaxation.

110. What are the commonly used tests to evaluate GER? Describe their roles in diagnosis and their limitations.
1. **Upper GI**
   - **Role:** Evaluate **anatomic or structural abnormalities** that predispose to GER.
   - **Limitations:** Not useful for diagnosing GER because it is performed over a short period of time (< 1 hour), under nonphysiologic conditions (being rolled around, with people pressing on the abdomen), with a nonphysiologic meal (barium).
2. **pH probe**
   - **Role:** The gold standard for **demonstrating and quantifying** the presence of acid in the esophagus. Most useful for silent GER. Enables calculation of various parameters including number of reflux episodes, total amount of time pH is below 4, and length of individual reflux episodes. Can be performed in conjunction with a multichannel thermistor, allowing correlation of GER with apnea, bradycardia, or other respiratory symptoms.
   - **Limitations:** If the patient is clinically refluxing, the test is not necessary. The utility can be limited by the lack of standardized norms for number of episodes. Anything

that buffers stomach acid will limit the probe's utility. Therefore, patients cannot be on acid suppression medication at the time of the study. Formula can also buffer acid, so the period after feedings may be falsely mistaken as normal.

3. **Gastroesophageal scintigraphy** (milk scan)
   - **Role: Demonstrates delayed gastric emptying, reflux, and aspiration.** The percentage of tracer remaining in the stomach at 1 and 2 hours can be quantified and compared to age-specific guidelines. The number of reflux episodes in those 2 hours can also be quantified, but this test should not be used to diagnose GER. The appearance of tracer in the lungs supports the diagnosis of aspiration.
   - **Limitations:** Because of a relatively short observation time, the test is a poor overall quantifier of reflux frequency. The results depend on the composition and volume of the formula being used, which may not necessarily reflect the patient's normal feeding regimen.

4. **Esophagogastroduodenoscopy** (EGD)
   - **Role:** Evaluates **visual and histologic mucosal abnormalities** of the esophagus, stomach, and duodenum. Identifies causes and degrees of esophagitis, gastritis, and duodenitis.
   - **Limitations:** EGD does not allow for the quantitation of the number of reflux episodes and cannot be used to evaluate malrotation or gastrointestinal dysmotility. EGD is more invasive and costly than the above tests.

111. What places premature infants at increased risk of side effects from cisapride?
- Immaturity of cytochrome P450 system
- Increased risk of uncorrected electrolyte abnormalities involving potassium, calcium, and magnesium
- Increased risk of intracranial hemorrhage

112. What treatments are available for GER in infants?
Nonpharmacologic:
- Smaller volume feeds given more frequently
- Thickened formula
- Avoidance of seated or supine positions after feeding
- Elevation of the head of the crib
- Elimination of second-hand smoke (which causes LES relaxation)

Pharmacologic:
- Antacids
- Prokinetic agents (metoclopramide, bethanechol, erythromycin)
- H_2-receptor antagonists (ranitidine, cimetidine, famotidine)
- Proton-pump inhibitors (omeprazole, lansoprazole)

Surgical:
- Transpyloric feeding tubes
- Fundoplication
- Pyloroplasty

113. What is the ideal position for infants with GER?
In the past, the prone position (with head elevated 30–45° was shown to decrease the frequency and severity of GER in infants. However, the use of this position has become controversial because of the recent American Academy of Pediatrics (AAP) statement that the prone position has been linked to sudden infant death syndrome (SIDS). Infants whose reflux can be controlled with conservative measures should follow the AAP guidelines and continue to be placed supine for sleep. However, in infants with complicated GER, the lateral decubitus or prone position provides a useful adjunct to medical therapy.

Orenstein SR: The prone alternative. Pediatrics 94:104–105, 1994.

ESOPHAGEAL ATRESIA AND TRACHEOESOPHAGEAL FISTULA

114. What are the most reliable findings in the prenatal detection of esophageal atresia by ultrasound?

Maternal hydramnios and an absent stomach bubble are the most reliable signs. However, the sensitivity and positive predictive value of prenatal ultrasound for esophageal atresia is only 50%.

115. What are the defects in the VACTERL associations?

V   Vertebral (hemivertebrae)
A   Anal (imperforate anus)
C   Cardiac (tetralogy of Fallot)
T   Trachea (tracheo-esophageal fistula)
E   Esophagus (esophageal atresia)
R   Renal (solitary kidney or vesicoureteral reflux)
L   Limb (absence of the radius)

116. What are the two most significant predictors of survival in infants with esophageal atresia?

GROUP	PREDICTORS	SURVIVAL
I	Birth weight > 1500 g *without* major cardiac defect	97%
II	Birth weight < 1500 g *or* major cardiac defect	59%
III	Birth weight < 1500 g *and* major cardiac defect	22%

117. What is the incidence of the three most common early complications following repair of esophageal atresia?

Anastomotic leak   10–15%
Esophageal stricture   30–40%
Recurrent transesophageal fistula (TEF)   5–10%

118. What are the most frequent causes of "dying" spells after repair of esophageal atresia/TEF?

Gastroesophageal reflux
Tracheomalacia
Esophageal stricture with distention of the proximal esophagus
Congenital heart disease

MALABSORPTION

119. What is an easy method of differentiating between the osmotic and secretory diarrhea?

Patients with secretory diarrhea continue to have diarrhea even after they are not fed enterally. The laboratory method of differentiating between osmotic and secretory diarrhea is the measurement of the osmotic gap in the stool, which is achieved by measuring the stool osmolality and sodium and potassium concentrations in a random sample of stool. Normal fecal osmolality is 290 mOsm/kg H_2O and normal osmotic gap is < 40 mEq/L.

$$\text{Osmotic gap} = \text{fecal osmolality} - 2 \times ([Na] + [K])$$

Osmotic gap and Na and K concentrations are expressed as mEq/L and fecal osmolality as mOsm/kg H_2O.

120. What are the most common causes of lactose malabsorption?

Almost any process damaging the mucosa of the small intestine can result in malabsorption of lactose due to secondary lactase deficiency. The most common cause of secondary lactase deficiency is mucosal damage due to infection (e.g., postviral damage). Lactase enzyme has the lowest activity of any brush border disaccharidases and is localized at the tip of the villus, thus making it vulnerable in a brush border injury during the time of infection. It is the first enzyme to be affected and the last one to recover following mucosal damage.

121. In carbohydrate malabsorption what are the stool characteristics, and why does diarrhea occur?

Stools in carbohydrate malabsorption are acidic, with a pH of less than 5.5 (due to the fermentation), and are positive for reducing substances (sugar). Reducing substances will be negative in the stool in the face of carbohydrate malabsorption, if the sugar is not a reducing sugar (e.g., sucrose). In that situation, the stool sample will need to be hydrolyzed with 0.1 N HCl and boiled briefly to break up the sucrose before being tested.

The malabsorbed carbohydrate induces an osmotic fluid shift in the small intestine resulting in increase in fluid delivery to the colon. There, the carbohydrate is fermented by colonic bacterial flora to organic acids such as lactic acid, yielding increase in the osmolality beyond the colon's salvage capacity. Colonic bacteria ferment carbohydrate in a process known as **colonic scavenging**. The main by-products of fermentation are short chain fatty acids, which can be used as a source of energy by the epithelial cells of the colon.

122. Is a 72-hour fecal fat collection useful for detecting fat malabsorption in the neonate?

The 72-hour fecal fat collection is only useful if patients are receiving a diet containing long chain fat as the only source of fat in the diet. The standard method used for quantitation of fat does not detect medium chain triglycerides. A 72-hour dietary record must be obtained simultaneously so that the coefficient of fat absorption can be obtained.

123. What is the coefficient of fat absorption in infants less than 6 months of age?

The coefficient of fat absorption in infants less than 6 months of age is 85%.

124. How does one detect protein malabsorption?

Protein malabsorption can be detected by the determination of a 24-hour fecal alpha$_1$-antitrypsin clearance. Alpha$_1$-antitrypsin is a normal, low–molecular weight body protein that leaks into the gut concomitantly with albumin. Wherever bowel damage, significant inflammation, or malabsorption of protein occurs, elevated amounts of alpha$_1$-antitrypsin will be lost in the stool. A 24-hour quantitative stool collection kept frozen and a single red top tube for serum alpha$_1$-antitrypsin levels are necessary for the interpretation.

125. How common is primary lactase deficiency in the neonate?

Contrary to common belief, primary or congenital lactase deficiency is a very rare disease with only a few dozen cases reported in the literature. The disease is manifested by severe diarrhea while the infant is on a lactose-containing formula or breast-feeding, and it starts within the first few hours or days of life.

126. What is microvillus inclusion disease?

This very rare congenital disease is often quoted as a common cause of neonatal diarrhea. The major manifestation is severe secretory diarrhea unresponsive to withdrawal of oral diet. Diagnosis is based on a small bowel biopsy where shortened enterocyte microvilli with microvillus inclusions are seen on electron microscopy. The etiology is unknown, and prognosis is poor.

Other uncommon causes of congenital diarrhea include autoimmune enteropathy, enterocolitis associated with Hirschsprung disease, necrotizing enterocolitis stricture, primary lactase deficiency, chloride diarrhea, microvillus atrophy, bile acid malabsorption, and enterokinase deficiency.

127. What is the cause of diarrhea in a neonate fed exclusively Pedialyte?

If other causes of diarrhea (e.g., infections) are excluded, glucose/galactose malabsorption (GGM) is a possibility since the carbohydrate in Pedialyte is dextrose (form of glucose monohydrate).

GGM is an autosomal recessive disease caused by a missense mutation in SGLT1 gene resulting in a complete loss of Na+-dependent glucose transporter, which mediates glucose absorption in the brush border of the intestine. The treatment is elimination of glucose and galactose from the diet.

128. Is there a test to assess the absorptive integrity of the small intestine?

D-xylose absorption test is a useful tool frequently used for the evaluation of small intestine integrity and to screen for carbohydrate malabsorption. D-xylose is a 5-carbon sugar handled similarly to natural 6-carbon sugars via high-efficiency proximal small bowel uptake. It is not metabolized and is rapidly excreted in the urine. Thus, it is ideally suited to test the most basic of carbohydrate pathways. The test is performed in a fasting patient who is given 14.5 g/m^2 of D-xylose orally as a 10 gm% solution. One hour later, a serum level of the D-xylose is measured. Alternatively, intestinal biopsies can be obtained and sent for histopathology and disaccharidase measurements.

129. A 21-year-old pregnant woman was diagnosed with polyhydramnios. A prenatal ultrasound study demonstrated distended loops of small intestine. The baby was delivered at 33 weeks' gestation by cesarean section, and at the time of delivery the amniotic fluid was noted to contain yellow-green stool. On day 2 of life, the infant developed a hypochloremic metabolic alkalosis and loose stools. A stool sample contained high concentrations of chloride. What is the most likely diagnosis in this case?

The following features of this case suggest a diagnosis of congenital chloride diarrhea:
• High concentrations of fecal chloride (exceeding the sum of sodium and potassium)
• Polyhydramnios
• Distended loops of bowel on a prenatal ultrasound
• Prematurity

This is an autosomal recessive disease caused by a defect in chloride-bicarbonate exchange transport system in the ileum and colon resulting in a life-long secretory diarrhea. The diagnosis is made by high concentration of fecal chloride. Treatment consists of fluid and electrolyte replacement—initially intravenously and then orally. If diagnosed and treated early, the prognosis is excellent.

130. What are the mechanisms responsible for diarrhea in short gut syndrome?

• Decreased absorptive surface area
• Rapid transit time
• Bacterial overgrowth
• Hypersecretion of motility hormones and impaired regulation of gut motility
• Decreased absorption of bile salts (the unabsorbed bile salts are deconjugated by anaerobic bacteria causing inhibition and even net secretion of water and electrolytes)
• Steatorrhea (secondary to decreased availability of bile salts)
• Loss of the ileocecal valve (this permits reflux of colonic bacteria contributing to bacterial overgrowth)
• Colonic resection (the colon is where most fluid reabsorption occurs)

131. What are the anatomic causes of gastric outlet obstruction in the neonate and infant?

• Hypertrophic pyloric stenosis
• Antral and pyloric membranes
• Eosinophilic gastroenteritis
• Aberrant pancreatic tissue
• Duplication cyst of antrum or duodenum
• Pyloric channel ulcer
• Pyloric atresia

132. What are the radiographic findings of pyloric stenosis?

Signs (British terminology in parentheses) that indirectly image the pyloric mass include:
• Shoulder = mass effect on the lesser curvature of the gastric antrum
• Teat (nipple) = peristaltic waves encroaching on the mass and the shoulder

- Beak = barium entering only the entrance of the pyloric canal
- String = barium extending into the narrowed and elongated pyloric canal
- U (string) = upturned course of the pyloric canal towards the duodenum
- Track (tram) = parallel columns of barium in the pyloric canal produced by longitudinal infolding of the pyloric mucosa
- Caterpillar = gastric contour distorted by multiple deep peristaltic waves
- Mushroom = encroachment of the base of the duodenal bulb by the hypertrophic muscle mass
- String and beak together (umbrella)

HIRSCHSPRUNG DISEASE

133. What is Hirschsprung disease?

Hirschsprung disease results from the failure of the parasympathetic nervous system to fully invest the digestive tract. Because the parasympathetic ganglion cells migrate from cranial to caudal, arrest of this migration results in the intestine beyond the arrest being unable to relax and propagate a peristaltic wave. Despite anatomic continuity of the intestine, there is a functional obstruction at the point of farthest migration of the ganglion cells. The ganglion cells are supposed to live between the muscular coats of the bowel (Meissner's plexus) and the submucosa (Auerbach's plexus).

134. Who gets Hirschsprung disease?

Hirschsprung disease is the most common form of neonatal intestinal obstruction. It typically occurs in term white males. The transition zone is usually in the sigmoid colon. The disease can occur in families and have other stigmata associated with it. The many exceptions to the typical case (term white males) often have more extensive (more proximal) transition zones.

135. How is the diagnosis made?

The typical newborn with Hirschsprung disease fails to pass meconium in the first 24 hours of life. A distended abdomen and sepsis secondary to enterocolitis may compound this. The diagnosis may be *suggested* by a contrast enema showing a change in colonic caliber. Only a rectal biopsy showing no ganglion cells in either Auerbach's or Meissner's plexus makes the diagnosis. The biopsy may show hypertrophied parasympathetic nerve bundle, which stain very intensely for acetylcholinesterase. The diagnosis can be ruled out by a suction rectal biopsy that shows ganglion cells in the submucosa.

136. What is the treatment?

The treatment for any surgical patient begins with resuscitation, particularly if the infant has enterocolitis. The treatment for enterocolitis consists of rectal irrigation with warm saline and intravenous antibiotics such as those used for necrotizing enterocolitis.

When the infant is resuscitated, he or she is ready for an operation. The traditional surgical treatment is a two or three stage operation. In the newborn period, a diverting colostomy is constructed at the transition zone. This site is determined intraoperatively with the help of pathologists interpreting frozen sections. Several months later, a "pull-through" operation is done to bring normally ganglionated bowel to the anoderm. There are a variety of ways to do this. The most common is the **Soave endorectal pull-through**, which removes the mucosa from the rectum that is aganglionic anteriorly and ganglionic posteriorly. The **Swenson procedure** resects the entire aganglionic rectum and brings the ganglionic bowel to the anoderm. All of these operations can work and have their proponents. Sometimes the pull-through is protected by a colostomy, which is closed as a third procedure.

More current treatment of Hirschsprung disease diagnosed in infancy is to do the pull-through when the diagnosis is made resulting in a single-stage operation. This single operation can be done with laparoscopic assistance or entirely transanally.

137. What are the early and late complications?

The immediate postoperative complications unique to Hirschsprung disease are enterocolitis and an abscess within the pull-through (cuff abscess). The abscess is drained and the fecal stream diverted (if it is not already). Enterocolitis is treated as described above.

Enterocolitis can occur almost anytime despite a technically perfect pull-through (no surgeon will admit to anything but a technically perfect result!). When it becomes a chronic problem, it may be associated with bacterial translocation. Although usually self-limited, it may be useful to rebiopsy the end of the GI tract to ensure the presence of ganglion cells.

138. What disorders are associated with Hirschsprung disease?

Down syndrome (2.9%)	Neuroblastoma
Waardenburg syndrome	Neurofibromatosis
Laurence-Moon-Biedl syndrome	Medullary carcinoma of the thyroid
Smith-Lemli-Opitz syndrome	Carcinoid tumors
Ondine's curse	Paragangliomas
Pheochromocytoma	

139. How should a family with Hirschsprung disease be counseled?
• The exact hereditary pattern is unclear.
• More than one-third of patients have a relative with a similar condition.
• Familial occurrence increases the length of the aganglionic segment.

140. What screening test should be done in every infant with Hirschsprung disease?

Sensorineural hearing loss is more common in infants with Hirschsprung disease, and all infants should be screened.

141. What are the clinical presentations of Hirschsprung disease?
• Failure to pass meconium in the first 24 hours of life
• Progressive constipation
• Abdominal distention
• Bilious vomiting
• Foul-smelling liquid stools associated with abdominal distention
• Urinary obstruction with hydronephrosis
• Protein losing enteropathy and failure to thrive
• Enterocolitis

142. What other medical conditions are associated with delayed passage of stool?

Sepsis	Maternal narcotic administration
Hypermagnesemia	Adrenal insufficiency
Hypothyroidism	Central nervous system (CNS) disorders

MALROTATION AND MIDGUT VOLVULUS

143. What are malrotation and nonrotation?

Normal rotation is 270°; any rotation that is less than complete has some element of malrotation. Nonrotation, or return of the gut to the abdomen without rotation, is reported in 0.5–2.0% of patients at autopsy or during contrast GI studies. Rarely is nonrotation pathologic. Because malrotation can occur with varying degrees of rotation, the exact placement of the GI tract as found during surgery is variable. However, the most common findings are a duodenum that does not cross the midline on upper GI studies and a cecum that is high-riding or superior to the transverse colon in the right upper quadrant (see figure, top of next page.

144. Do all patients with malrotation become symptomatic?

No, but most do so at a very young age.

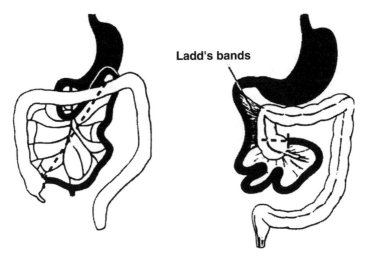

Ladd's bands

Left, The cecum descends into the right lower quadrant. Note the normal broadness of the small bowel mesentery (*dashed line*). *Right*, In malrotation, the duodenal loop typically lacks 90° of its normal 270° rotation, and the cecocolic loop lacks 180° of its normal rotation.

145. What causes the symptoms?

A midgut volvulus is the most common and catastrophic cause of symptoms in patients with malrotation; 30% occur in the first week of life, and 50% occur before 1 month of age. Midgut volvulus results from the narrow mesenteric base (see figure in question 144, right image). The small bowel hangs down in the abdomen like a bell clapper. This position allows the bowel to twist, become obstructed, and cause symptoms.

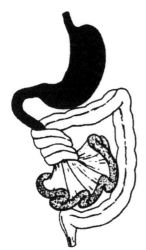

In midgut volvulus, the small bowel becomes supported only by a narrow pedicle containing the superior mesenteric artery. As a result, the small bowel may twist in a clockwise direction about this narrow axis.

146. How do patients with malrotation and midgut volvulus present?

Bilious (green) vomiting is the sentinel event, occurring in > 95% of patients with malrotation and midgut volvulus. The most common scenario is green vomiting for no reason in an infant who has a flat abdomen (initially), is afebrile, and has not been previously ill. The infant may become jittery, tachycardic, pale, and diaphoretic. Abdominal distress and rectal bleeding may occur, although they are late and ominous signs.

147. If an infant has bilious vomiting, what should be done?

If no other explanation is apparent (e.g., bilious vomiting with profuse diarrhea and fever may identify a systemic infection, such as gastroenteritis), an immediate evaluation for malrotation should be done. *Unexplained bilious vomiting in an infant is a surgical emergency until proved otherwise.* An immediate upper GI contrast study is ordered to determine the position of the duodenojejunal junction (ligament of Treitz), or a contrast enema is done to determine the position of the cecum in the right lower quadrant. Most pediatric surgeons prefer the upper GI series.

148. If the diagnosis is delayed, what may occur?

Dead bowel may mean a dead baby in as little as 6 hours. Midgut volvulus is characterized by a 720° twist of the bowel around the axis of the superior mesenteric artery (SMA). This twist, caused by the narrow mesenteric base created by the malrotation, occludes first venous outflow, then arterial inflow to the gut. Ischemia, bleeding, necrosis, and perforation relentlessly and quickly ensue.

149. Besides upper GI and contrast enema, what other studies help to diagnose malrotation and midgut volvulus?

Ultrasound may suggest malrotation by picking up the relationship of the SMA, superior mesenteric vein (SMV), and duodenum. Normally the SMV lies to the right of the SMA. If their relationship is different (left or anterior), malrotation may be the cause. However, this test is not as specific or accurate as GI contrast studies.

150. What other diagnoses can be confused with malrotation?

Any anomaly or disease that causes obstruction of the upper GI tract can be confused with malrotation, including:
- Duodenal atresia
- Gastric or duodenal web (windsock deformity)
- Proximal jejunal atresia
- Duplication of the duodenum and proximal jejunum with compression and obstruction
- Necrotizing enterocolitis

INTESTINAL ATRESIAS

151. What is the etiology of intestinal atresia?

Jejunal and ileal atresia are believed due to an intrauterine vascular accident (which would include an intrauterine intussusception with infarction). However, in duodenal atresia, the etiology is thought to be failure of recanalization of the bowel lumen at the second portion of the duodenum. Therefore, duodenal atresia is a true malformation and is commonly associated with other extraintestinal malformations.

152. Can intestinal atresias be diagnosed prenatally?

In the case of duodenal atresia, there is a well-described pathognomonic finding of a "double bubble." This finding was first described in abdominal radiographs obtained postnatally. However, this imaging sign is frequently present on prenatal ultrasound studies. Prenatal diagnosis of jejunal and ileal atresia is more difficult, and ultrasound is unreliable.

153. Is there a role for fetal intervention in the correction of intestinal atresia?

Because there are no progressive adverse effects from intestinal obstruction in utero and the postnatal correction of intestinal atresia has an excellent prognosis, there is no defined role for prenatal intervention.

154. What are the two most common clinical symptoms or signs of intestinal atresia?

For duodenal atresia—bilious emesis and a scaphoid (flat) abdomen
For jejunal atresia—bilious emesis and mild abdominal distention
For ileal atresia—bilious emesis and significant abdominal distention

155. Which type of intestinal atresia is associated with trisomy 21?

Infants with duodenal atresia have a significant (approximately 30%) incidence of Down syndrome. In addition, it is important to look for associated anomalies that include a more distal intestinal obstruction (atresia, web), congenital cardiac anomalies, and imperforate anus.

156. What is the optimal radiographic study to make the diagnosis of jejunal atresia?

Plain abdominal radiographs will demonstrate dilated small bowel loops indicative of a proximal to mid small intestine obstruction. There is no advantage to performing an upper GI contrast study.

157. What is the optimum imaging study in an infant with significant abdominal distention and multiple dilated small intestine loops on a plain abdominal radiograph?

The description may be suggestive of ileal atresia. However, meconium ileus and total colonic Hirschsprung disease can produce similar abdominal radiographic findings. Thus, the optimum imaging study to define the etiology of apparent distal intestinal obstruction is a contrast enema.

158. Why is it important to differentiate between ileal atresia and meconium ileus?

Many infants with meconium ileus can be managed nonoperatively with Gastrografin enemas. The presence of meconium ileus strongly suggests cystic fibrosis.

159. What nongastrointestinal anomaly is associated with jejunal atresia?

There are none.

160. Do infants with intestinal atresia require immediate surgery?

Unless there is evidence of bowel perforation at the time of birth, there is no benefit from urgent surgical intervention. These infants do require intravenous fluids and nasogastric decompression. Most neonatal centers also institute preoperative intravenous antibiotics. Surgical correction should be undertaken within 12–24 hours of birth.

161. What is the prognosis for newborns with intestinal atresia?

In the recent past, the outcome for surgical correction of duodenal, jejunal, or ileal atresia has been excellent. Mortality is rare and morbidity is uncommon.

162. What are the congenital gastrointestinal anomalies associated with trisomy 21?

As many as 22–30% of patients with duodenal atresia and duodenal stenosis have Down syndrome. Annular pancreas has a high frequency of association with duodenal stenosis, duodenal atresia, and therefore Down syndrome. Other associated anomalies include malrotation, esophageal atresia, imperforate anus, small bowel atresia, and biliary atresia. Two percent to 15% of patients with Hirschsprung disease also have Down syndrome.

GASTROSCHISIS AND OMPHALOCELE

163. What is the incidence of omphalocele and gastroschisis?

The incidence of gastroschisis and omphalocele is approximately 1 in 2000 births. Over the past several decades, the incidence of gastroschisis has increased, whereas the incidence of omphalocele has remained unchanged.

164. What syndromes are associated with omphalocele?

Several genetic syndromes are associated with omphaloceles:

1. Pentalogy of Cantrell
2. Lower midline syndrome (bladder or cloacal extrophy)
3. Beckwith-Wiedemann syndrome
4. Several trisomies (e.g., trisomy 13 and 18)
5. Charge association
6. Prune-belly syndrome
7. Meckel-Gruber syndrome

In addition, cardiac anomalies are common in infants with omphalocele, particularly tetralogy of Fallot and atrial septal defects.

165. What syndromes are associated with gastroschisis?

Gastroschisis is not associated with genetic syndromes. However, approximately 10% of cases of gastroschisis are associated with intestinal atresia.

166. What is the importance of prenatal diagnosis?

Detection of abdominal wall defects in utero is important for several reasons. In the case of omphaloceles, a search for associated anomalies is made. Results affect prenatal care, timing and mode of delivery, and, in the case of multiple severe anomalies, potential termination of pregnancy. In addition, early parental counseling can be initiated with perinatologists, obstetricians, neonatologists, pediatric surgeons, ethicists. Such a team approach optimizes prenatal, perinatal, and postnatal care by involving all caregivers who understand the therapeutic options and natural history of the birth defect.

167. What is the best method for delivering a child with an abdominal wall defect?

Most studies show that cesarean section provides no significant advantage over vaginal delivery. One exception is the fetus with a large omphalocele. Several reports have documented dystocia and liver damage during vaginal delivery.

168. Define the principles of immediate postnatal management in infants with abdominal wall defects.

Infants born with abdominal wall defects are subject to three serious problems at birth. Management is directed at correcting **hypovolemia**, preventing **hypothermia**, and monitoring for signs of **sepsis**. Exposed bowel leads to increased loss of insensible fluid as well as heat loss. Immediate management includes placing the lower half of the infant, including exposed viscera, in a bowel bag ("turkey bag") or wrapping the viscera in sterile gauze; placing the infant in a warmer; initiating intravenous access and fluids; obtaining an airway in cases of respiratory distress; and placement of an orogastric tube to decompress the bowel and decrease the risk of aspiration. Parenteral antibiotics also are initiated soon after delivery to decrease the risk of sepsis.

169. What are the options for surgical closure? How do you choose between them?

There are essentially two options: primary closure or staged closure. Most infants with gastroschisis can be closed primarily (80–90%), but primary closure should not be performed if it will significantly compromise ventilation or abdominal viscera. Reduction usually is performed under general anesthesia with careful attention to ventilation. A maximal ventilatory pressure of 25 cm can be used as a safe guideline to determine whether primary closure is feasible. If primary closure is not deemed safe, a staged procedure is performed (i.e., silo formation).

170. What is staged closure?

Staged closure involves placing a reinforced silastic silo over the exposed viscera and attaching it to the fascia. Silos come in prefabricated versions or can be custom fabricated using sheets of reinforced silastic (0.03-inch thickness). Slowly the silo contents are reduced into the abdominal cavity. Most infants can be closed within 7–10 days using this method. The silo protects the herniated bowel and redirects the pressure in the abdomen to promote enlargement of the abdominal cavity.

171. How can one distinguish an omphalocele from a gastroschisis by visual inspection?

- **Location of defect.** A gastroschisis is located lateral to the cord (usually on the right), whereas omphaloceles are defects of the umbilical ring.
- **Cord.** The cord inserts into the sac in an omphalocele and is inserted normally in a gastroschisis.

- **Sac.** A gastroschisis has no sac. An omphalocele usually has a sac or, if it ruptures in utero, a remnant of a sac.
- **Defect size.** Omphaloceles normally have larger defects.
- **Content of defect.** Gastroschisis contains hollow viscera and occasionally tubes and ovaries, but never liver. Omphaloceles, on the other hand, commonly contain liver as well as all of the above.

172. What is the long-term outlook for children with abdominal wall defects?

Studies have shown that such children are prone to growth delay and lower IQ, even with normal bowel function.

MECONIUM ILEUS AND MECONIUM PLUG

173. What are meconium ileus and meconium plug? What is the relationship to cystic fibrosis?

Meconium ileus is a form of distal small bowel obstruction secondary to thick and viscid meconium. Approximately 10–20% of neonates with cystic fibrosis will present with meconium ileus. All neonates diagnosed with meconium ileus must be considered as having cystic fibrosis until proven otherwise. In cystic fibrosis, pancreatic and intestinal secretions are abnormal leading to a meconium that has a high protein content. The abnormal composition, combined with intestinal glandular dysfunction and an abnormal concentrating process in the proximal small bowel, leads to the formation of a highly viscid tenacious meconium in utero. This thickened substance fills the lumen of the small bowel and causes a mechanical bowel obstruction. Typically the distal ileum and proximal colon contain inspissated pellets of meconium whereas the proximal dilated small bowel contains thick and tenacious meconium. The entire colon is of small caliber (also known as **microcolon**) because of lack of use.

Meconium plug is a form of neonatal intestinal obstruction caused by an obstructing plug of meconium, typically at the level of the sigmoid and descending colon. The pathogenesis is poorly understood but is believed to be secondary to immature myenteric nervous system causing ineffective peristalsis, followed by excessive water absorption from the colon, which results in the development of segments of thick meconium that plugs and obstructs the colon. It is not associated with cystic fibrosis although it is possible to have a patient with cystic fibrosis present with meconium plug syndrome. Since the plug is usually located in the left colon, it is not associated with microcolon. However, the obstructed portion of the colon is of small caliber and it may resemble **small left colon syndrome** (see question 175).

174. List the main differences between meconium ileus and meconium plug.

Both meconium ileus and meconium plug can be a cause of intestinal obstruction in neonates. The clinical presentation is typically similar, with bilious vomiting, abdominal distention, and failure to pass meconium as the hallmark findings. The pediatrician must be able to differentiate between the two because management strategies and long-term outcome are quite different. The following table is a useful guideline:

	MECONIUM PLUG	MECONIUM ILEUS
Bilious vomiting	Yes	Yes
Abdominal distention	Yes	Yes
Abdominal x-ray appearance	Diffuse gas distention with lack of gas in the rectum	Soap-bubble or ground-glass appearance*
Associated with cystic fibrosis	No (rarely)	Yes
Associated with Hirschsprung disease	Yes	No
Usually resolves after contrast enema	No (success rate of 50–60%)	Yes (success rate > 90%)

* Also known as Neuhauser's sign (secondary to the mixing of air in the dilated loops of small bowel with the thick meconium, usually in the right lower quadrant of the abdomen).

175. What is small left colon syndrome?

Although meconium plug and meconium ileus are frequently associated with the presence of a small and unused colon (microcolon), this should not be confused with small left colon syndrome. Small left colon syndrome is a dysfunctional, atrophied left colon that causes transient obstructive symptoms and can be rarely associated with complications such as an intestinal perforation. Approximately 50% of infants with this disorder are born to diabetic mothers, almost all of whom are insulin dependent. The obstruction is typically partial and involves the descending and sigmoid colon distal to the splenic flexure. The degree of obstruction varies. Proximal perforation, especially of the cecum, has been described. One hypothesis suggests that the pathogenesis is related to hypoglycemia-induced release of glucagon in the infant. Glucagon acts as a smooth muscle constrictive chemical. The obstructive symptoms usually resolve within 48 hours as the infants' endogenous insulin output normalizes in the postpartum period.

176. What is the treatment of meconium ileus and meconium plug?

In the presence of any suspected distal intestinal obstruction in a neonate, a contrast enema with water-soluble contrast (Gastrografin) is indicated. If the patient is found to have meconium ileus or meconium plug, the radiographic test can often be therapeutic. More than 90% of neonates with meconium plug will have resolution of their symptoms within 24–48 hours after the study with passage of several meconium plugs and rapid improvement of the abdominal distention. In cases of meconium ileus, the success rate of the contrast enema is not as good. Because the obstruction is caused by a significant amount of inspissated meconium and meconium pellets, repeat contrast enemas with hyperosmolar dye (using 2:1 or 3:1 dilutions of Gastrografin) are frequently necessary. Such method of intermittent retrograde colonic irrigation, combined with aggressive fluid resuscitation, and the use of N-acetylcysteine by orogastric tube, has a reported success rate of 50–60% in cases of uncomplicated meconium ileus.

177. What is *complicated meconium ileus* and what is the treatment?

Complicated meconium ileus refers to the condition in which the initial intestinal obstruction has resulted in intra-abdominal problems such as intestinal perforation, peritonitis (with or without calcification), volvulus, intestinal atresia, ascites, and abdominal pseudocyst (also known as giant meconium cyst). Under such circumstances, treatment will always include an operative exploration (laparotomy).

178. What are the indications for surgery in patients with meconium ileus?

Neonates with uncomplicated meconium ileus that have failed two or three therapeutic enemas and *all* neonates with complicated meconium ileus (as listed above) require operative intervention. It is important to remember that meconium ileus was generally a fatal condition until 1948, when Hiatt and Wilson described the successful management with enterotomy and saline irrigation of the obstructing meconium pellets.

179. What type of surgery is typically performed in complicated cases of meconium ileus?

In 1957, Bishop and Koop described the technique of resection of the dilated ileal segment and proximal end-to-distal side ileal anastomosis with distal ostomy, also known as the **Bishop-Koop ileostomy**. This procedure minimizes contamination, allows for anastomosis between appropriately sized bowel, provides access to the distal bowel for decompression and irrigation, and allows for bedside closure of the stoma once the obstruction has resolved. Various irrigating solutions have been used, including normal saline, Gastrografin, hydrogen peroxide, and 2% to 4% solutions of N-acetylcysteine. The figures (next page) illustrate the typical findings of meconium ileus with obstruction and the technique of the Bishop-Koop ileostomy.

180. What is the operative approach if the patient has meconium ileus with suspected intestinal perforation?

If the infant has had a perforation with peritonitis, one must determine the degree of peritonitis. If perforation occurs just before delivery, meconium ascites without calcification is present,

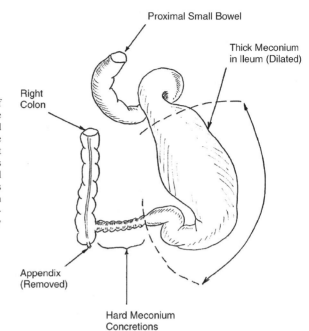

Typical appearance, at the time of operative exploration, of a neonate with meconium ileus that failed nonoperative management. Note the dilated ileum proximal to the point of obstruction. Thick and viscous meconium is found in the dilated segment, and hard meconium pellets are found on the segment of ileum that is causing the complete mechanical obstruction. The massively dilated bowel must be resected.

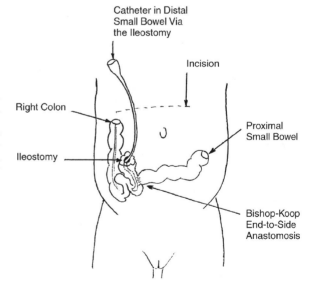

Creation of the Bishop-Koop ileostomy after segmental ileal resection for management of meconium ileus. A catheter can be placed in the ileostomy for postoperative irrigation of the distal ileum and colon that still contain thick and partially obstructing meconium.

whereas if it occurs several weeks or months before delivery, calcification and dense adhesions develop. Occasionally a fibrous wall forms around the meconium leading to a pseudocyst, often referred to as **giant cystic meconium peritonitis.** Operative repair of the obstruction can be difficult because of the adhesions, which are usually quite vascular. The goal is relief of the obstruction and, if possible, restoration of bowel continuity or creation of a Bishop-Koop ileostomy (temporary). Ostomy closure is usually safe 6–8 weeks later. TPN may be necessary if inadequate bowel length is available for feeding.

181. In the newborn, what are the three most common gastrointestinal manifestations of cystic fibrosis?

1. **Meconium ileus** is the earliest clinical manifestation of cystic fibrosis. Between 10% and 20% of patients with cystic fibrosis develop intestinal obstruction in utero during the last trimester of development. Abdominal distention is marked with no passage of meconium. The obstruction is secondary to mass of extremely thick, tenacious meconium, which adheres to the wall of the distal small bowel and impacts the lumen.

2. The most common complication is **volvulus** of meconium-laden loops, frequently associated with ischemia, necrosis, perforation, and peritonitis. Twisted devitalized loops may become adherent, lose their continuity with the intestinal lumen, and form a gelatinous pseudocyst.

3. Spillage of meconium into the peritoneal cavity following antenatal intestinal perforation results in the development of **meconium peritonitis**. Meconium peritonitis may be seen before birth on ultrasound and presents as calcifications of the abdomen during the newborn period.

IMPERFORATE ANUS

182. How is imperforate anus diagnosed?

One of the simpler anomalies to diagnose, one need only look! Part of the newborn examination, verification of a patent and functioning anus is the standard of care prior to discharge. Rectal atresia might be missed during a cursory exam because the anus can appear normal, but failure to pass meconium and increasing distention would bring this related, unusual condition to attention.

183. How frequently is imperforate anus associated with other anomalies?

Associated spinal and genitourinary anomalies are rather common, occurring in 20% to over 50% of imperforate anus cases. Part of the VATER or VACTERL association, imperforate anus may be accompanied by TEF, ventricular septal defects, renal abnormalities, or radial limb anomalies. Part of the work-up of imperforate anus is the search for its commonly associated anomalies.

184. In contemporary parlance, how is imperforate anus classified?

Until recently, imperforate anus was classified into "high" and "low" based on the distal extent of the rectum relative to a line connecting the pubis and the coccyx (the levator muscle). This classification is not useful in that it does not readily translate into an operative plan or a prognosis. The following chart details the anatomy by patient sex, operative strategy, and prognosis for voluntary bowel movement.

SEX	FISTULA ENDS	OPERATIVE STRATEGY	PROGNOSIS FOR VOLUNTARY BOWEL MOVEMENT
Male	Perineum*	Newborn anoplasty No colostomy	100%
	Bulbar urethra	Colostomy, PSARP	About 80%
	Prostatic urethra	Colostomy, PSARP	About 65%
	Bladder neck	Colostomy, PSARP	About 15%
Female	Perineum*	Newborn anoplasty No colostomy	100%
	Vaginal fourchette	Colostomy, PSARP	About 90%
	Vagina	Colostomy, PSARP	About 70%
	Cloaca	Colostomy, PSARVUP	About 70%

* Includes anal stenosis and anal membrane
PSARP = posterior sagittal anorectalplasty; PSARVUP = anorectalvaginourethroplasty

185. What factors determine the initial management of an infant with imperforate anus?

Inspection and **urinalysis** are able to determine the initial therapy in about 90% of cases. If the baby has a flat bottom without a well-developed gluteal fold or has meconium in the urine, a colostomy is indicated. Conversely, in the setting of a bucket handle deformity or meconium staining in the perineal midline, a newborn minimal PSARP is indicated without colostomy. In girls, only demonstration of a perineal fistula will avoid a colostomy. These decisions are all made after 16–24 hours in order to permit increased luminal pressure to force meconium through a fistula so that it is noted on exam. In all cases, an abdominal ultrasound is obtained to exclude other anomalies.

The invertogram is passé and no longer needed. In the few cases (< 10% of the time) where inspection and urinalysis cannot provide a provisional diagnosis and plan, a cross-table lateral film with the baby in the prone position can determine the extent of the fistula relative to a marker placed on the perineum. this film should be taken at 24 hours of life to allow building of intraluminal pressure to force gas into the most distal aspect of the rectum, wherever it may lie.

186. For those infants requiring colostomy, what key features must be kept in mind?

1. The colostomy should be completely diverting. A loop colostomy permits the rectum to become distended with spillover, and this will make reconstruction problematic. Furthermore, urinary contamination continues.

2. The colostomy should be accompanied by a mucus fistula that permits future study of the distal rectal fistula; the formation of a Hartmann's pouch is absolutely contraindicated.

3. The mucus fistula should be fashioned at the redundant portion of the sigmoid and placed in the left lower quadrant to allow for pull down during a perineal operation. Other arrangements may place the distal segment under undue tension and make a perineal operation impossible without a simultaneous abdominal-pelvic operation.

187. After newborn colostomy, what key elements comprise the management of the infant with imperforate anus prior to anoplasty?

1. Complete evaluation for concomitant anomalies, particularly genitourinary and sacral. Tethered cord must also be excluded.

2. Three to 6 month waiting period to ensure growth and development.

3. "Distal colostogram" to identify the distal fistula. This permits planning the final reconstruction and allows counseling of the family about continence.

188. What should the parents be told about continence?

Continence is the ability to control bowel movements so that bowel movements are voluntary and there is no soiling between movements. The potential for voluntary bowel movements is excellent for most infants as seen in the table above. Soiling is fairly frequent, however, and true continence is not obtained in many cases.

ANATOMY	VOLUNTARY MOVEMENTS (%)	SOILING (%)	CONTINENCE (%)
Perineal fistula	100	0	100
Bulbar	80	65	35
Prostatic	65	75	25
Bladder neck	15	80	0
Vestibular	95	40	60
Vaginal	75	100	0
Cloaca	70	70	30

189. What are the most common causes of a relatively airless abdomen in the neonate?

• Esophageal atresia with no fistula
• Orotracheal intubation (prevention of air swallowing)

• Gastric suction or forceful vomiting (removal of bowel gas)
• Marked electrolyte imbalance (fluid containing loops of bowel)
• Paralytic therapy (pavulon) (elimination of swallowing mechanism)
• Severe neonatal sepsis

GASTROINTESTINAL HEMORRHAGE

190. How does one determine if swallowed maternal blood is the cause for GI bleeding in the neonate?
Using the Apt-Downey test. For this test, 1 part stool is mixed with 5 parts water in a test tube and centrifuged for 2 minutes to separate out fecal material. The supernatant is removed, and 1 ml of 0.25 N (1%) sodium hydroxide is mixed with 5 ml of the supernatant. After 2 minutes there is a color change; if the hemoglobin is fetal, the color stays pink, and if it is adult in origin, it turns a yellow-brown color.

191. What are the common causes of acute upper GI bleeding in the critically ill newborn?
Stress ulcers and gastritis occur more frequently in the critically ill newborn and can be associated with significant blood loss and (on rare occasions) gastric perforation.

192. Describe the different characteristics of rectal bleeding in the newborn and the diseases associated.

Characteristics	Associated diseases
Normal stools with blood flecks or streaks (focal bleeding site)	Rectal fissure
Bloody diarrhea (colitis)	Dietary protein-induced colitis, necrotizing enterocolitis (NEC), Hirschsprung enterocolitis, infectious colitis
Passage of large quantities of red or black blood	Swallowed maternal blood, upper GI bleeding, hemorrhagic disorder (vitamin K deficiency, hemophilia, thrombocytopenia), Meckel's diverticulum

193. What are some of the risk factors and clinical features that help distinguish NEC from other causes of gastrointestinal bleeding in a neonate?
NEC tends to be more common in premature infants and often occurs in those who have experienced some type of perinatal stress such as hypoxic injury, need for mechanical ventilation, and sepsis. In addition to the presence of gross or occult blood in the stools, feeding intolerance, abdominal distention, bilious emesis, and lethargy should all lead to consideration of NEC in the differential diagnosis.

194. What should be the first step in the management of an acutely ill infant with significant GI bleeding?
The key first step is obtaining adequate, sustainable intravenous access. Because of the smaller blood volume of the newborn, significant bleeding can be associated with hypotension of rapid onset, requiring aggressive fluid management and volume-replacement therapy.

NECROTIZING ENTEROCOLITIS

It is said that faith can move mountains, but how do we get to move the bowels of the extremely low birth weight infants?
                                                                Avroy A. Fanaroff

195. What is necrotizing enterocolitis (NEC)?
NEC is a disease of unknown origin that affects premature infants after the onset of enteral alimentation during convalescence from the common cardiopulmonary disorders associated with

prematurity. Manifestations cover a broad spectrum from mild abdominal distention with hema-
tochezia to a fulminant septic shock-like picture with transmural necrosis of the entire gastrointestinal tract (NEC totalis).

196. Which infants are at risk for developing NEC?

NEC typically occurs in infants with a corrected-gestational age of 30–32 weeks when
most premature infants are on progressive enteral feedings. Onset of NEC is unusual on the first
day of life and highly uncommon among infants who have not received enteral feeds. NEC may
occur sporadically, but often affected patients are clustered in place and time. Although an infectious etiology is often sought, no consistent agent has been isolated from all reported epidemics.

Many associated risk factors have been suggested, which are not necessarily associated
with the pathogenesis of NEC. Thus, when investigated in carefully controlled studies, risk factors such as perinatal asphyxia, respiratory distress syndrome, umbilical catheters, patent ductus
arteriosus, hypotension, and anemia have not been demonstrated to be more common among patients who developed NEC than among unaffected age-matched controls. The most dominant risk
factor for NEC is the degree of immaturity.

197. How are breast-milk–fed infants thought to be protected from NEC?

Breast milk may reduce the risk of NEC. Breast milk offers many nutritive advantages in
addition to non-nutritive advantages. Milk macrophages and phagocytes, immunoglobulins IgA
and IgG, and immunocompetent T and B lymphocytes may offer a protective advantage to the
mucosa. These components potentiate the effect of complements (C3 and C4), lysozyme, lactoferrin, and secretory IgA. Breast milk contains hormones (thyroid, TSH, prolactin, steroid), enzymes (amylase, lipase), and growth factors (EGF). Breast milk also favors the growth of
Lactobacillus bifidus and promotes a healthy gut flora.

198. What feeding risk factors have been associated with the development of NEC?

The absence of NEC in utero suggests an absolute requirement for gut colonization in its
pathogenesis. Host luminal pH, proteases, oxygen tension, temperature, and osmolarity of enteral
feedings have been implicated in the pathogenesis of NEC. The volume of milk fed to infants
may also predispose to NEC. Excessively rapid increments of milk feeding may overcome the
infant's intestinal absorptive capability especially in the presence of altered motility, resulting
in malabsorption.

Large-volume milk feedings that are increased too rapidly during the feeding schedule may
place undue stress on a previously injured or immature intestine. Two studies have shown that
volume increments in excess of 20–25 ml/kg/day have been associated with NEC, whereas another two studies have shown safety of 30–35 ml/kg/day increments. Therefore, volume increments should not be more than 20–35 ml/kg/day and should be based on normal clinical
examination, physiologic stability, and absence of feeding intolerance.

199. What is the gas in pneumatosis intestinalis?

Malabsorbed carbohydrates contribute to enhanced intestinal bacterial gas production, resulting in abdominal distention. This gas dissects into the submucosa and subserosa producing
pneumatosis intestinalis; it is 30–40% hydrogen gas. High intraluminal pressure from gaseous
distention may reduce mucosal blood flow, producing secondary intestinal ischemia.

200. What infective agents are associated with NEC?

In many cases of NEC, no infective agent is identifiable. Bacteria identified by positive
blood cultures are seen in only 20–30% of patients with NEC. *Staphylococcus epidermidis* is the
most common organism, followed by gram-negative bacilli such as *Escherichia coli* and
Klebsiella. Epidemics have been associated with a single pathogen such as *E. coli*, *Klebsiella*,
Salmonella, *Staphylococcus epidermidis*, *Clostridium butyricum*, *Coronavirus*, *Rotavirus*, and
enteroviruses. NEC has also been associated with fungal sepsis. NEC may also result from an

enterotoxin-mediated illness, such as toxins produced by *Clostridium* or *S. epidermidis*. It may be noted that, unlike in adults, *C. difficile* and associated toxins are found in the intestinal tracts of many neonates who are entirely asymptomatic. The asymptomatic carrier state in some infants may be due to differences in intestinal immaturity, local differences in the intestinal milieu, absence of toxin-related receptors, or undescribed protective factors.

201. What are the criteria for considering the diagnosis of NEC?

NEC is a common cause of the systemic inflammatory response syndrome (SIRS) in neonates. Based on systemic signs, intestinal signs, and radiologic signs, staging of NEC is done as shown in the table below.

STAGE	SYSTEMIC SIGNS	INTESTINAL SIGNS	RADIOLOGIC SIGNS
IA (suspected NEC)	Temperature instability, apnea, bradycardia, lethargy	Increased pregavage residuals, mild abdominal distention, emesis, guaiac-positive stool	Normal or intestinal dilatation, mild ileus
IB (suspected NEC)	Same as IA	Bright red blood per rectum	Same as IA
IIA (definite NEC, mildly ill)	Same as IA	Same as IA and IB plus diminished or absent bowel sounds ± abdominal tenderness	Intestinal dilatation, ileus, pneumatosis intestinalis
IIB (definite NEC, moderately ill)	Same as IIA plus mild metabolic acidosis and mild thrombocytopenia	Same as IIA plus definite abdominal tenderness, ± abdominal cellulitis, or right lower quadrant mass, absent bowel sounds	Same as IIA ± portal vein gas ± ascites
IIIA (advanced NEC, severely ill,	Same as IIB, plus hypotension, bradycardia, severe apnea, combined respiratory and metabolic acidosis, DIC, neutropenia, anuria	Same as IIB plus signs of generalized peritonitis, marked tenderness, distention, and abdominal wall erythema	Same as IIB, definite ascites
IIIB (advanced NEC, severely ill, bowel perforated)	Same as IIIA, sudden perforation	Same as IIIA, sudden increased distention	Same as IIB plus pneumoperitoneum

Modified from Kliegman R: Necrotizing enterocolitis. In Burg FD, Ingelfinger JR, Wald ER, Polin RA (eds): Gellis and Kagan's Current Pediatric Therapy, 15th ed. Philadelphia, W.B. Saunders, 1996, with permission.

202. *Case.* A 1000-g infant, born at 28 weeks' gestation, had an initial course characterized by respiratory distress syndrome (RDS) and suspected sepsis. He was initially treated with surfactant and mechanical ventilation. The antibiotics were stopped after 3 days because the blood cultures were negative. On day 5, he was placed on nasal continuous positive airway pressure (CPAP) until day 18. He began enteral gavage feeds on day 5, at 20-cc/kg/day increments, and finally achieved "full feeds" (150 cc/kg/day) by day 20. He then developed an increased frequency of apnea and bradycardia associated with temperature instability. The gavage feeds were held because of increasing gastric residuals, presence of blood in stools, and abdominal distention. What is the approach to management of this infant?

This infant falls in stage IB, because of the temperature instability, apnea and bradycardia, increased gastric residuals, presence of blood in stools, and abdominal distention. An abdominal x-ray is recommended to view bowel gas pattern. We expect to see dilated bowel loops. Management includes withdrawing all enteral feeds, gastric decompression by placing an orogastric tube to suction, and ruling out sepsis. Appropriate antibiotic coverage for at least 3 days pending cultures is imperative. Meanwhile total parenteral nutrition is necessary. It is important to carefully follow this infant for progression to NEC and to exclude other diagnostic possibilities that may mimic NEC at this age.

203. One day after beginning appropriate management, the same infant develops persistent abdominal distention, right lower quadrant tenderness, and diminished bowel sounds. The abdominal x-rays are shown in the figures. How do you interpret these signs? What is the approach to the management of this infant?

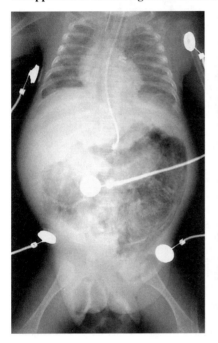
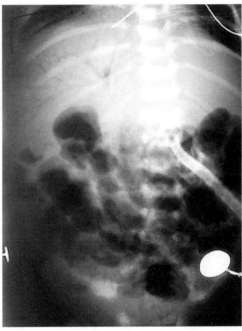

Left, Abdominal x-ray 1 day after treatment for NEC stage IB. *Right*, Abdominal x-ray of same infant 8 hours later. (Courtesy of Dr. Jack Sty, Department of Pediatric Radiology, Children's Hospital of Wisconsin, Medical College of Wisconsin, Milwaukee, WI.)

At this stage, the infant is showing definite signs of NEC, as in stage II. This is evidenced by failure to recover from earlier stage and worsening intestinal signs such as diminished bowel sounds, distention of abdomen, guarding, and abdominal tenderness. These clinical findings may herald the beginning of dilated viscus, submucosal or subserosal dissection of air, and peritonitis. Such an infant should be regarded as having NEC and is moderately ill. The x-ray in the first figure shows grossly dilated bowel loops and submucosal and subserosal pneumatosis intestinalis. Management at this stage includes careful monitoring for worsening of clinical status (metabolic acidosis and thrombocytopenia) and continuing appropriate antibiotics for 7–10 days *if* the clinical examination returns to normal in the next 24–48 hours.

However the second x-ray in figure 2 confirms the worsening status, manifested by portal vein gas (within the liver). NEC in this infant is progressing. At this stage, it is imperative to anticipate the possible future intestinal perforation. Management at this stage includes correction of hypovolemia and metabolic acidosis using colloids and sodium bicarbonate, respectively. If NEC does not progress further, then 2 weeks of appropriate antibiotics would suffice.

204. Twenty-four hours later, the infant deteriorates suddenly. He develops generalized abdominal tenderness and periumbilical erythema. An arterial blood gas determination shows a pH of 7.10, pCO_2 of 80 mmHg, pO_2 32 mmHg, HCO_3^- of 12 mEq/L, and a base deficit of 16. The blood count is remarkable for a platelet count of 22,000/uL. The abdominal x-ray is shown. How do you interpret these signs? What is the approach to the management of this infant?

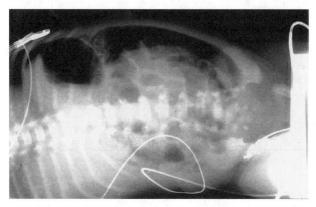

Courtesy of Dr. Jack Sty, Department of Pediatric Radiology, Children's Hospital of Wisconsin, Medical College of Wisconsin, Milwaukee, WI.

The infant at this stage has advanced NEC and is severely ill. This condition is characterized by worsening hypotension, a combined respiratory and metabolic acidosis, thrombocytopenia, and anuria. Thrombocytopenia may be an indication of evolving disseminated intravascular coagulation (DIC) with or without intestinal perforation. The sudden deterioration is ominous for a bowel perforation, and progressive abdominal distention with erythema signifies worsening peritonitis and pneumoperitoneum. The lateral decubitus abdominal x-ray is remarkable for worsening pneumatosis and free air (see figure). Another commonly used abdominal x-ray for identifying free air is cross-table lateral view.

This infant needs vigorous fluid resuscitation with colloids (fresh frozen plasma, albumin) and cellular products (packed red cells and platelets). Inotropic support using dopamine and epinephrine drips may be needed. Surgical support using dopamine and epinephrine drips may be needed. Surgical exploration is indicated in this setting to facilitate abdominal decompression and salvage the viable bowel. If it is difficult to ventilate the infant at this stage, an abdominal paracentesis may be helpful.

205. When is surgery indicated in an infant with NEC? What are the complications of performing surgery on an infant with advanced NEC with bowel perforation?

Absolute indications for surgery include pneumoperitoneum and intestinal gangrene (as evidenced by positive results of abdominal paracentesis). Relative indications include progressive clinical deterioration (metabolic acidosis, ventilatory failure, oliguria, thrombocytopenia), fixed abdominal mass, abdominal wall erythema, portal vein gas, and persistently dilated bowel loop.

The postoperative complications occurring immediately after surgery are usually related to the stoma (retraction, prolapse, or peristomal hernia) or wound (infection, dehiscence, enterocutaneous fistula). Rarely, intra-abdominal abscesses, recurrence of NEC, and bowel obstruction can develop. Chronic complications result from the dysfunctional ostomies, strictures, or short gut syndrome.

206. What are considerations for *not* operating on an infant with NEC?

It may be less useful to operate when NEC is still evolving. Some cases recover by effective medical management alone. Other situations where acute surgery can be avoided include severe GI hemorrhage, abdominal tenderness (may occur from distended viscus or peritonitis), intestinal obstruction (may simply be an ileus), or a gasless abdomen with ascites.

207. *Case.* A 30-week gestation male infant had been diagnosed with stage IIA NEC and appropriately managed medically for 10 days. He subsequently tolerated feeds poorly. The stooling pattern was reported as normal (small green stools). Different formulas and prokinetics were tried without any positive result. An abdominal x-ray was reported as a "gassy abdomen." Antibiotics were begun again, and feedings were held for 3 days. A sepsis work-up was negative at 3 days. Feedings were then resumed with an elemental formula. The same feeding-intolerance pattern prevailed. What are the diagnostic considerations in this infant?

Recovery after NEC occurs by second intention. Areas of patchy necrosis often heal by fibrosis and stricture formation. The repair process also involves the peritoneum, resulting in adhesions. An upper GI contrast x-ray may show a prolonged transit time and gross dilation of jejunum consistent with more distal stricture formation. A lower GI contrast x-ray may be necessary to identify strictures in the large bowel. At laparotomy, he was found to have multiple strictures, which were resected and ultimately resulted in a short bowel syndrome.

208. *Case.* A 3500-g full-term female infant born after an uncomplicated pregnancy was discharged home from the newborn nursery after a normal transition. She was fed exclusively with breast milk. On the 7th day of life, she presented acutely with bilious emesis. Clinical examination was remarkable for a pulse rate 180 beats per minute, respiratory rate of 70/min, mean blood pressure of 30 mmHg, abdominal distention, and marked tenderness with diminished bowel sounds. She passed a dark bloody stool. Laboratory studies were notable for an arterial blood gas of pH 7.15, pCO_2 of 30 mmHg, pO_2 of 120 mmHg, and HCO_3^- of 10 mEq/L. The complete blood count was remarkable for a hematocrit of 24 and platelet count of 400,000/uL. What is the approach to management in this infant? How do you establish a diagnosis in this infant?

The infant's exam is compatible with "acute abdomen," and she has signs of hypovolemia and shock. She needs fluid resuscitation and correction of metabolic acidosis. Because sepsis is a common entity in the neonatal period, antibiotics are indicated after obtaining blood cultures. A nasogastric tube should be placed and stomach decompressed. An abdominal x-ray reveals gassy distended bowel loops with fluid levels. An upper GI contrast x-ray is shown in the figure.

The contrast fails to flow distally, suggesting intestinal obstruction, and in this case it looks like a pig-tail. A diagnosis of volvulus is highly likely in this infant, and surgical exploration should be considered.

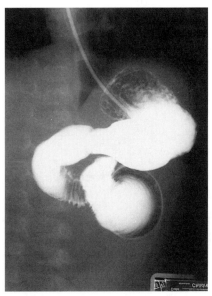

Upper GI contrast x-ray. (Courtesy of Dr. Jack Sty, Department of Pediatric Radiology, Children's Hospital of Wisconsin, Medical College of Wisconsin, Milwaukee, WI.)

209. How do you differentiate NEC from volvulus? In what conditions is pneumatosis intestinalis seen?

NEC Differentiated from Volvulus

CHARACTERISTICS	NEC	VOLVULUS
Preterm	90%	30%
Onset by 2 wks	90%	60%
Male:female ratio	1:1	2:1
Associated anomalies	Rare	25–40%
Bilious emesis	Unusual	75%
Grossly bloody stools	Common	Less common
Pneumatosis intestinalis	90%	2%
Marked proximal obstruction	Rare	Common
Thrombocytopenia without DIC	Common	Rare

Modified from Kliegman R: Necrotizing enterocolitis: Differential diagnosis and management. In Polin RA, Yoder MC, Burg FD (eds): Workbook in Practical Neonatology, 2nd ed. Philadelphia, W.B. Saunders, 1993, with permission.

Apart from NEC, pneumatosis intestinalis is also seen in midgut volvulus, acute or chronic diarrhea, postoperative gastrointestinal surgery, Hirschsprung disease, short bowel syndrome, mesenteric thrombosis, post cardiac catheterization, structural disease of hindgut (colonic atresias and stricture, imperforate anus), and congenital malignancy.

NEONATAL ASCITES

210. What is the most common etiology of neonatal ascites? What other etiologies should be considered?

Extravasation from the urinary tract accounts for 25% of all cases of ascites, although many other etiologies have been identified (see table). In 15% of neonates, no identifiable cause is found.

Differential Diagnosis of Neonatal Ascites

TYPE	CAUSE
Genitourinary	Posterior urethral valves
	Bladder obstruction or rupture
	Congenital nephrosis
Gastrointestinal	Intestinal obstruction or perforation
Hepatobiliary	Hepatitis
	Biliary atresia
	Metabolic disease
	Bile duct perforation
Cardiac	Congenital heart disease
	Arteriovenous malformation
	Arrhythmia
Infectious	Cytomegalovirus infection
	Toxoplasmosis
	Syphilis
Chylous	Obstruction or disruption of thoracic duct lymphatics
Miscellaneous	Ovarian cyst
	Trauma: Urachal transection
	Thoracic duct perforation

From Harris MC: Neonatal ascites. In Burg FD, Inglefinger JR, Wald ER, Polin RA (eds): Gellis & Kagan's Current Pediatric Therapy, 16th ed. Philadelphia, W.B. Saunders, 1999, p 269, with permission.

211. What is the difference between a transudate and an exudate?

Peritoneal fluid can usually be classified as a transudate or an exudate. A transudate is usually clear fluid with a low specific gravity (< 1.015) and protein content (< 2.5 g/dl). The cellular content is also low (< 20 cells/nm^3) with a predominance of lymphocytes. An exudate usually represents lymph exudation from the liver or inflammation of abdominal viscera or peritoneum. Exudative fluid is usually turbid with a high cell count, protein content, and specific gravity.

212. Which tests or procedures aid in the accurate diagnosis of ascites?

Abdominal ultrasound is the preferred imaging modality for identifying and localizing ascites in neonates and will differentiate intra-abdominal fluid from masses and dilated fluid-filled loops of bowel. An abdominal paracentesis, however, will establish the diagnosis in most cases. Clear or light yellow fluid suggests a renal origin, golden fluid suggests bile, and green fluid suggests intestinal perforation and peritonitis. Laboratory studies performed on the ascitic fluid should include chemical, microscopic, and bacteriologic analyses.

Laboratory Analysis of Ascitic Fluid

MICROSCOPIC	CHEMICAL	CULTURE
Red cell count	Specific gravity	Bacterial
White cell count/	Total protein	Fungal
differential	Glucose	Viral
Hematocrit	Triglycerides	
Cytology	Bilirubin	
Fat globules	Creatinine/urea nitrogen	
Gram stain, fungal stain	Amylase	
	Lactate dehydrogenase	

From Harris MC: Neonatal ascites. In Burg FD, Inglefinger JR, Wald ER, Polin RA (eds): Gellis & Kagan's Current Pediatric Therapy, 16th ed. Philadelphia, W.B. Saunders, 1999, p 270, with permission.

213. In the jaundiced infant with a distended abdomen, what are the most likely causes of ascites?

1. **Bile duct perforation.** Although an uncommon cause of ascites in the neonatal period, perforation may occur at the junction of the cystic and common bile ducts. The infant presents with a distended abdomen, with or without signs of peritoneal inflammation. The paracentesis fluid is golden in color, and operative exploration is indicated.

2. **Necrotizing enterocolitis.** Ascites is a frequent finding in NEC, and may represent peritoneal inflammation or frank perforation of an abdominal viscus. The infant presents with abdominal distention, often with signs of peritoneal irritation. Abdominal paracentesis reveals either clear fluid (inflammation) or green fecal material (perforation), whose culture is reflective of gram-negative enteric flora.

214. Why are medium chain triglycerides the recommended source of fat in cases of chylous ascites?

Chylous ascites results from a leak of lymphatic fluid en route from the GI tract to the thoracic duct. Medium chain triglycerides are transported directly from the intestine into the portal venous system, thus bypassing lymphatic channels.

BILE DUCT DISORDERS AND BILIARY ATRESIA

215. What are the components of neonatal biliary disease?

Any disease process in the neonate with altered bile acid transport or biliary structure is a biliary disease. The clues to its presence include cholestasis (elevated serum bile acids), conjugated hyperbilirubinemia, and altered serum levels of enzymes from biliary inflammation or obstruction (e.g., gamma glutamyl transferase [GTT] and alkaline phosphatase).

216. What is cholestatic jaundice?

Conjugated bilirubin > 2.0 mg/dl or exceeding 15% of the total bilirubin is referred to as cholestatic jaundice. Cholestatic jaundice is always physiologically abnormal and warrants a medical evaluation. Note that biliary disease can present with or without cholestatic jaundice.

217. What are the causes of direct hyperbilirubinemia?

The mechanisms include:
1. Impaired bilirubin metabolism secondary to liver parenchyma disease
2. Inherited disorders of bilirubin excretion.
3. Mechanical obstruction to biliary flow, both intra- and extrahepatic
4. Excessive bilirubin loads such as may occur in massive hemolysis

218. When should an infant's fractionated bilirubin be obtained?

Evaluation of jaundice persisting beyond the normal physiologic period (2 weeks) in newborns must always include a fractionation of bilirubin.

219. How should the evaluation of cholestatic jaundice in infants be approached?

Neonatal cholestasis can be a manifestation of (1) extrahepatic biliary disease, (2) intrahepatic biliary disease, and (3) hepatocellular disease. All can present with similar symptoms. Therefore, differentiation based on history and physical examination alone is not helpful.

The physician should embark on a diagnostic evaluation that will promptly identify clinical conditions amenable to therapy and where delay in treatment could be tragic (e.g., sepsis, urinary tract infection (UTI), hypothyroidism, biliary atresia, and congenital metabolic disorders treated with special diets such as galactosemia, hereditary fructose intolerance [HFI], and tyrosinemia).

Treatable Causes of Neonatal Cholestasis

INFECTIOUS	SURGICAL	METABOLIC	OTHER
UTI	Biliary atresia	Galactosemia	Hypothyroidism
Sepsis	Choledochal cyst	HFI	Neonatal iron storage
	Cholelithiasis	Tyrosinemia	TPN
	Biliary strictures		Bile acid synthetic disorders
	Duct perforation		Histiocytosis X
	Congenital duct anomalies		
	Mass (neoplasia)		
	Intestinal obstruction		

220. What tests should be obtained during the initial evaluation of neonatal cholestasis?

TEST	INDICATION
Blood	
Fractionation of bilirubin	Detect cholestatic jaundice
CBC	
Blood cultures (as clinically indicated)	To rule out sepsis
Hepatic function panel	Abnormal in hepatobiliary disease
TSH/T4	To rule out hypothyroidism
Urine	
Urinalysis and culture	(+) reducing sugar: galactosemia
	(±) protein: galactosemia, HFI, tyrosinemia
	(+) culture: UTI, sepsis
Abdominal ultrasound	(+) choledocal cyst, stones, masses, and stricture
DISIDA scan	Nonexcreting in biliary atresia, delayed uptake and (+) excreting in neonatal hepatitis

221. When should the infant be referred to the hepatologist?

As soon as cholestatic jaundice is diagnosed and sepsis ruled out, the infant should be promptly referred to the hepatologist. The above tests can be scheduled, but no time should be spent waiting for results. In most cases the final diagnosis requires that a liver biopsy be performed. The hepatologist will conduct a broad laboratory evaluation in order to make a diagnosis so that therapy can be initiated. In addition to medical therapy, preventative therapy can be provided through genetic counseling.

222. A 6-week-old healthy, term breast-fed infant was noted to be jaundiced at the routine well-care visit. She was growing well. Examination of the abdomen revealed a palpable liver (1 cm below right costal margin) and spleen (2 cm below left costal margin). By history she had pigmented stools. Total and direct bilirubin were 6.9 and 4.3 mg/dl, respectively. Other findings include: alanine aminotransferase (ALT), 138 U/L; aspartate aminotransferase (AST), 120 U/L; alkaline phosphatase (ALK), 205 U/L; gamma-glutamyl transferase (GGT), 420 U/L; albumin, 3.0 g/dl; and prothrombin time (PT) 13.9 sec. Ca, PO_4, and Mg were normal; complete blood count, urinalysis, and culture were normal. What do the lab results suggest and which further tests need to be performed?

Apart from ruling out sepsis and UTI, the above tests are nondiagnostic. The liver enzymes and PT are useful for following the course of hepatic function. Other tests should be performed:

- **Ultrasound** is a quick noninvasive test for detecting causes of extrahepatic cholestasis (e.g., choledochal cysts, biliary stones, tumor). Finding a gallbladder on ultrasound does not rule out biliary atresia.
- **Radionuclide scans (DISIDA):** Good hepatic uptake of radionuclide with absence of excretion into the gut lumen is suggestive of an obstructive process such as biliary atresia. Delayed excretion may also occur in hepatitis.

223. The ultrasound revealed hepatosplenomegaly, and no gallbladder was seen. The DISIDA scan showed normal uptake but no excretion at 24 hours. A liver biopsy was obtained, which showed intrahepatic cholestasis with proliferation of the bile ducts. Is the evaluation now complete for making a definitive diagnosis?

No. The evaluation is very suggestive of biliary atresia; however, this can be confirmed only by performing an intraoperative cholangiogram. Other causes of neonatal cholestasis such as Alagille syndrome may clinically mimic biliary atresia and may only be differentiated by intraoperative cholangiogram.

224. Is it critical to make an early diagnosis of biliary atresia?

Yes. The outcome of surgical therapy (Kasai operation) for biliary atresia is dependent on age at surgery, with best outcome when intervention is before 8–10 weeks. Biliary atresia is the leading indication for liver transplantation in children.

225. A 10-week-old former 34-week premature, breast-fed boy was referred for evaluation of jaundice and elevated liver enzymes. His test results indicated a conjugated bilirubin, 3.8 mg/dl; ALK 650 U/L; AST, 120 U/L; ALT, 138 U/L; and GGT, 1200 U/L. During the newborn period, he had mild RDS, was treated for sepsis, and received TPN for 7 days. He was discharged home on breast-milk feeds at age 3 weeks. How should the evaluation proceed?

The laboratory results show a disproportionately elevated serum GGT and ALK, suggesting biliary disease. However, because the clinical manifestations of neonatal cholestasis are independent of etiology, the initial basic evaluation should be as described in the table in question 220.

226. A careful physical exam revealed he had a prominent forehead, small chin, and a systolic heart murmur consistent with peripheral pulmonary stenosis. The ultrasound was normal. The DISIDA scan showed excretion at 24 hours. Is this sufficient for making the diagnosis of Alagille syndrome?

No! A liver biopsy is necessary to confirm the diagnosis. Alagille syndrome is also referred to as **syndromic bile duct paucity**. It needs to be differentiated from biliary atresia. It is characterized by chronic cholestasis and extrahepatic features such as characteristic facies, heart murmur, vertebral anomalies (winged vertebrae), and posterior embryotoxon. During infancy, histology may show bile duct proliferation. However, in later childhood and adulthood, the liver histology commonly shows bile duct paucity. The genetic defect has been localized on chromosome 20p12.

227. What clinical conditions are associated with cholelithiasis?

Congenital stones	Short bowel syndrome
TPN	Small bowel bacterial overgrowth
Diuretic use	Sepsis

228. What are common mistakes in evaluation of an infant with neonatal cholestasis?
- Attributing all jaundice beyond the physiologic period in healthy infants to breast milk
- Not fractionating bilirubin
- Not performing the basic evaluation in an expedited fashion
- Relying on clinical history and physical exam to make diagnosis
- Delayed referral to specialist

229. What is extrahepatic biliary atresia?

Extrahepatic biliary atresia is the term given to idiopathic progressive obliteration or discontinuity of the extrahepatic biliary tree in infancy.

230. What are the demographics of extrahepatic biliary atresia?

Biliary atresia occurs in 1 in 10,000–15,000 live births with females affected 1.4 times more frequently than males. Approximately 10% of infants with biliary atresia will have associated anomalies (syndromic biliary atresia) including splenic abnormalities (polysplenia or asplenia), malrotation, and situs inversus.

231. What are the typical presenting clinical features of an infant with extrahepatic biliary atresia?

The usual presentation is that of an otherwise healthy infant with jaundice and acholic stools developing between 3 and 6 weeks of age. If an infant is ill appearing (vomiting, acidosis, failure to thrive), metabolic (nonobstructive) causes of jaundice should be considered promptly.

232. What are the typical radiographic findings in extrahepatic biliary atresia?

Ultrasound. Hepatic parenchyma may be normal, and the gallbladder and common bile duct are generally not visualized. It is important to note that the gallbladder may not be visualized in normal infants because of contraction; nonvisualization of the gallbladder should not be considered diagnostic of biliary atresia. The main purpose of ultrasound in this setting is to rule out an obstructing choledochal cyst.

DISIDA scan. There should be uptake of the radiotracer by the hepatic parenchyma, although uptake may be delayed (due to associated hepatocyte injury). In biliary atresia, absolutely no contrast will reach the bowel even after 12 to 24 hours; contrast will ultimately appear in the kidneys and urinary bladder as it is cleared through the urinary tract.

233. What are the typical histopathologic findings in extrahepatic biliary atresia?

Liver biopsy is the final step in preoperative diagnosis of biliary atresia. The biopsy will demonstrate proliferation of bile ducts in response to extrahepatic obstruction. A variable amount of fibrosis will also be present, depending on the age of the infant and the rapidity of progression of the disease process.

234. How do the radiologic and histopathologic findings in biliary atresia compare to those of neonatal hepatitis?

STUDY	BILIARY ATRESIA	NEONATAL HEPATITIS	OTHER DISORDERS OF INTEREST
Ultrasound	Nonvisualization of gall-bladder, common bile duct	Normal gallbladder and common bile duct, occa-sional nonvisualization of gallbladder and common bile duct	Choledochal cyst
DISIDA scan	Good or delayed uptake of tracer with no excretion into bowel	Delayed uptake of tracer, excretion of tracer into bowel occurs	Will detect bile leak in rare setting of spon-taneous rupture of biliary tree
Liver biopsy	Proliferation of bile ducts, bile plugs in ducts, fibrosis of portal tracts or cirrhosis, formation of hepatic acini (rosettes), and variable inflammation	Inflammation of hepatic parenchyma, giant cell transformation of hepatocytes is common in infants, cholestasis	Wide variety of specific abnormalities sug-gestive of other specific diseases

235. What is the natural history of untreated biliary atresia?

Untreated biliary atresia is uniformly fatal within 2 years with a median survival of 8 months. Untreated biliary atresia leads to biliary cirrhosis, portal hypertension, esophageal varices, failure to thrive, and liver failure, and death can occur due to any of a number of complications.

236. What is appropriate surgical and medical therapy for biliary atresia and how does therapy impact survival?

Surgical. If the liver biopsy is suggestive of biliary atresia, the infant undergoes exploratory laparotomy and intraoperative cholangiogram. If biliary atresia is confirmed, an attempt to restore biliary drainage by the Kasai procedure (hepatic portoenterostomy) is made. A loop of bowel is anastomosed directly to the hepatic capsule at the porta hepatis after resection of the fibrous bil-iary remnants. Bowel continuity is restored by formation of a Roux-en-Y intestinal anastomosis. The success of the procedure depends on the age of the infant at operation and the experience of the surgeon. Long-term survival may exceed 60% for infants younger than 2 months of age at the time of portoenterostomy, compared with only 25% for those over 2 months of age. The first sign of a successful portoenterostomy is the passage of green (bile stained) rather than acholic stools.

Medical. Any child with biliary atresia regardless of the status of portoenterostomy should be treated for chronic liver disease and its potential complications. Infants should receive oral ur-sodeoxycholate (a bile acid that stimulates bile flow) and fat-soluble vitamin supplementation. Many infants require supplemental tube feedings, particularly if the portoenterostomy is unsuc-cessful. Good nutritional status will optimize the infant's survival if liver transplantation be-comes necessary.

237. What are the potential complications of the Kasai portoenterostomy?

Specific complications include failure to achieve drainage, ascending cholangitis where drainage is achieved, and biliary cysts at the portoenterostomy site. Other nonspecific surgical complications can also occur.

238. What are the therapeutic options exist for children who do not undergo portoenteros-tomy or in whom drainage is not achieved?

Liver transplantation is the only definitive therapy and has an approximately 80% expected 5-year survival.

239. Other than biliary atresia, what are causes of obstructive jaundice in infancy?

Choledochal cyst and spontaneous perforation of the extrahepatic biliary tree are two causes of obstructive jaundice in infancy. Cholelithiasis is not a major cause of biliary obstruction in infancy, although gallstones may be seen as incidental findings on ultrasound of premature infants and occasionally even on prenatal ultrasound.

240. What are the demographics and presentation of choledochal cyst?

Choledochal cysts are rarer than biliary atresia with estimates of incidence ranging from 1 in 13,000 to 1 in 2,000,000 live births. Girls are affected 4 times more frequently than males. The classic triad of abdominal pain, mass, and jaundice occurs in fewer than 20% of cases. Choledochal cyst may present as jaundice, mass, vomiting, fever, and even pancreatitis. Less than half of choledochal cysts present in infancy.

241. What are the types of choledochal cyst?

Type I—diffuse enlargement of the common bile duct (the majority fall in this category)
Type II—diverticular cyst
Type III—choledochocele
Type IV—multiple cysts of the intra- and extrahepatic biliary tree
Type V—Caroli's disease

UNCONJUGATED HYPERBILIRUBINEMIA

242. How common is hyperbilirubinemia and how do we define its severity?

Neonatal hyperbilirubinemia, defined as a total serum bilirubin value > 12.9 mg/dl in a term infant, is one of the most frequent neonatal diagnoses. Usually benign and considered physiologic, it has a myriad of pathologic etiologies and potential deleterious sequelae. Nearly 50% of term and near-term babies deemed healthy and discharged from the well-baby nurseries may develop neonatal hyperbilirubinemia during the first week after birth. In about 5% of newborns, the total serum bilirubin (TSB) level will be above 17 mg/dl (the definition of significant hyperbilirubinemia for a term infant > 95th percentile at 72 hours old).

243. What are the cause of neonatal hyperbilirubinemia?

- Increased bilirubin production
- Decreased bilirubin clearance:
    Decreased hepatic clearance
    Increased enterohepatic circulation

244. What are the usual causes of increased bilirubin production?

Bilirubin is the end product of the catabolism of heme (from circulating hemoglobin). In newborns, normal destruction of senescent red blood cells (RBCs) accounts for about 75% of bilirubin production. The remaining 25% are from other sources: nonerythropoietic (nonhemoglobin sources such as cytochromes, catalases), and erythropoietic component (products of ineffective erythropoiesis). Bilirubin production can be exacerbated by:

- Prematurity
- Blood group incompatibility
- Breakdown of extravascular blood
- Maternal diabetes
- Ethnicity, especially East Asians
- RBC enzyme defects, such as glucose-6-phosphate dehydrogenase (G6PD) deficiency
- RBC membrane defects
- Hemoglobinopathies

245. What are the common causes of delayed clearance of bilirubin?

Bilirubin clearance from the body usually requires fecal or urinary losses of the water-soluble conjugated bilirubin. Delay may occur due to conditions that include:

- Decreased glucoronyl transferase enzyme conjugating activity
- Delayed hepatic excretion with increasing levels of direct bilirubin
- Decreased gut transit and delayed passage of meconium
- Inadequate enteral intake
- Prematurity

246. What is excessive jaundice in a term or near term infant?
Excessive jaundice is defined as an hour-specific serum bilirubin value > 95th percentile track (see figure).

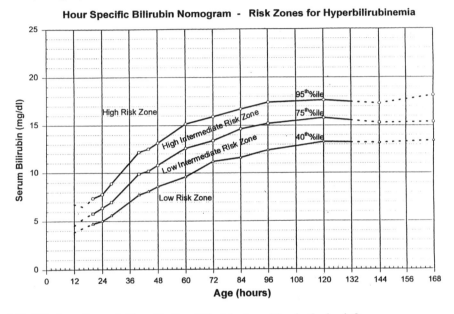

247. What are the variables affecting bilirubin deposition in the brain?
- Concentration of serum unconjugated (free) bilirubin
- Concentration of serum albumin
- Concentration of hydrogen ions
- Blood flow to the brain
- Affinity of albumin for bilirubin
- Blood-brain barrier integrity
- Neuronal susceptibility
- Other causes such as variations in brain bilirubin oxidase

248. What are the potential mechanisms of bilirubin neurotoxicity?
Based on studies in animals, bilirubin impairs the following activities in neuronal cells:
Oxidative phosphorylation, ATP levels
DNA synthesis
Protein synthesis
Protein phosphorylation
Neurotransmitter synthesis
Synaptic transmission

249. Which areas of the brain are stained by bilirubin during acute bilirubin encephalopathy?
The most commonly affected areas are the basal ganglia (particularly, globus pallidus and subthalamic nuclei), hippocampus (specifically, sectors H2–3), substantia nigra, cranial nerve nuclei (oculomotor, vestibular, cochlear and facial), reticular formation of pons, inferior olivary nuclei, cerebellar nuclei (especially the dentate), and anterior horn cells of the spinal cord. The yellow staining may last 7–10 days. The distribution of bilirubin staining often corresponds to the distribution of neuronal injury. However, damage to the basal ganglia and brain stem nuclei (oculomotor and cochlear) are most evident clinically. Involvement of cerebral cortical nuclei is not a prominent feature or kernicterus.

250. Why does a certain part of the brain have a predilection for bilirubin-related neuronal injury?

Neurons are more easily injured than glial cells, and there also appears to be a selective regional susceptibility. The neuronal surface (with abundance of gangliosides) readily binds to bilirubin and that may be the initial site of injury.

251. What is the tetrad of clinical signs of "kernicterus"?

These usually refer to the chronic sequelae of acute bilirubin encephalopathy:
- Motor: choreoathetoid cerebral palsy, motor delay
- Cochlear: sensorineural deafness (auditory aphasia)
- Oculo-motor: gaze abnormalities, upward gaze paresis
- Intellectual: minimal impairment, cognitive dysfunction

Dental dysplasia has been associated with these chronic sequelae.

252. What are the clinical manifestations of acute bilirubin encephalopathy?

Clinical manifestations of acute bilirubin encephalopathy can be insidious and progress rapidly to severe and life-threatening manifestations. The signs of bilirubin-induced neurologic dysfunction (BIND) can be grouped to (1) behavior or mental state, (2) muscle tone, and (3) cry pattern abnormalities.

Clinical Features of Bilirubin-induced Neurologic Dysfunction (BIND)

SIGNS	MILD	MODERATE	SEVERE
Behavior	Too sleepy Decreased feeding Decreased vigor	Lethargy and/or irritable (depending on arousal state) Very poor feeding	Semi-coma Apnea Extreme irritability Seizures Fever
Muscle tone	Slight but persistent decrease in tone	Mild to moderate Hypertonicity Mild nuchal or truncal arching	Severe hypo- or hypertonia Atonic Ophisthotonus Posturing, bicycling
Cry pattern	High pitched	Shrill and piercing (especially when stimulated)	Inconsolable, very weak, and cries only with stimulation

253. What is the risk of neurologic dysfunction in infants with high bilirubin levels?

Babies with excessive hyperbilirubinemia (who were a part of Collaborative Perinatal Project) were followed for 6–7 years and evaluated for extrapyramidal dysfunction. Of the 44,000 children evaluated from a study population, 16.7% of the babies with bilirubin values > 17 mg/dl showed suspicious neurologic signs:
- Awkwardness
- Gait abnormalities
- Upward gaze abnormalities
- Failure at fine stereognosis
- Nystagmus
- Exaggerated abdominal and cremasteric reflexes
- Vasomotor abnormalities
- Equivocal Babinski reflexes
- Questionable hypotonia

Newman TB, Klebanoff MA: Neonatal hyperbilirubinemia and long-term outcome: Another look at the Collaborative Perinatal Project. Pediatrics 92:651–657, 1993.

254. What is low-bilirubin kernicterus?
- **Displacement of unbound bilirubin** (the neurotoxic free bilirubin) from albumin by competing small molecules such as sulfa drugs or benzyl alcohol (a preservative in several drugs)
- **Injury to blood-brain barrier:** asphyxia/hypoxia, hyperosmolarity (use of hypertonic solutions), seizures, meningitis, sepsis with shock and hypercapnia. Loss of cerebral blood flow autoregulation may be an additional complicating variable.

255. What factors potentiate bilirubin toxicity with asphyxia?
- Impaired bilirubin–albumin binding and increased free bilirubin
- Increased proportion of bilirubin as bilirubin acid (acidosis)
- Increased blood-brain transport of bilirubin (hypercarbia)
- Increased neuronal susceptibility (hypoxemia-ischemia)
- Increased susceptibility to excitotoxic amino acids and reperfusion injury

256. Why is bilirubin more neurotoxic in the preterm neonate?
Preterm babies are known to be vulnerable to bilirubin-induced neurotoxicity, and several authors have reported low bilirubin kernicterus in preterm babies. Predisposing factors for bilirubin neurotoxicity in the preterm infant include:
- Injury to or potential disruption of the blood-brain barrier
- Hypoalbuminemia (serum albumin < 3.4 g/dl)
- Lessened ability of albumin to bind bilirubin (diminishes further with increasing prematurity)
- Illness (RDS, infection shock)
- Displacement of bilirubin from binding sites by competing small molecules

257. Is there a specific level of bilirubin or albumin that places the preterm infant at risk for kernicterus?
No precise data link a specific level of bilirubin or serum albumin to the neuronal entry of unbound bilirubin. However, the aggressive use of phototherapy in preterm babies (especially those with birth weight < 1000 g) has been associated with near elimination of low bilirubin kernicterus. In the at-risk or bruised VLBW baby, phototherapy is commonly initiated by 24 hours of age. An alternative approach has been to initiate phototherapy at 5% of body weight. For example, in a baby with a birth weight of 800 g (0.8 kg), phototherapy should be considered at a bilirubin level of ≥ 4 mg/dl. Until techniques are available to easily measure unbound bilirubin or objectively determine predictors of neurotoxicity, a practical but conservative approach for early treatment of jaundice needs to be clinically based.

258. At what level is bilirubin neurotoxic in the term newborn?
There are no precise data that correlate a specific bilirubin value to neurotoxicity. Therefore, the decisions for clinical interventions are based on potential risks. The infant's history, course, physical findings (especially, neurologic signs), and increasing levels of bilirubin temper clinical decisions. These are balanced by comparing potential benefits and risks of the intervention itself. The table below is that proposed by the American Academy of Pediatrics as a paradigm to consider intervention based on a serum bilirubin value.

Management of Hyperbilirubinemia in the Health Term Newborn

AGE (HOURS)	TSB LEVEL, mg/dL (µmol/L)			
	CONSIDER PHOTOTHERAPY*	PHOTOTHERAPY	EXCHANGE TRANSFUSION IF INTENSIVE PHOTO-THERAPY FAILS[†]	EXCHANGE TRANSFUSION AND INTENSIVE PHOTOTHERAPY
≤ 24[‡]	—	—	—	—
25–48	≥ 12 (170)	≥ 15 (160)	≥ 20 (340)	≥ 25 (430)
49–72	≥ 15 (260)	≥ 18 (310)	≥ 25 (430)	≥ 30 (510)
> 72	≥ 17 (290)	≥ 20 (340)	≥ 25 (430)	≥ 30 (510)

* Phototherapy at these TSB levels is a clinical option, meaning that the intervention is available and may be used on the basis of individual clinical judgment.

[†] Intensive phototherapy should produce a decline of TSB of 1–2 mg/dl within 4–6 hours, and the TSB level should continue to fall and remain below the threshold level for exchange transfusion. If this does not occur, it is considered a failure of phototherapy.

[‡] Term infants who are clinical jaundiced at ≤ 24 hours old are not considered healthy and require further evaluation.

259. At what level of predischarge serum bilirubin can one predict significant hyperbiliru-binemia (≥ 17 mg/dl)?

Referring to the figure in question 246, hyperbilirubinemia can be predicted as follows:

Risk of Excessive Hyperbilirubinemia Using Serum Bilirubin as Vector

PREDISCHARGE TOTAL SERUM BILIRUBIN (MEASURED < 72 HOURS AGE)	PROBABILITY OF SIGNIFICANT HYPERBILIRUBINEMIA
Values < 40th percentile track	< 1:46 (most likely 0)
Values 40th–75th percentile track	1:46
Values 75th–95th percentile track	1:8
Values > 95th percentile track	2:5

260. At what serum albumin value should there be a concern of bilirubin neurotoxicity?

The bilirubin-to-albumin (B:A) ratio has been shown by Japanese investigators to predict abnormalities in the auditory brain stem evoked responses related to hyperbilirubinemia. In an ideal situation, the B:A ratio should be a molar equivalent. However, because of the available binding sites on albumin, free bilirubin is anticipated when the B:A ratio exceeds a 0.80 molar ratio. This value translates to 7.0 mg of bilirubin to 1.0 g of albumin. A molar ratio of < 0.65 (5.5 mg of bilirubin : 1 g of albumin) could be considered safe in term and near-term babies. Thus, a baby with serum albumin of 3.0 g/dl who has a bilirubin value > 21 mg/dl is likely to exceed the albumin-binding sites for bilirubin. In preterm and sick babies, the B:A ratio may underestimate the risk of irreversible injury because the binding affinity of albumin for bilirubin is compromised. In such instances, an actual measure of the unbound bilirubin could be predictive.

261. What are the common drugs that displace bilirubin from the albumin binding sites?

Common drugs that displace bilirubin from the binding sites on albumin, in descending order of effect, include:

Ceftriaxone	Salicylates
Sulfisoxazole	Carbenicillin
Cefmetazole	Ethacrynic acid
Sulfamethoxazole	Aminophylline
Cefonicid	Ibuprofen
Cefotetan	Ampicillin, cefotaxime, and vancomycin can be
Moxalactam	safely given to a jaundiced infant.

262. Why is a near-term newborn more likely to have excessive hyperbilirubinemia?

Near-term infants weighing more than 2000 g are generally cared for in "well baby" nurseries. However, because of their biologic immaturity, they are likely to tolerate feedings more slowly and exhibit slower maturation of hepatic glucoronyl transferase enzyme activity. Passage of meconium may also be delayed. All of these factors contribute to the severity of hyperbilirubinemia.

Near-term babies are often discharged by 48 hours of age (like term babies) and are more likely to be readmitted with dehydration, excessive hyperbilirubinemia, and even kernicterus. Predischarge evaluation, risk assessment, nutritional support, diligent plans for follow-up, and mandatory revisits are crucial to ensure the baby's well-being.

263. Does exchange transfusion prevent kernicterus?

The controlled clinical trial reported by Mollison and Walker established exchange transfusion as the standard treatment for preventing kernicterus in neonatal Rh hemolytic disease. Furthermore, this trial and subsequent clinical experience confirmed that kernicterus was unlikely if serum bilirubin concentrations were kept below 20 mg/dl (342 μmol/L).

Based on the pathophysiology of Rh disease, the extrapolation of these data to babies with non-Rh disease–related jaundice is inappropriate. Currently, the AAP Practice Parameters recommends an exchange transfusion upon failure of intensive phototherapy in newborns ≤ 48 hours of age for a TSB > 20 mg/dl (342 μmol/L). For babies > 48 hours age who have TSB values > 25 mg/dl (430 μmol/L), an exchange transfusion is recommended upon failure of intensive phototherapy.

Mollison PL, Walker W: Controlled trials of the treatment of haemolytic disease of the newborn. Lancet 1:429–433, 1952.

264. How does phototherapy work?

The goal of phototherapy is to reduce the amount of bilirubin in the jaundiced infant. In contrast to the effect of sunlight in reducing jaundice (heliotherapy), photodestruction of bilirubin can be predictable and controlled and is not seasonal dependent. Phototherapy is accomplished by (1) absorption of light by the bilirubin molecule, (2) photoconversion of bilirubin, and (3) excretion of photoproducts.

- **Chemical process.** The absorption by the bilirubin of a photon from a light source is the initial step that commences the process of photoelimination. A photon with a wavelength of 450 nm (blue photon) has the highest probability of being absorbed by the bilirubin molecule in vitro. However, in vivo the actual spectral wavelength is dependent on the albumin-binding characteristics and the photon's ability to penetrate the skin. Longer wavelength light penetrates more deeply.
- **Photon effect.** The photon's energy produces an excited state of bilirubin that leads to heat production, fluorescence, or a photochemical reaction that changes the structure of the bilirubin molecule (photoisomerization) or destroys the bilirubin molecule (photo-oxidation). Photoisomerization is the main pathway of bilirubin elimination. There are two known pathways of photoisomerization: configurational isomerization (formation of 4Z,15E isomer) and structural isomerization (formation of lumirubin). Lumirubin, but not the 4Z,15E isomer, is rapidly excreted from the body and accounts for the effectiveness of phototherapy.
- **Excretion.** These photoproducts are generally water soluble and are excreted through the urine and stools.

265. What variables control the effectiveness of phototherapy?

The intensity of phototherapy is determined by the energy output of the light source (irradiance), the spectral output of the light source, and the baby's skin surface area. When using more than one light source, caution must be exercised not to over heat or burn the skin.

266. What are the clinical manifestations of neonatal hemolysis other than jaundice?

Hematologic
Decrease in hemoglobin
Reticulocytosis (> 8% at birth, > 5% in first 2–3 days, and > 2% after first week)
Changes in the peripheral smear: microspherocytosis, anisocytosis, target cells
Elevated carboxyhemoglobin levels

Respiratory
Increased levels of end-tidal carbon monoxide

267. What are the side-effects of phototherapy?

After nearly 40 years of clinical use and experience, phototherapy is believed to be relatively benign. The following side effects have been investigated and are listed along with the reported likelihood of occurrence:

SIDE-EFFECTS INVESTIGATED	REPORTED OUTCOMES
Albumin binding	No effect on albumin's ability to bind bilirubin
Insensible water loss	Increased, especially in preterm neonates and those cared for under radiant warmers

(Table continued on next page.)

SIDE-EFFECTS INVESTIGATED	REPORTED OUTCOMES
Effect on growth	No demonstrable effect on long-term body weight, length, and head circumference
GI effects	Gut transit time is reduced but does not seem to be related to the type of milk intake, but is related to the increased bilirubin and photoproducts in the gut
Platelet counts	Platelet counts < 150,000/mm^3 in babies with BW < 2 kg as reported in a single study. Associated with increased turnover.
Patent ductus arteriosus (PDA)	Based on clinical diagnosis of PDA, no effect has been demonstrated or observed.
Riboflavin status	May lead to short-term and transient deficiency that corrects within 24 hours of discontinuation of phototherapy
Mortality	None reported

268. Do events during labor and delivery influence the occurrence of hyperbilirubinemia?

No! The following events have *not* been shown to affect the severity or incidence of hyperbilirubinemia:

Pitocin induction
Epidural anesthesia and maternal anesthetic agents
Maternal vitamin K
Tocolytic agents
Mode of delivery (no known effect unless associated with bruising)

269. Should phototherapy be discontinued in babies with both unconjugated and conjugated hyperbilirubinemia?

Babies with a combined indirect and direct hyperbilirubinemia are prone to acquire long-term "bronzing" of the skin as a result of exposure to phototherapy and accumulation of lumirubin. However, although these infants look unwell, bronzing is not a reason to discontinue phototherapy. Direct bilirubin may compete with indirect bilirubin for albumin-binding sites and increase the risk of kernicterus, although it is not by itself neurotoxic. Furthermore, the concentration of direct reacting bilirubin should not be subtracted from the TSB value to ascertain the potential neurotoxicity of indirect bilirubin. The validity of that practice has never been substantiated.

270. When should phototherapy be stopped in term and near-term babies?

When phototherapy is discontinued in a term or near-term baby with nonhemolytic disease, the "rebound hyperbilirubinemia" is generally modest. Some arbitrary recommendations for discontinuing phototherapy are based on serum bilirubin values ranging from 12 to 15 mg/dl, but it may be more prudent to continue phototherapy until the values have reached to < 40th percentile track for the hour-specific bilirubin level. Similar recommendations may also be used for babies with hemolytic disease. When using intensive phototherapy, the clinician is advised to account for the impact of the high dosage of light and consider weaning slowly to avoid a more significant rebound effect.

271. When should phototherapy be stopped in preterm infants?

There is no consensus or adequate clinical data that address this issue. From a practical perspective, phototherapy should be discontinued at the level at which it was considered appropriate to initiate the intervention.

272. Should exposing the term newborn with hyperbilirubinemia to sunlight (heliotherapy) be encouraged as the natural source of phototherapy?

This recommendation stems from the original observation by Sister Ward in 1956 that led to the subsequent development of phototherapy. However, the confounding issues of heat, excessive water loss and dehydration, and unnecessary exposure to ultraviolet light (prevented by window glass) need to be considered. Furthermore, the clinical evaluation of jaundice can no longer be based on visual impression because the skin bilirubin content would change before the serum.

273. Who was Sister Ward?

In the early 1950s, Sister Ward was the nurse in charge of the unit for premature infants at Rochford General Hospital in Essex, England. On warm summer days, Sister Ward would take her infants to the courtyard to give them a little fresh air and sunshine. It was following such an afternoon of sunshine that Sister Ward observed that sunlight was able to "bleach" the skin of jaundiced neonates. The account of her discovery, as recorded by R. H. Dobbs, follows:

> One particularly fine summer's day in 1956, during a ward routine, Sister Ward diffidently showed us a premature baby, carefully undressed and with fully exposed abdomen. The infant was pale yellow except for a strongly demarcated triangle of skin very much yellower than the rest of the body. I asked her, "Sister, what did you paint it with—iodine or flavine—and why?" But she replied that she thought it must have been the sun. "What do you mean Sister? Suntan takes days to develop after the erythema has faded." Sister Ward looked increasingly uncomfortable, and explained that she thought it was a jaundiced baby, much darker where a corner of the sheet had covered the area. "It's the rest of the body that seems to have faded." We left it at that, and as the infant did well and went home, fresh air treatment of prematurity continued.

274. What is irradiance of phototherapy?

Irradiance is the dosage of light (uwatts/cm^2/nm) at the skin surface. The rate of bilirubin decline is proportional to the dose of phototherapy. Devices that measure irradiance accurately are easy to operate. The maximal achievable irradiance is generally between 30 and 40 uwatts/cm^2/nm. The minimally effective irradiance is ~ 5 uwatts/cm^2/nm.

275. Can phototherapy be administered at home?

Home phototherapy is an acceptable alternative for "healthy" term jaundiced infants who are feeding well if:
- Follow-up mechanisms are in place for both the baby and the mother.
- Comprehensive discharge education has been provided to parents with informed consent.
- Adequate monitoring of the newborn's intake and output are established.

276. Should albumin administration be considered in babies with excessive hyperbilirubinemia prior to exchange transfusion?

Albumin administration has been considered as a means to temporize the rising level of serum bilirubin prior to exchange transfusion. Although the rationale may have merit, it has not been proven in a clinical setting. Its use needs to be considered in the context of potential benefits and risks.

277. Should exchange transfusion be avoided because of the life-threatening side effects?

When performed by skilled and credentialed personnel, exchange transfusion can be a safe and effective procedure that will prevent long-term neurologic consequences. However, intensive phototherapy has largely supplanted exchange transfusions except when bilirubin levels do not decline or continue to increase despite intensive treatment. In babies with Rh hemolytic disease, an exchange transfusion provides an added advantage of antibody reduction. It is important to remember, however, that the risks of exchange transfusion are very great in small preterm infants.

278. Through which routes can an exchange transfusion be performed?

Traditionally, an exchange transfusion has been done through an umbilical venous catheter that has been placed in the inferior vena cava. Blood is removed in aliquots of about 5–8 ml/kg over a 1-minute duration and reinfused with fresh donor blood at the same volume and rate while continuous cardiorespiratory monitoring is maintained.

Alternatively, isovolumic exchange transfusions have also been recommended using centrally or peripherally placed catheters. For a central site, catheters are placed in the umbilical artery (low position) and in the umbilical vein (inferior vena cava) for withdrawal and infusion, respectively. The radial artery and antecubital vein are acceptable peripheral sites. Withdrawal and infusion are done concurrently at the same rate either by a manual mechanism or with the use of timed pumps.

279. Why has double-volume exchange transfusion been recommended instead of a single-volume or triple-volume exchange transfusion?

An effective double-volume exchange transfusion (160 ml/kg) reduces the serum bilirubin by two time constants (84.5% reduction). With a one-volume exchange transfusion (80 ml/kg) bilirubin is reduced one time constant (63%), and with a three-volume exchange it is reduced by 95%. The three-volume exchange transfusion is not used because it prolongs the procedure and increases the risk of a complication.

280. What are the indications for readmission of an infant with hyperbilirubinemia?
- Rate of rise in total serum bilirubin > 6 mg/24 hours
- Level of bilirubin > 95th percentile track (persistent) *or* any value above 98th percentile track
- Level of bilirubin that has jumped tracks from < 75th percentile track to > 95th percentile track
- Clinical signs of neurotoxicity (see BIND evaluation)
- B:A ratio (mg/g) > 6.0

A baby needs hospital admission to receive intensive phototherapy. The bilirubin in such infants should be persistently > 95th percentile track. Clinical judgment is enhanced by measuring the serum albumin value. In babies with B:A ratio (mg/g) of < 5.5, the decision to administer intensive phototherapy can be delayed as long as the baby is closely watched for clinical signs of BIND and is feeding, urinating, and stooling normally. On the other hand, in babies with low serum albumin (values < 3.4 g/dl), one needs to be more aggressive in implementing therapy.

281. What is the value of routinely administering fluids when an infant is admitted for excessive hyperbilirubinemia?

The clinical goal in the management of hyperbilirubinemia is to reduce the total bilirubin load of the body and facilitate the natural modes of excretion (stools, urine, skin). Dilution is not a true option. The need for intravenous fluids is indicated in the event of dehydration with oliguria or poor feeding by the baby. Continuing oral feedings significantly decreases enterohepatic circulation of bilirubin.

282. Should a sepsis evaluation be done routinely when an infant is admitted for excessive hyperbilirubinemia?

Evaluation for sepsis and need of antibiotics are based on the usual indications for assessment of perinatal sepsis; there is no indication for prophylactic antibiotics in jaundiced infants. In the event of neurologic manifestations or suspected galactosemia, a heightened concern for sepsis warrants an aggressive approach.

283. What are the indications to discontinue breast-feeding in an excessively jaundiced baby?

None. At times, however, it is helpful to discontinue breast-feeding to diagnose breast milk jaundice. In such cases, the bilirubin levels drop precipitously, but may rebound when breast-feeding resumes.

284. What advice should be given to a mother who is breast-feeding her excessively jaundiced baby?
- Continue breast-feeding. Evaluate for adequate latching and audible swallowing of milk by baby and assess infant's consolability after a feed.

- Use an electrical breast pump to facilitate "let down of milk" and to collect expressed breast milk for extra supplementation.
- Avoid use of opioid analgesics (Percocet, Tylenol III, and other codeine preparations) that could impact on newborn's feeding and stooling.
- Identify ways to reduce the stress and anxiety to promote lactation.

ABDOMINAL MASSES

285. What is the origin of most neonatal abdominal masses?

Over half of all abdominal masses in the neonate arise from the urinary tract.

286. List the two most common causes of abdominal masses of urologic origin in the neonate.

1. Hydronephrosis secondary to ureteropelvic junction (UPJ) obstruction
2. Multicystic kidney disease

287. A pregnant mother-to-be has an antenatal ultrasound that reveals an intra-abdominal mass in the fetus. Are any special arrangements necessary for the timing and mode of delivery?

No.

288. How do the location and other physical examination characteristics of the common abdominal masses in newborn infants provide clues for their identification?

Physical examination may significantly narrow the diagnostic possibilities, even if it does not provide an absolute answer. Of note:

- Large masses may fill the entire abdomen, making it impossible to determine the site of origin on examination.
- Hard, nodular masses are usually malignant tumors.
- A highly mobile mass is usually a mesenteric cyst, a duplication, or an ovarian cyst.

MASS LOCATION	TYPE	CHARACTERISTICS
Lateral mass	Multicystic kidney or hydronephrosis	Smooth, moderate mobility, transilluminates
	Renal tumor (Wilms' or mesoblastic nephroma)	Smooth, minimal mobility, does not transilluminate
	Neuroblastoma	Irregular contour, minimally mobile, frequently crosses the midline, does not transilluminate
Midabdominal mass	Mesenteric cyst	Smooth, mobile, transilluminates
	Gastrointestinal duplication cyst	Smooth, mobile, does not transilluminate; may be associated with obstruction
	Ovarian cyst	Smooth, mobile, transilluminates
Upper abdominal mass	Hepatic tumors	Hard, immobile, does not transilluminate
	Choledochal cyst	Smooth, immobile, does not transilluminate; may be associated with jaundice
Lower abdominal mass	Hydrometrocolpos	Smooth, immobile, does not transilluminate; may be associated with imperforate hymen
Lower abdominal mass	Bladder	Smooth fixed; associated with lower urinary obstruction
	Urachal cyst	Smooth, fixed to abdominal wall, extends to umbilicus
	Sacrococcygeal teratoma	Hard, fixed, does not transilluminate; often associated with external sacral component

289. What is the recommended treatment for a newborn girl with an ovarian cyst that has been detected on antenatal ultrasound?

The management of ovarian cysts in the neonate is somewhat controversial. Most arise in response to antenatal hormonal stimulation and may subsequently resolve after birth. Potential complications, such as torsion, hemorrhage into the cyst, and rupture, are somewhat related to the size of the cyst; the risk of malignancy depends on whether the cyst is simple (homogeneous) or complex.

Most authorities recommend carefully following asymptomatic cysts by serial ultrasonography for several months if they are ECHO-free and less than 5 cm in diameter. If the cysts causes compressive symptoms, has any solid components, or is greater than 5 cm, it should be excised. The roles of laparoscopic resection and percutaneous drainage versus open surgery are not yet well defined.

Even more controversial and as yet of unproven utility is a suggestion that in-utero ovarian cyst decompression be considered for anechoic cysts that are greater than 4 cm, wander about the abdomen, or enlarge rapidly in an effort to prevent potential fetal ovarian torsion.

290. What imaging studies are most useful in a newborn with an abdominal mass?

A **plain abdominal radiograph** might reveal a mass effect or bowel obstruction, can help localize the mass, and can sometimes provide useful information about the mass itself, such as the presence of calcifications or stool. An **abdominal ultrasound** is the most useful study in the majority of cases because it can show whether the mass is cystic or solid, the effect on adjacent anatomic structures, and often the exact anatomic location of the mass. Rarely, more information is required and can be provided with **abdominal computed tomography** (CT), **magnetic resonance imaging** (MRI), or **urologic imaging.**

291. What is the differential diagnosis of a solid mass arising from the liver?
1. Hemangioma (benign)
2. Hemangioendothelioma (benign)
3. Hepatoblastoma (malignant)

Ultrasound appearance is characteristic and often diagnostic. Serum alpha-fetoprotein (AFP) is usually elevated in hepatoblastoma. Small to moderate hemangiomas can be observed or treated medically with corticosteroids or alpha-interferon. Most large or symptomatic (pain, heart failure, thrombocytopenia) hemangiomas and all hemangioendotheliomas and hepatoblastomas require hepatic resection.

292. What is the most common cause of bilateral abdominal masses in the neonate?

Hydronephrosis secondary to UPJ obstruction.

293. What is the percentage of contralateral renal anomalies in patients with hydronephrosis secondary to UPJ obstruction?
- 10–40% have contralateral hydronephrosis secondary to UPJ obstruction
- 10–15% have a contralateral multicystic kidney
- 5% have contralateral renal agenesis

294. What are the etiologies of presacral masses in the neonate?
- Congenital
    Anterior meningocele, teratoma, lipoma, neuroenteric cyst, rectal duplication
    Chordoma
- Neurogenic tumors—neuroblastoma, presacral glioma
- Currarino triad—sacral bony defect, presacral mass, and anorectal malformation

ACKNOWLEDGMENT

Dr. Schanler is supported by the National Institute of Child Health and Human Development, Grant No. RO-1-HD-28140 and the General Clinical Research Center, Baylor College of Medicine/Texas

Children's Hospital Clinical Research Center, Grant No. MO-1-RR-00188, National Institutes of Health. Partial funding also has been provided from the USDA/ARS under Cooperative Agreement No. 58-6250-6-001. The contents of this publication do not necessarily reflect the views or policies of the USDA, nor does mention of trade names, commercial products, or organizations imply endorsement by the US Government.

BIBLIOGRAPHY

Fetal Growth Assessment
1. Adeniyi-Jones S: Intrauterine growth retardation. In Spitzer AR (ed): Intensive Care of the Fetus and Neonate. Philadelphia, W.B. Saunders, 1996, p 137.
2. Hacket GA, et al: Doppler studies in growth retarded fetus and prediction of neonatal necrotizing enterocolitis, hemorrhage, and neonatal morbidity. BMJ 294:13, 1987.
3. Sparks JW: Intrauterine growth and nutrition. In Polin RA, Fox WW (eds): Fetal and Neonatal Physiology, 2nd ed. Philadelphia, W.B. Saunders, 1998, p 267.
4. Walther FJ: Growth and development of term-disproportionate small-for-gestational-age infants at age of 7 years. Early Hum Dev 18:1, 1988.

Medical Problems of the Growth-Retarded Infant
5. Whyte RK, Sinclair JC, Bayley HS, et al: Energy cost of growth of premature infants. Acta Paediatr Acad Sci Hung 23:85-98, 1982.

Caloric Requirements
6. Chessex P, Reichman BL, Verellen GJ, et al: Influence of postnatal age, energy intake, and weight gain on energy metabolism in the very low-birth-weight infant. J Pediatr 99:761–766, 1981.
7. Denne SC, Kalhan SC: Glucose carbon cycling and oxidation in human newborns. Am J Physiol 251:E71-E77, 1986.
8. Hey EN, O'Connell B: Oxygen consumption and heat balance in cot-nursed baby. Arch Dis Child 45:335–343, 1970.
9. Mestyan J, Jarai I, Fekete M: The total energy expenditure and its components in premature infants maintained under different nursing and environmental conditions. Pediatr Res 2:161–167, 1968.
10. Putet G, Senterre J, Rigo J, Salle B: Energy balance and composition of body weight: Energy metabolism, nutrition, and growth in premature infants. Biol Neonate 52(suppl 1):17–24, 1987.
11. Roberts SB, Young VR: Energy costs of fat and protein deposition in human infants. Am J Clin Nutr 48:951–955, 1988.
12. Schofield WN: Predicting basal metabolic rate: New standards and review of previous work. Hum Nutr Clin Nutr 39(suppl 1):5–41, 1985.
13. Schulze K, Kairam R, Stefanski M, et al: Spontaneous variability in minute ventilation, oxygen consumption, and heart rate of low birth weight infants. Pediatr Res 15:1111–1116, 1981.
14. Sinclair JC, Driscoll JM, Heird WC, Winters RW: Supportive management of the sick neonate. Pediatr Clin North Am 17:863–893, 1970.

Carbohydrate Requirements
15. Anderson GH: Human milk feeding. Pediatr Clin North Am 32:335, 1988.
16. Bresson JL, et al: Energy substrate utilization in infants receiving parenteral nutrition with different glucose to fat ratios. Pediatr Res 25:645, 1989.
17. Denne SC: Carbohydrate requirements. In Polin RA, Fox WW (eds): Fetal and Neonatal Physiology, 2nd ed. Philadelphia, W.B. Saunders, 1998, pp 325–327.
18. Grand RJ, et al: Development of the human gastrointestinal tract. Gastroenterology 70:790, 1976.
19. Kalhan SC, et al: Measurement of glucose turnover in the human newborn with (1-13C) glucose. J Clin Endocrinol Metabol 43:704, 1976.
20. Kien CL, Liechty EA, Myerberg DZ, et al: Dietary carbohydrate assimilation in the preterm infant. Evidence for a nutritionally significant bacterial ecosystem in the colon. Am J Clin Nutr 46:456–460, 1987.
21. Sauer PJ, et al: Glucose oxidation rates in newborn infants measured with indirect calorimetry and U-13C glucose. Clin Sci (Colch) 70:587, 1986.

Protein Requirements
22. American Academy of Pediatrics, Committee on Nutrition: Protein. In Kleinman RE (ed): Pediatric Nutrition Handbook, 4th ed. Elk Grove Village, IL, AAP, 1998, pp 185–196.
23. Denne SC: Protein requirements. In Polin RA, Fox WW (eds): Fetal and Neonatal Physiology, 2nd ed. Philadelphia, W.B. Saunders, 1998, pp 315–325.
24. Heird WC, Kashyap S: Protein and amino acid requirements. In Polin RA, Fox WW (eds): Fetal and Neonatal Physiology, 2nd ed. Philadelphia, W.B. Saunders, 1998, pp 654–665.

25. Kashyap S, Heird WC: Protein requirements of low birth weight, very low birth weight, and small for gestational age infants. In Raiha NCR (ed): Protein Metabolism during Infancy. Nestle Nutrition Workshop Series, Vol. 33. New York, Raven Press, 1994, pp 133–146.
26. Silverio J: Lactobezoar risk. Pediatrics 81:177–178, 1988.

Lipid Requirements
27. Bresson JL, et al: Energy substrate utilization in infants receiving parenteral nutrition with different glucose to fat ratios. Pediatr Res 25:645, 1989.
28. Kleinman RE (ed): Pediatric Nutrition Handbook, 4th ed. Elk Grove Village, IL, AAP, 1998.
29. Roberts SB, Young VR: Energy costs of fat and protein deposition in human infant. Am J Clin Nutr 48:951–955, 1988.

Total Parenteral Nutrition
30. Koo WWK, Tsang RC, Steichen JJ, et al: Parenteral nutrition in infants: The effect of high versus low calcium and phosphorus content. J Pediatr Gastroent Nutr 6:96–104, 1980.
31. Neuzil J, Darlow BA: Oxidation of parenteral lipid emulsions by ambient and phototherapy lights: Potential toxicity of routine parenteral feeding. J Pediatr 126:785–790, 1995.
32. Nose O, Tipton JR, Ament ME, Yabuuchi H: Effect of energy source on changes in energy expenditure, respiratory quotient, and nitrogen balance during TPN in children. Pediatr Res 21:538–541, 1987.
33. Pereira GR, Glassman M: Parenteral nutrition in the neonate. In Rombeau JL, et al (eds): Parenteral Nutrition. Philadelphia, W.B. Saunders, 1986, pp 702–720.
34. Reifen RM, Zlotkin S: Microminerals. In Nutritional Needs of Preterm Infants. Philadelphia, Lippincott Williams & Wilkins, 1993, pp 195–207.
35. Wilson DC, Cairns P, Halliday HL, et al: Randomized, controlled trial of aggressive nutritional regimen in sick very low birth weight infants. Arch Dis Child 77:4F–11F, 1997.

Enteral Nutrition
36. American Academy of Pediatrics, Committee on Nutrition: Formula feeding of term infants. In Kleinman RE (ed): Pediatric Nutrition Handbook, 4th ed. Elk Grove Village, IL, AAP, 1998, pp 36–38.
37. Kashyap S, Heird WC: Nutritional requirements for preterm infants. In Burg FD, Ingelfinger JR, Polin RA, Wald ER (eds): Current Pediatric Therapy, 16th ed. Philadelphia, W.B. Saunders, 1999, pp 275–278.
38. Lucas A, Bloom SR, Aynsley-Green A: Gut hormones and "minimal enteral feeding." Acta Paediatr Scand 75:719–723, 1986.
39. Raiten DJ, Talbot JM, Waters JH: Assessment of nutritional requirements for infant formulas. J Nutr 128:2059–2293, 1998.

Breast-feeding
40. American Academy of Pediatrics, Work Group on Breastfeeding: Breastfeeding and the use of human milk. Pediatrics 100:1035–1039, 1997.
41. Briggs GG, Freeman RK, Yaffe SJ, Mitchell CW: Drugs in Pregnancy and Lactation, 5th ed. Baltimore, Williams & Wilkins, 1998.
42. Gartner LM, Lee K: Jaundice in the breastfed infant. Clin Perinatol 26:431–445, 1999.
43. Hale T: Medications and Mothers' Milk, 6th ed. Amarillo, TX, Pharmasoft Medical Publishing, 1997.
44. Howard CR, Lawrence RA: Drugs and breastfeeding. Clin Perinatol 26:447–478, 1999.
45. Labbok MH: Health sequelae of breastfeeding for the mother. Clin Perinatol 26:491–503, 1999.
46. Lawrence RA: Breastfeeding, 4th ed. St. Louis, Mosby, 1994.
47. Lawrence RA, Howard CR: Given the benefits of breastfeeding, are there any contraindications? Clin Perinatol 26:479–490, 1999.
48. Neifert MR: Clinical aspects of lactation: Promoting breastfeeding success. Clin Perinatol 26:281–306, 1999.
49. Powers NG: Slow weight gain and low milk supply in the breastfeeding dyad. Clin Perinatol 26:399–430, 1999.
50. Riordan J, Auerback KG: Breastfeeding and Human Lactation, 2nd ed. Sudbury, Jones & Bartlett Publishers, 1999.

Vitamins and Trace Minerals
51. Atkinson SA, Zlotkin S: Recognizing deficiencies and excesses of zinc, copper, and other trace elements. In Tsang RC, Zlotkin SH, Nichols BL, Hansen JW (eds): Nutrition during Infancy. Cincinnati, Digital Educational Publishing.
52. Koo WWK, Tsang RC: Calcium, magnesium, phosphorus, and vitamin D. In Tsang RC, Lucas A, Uauy R, Zlotkin S (eds): Nutritional Needs of the Preterm Infant. Pawling, NY, Caduceus Medical Publishers, 1993, pp 135–156.
53. Mahoney CP, Margolis MT, Knauss TA, Labbe RF: Chronic vitamin A intoxication in infants fed chicken liver. Pediatrics 65:893–896, 1980.

54. Raiten DJ, Talbot JM, Waters JH: Assessment of nutritional requirements for infant formulas. J Nutr 128:2059–2293, 1998.
55. Schanler RD: Water-soluble vitamins: C, B1, B2, B6, niacin, biotin, and pantothenic acid. In Tsang RC, Nichols BL (eds): Nutrition During Infancy. Philadelphia, Mosby, 1988, pp 236–252.
56. Schlaner RJ: Who needs water-soluble vitamins? In Tsang RC, Zlotkin SH, Nichols BL, Hansen JW (eds): Nutrition during Infancy. Cincinnati, Digital Educational Publishing.
57. Shenai JP: Vitamin A. In Tsang RC, Lucas A, Uauy R, Zlotkin S (eds): Nutritional Needs of the Preterm Infant. Pawling, NY, Caduceus Medical Publishers, 1993, pp 87–100.

Iron Requirements
58. American Academy of Pediatrics, Committee on Nutrition: Iron deficiency. In Kleinman RE (ed): Pediatric Nutrition Handbook, 4th ed. Elk Grove Village, IL, AAP, 1998, pp 233–246.
59. American Academy of Pediatrics, Committee on Nutrition: Iron fortification of infant formulas. Pediatrics 104:119–123, 1999.
60. Chockalingam UM, Murphy E, Ophoven JC, et al: Cord transferrin and ferritin values in newborn infants at risk for prenatal uteroplacental insufficiency and chronic hypoxia. J Pediatr 111:283–286, 1987.
61. Guiang SF 3d, Georgieff MK: Fetal and neonatal iron metabolism. In Polin RA, Fox WW (eds): Fetal and Neonatal Physiology, 2nd ed. Philadelphia, W.B. Saunders, 1998, pp 401–409.
62. Siimes MA, Jarvenpaa AL: Prevention of anemia and iron deficiency in very-low-birth-weight infants. J Pediatr 101:277–282, 1982.

Gastroesophageal Reflux
63. Hyman PE: Gastroesophageal reflux: One reason why baby won't eat. J Pediatr 125:S103–S109, 1994.
64. Orenstein SR: Gastroesophageal reflux. Pediatr Rev 20:24–28, 1999.
65. Orenstein SR: Infantile reflux: Different from adult reflux. Am J Med 103:114S–119S, 1997.
66. Orenstein SR: The prone alternative. Pediatrics 94:104–105, 1994.
67. Vandenplas Y, Bell DC, Benatar A, et al: The role of cisapride in the treatment of pediatric gastroesophageal reflux. J Pediatr Gastroenterol Nutr 28:518–528, 1999.

Esophageal Atresia and Tracheoesophageal Fistula
68. Harmon CM, Coran AG: Congenital anomalies of the esophagus. In O'Neill JA, Rowe MI, Grosfeld JL, et al (eds): Pediatric Surgery, 5th ed. St. Louis, Mosby, 1998, pp 941–967.
69. Spitz L, Kiely EM, Morecroft JA, et al: Esophageal atresia: At-risk groups for the 1990s. J Pediatr Surg 29:723–725, 1994.
70. Stringer MD, McKenna KM, Goldstein RB, et al: Prenatal diagnosis of esophageal atresia. J Pediatr Surg 30:1258–1263, 1995.

Malabsorption
71. Altschuler SM, Liacouras CA: Clinical Pediatric Gastroenterology. Philadelphia, Churchill Livingstone, 1998.
72. Ducker DA, Hughes CA, Warren I, McNeish AS: Neonatal gut function, measured by the one-hour blood + D-xylose test: Influence of gestational age and size. Gut 21:133–136, 1980.
73. Foman SJ, et al: Excretion of fat by normal full-term infants fed various milks and formulas. Am J Clin Nutr 23:1299–1313, 1970.
74. Liefaard G, Heineman E, Molenaar JC, Tibboel D: Prospective evaluation of the absorptive capacity of the bowel after major and minor resections in the neonate. J Pediatr Surg 30:388–391, 1995.
75. Lifschitz C: Role of colonic scavengers of unabsorbed carbohydrates in infants and children. J Am Coll Nutr 15:30S–34S, 1996.
76. Shearman DJC, Finlayson N, Camilleri M, Carter D: Diseases of the Gastrointestinal Tract and Liver, 3rd ed. New York, Churchill Livingstone, 1997.
77. Turk E, Zabel B, Mundlos S, et al: Glucose/galactose malabsorption caused by a defect in the Na+/glucose cotransporter. Nature 350:355–357, 1991.
78. Walker WA, Drurie PR, Hamilton JR, et al: Pediatric Gastrointestinal Disease, 2nd ed. Philadelphia, Mosby, 1991.

Intestinal Atresias
79. Fonkalsrud EW, DeLorimier AA, Hays DM: Congenital atresia and stenosis of the duodenum. Pediatrics 43:79–83, 1969.
80. Moore SW, Johnson AG: Hirschsprung disease: Genetic and functional associates of Down and Waardenburg syndromes. Semin Pediatr Surg 7:156–161, 1998.

Meconium Ileus and Meconium Plug
81. Gross K, Desant A, Grosfeld JL, et al: Intra-abdominal complications of cystic fibrosis. J Pediatr Surg 20:431–435, 1985.
82. Olsen MM, Luck SR, Lloyd-Still J, Raffensperger JG: The spectrum of meconium disease in infancy. J Pediatr Surg 17:479–481, 1982.

83. Rescorla FJ, Grosfeld JL: Contemporary management of meconium ileus. World J Surg 17:318-325, 1993.
84. Wagget J, Johnson DG, Borns P, Bishop HC: The nonoperative treatment of meconium ileus by Gastrografin enema. Pediatrics 77:407–411, 1970.

Imperforate Anus
85. Kiely EM, Peña A: Anorectal malformations. In O'Neill JA, Rowe MI, Grosfeld JL, et al (eds): Pediatric Surgery, 5th ed. St. Louis, Mosby, 1998, pp 1425–1428.
86. Peña A: Atlas of Surgical Management of Anorectal Malformations. New York, Springer-Verlag, 1990.

Gastrointestinal Hemorrhage
87. Heitlinger LA, McClung HJ: Gastrointestinal hemorrhage. In Wyllie R, Hyams JS (eds): Pediatric Gastrointestinal Disease. Philadelphia, W.B. Saunders, 1999, pp 64–72.
88. Perrault JF, Berry R: Gastrointestinal bleeding. In Walker WA, Durie PR, Hamilton JR, et al (eds): Pediatric Gastrointestinal Disease. St. Louis, Mosby, 1996, pp 323–342.

Necrotizing Enterocolitis
89. Kliegman R: Necrotizing enterocolitis. In Burg FD, Ingelfinger JR, Wald ER, Polin RA (eds): Gellis & Kagan's Current Pediatric Therapy, 15th ed. Philadelphia, W.B. Saunders, 1996.
90. Kliegman R: Necrotizing enterocolitis: Differential diagnosis and management. In Polin RA, Yoder MC, Burg FD (eds): Workbook in Practical Neonatology, 2nd ed. Philadelphia, W.B. Saunders, 1993.
91. Neu J (ed): Neonatal Gastroenterology: Clinics in Perinatology. Philadelphia, W.B. Saunders, 1996.
92. Stoll BJ, Kliegman RM (eds): Necrotizing Enterocolitis: Clinics in Perinatology. Philadelphia, W.B. Saunders, 1994.

Neonatal Ascites
93. Harris MC: Neonatal ascites. In Burg FD, Ingelfinger JR, Wald ER, Polin RA (eds): Gellis & Kagan's Current Pediatric Therapy, 16th ed. Philadelphia, W.B. Saunders, 1999, pp 269–272.
94. Raffensperger JG: Neonatal ascites. In Raffensperger JG (ed): Swenson's Pediatric Surgery, 5th ed. Norwalk, CT, Appleton & Lange, 1990, pp 641–645.
95. Unger SW, Chandler JG: Chylous ascites in infants and children. Surgery 93:455–461, 1983.
96. Wyllie R, Arasu TS, Fitzgerald JF: Ascites: Pathophysiology and management. J Pediatr 97:167–176, 1980.

Bile Duct Disorders and Biliary Atresia
97. Bates MD, Bucuvalas JC, Alonso MH, Ryckman FC: Biliary atresia: Pathogenesis and treatment. Semin Liver Dis 18:281–293, 1998.
98. Stein JE, Vacanti JP: Biliary atresia and other disorders of the extrahepatic biliary tree. In Suchy FJ (ed): Liver Disease in Children. St. Louis, Mosby, 1994, pp 426–442.

Unconjugated Hyperbilirubinemia
99. Newman TB, Klebanoff MA: Neonatal hyperbilirubinemai and long-term outcome: Another look at the Collaborative Perinatal Project. Pediatrics 92:651–657, 1993.

Abdominal Masses
100. Bauer SB: Anomalies of the kidneys and ureteropelvic junction. In Walsh PC, Retik AB, Vaughn ED, Wein AJ (eds): Campbell's Urology, 7th ed. Philadelphia, W.B. Saunders, 1999, pp 1708–1755.
101. Crombleholme TM, Craigo SD, Garmel S, D'Alton ME: Fetal ovarian cyst decompression to prevent torsion. J Pediatr Surg 32:1447–1449, 1997.
102. Filston HC, Izant RJ: The Surgical Neonate. Norwalk, CT, Appleton-Century-Crofts, 1985.
103. Glassberg KI: Renal dysplasia and cystic disease of the kidney. In Walsh PC, Retik AB, Vaughn ED, Wein AJ (eds): Campbell's Urology, 7th ed. Philadelphia, W.B. Saunders, 1999, pp 1757–1813.
104. Leape LL: Pediatric Care in Pediatric Surgery. Boston, Little, Brown, 1987.
105. Tank ES: Evaluation and Treatment of Abdominal Masses in Infancy and Childhood. American Urological Association Update Series, Volume III, Lesson 3. Baltimore, AUA, 1983.

9. GENETICS AND GENE THERAPY

1. What are the most common major congenital anomalies in the United States?

Anencephaly and spina bifida, occurring with a prevalence of about 0.5–2.0/1000 live births.

2. Should an asymptomatic infant with a single umbilical artery have a screening ultrasound done for renal anomalies?

This point has been argued for years. A single umbilical artery is a rare phenomenon. In one study of nearly 35,000 infants, examination of the placenta showed that only 112 (0.32%) had a single umbilical artery. All 112 underwent renal ultrasonography, and 17% had abnormalities (45% of which persisted). A more recent study demonstrated that left umbilical arteries tend to be absent more often than right when only a single artery is present. In addition, there was a high incidence of associated congenital malformations in nearly 25% of the infants diagnosed prenatally with a single umbilical artery. Because of the rarity of the condition and the increased association of abnormalities, patients with single umbilical arteries probably should receive a screening renal ultrasound.

Burke WG, et al: Isolated single umbilical artery: The case for routine renal screening. Arch Dis Child 68:600–601, 1993.

Geipel A, et al: Prenatal diagnosis of single umbilical artery: Determination of absent side, associated anomalies, Doppler findings, and perinatal outcome. Ultrasound Obstet Gynecol 15:114–117, 2000.

3. The maternal serum screening test or "triple screen" is done between 14 and 22 weeks gestation. What markers are included on this screen?

The following tests comprise the "triple screen":

- Alpha-fetoprotein (AFP)
- Human chorionic gonadotropin (hCG)
- Unconjugated estriol
  (free 13-subunit)

4. Name the major conditions screened using the "triple screen." What is the detection rate and false-positive rate?

The major conditions screened are:

- Down syndrome (trisomy 21)
- Trisomy 18
- Open neural tube defects
  (high AFP only)

There is a 60% detection rate and a 5% false-positive rate for Down syndrome. The detection rate is 80% for open neural tube defects (high AFP).

5. A new marker has been added to the "triple screen" in some laboratories; what is it?

Inhibin-A, a subunit of the heterodimeric glycoprotein secreted mainly from the corpus luteum and placenta, is elevated in pregnancies affected by Down syndrome.

6. Which other conditions may be detected by raised amniotic fluid AFP?

Multiple gestation	Congenital nephrosis (Finnish type)
Intrauterine fetal death	Sacrococcygeal teratoma
Omphalocele and gastroschisis	Bladder exstrophy
Bowel and esophageal atresias	Focal dermal hypoplasia/aplasia cutis congenita
Turner syndrome (cystic hygroma)	Meckel syndrome

7. A woman who had a positive triple screen in the second trimester and normal fetal ultrasound but declined amniocentesis delivers a healthy-appearing infant. What further studies are indicated based on the "triple screen"?

None. A positive triple screen is a screening test, *not* a diagnostic test. If the infant looks healthy without features of Down syndrome or other anomalies, no further testing is necessary.

Chromosome tests do not need to be done on a normal-appearing infant just because the triple test was abnormal.

8. First trimester screening for aneuploidy is becoming available. What is being measured and how reliable is this new method?

Pregnancy-associated plasma protein (PAPP-A), free hCG, and ultrasound nuchal translucency are being used. PAPP-A is the single best serum marker in early pregnancy found to date. Its levels decrease by more than one half on average in a Down syndrome pregnancy. Low PAPP-A may also be associated with trisomy 18. hCG levels are approximately doubled in Down syndrome.

Measurement of nuchal translucency thickness between 10 and 13 weeks gestation has been shown to identify about 75% of fetuses with Down syndrome. Higher detection rates are obtained by combining free hCG, PAPP-A, and nuchal thickness—up to 85% detection of Down syndrome with a 3.3% false-positive rate.

9. How would you evaluate a newborn with Down syndrome (DS) to ensure you are discharging a healthy infant? What serious abnormalities could one expect to find?
- Order a chromosome study on peripheral blood (G-banding), to rule out translocation or mosaicism.
- Perform a cardiac evaluation (40% of infants with DS have congenital heart disease, with the most common defect being an A-V canal).
- Ensure there is no bowel obstruction. Duodenal atresia, duodenal web, and Hirschsprung disease are more common in DS. Anal stenosis may mimic Hirschsprung disease.
- Assess hearing.
- Check eyes for cataracts, nystagmus, and strabismus.
- Monitor feeding and sucking.
- Perform a thyroid screen (state screen).
- Refer for genetic counseling and early intervention.

10. A macrosomic infant is born with an omphalocele and large tongue. What would you anticipate monitoring closely in this baby and why?

This baby may have Beckwith-Wiedemann syndrome and be at risk for hypoglycemia. Other signs of Beckwith-Wiedemann syndrome include grooves on the ear lobes, hemihypertrophy, and visceromegaly. These children are at risk for Wilms tumor and hepatoma and should be monitored with an abdominal ultrasound every 3 months for the first 3 years of life. The serum AFP should be measured regularly.

11. What is the difference between an omphalocele and gastroschisis?
Omphalocele
- This midline anterior abdominal well defect is covered by a transparent sac consisting of amnion and peritoneum with Wharton's jelly between them.
- Intra-abdominal viscera is herniated through the umbilical ring. The size varies with contents.
- Umbilical cord inserts into the sac.
- Other malformations are present in 67% of cases.
- Frequently associated with chromosome abnormalities, especially trisomy 13.
Gastroschisis
- Umbilical cord is attached to abdominal wall to the left of the defect. There is a normal umbilical cord insertion.
- Herniated organs usually consist of thickened loops of small intestine with no membranous covering and float freely in the amniotic fluid in utero.
- 15% of cases of gastroschisis are associated with other major malformations.
- It is not commonly found in fetuses with chromosome abnormalities.

12. What are the most common causes of congenital diaphragmatic hernia (CDH)?

CDH is an associated inherited condition in the following syndromes:

- Fryns syndrome
- Cornelia de Lange syndrome
- Simpson-Golabi-Behmel syndrome
- Pallister-Killian syndrome
  (mosaic tetrasomy 12p)
- Donnai syndrome
- Beckwith-Wiedemann syndrome
- Denys-Drash syndrome
- Perlman syndrome

The estimated prevalence is 1/2000–1/3000. Isolated CDH may be sporadic. Several multiple malformation syndromes and abnormalities are associated with CDH as seen above.

13. An infant is born with the following features: puffiness of dorsum of hands and feet, excessive skin at nape of neck with low posterior hairline, broad chest and widely spaced nipples, cardiac and aortic defect, cubitus valgus, and renal anomaly. What is your differential diagnosis?

Turner syndrome
Noonan syndrome

14. How would you work up this baby?

- Chromosome study on peripheral
  blood (G-banding)
- Cardiac evaluation
- Renal ultrasound
- Hearing evaluation
- Referral to endocrinologist
- Refer for genetic counseling and
  early intervention

15. How do you define fetal growth retardation?

Fetal growth retardation is the failure of a fetus to achieve its growth potential. In practice, measures of size relative to the population mean for gestational age and sex are used. Fetal growth retardation is variably defined as an infant who is either below the tenth percentile or less than two standard deviations (SD) below the population mean for that gestational age and sex.

16. Intrauterine growth retardation (IUGR) has many causes. What approach would you use to evaluate a newborn with IUGR?

- Establish whether the growth retardation is proportionate or disproportionate.
- Perform a detailed physical examination for anomalies or dysmorphic features.
- If dysmorphic or multiple anomalies, chromosome studies are indicated.
- Take a detailed pregnancy history to look for teratogenic exposures, infection history, or maternal illness (hypertension and preeclampsia).
- Viral studies and antibody titers should be ordered as indicated.
- Uncontrolled maternal phenylketonuria (PKU) can be associated with IUGR and microcephaly.
- An infant with disproportionate IUGR should be worked up for skeletal dysplasia or metabolic bone disease.
- Proportionate IUGR may be associated with many dysmorphic syndromes that may be recognized by a geneticist.
- Placental studies should be performed for confined placental mosaicism and uniparental disomy (UPD).

17. What is confined placental mosaicism (CPM)?

The abnormal cell line in this condition is "confined" either to the cytotrophoblast or chorionic stroma cells of the placenta and is not present in the fetus itself. This situation may be discovered when, on chorionic villous sampling (CVS), there is an abnormal chromosome result (reflecting the placenta), but the fetus appears to be healthy and amniocentesis is normal. The diagnosis of CPM postnatally is usually made retrospectively by follow-up studies on the infant or fetus, placenta, and membranes. The clinical significant of CPM is not yet clear. It has been suggested that CPM may be associated with growth retardation in chromosomally normal fetuses. It may increase the risk of a spontaneous abortion. However, a diploid cell line in the placenta of a fetus with trisomy 18 or 13 may help ensure viability of a fetus with full trisomy 18 or 13. Overall there appears to be a low risk of adverse pregnancy outcome with CPM.

18. What is uniparental disomy (UPD)?

UPD occurs when both members of a chromosome pair are derived solely from one parent in a diploid offspring. Many cases of UPD are the result of resolved trisomies where the individual was initially trisomic but lost one of the extra chromosomes and ended up with two chromosomes from the same parent. The disomy may be two copies of the same chromosome (isodisomy) or one copy of each of the given parent's chromosomes (heterodisomy).

19. What conditions are associated with UPD?
- Prader-Willi syndrome is associated with maternal UPD 15, whereas Angelman syndrome is associated with paternal UPD 15.
- Paternal UPD 11 is associated with Beckwith-Wiedemann syndrome.
- Maternal UPD 7 has been seen in some cases of Russell-Silver syndrome.
- Paternal UPD 6 causes growth retardation (sometimes severe) and transient neonatal diabetes.
- Maternal UPD 16 is associated with growth retardation and variable congenital anomalies but a generally good prognosis.

20. What is FISH and when is it useful?

Fluorescence in situ hybridization (FISH) is a molecular cytogenetic technique used to identify abnormalities of chromosome number or structure using a single-stranded DNA probe (for a known piece of DNA or chromosome segment). The probe is labeled with a fluorescent tag and targeted to a single-strand DNA that has been denatured in place on a microscope slide. The use of fluorescent microscopy enables the detection of more than one probe, each labeled with a different color. An example of the use of FISH is for rapid prenatal diagnosis of trisomies on amniotic fluid or chorionic villi, utilizing interphase cells from cultured specimens and probes for the most common chromosomal abnormalities (13, 18, 21, X, and Y). Although interphase FISH for prenatal diagnosis has low false-positive and false-negative rates, it is considered investigational and is used only in conjunction with standard cytogenetic analysis.

21. The geneticist cannot be reached and you have to evaluate an intrauterine fetal demise. What do you do?
- Obtain a history of the pregnancy and a family history.
- Take photographs and obtain an x-ray (babygram) of the infant.
- Do a detailed clinical exam of the fetus.
- Obtain a skin biopsy for fibroblasts, to obtain chromosome studies and possible metabolic studies.
- Examine the placenta, and culture the placenta or fetal membranes if available.
- If possible, obtain blood samples from the cord or perform a cardiac stick for IgM and cultures if you suspect a congenital infection.
- Obtain autopsy permission (freeze liver or brain from autopsy for additional metabolic studies if indicated).

22. What is anophthalmia?

Anophthalmia is the medical term used to describe the absence of the globe and ocular tissue from the orbit. Anophthalmia and microphthalmia are often used interchangeably because in most cases, the magnetic resonance imaging (MRI) or computed tomography (CT) scan shows some remnants of either the globe or surrounding tissue. Anophthalmia may be unilateral or bilateral and is often associated with other anomalies. There are many causes of anophthalmia including single gene mutations, syndromes, chromosome abnormalities, and teratogenic exposures. Anophthalmia is rare, with an incidence of about 1/10,000.

23. How would you evaluate a newborn with anophthalmia?

- Ophthalmology evaluation and referral to an oculoplastic surgeon and ocularist
- CT scan or MRI of brain and globe to determine if any ocular tissue is present and whether optic nerve is present. Brain anomalies may help point to a specific diagnosis.
- Genetics evaluation
- Renal ultrasound
- Chromosome study, G-banding
- Referral to early intervention and nearest school for the blind
- Parent support group information can be obtained from the Alliance of Genetic Support Groups, (800)-336-GENE.

24. Excluding chromosomal analysis, what laboratory tests suggest that a woman is carrying a fetus with trisomy 21?

The combination of low levels of maternal serum AFP and unconjugated estriol and elevated levels of hCG (the so-called triple screen) can identify 60% of fetuses with Down syndrome with a false-positive rate of 5–7%. Abnormal screening tests can prompt definitive studies of chromosomal analysis.

25. What are the main advantages of CVS over amniocentesis?

CVS is the aspiration of chorionic villi via a transcervical catheter or transabdominal needle using ultrasound guidance. The main advantage of CVS is that is can be done between 10 and 12 weeks of gestation compared with the usual 16-week tinting of amniocentesis. Because of its equivalent accuracy, it permits termination of pregnancy at a significantly earlier date in the event of major chromosomal anomalies.

26. What are the major characteristics of the three major chromosomal malformations: trisomy 21, trisomy 18, and trisomy 13?

Common Autosomal Trisomies

FEATURE	TRISOMY 21	TRISOMY 18	TRISOMY 13
Eponym	Down syndrome	Edward syndrome	Patau syndrome
Tone	1/800	1/8000	1/15,000
Liveborn incidence	Hypotonia	Hypertonia	Hypo- or hypertonia
Cranium/brain	Mild microcephaly, flat occiput, 3 fontanels	Microcephaly, prominent occiput	Microcephaly, sloping forehead, occipital scalp defects, holoprosencephaly
Eyes	Upslanting, epicanthal folds. Speckled iris (Brushfield spots)	Small palpebral fissures, corneal opacity	Microphthalmia, hypotelorism, iris coloboma, retinal dysplasia
Ears	Small, low-set, over-folded upper helix	Low-set, malformed	Low-set, malformed
Facial features	Protruding tongue; large cheeks; low, flat nasal bridge	Small mouth, micrognathia	Cleft lip and palate
Skeletal	Clinodactyly 5th digit, gap between toes 1 and 2, excess nuchal skin, short stature	Clenched hand, absent 5th finger distal crease, hypoplastic nails, short stature, thin ribs	Postaxial polydactyly, hypoconvex finger-nails, clenched hands
Cardiac defect	40%	60%	80%

(Table continued on next page).

Common Autosomal Trisomies (Continued)

FEATURE	TRISOMY 21	TRISOMY 18	TRISOMY 13
Survival	Long-term	90% die in first year	80% die in first year
Other	Abnormal palate, single palmar crease (simian crease)	Rocker bottom feet, polycystic kidneys, dermatoglyphic arch pattern	Genetic anomalies, polycystic kidneys, increased nuclear projections

27. What is the chance that a newborn with a simian crease has Down syndrome?

A single transverse palmar crease is present in 4% of normal newborns. Bilateral palmar creases are found in 1%. These features occur twice as commonly in males than females. However, 50–55% of newborn infants with Down syndrome have a single transverse crease. Since Down syndrome occurs in 1/800 live births, the chance that a newborn with a simian crease has Down syndrome is only 1 in 60.

28. What is the expected intelligence and personality of a child with Down syndrome?

The IQ range is generally 35–65, with a mean reported IQ of 54. Occasionally, the IQ may be higher. Intelligence deteriorates in adulthood, with clinical and pathologic findings consistent with advanced Alzheimer disease. Autopsy results from brains of deceased adults with Down syndrome reveal both neurofibrillary tangles and senile plaques, as found in Alzheimer disease. By age 40, the mean IQ is 24. Children with Down syndrome are generally affectionate and docile. They tend toward mimicry and are noted usually to enjoy music, having a good sense of rhythm. However, 13% have serious emotional problems, and coordination is usually poor.

29. Why is maternal age of 35 at delivery chosen as the cutoff for recommending amniocentesis for chromosome analysis?

There is a well-known association between advanced maternal age and trisomies (including XXY, XXX, and trisomies 13, 18, and 21).

MATERNAL AGE	APPROXIMATE RISK OF TRISOMY 21
30	1/1000
35	1/365
40	1/100
45	1/50

Most cases of Down syndrome involve nondisjunction at meiosis I in the mother. This may be related to the lengthy stage of meiotic arrest between oocyte development in the fetus until ovulation, which may occur as much as 40 years later.

30. What percentage of all babies with Down syndrome are born to women over the age of 35?

Only 20% of babies are born to mothers with advanced maternal age. While their individual risk is higher, women in this age bracket account for only 5% of all pregnancies in the United States.

Haddew JE, et al: Prenatal screening for Down syndrome with use of maternal serum markers. N Engl J Med 327:588–593, 1992.

31. What percentage of cases of Down syndrome are due to translocations?

3.3% of all cases of Down syndrome are due to unbalanced robertsonian translocations in which a third copy of chromosome 21 is present, attached to an acrocentric chromosome. The chance of translocation Down syndrome is two to three times greater in children of younger mothers (6–8% of mothers under 30). One of three infants with translocation Down syndrome will have a parent with a robertsonian translocation. Two-thirds of the time, translocation Down syndrome occurs as a de novo event in the infant.

32. What is the overall recurrence risk of Down syndrome?

In chromosomally normal women under age 40, the recurrence risk for Down syndrome is 1% (assuming the father's chromosomes are also normal). Above age 40, the risk of having a child with Down syndrome increases, primarily as a function of maternal age. If the mother carries a translocation, the recurrence risk is 10%. If the father carries a translocation, the recurrence risk is 3–3.5%. One theory for this observed discrepancy between maternal and paternal rates of translocation Down syndrome is hindered motility of chromosomally abnormal sperm.

33. Does advanced paternal age increase the risk of having a child with trisomy 21?

There does not appear to be an increased risk of Down syndrome associated with paternal age until after age 55. Some studies have noted an increased risk of Down syndrome after this age, although others have not. The reports are controversial, and the statistical analysis needed to perform such a study is cumbersome. It is known that approximately 10% of all trisomy 21 cases derive the extra chromosome 21 from the father.

34. Why has the incidence of Down syndrome decreased from 1.6/1000 live births to 1.0–1.2/1000 live births over the past 25 years?

The decrease in incidence is a result of the reduction of births in older women and the improvements in prenatal diagnosis. The risk for older women has not changed, but, at the present time, only 20% of children with Down syndrome are born to mothers over 35 years of age, whereas 25 years ago 50% of the children with Down syndrome were born to older mothers. Even though women are now giving birth at a later time in their live because of career obligations, the improvements in prenatal diagnosis for Down syndrome have prevented trisomy 21 from being the surprise at birth that it once was.

35. Which is technically correct: Down's syndrome or Down syndrome?

In 1866, John Langdon Down, physician at the Earlswood Asylum in Surrey, England, described the phenotype of a syndrome that now bears his name. However, it was not until 1959 that it was determined that this disorder is caused by an extra chromosome 21. The correct designation is Down syndrome.

36. What genetically inherited disease has the highest known mutation rate per gamete per generation?

Neurofibromatosis. The estimated mutation rate for this disorder is 1×10^{-4} per haploid genome. The clinical features are café-au-lait spots and axillary freckling in childhood followed by development of neurofibromas in later years. There is approximately a 10% risk of malignancy with this condition, and mental deficiency is common.

37. Which disorders with ethnic and racial predilections most commonly warrant maternal screening for carrier status?

DISORDER	ETHNIC/RACIAL GROUP	SCREENING MARKER
Tay-Sachs disease	Ashkenazi Jewish, French Canadian	Decreased serum hexosaminidase A concentration
Sickle cell anemia	Black African, Mediterranean, Arab, Indian, Pakistani	Presence of sickling of cells in hemolysate, followed by confirmatory hemoglobin electrophoresis
Alpha- and beta-thalassemia	Mediterranean, southern and southeastern Chinese, Chinese	MCV < 80 µm³, followed by hemoglobin electrophoresis

From D'Alton ME, DeCherney AH: Prenatal diagnosis. N Engl J Med 328:115, 1993, with permission.

38. Why are mitochondrial disorders transmitted from generation to generation by the mother and not the father?

Mitochondrial DNA abnormalities (e.g., many cases of ragged red fiber myopathies) are passed on from the mother because mitochondria are present in the cytoplasm of the egg and not the sperm. Transmission to males or females is equally likely; however, expression is variable because mosaicism with normal and abnormal mitochondria in varying proportions is very common.

Johns DR: Mitochondrial DNA and disease. N Engl J Med 333:638–644, 1995.

39. Which syndromes are associated with advanced paternal age?

Advanced paternal age is well documented to be associated with new dominant mutations. The assumption is that the increased mutation rate is due to accumulation of new mutations from many cell divisions. The more cell divisions, the more likely an error (mutation) will occur. The mutation rate in fathers > 50 years is five times higher than the mutation rate in fathers < 20 years of age. New, common autosomal dominant mutations that have been recently mapped and identified are achondroplasia (Shiang et al., 1994), Apert syndrome (Wilkie et al., 1995), and Marfan syndrome (Dietz et al., 1991).

Dietz HC, Cutting GR, Pyeritz RE, et al: Marfan syndrome caused by a recurrent de novo missense mutation in the fibrillin gene. Nature 352:337_339, 1991.

Shiang R, Thompson LM, Zhu YZ, et al: Mutations in the transmembrane domain of FGFR3 cause the most common genetic form of dwarfism, achondroplasia. Cell 78:335–342, 1994.

Wilkie AO, Slaney SF, Oldridge M, et al: Apert syndrome results from localized mutations of FGFR2 and is allelic with Crouzon syndrome. Nature Gen 9:165–172, 1995.

40. What is the most common genetic-lethal disease?

Cystic fibrosis (CF). A genetic-lethal disease is one that interferes with a person's ability to reproduce due to early death (before childbearing age) or impaired sexual function. CF is the most common autosomal recessive disorder in whites, occurring in 1/1600 (1 of every 20 individuals is a carrier for this condition). CF is characterized by widespread dysfunction of exocrine glands, chronic pulmonary disease, pancreatic insufficiency, and intestinal obstructions. Presentation during the newborn period can include meconium ileus with intestinal obstruction, nonspecific pulmonary disease of a recurring nature, rectal prolapse, malabsorption, and failure to thrive. Males are azoospermic later in life. The median survival is approximately 29 years.

Much work, however, is currently underway using CF as the prototypical disease that should be amenable to genetic therapy. It is hoped that genetic treatment will add immeasurably to the life expectancy of these patients.

41. What are the "fat baby" syndromes, in which the appearance of obesity is prominent?

• Prader-Willi syndrome (obesity, hypotonia, small hands and feet)
• Beckwith-Wiedemann syndrome (macrosomia, omphalocele, macroglossia, ear creases)
• Sotos syndrome (macrosomia, macrocephaly, large hands and feet)
• Weaver syndrome (macrosomia, accelerated skeletal maturation, camptodactyly)
• Laurence-Moon-Biedl syndrome (obesity, retinal pigmentation, polydactyly)
• Infants of diabetic mothers syndrome

42. What is the H_3O of Prader-Willi syndrome?

Hyperphagia, **h**ypotonia, **h**ypopigmentation, and **o**besity. Up to 50% of patients, most with mental retardation, have a deletion on the long arm of chromosome 15. The gene(s) responsible for Prader-Willi syndrome are subject to parental imprinting. Imprinting is the process by which expression of a gene depends on whether it has been inherited from the mother or the father (Deal, 1995). The gene(s) associated with Prader-Willi syndrome are paternally imprinted, meaning that loss of the paternal copy will result in the phenotype of Prader-Willi (Knoll et al., 1989; Robinson et al., 1991). A closely related area of the long arm of chromosome 15 is maternally imprinted, and loss of the maternal copy leads to Angelman syndrome (Chan et al., 1993).

Angelman syndrome is characterized by severe developmental delay, abnormal gait, inappropriate laughter, and excessive movements, especially of the arms.

Chan CTJ, Clayton-Smith J, Cheng XJ, et al: Molecular mechanisms in Angelman syndrome: A survey of 93 patients. Am J Med Genet 30:895–902, 1993.

Deal CL: Parental genomic imprinting. Curr Opin Pediatr 7:445–458, 1995.

Knoll JHM, Nicholls RD, Magenis RE, et al: Angelman and Prader-Willi syndromes have a chromosome 15 deletion but differ in parental origin of the deletion. Am J Med Genet 32:285–290, 1989.

Robinson WP, Bottani A, Xie YG, et al: Molecular, cytogenetic, and clinical investigations of Prader-Willi syndrome patients. Am J Hum Genet 49:1219–1234, 1991.

43. Name the two most common forms of dwarfism recognizable at birth.

Twenty-one different skeletal dysplasia syndromes were classified at the International Nomenclature of Constitutional Diseases of Bone meeting as "recognizable at birth." The most common is **thanatophoric dwarfism**, a lethal chondrodysplasia characterized by flattened, U-shaped vertebral bodies, telephone-receiver-shaped femurs, macrocephaly, and redundant skin folds causing a pug-like appearance. Thanatophoric means "death-loving" (an apt description). The incidence is 1 in 6400 births.

Achondroplasia is the most common viable skeletal dysplasia, occurring 1 in 26,000 live births. Its features are small stature (mean adult height 4 feet, 2 inches), macrocephaly, depressed nasal bridge, lordosis, and a trident hand. Some patients develop hydrocephalus due to a small foramen magnum. Radiographic findings include narrowing of the interpedicular distance as one proceeds caudally. Both achondroplasia and thanatophoric dysplasia are due to mutations in fibroblast growth factor receptor 3. In achondroplasia, the mutation is in the transmembrane domain, while the mutation in thanatophoric dysplasia is either in the intracellular domain (type 11) or in the extracellular domain (type 1).

Tavormina PL, Shiang R, Thompson LM, et al: Thanatophoric dysplasia (types I and 11) caused by mutations in fibroblast growth factor receptor 3. Nature Genetics 9:321–328, 1995.

44. What chromosomal abnormality is found in cri du chat syndrome?

Cri du chat syndrome is due to a deletion of material from the short arm of chromosome 5 (i.e., 5p–) that causes many problems including growth retardation, microcephaly, and severe mental retardation. Patients have a characteristic cat-like cry in infancy from which the syndrome derives its name. In 85% of cases, the deletion is a de novo event. In 15%, it is due to malsegregation from a balanced parental translocation.

45. List the syndromes and malformations associated with congenital limb hemihypertrophy.

- Russell-Silver syndrome
- Conradi-Hünermann syndrome
- Klippel-Trénaunay-Weber syndrome
- Beckwith-Wiedemann syndrome
- Wilms tumor
- Hypomelanosis of Ito
- CHILD syndrome (**c**ongenital **h**emidysplasia, **i**chthyosiform erythroderma, **l**imb **d**efects)
- Neurofibromatosis

One of every 32 patients with isolated hemihypertrophy is at risk for developing Wilms tumor. For this reason, renal and abdominal ultrasound should be offered periodically in childhood as a screening device for patients with hemihypertrophy.

46. Which genetic disorders are associated with hypoplastic left heart syndrome?

Most newborns with hypoplastic left heart syndrome have this defect as an isolated abnormality, but several syndromes of which this congenital heart malformation is a component have been identified: Down syndrome, Turner syndrome, Smith-Lemli-Opitz syndrome, trisomy 13, trisomy 18, and Ivemark syndrome. Before extensive reconstructive surgery is attempted, it may be prudent to obtain a chromosomal analysis in cases where malformations are noted. There is no question, however, that one of the major ethical dilemmas that confronts all neonatologists is the extent to which one embarks on surgical repair of a variety of defects when one has chromosomal aberrations, especially those with known limited life expectancy.

47. In the evaluation of a stillborn infant, how does the general appearance of the fetus suggest a likely etiology?

A fresh embryo or fetus implies a rapid expulsion after intrauterine or intrapartum death. These fetuses are usually without major anomalies and have normal karyotypes. Common causes of death are placental abruption, cord accidents, and infection. A macerated fetus indicates prolonged retention and is more likely to be associated with structural malformations or chromosomal anomalies.

48. In which fetal and infant deaths are autopsies strongly advised?

- Infants with external or suspected internal structural abnormalities
- Infants with IUGR
- Infants with nonimmune hydrops
- Families with a previous unexplained loss
- Infants with no obvious cause of death
- Macerated fetuses
- Infants who have participated in research investigations

In addition to an autopsy, other studies that should be considered include chromosomal analysis, skeletal radiographs, placental and cord histologic studies, titers for congenital infection, and, if hydropic, evaluation for a hemoglobinopathy (e.g., alpha thalassemia), or possible metabolic storage disease.

Curry CJR: Pregnancy loss, stillbirth, and neonatal death. Pediatr Clin North Am 39:157–192, 1992.

49. How should women with recurrent pregnancy loss be evaluated?

Couples with recurrent pregnancy loss, variably defined as either two or three losses, should be considered for the following evaluations:

- Cytogenic analysis of both parents to rule out mosaicism or a balanced translocation
- Hysterosalpingography to rule out malformations of the uterine cavity (congenital, diethylstilbestrol [DES]-induced, myomas, and intrauterine synechiae)
- Infectious work-up for *Mycoplasma, Chlamydia*, and other pathogens
- Immunologic evaluation for antiphospholipid antibody, anticardiolipin antibody, and antinuclear antibody (e.g., systemic lupus erythematosus)
- Hormonal-endometrial biopsy or progesterone level analysis to rule out a luteal phase defect
- Thyroid function tests
- Evaluation of any suspected systemic illnesses

It is particularly important to initiate these studies prior to pursuit of any in vitro fertilization approach, because the pregnancy may be adversely impacted again with a number of these problems.

50. How are structural dysmorphisms categorized?

- **Malformation:** a problem of poor formation (likely genetically based) in which the abnormality is present at the onset of development (e.g., hypoplastic thumbs of Fanconi syndrome)
- **Disruption:** an extrinsic destructive process interferes with previously normal development (e.g., thalidomide causing limb abnormalities)
- **Deformation:** an extrinsic mechanical force causes abnormalities, which are usually asymmetrical (e.g., breech position causing tibial bowing and positional club feet)
- **Dysplasia:** an abnormal cellular organization or function that generally affects only a single tissue type (e.g., cartilage abnormalities that result in achondroplasia)

51. What is the difference between a major and a minor malformation?

Major malformations are unusual morphologic features that cause cosmetic, medical, or developmental consequences for the patient. **Minor** anomalies are features that do not have associated medical or cosmetic problems. Approximately 14% of newborn babies will have a minor malformation, whereas only about 2–3% will have a major malformation. As we unravel more of the genetic code, it is remarkable that relatively so few neonates are affected by malformations.

52. What are the three principal types of sequences?
1. Malformation sequences (resulting from poor formation of tissues)
2. Deformation sequences (resulting from mechanical factors)
3. Disruptive sequences (initiated by a disruptive process)

Examples include:
- DiGeorge sequence
- Pierre Robin sequence
- Early urethral obstruction sequence
- Extrophy of bladder sequence
- Extrophy of cloaca sequence
- Rokitansky sequence
- Oligohydramnios sequence
- Sirenomelia sequence
- Caudal dysplasia sequence
- Early amnion rupture sequence
- Jugular lymphatic obstruction sequence

53. Describe the most common associations.
- CHARGE—**c**oloboma of the eye, **h**eart defects, **a**tresia of the choanae, **r**etardation (mental and growth), **g**enital anomalies (in males), **e**ar anomalies
- MURCS—**mu**llerian duct aplasia, **r**enal aplasia, **c**ervicothoracic **s**omite dysplasia
- VATER—**v**ertebral, **a**nal, **t**racheoesophageal, **r**enal or **r**adial anomalies
- VACTERL—VATER anomalies plus **c**ardiac and **l**imb anomalies

54. What are the major vascular disruption sequences?
- **Poland anomaly**—unilateral defect of the pectoralis muscle and syndactyly of the hand. This is thought to be due to an early deficit of blood flow through the subclavian artery to the distal limb and pectoral region.
- **Hydranencephaly**—congenital absence of the cerebral hemispheres. Although the cause of this devastating defect is not certain, bilateral internal carotid artery occlusion has been commonly postulated.
- **Proximal focal femoral hypoplasia**—unilateral dysgenesis of the proximal femur. Etiologies for this defect include familial genetic disorders, teratogenic influences, viral agents, maternal diabetes, trauma, and ischemia caused by vascular disruption.
- **Oromandibular-limb hypogenesis spectrum**—craniofacial, limb, and often brain defects. This spectrum of anomalies suggests a diffuse disruptive vascular occlusion or hemorrhagic etiology.

55. What malformations are associated with oligohydramnios and polyhydramnios?
In early pregnancy (< 4 mos), the majority of amniotic fluid is produced by transudation through the placental membranes and fetal skin. Later in pregnancy, the bulk of amniotic fluid arises as a product of fetal urination. At term, the fetus swallows approximately 500 ml of amniotic fluid per day and urinates an equivalent amount. Fetal urine production increases rapidly from 3.5 ml/hr at 25 weeks to 25 ml/hr at term. Any malformation that leads to impaired urine production will cause oligohydramnios, including renal dysplasia, renal agenesis, and bladder outlet obstruction. When uteroplacental insufficiency occurs, the fetus is often faced with poor nutritive and volume support. The fetus becomes intravascularly depleted, leading to increased fluid conservation and decreased urine output, causing oligohydramnios. Oligohydramnios is often associated with IUGR.

The etiology of polyhydramnios may be broken down into maternal causes (30%), fetal causes (30%), and idiopathic causes (40%). Maternal disorders, such as diabetes, erythroblastosis fetalis, and preeclampsia, are often associated with excess amniotic fluid. Fetal disorders that commonly predispose to polyhydramnios are central nervous system (CNS) anomalies (e.g., anencephaly, hydrocephaly, neurologic disorders), gastrointestinal (GI) disorders (tracheoesophageal fistula, duodenal atresia), fetal circulatory disorders, and multiple gestation. The etiology for polyhydramnios in fetuses with CNS and upper GI anomalies is presumed to be impaired fetal swallowing ability.

56. What causes Potter syndrome?

Potter syndrome has come to be synonymous with fetal malformations caused by extreme oligohydramnios. Lack of amniotic fluid leads to fetal compression, a squashed, flat face, clubbing of the feet, pulmonary hypoplasia, and, commonly, breech presentation. Normal fetal lung development is dependent on in utero "breathing" and production of fetal lung fluid. In the absence of amniotic fluid, pulmonary hypoplasia occurs and is the cause of death for most fetuses with Potter syndrome. The underlying mechanism in Potter syndrome was initially reported to be renal agenesis or renal dysplasia. However, bladder outlet obstruction and prolonged premature rupture of the membranes may also cause this sequence. Some prefer that Potter syndrome be defined solely as renal agenesis.

Often, these children present in the neonatal period with severe respiratory distress beginning shortly after birth. Pneumothorax is common, because high ventilatory pressures are often used in an attempt to initiate gas exchange, usually with little success. Survival rarely lasts longer than a few hours in the most severe cases.

57. If an infant is born with Potter syndrome, why should the parents undergo a renal ultrasound?

Renal agenesis is thought to be a sporadic or multifactorial condition, although autosomal dominant inheritance with variable expression (i.e., unilateral renal agenesis in a parent) has also been postulated. For this reason, obtaining a renal ultrasound on parents of a child with renal agenesis is advised. If the parents have normal renal evaluations, the empirically determined recurrence risk is approximately 3%. If one of the parents has unilateral renal agenesis, the recurrence risk may be as high as 50% because of a presumed autosomal dominant gene.

58. How do clinodactyly, syndactyly, and camptodactyly differ?

- **Clinodactyly:** curvature of a toe or finger (usually the fifth) due to hypoplasia of the middle phalanx, which is the last fetal bone to develop in the hands and feet. Normal curvature can consist of up to 8° of in-turning. Curvature beyond this is considered a minor anomaly.
- **Syndactyly:** an incomplete separation of fingers (usually 3rd and 4th) or toes (usually 2nd or 3rd)
- **Camptodactyly:** abnormal persistent flexion of fingers or toes

59. Are preauricular ear tags a significant finding?

Preauricular pits and tags are minor anomalies that occur in about 0.3–1.0% of individuals, with a wide variance in frequency among racial groups. They are twice as common in females as in males and can be inherited as an autosomal dominant trait. They are believed to represent remnants of early embryonic bronchial cleft or arch structures. As isolated findings, they do not warrant additional evaluations.

60. What is the proper way to test for low-set ears?

This designation is made when the upper portion of the ear (helix) meets the head at a level below a horizontal line drawn from the lateral aspect of the palpebral fissure. The best way to measure is to align a straight edge between the two inner canthi and determine whether the ears lie completely below this plane. In normal individuals, approximately 10% of the ear is above this plane.

Feingold M, Bossert VM: Normal values for selected physical parameters: An aid to syndrome delineation. In Bergsma D (ed): The National Foundation-March of Dimes Birth Defects Series 10:9. White Plains, NY, March of Dimes Birth Defects Foundation, 1974.

61. Why do the sclerae of patients with osteogenesis imperfecta appear blue?

Osteogenesis imperfecta is an often devastating disease of bone, in which the affected neonate often manifests severe fractures shortly after birth. Although the disease has several levels of severity, in its most problematic forms, growth is significantly impaired and life expectancy is very short. Phylogenetically, the sclerae are closely related to the skeleton. In many animals, the sclera contains cartilage and osseous material. The primary component of sclera in humans is collagen. It is not surprising that in osteogenesis imperfecta and many other connective tissue diseases, the sclerae are abnormally thin and transparent, because abnormal collagen formation is the underlying defect in many of these disorders. The bluish color of the sclera in patients with connective tissue (especially collagen) diseases is thought to be due to visualization of the bluish-colored uvea (the eye layer behind the retina) as seen through a more transparent sclera. *Uvea* literally means "grape," the name being derived from the similarity in their colors.

62. What is the inheritance pattern of cleft lip and palate?

Most cases of cleft lip and palate are inherited in a polygenic or multifactorial pattern. The male-to-female ratio is 3:2, and the incidence in the general population is approximately 1/1000. Recurrence risk after one affected child is 3–4%; after two affected children, 8–9%.

63. How can hypertelorism be rapidly assessed?

If an imaginary third eye would fit between the eyes, hypertelorism is possible. Precise measurement involves measuring the distance between the center of each eye's pupil. This is a difficult measurement in newborns and uncooperative patients because of eye movement. In practice, the best way to determine hypotelorism or hypertelorism is to measure the inner and outer canthal distances, then plot these measurements on standardized tables of norms.

64. Which syndromes are associated with iris colobomas?

Colobomas of the iris are due to abnormal ocular development and embryogenesis. They are frequently associated with chromosomal syndromes, most commonly trisomy 13, 4p–, 13q–, and triploidy. In addition, they may be commonly found in the CHARGE association, Goltz syndrome, and Rieger syndrome. Whenever iris colobomas are noted, chromosome analysis is recommended. The special case of complete absence of the iris (aniridia) is associated with the development of Wilms tumor and may be caused by an interstitial deletion of the short arm of chromosome 11.

65. How large is the posterior fontanel in the healthy term infant?

In 97% of full-term infants, the posterior fontanel is normally fingertip size or smaller. Large posterior fontanels can be seen in infants with congenital hypothyroidism, skeletal dysplasias, or increased intracranial pressure.

66. On which side does the newborn "crown" usually sit?

In the fetus, hair follicles on the skin surface grow downward during weeks 10–16. During this time, the brain and scalp expand outward in a dome-like fashion, pulling the follicles in different directions, and at 18 weeks, when the hair erupts, patterns are set. The "crown," or parietal hair whorl, is the focal point of this outgrowth. At birth, it is usually a few centimeters anterior to the posterior fontanel. Fifty-five percent of single parietal scalp whorls are left of midline (presumably secondary to the larger size of the left brain), 30% are right-sided, and 15% are midline. Five percent of normal individuals have bilateral hair whorls. Abnormal positioning of the hair whorl (particularly a posterior location) can be seen in microcephaly.

67. Why is chromosomal banding such a valuable asset?

Chromosome banding was introduced in the early 1970s and has revolutionized cytogenetics. Prior to banding, all chromosomes appeared as solid, dark figures and could not be individually identified. Stains such as Giemsa and quinacrine can now be used to differentially stain certain chromosome regions, producing a characteristic striped pattern that can accurately identify each chromosome. Even small chromosome fragments often can be identified on the basis of their banding patterns. Contiguous gene disorders are syndromes due to a microdeletion of specific chromosomal regions. Examples of microdeletion syndromes include Prader-Willi syndrome, Angelman syndrome, Miller-Dieker syndrome, DiGeorge syndrome, and velocardio-facial syndrome. Whereas the deletions are sometimes detectable on a karyotype, submicroscopic deletions cannot be visualized even on high-resolution chromosome banding. These deletions cannot be visualized even on high-resolution chromosome banding. These deletions can be detected by fluorescent in situ hybridization (FISH). In this technique, a DNA probe specific for the chromosomal region of interest is hybridized to the chromosomes. A fluorescent signal is attached to the probe so that the number of copies of the DNA corresponding to the probe can be determined for each cell. Normally, two copies of each region, one on each chromosome, should be present. If a deletion has occurred, only one of the copies will be seen. This technique has aided in the diagnosis of microdeletion syndromes that were formerly difficult to detect because of their small size.

68. Why has the polymerase chain reaction (PCR) revolutionized molecular genetics?

Most DNA techniques require a microgram of DNA, and this amount is often difficult to obtain. The PCR technique allows a million-fold amplification of a specific DNA fragment from a sample as small as a billionth of a microgram. The DNA to be amplified is denatured by heating the sample. In the presence of DNA polymerase and excess deoxynucleotide triphosphates, oligonucleotides that hybridize specifically to the target sequence prime new DNA synthesis.

The first cycle is characterized by a product of indeterminate length. However, the second cycle produces the discrete short product, which accumulates exponentially with each successive round of amplification. This leads to the million-fold amplification of the discrete fragment over the course of 20–30 cycles. PCR and other recently developed molecular techniques have led to a boom in the identification of genes associated with clinical disorders.

69. What is a linkage map?

Linkage is the coinheritance of two or more nonallelic genes because their loci are in close proximity on the same chromosome. A linkage map is a chromosome map showing the relative positions of genetic markers of a given species, as determined by linkage analysis.

70. How does mosaicism develop?

Mosaicism is the possession of multiple chromosomally different cell lines in a single individual. Most mosaicism involves the sex chromosomes and occurs because of defects in mitosis in an early embryo. Normally, chromosomes duplicate and separate equally in mitotic division. Mosaicism occurs when the chromosomes fail to separate (mitotic nondisjunction) or fail to migrate (anaphase lag). In general, the greater the proportion of abnormal cell lines, the more abnormal the phenotype. The earlier in embryonic development an abnormal cell is established, the higher the percentage of abnormal cells in that individual.

71. What causes chimerism in infants?

The term *chimera* is derived from the Greek mythological monster that, according to Homer, had the head of a lion, body of a goat, and tail of a dragon. In cytogenetic parlance, chimerism is the presence of two or more cell lines in an individual that are derived from two separate zygotes. The most common cause of chimerism is the mixing of blood from unlike-sexed twins, resulting in a karyotype of 46,XX/46,XY. Chimerism can also result from the admixture of cells from a nonviable twin into a surviving fetus or, most rarely, from incorporation of two zygotes into a single embryo.

72. What is the risk of having a child with a recessive disorder when the parents are first or second cousins?

First cousins may share more than one deleterious recessive gene. They have $\frac{1}{8}$ of their genes in common, and their progeny are homozygous at $\frac{1}{16}$ of their gene loci. Second cousins have only $\frac{1}{32}$ of their genes in common. The risk that consanguineous parents will produce a child with a severe or lethal abnormality is 6% for first-cousin marriages and 1% for second-cousin marriages.

73. How does a reciprocal translocation differ from a robertsonian translocation?

A chromosome translocation is a transfer of chromosomal material between two (or more) nonhomologous chromosomes. The exchange is usually reciprocal (the two segments trading places). The genetic content of the individual is therefore complete but rearranged. Robertsonian translocation represents a special variety of chromosome translocation in which the long arms of two acrocentric chromosomes (#13, 14, 15, 21, or 22) fuse at their centromeres. The breaks may occur within, above, or below the centromeres. The short arms are usually lost, but this does not produce an abnormality because the genetic material on the short arms of acrocentric chromosomes occurs in multiple copies throughout the genome. A phenotypically normal individual with a robertsonian translocation has only 45 chromosomes inasmuch as the long arms of two acrocentric chromosomes are fused into one.

74. How can an autosomal recessive disease occur when only one parent is a carrier?

Uniparental disomy is an inheritance pattern in which a child receives two identical chromosomes from one parent and none from the other. The most likely explanation is an abnormality in meiosis whereby one gamete receives an extra copy of a homologous chromosome due to an error in separation. This gamete with two copies from one parent then unites with the gamete of the other parent. If the second gamete lacks that particular chromosome (i.e., nullisomic gamete), a normal karyotype results. If the second gamete contains that particular chromosome, a trisomic zygote results. During embryonic development, this trisomy may be lost, resulting in a normal karyotype. Uniparental disomy has been reported in some patients with Prader-Willi, Angelman, and Beckwith-Wiedemann syndromes as well as CF and hemophilia A.

75. How can the same genotype lead to different phenotypes?

In parental imprinting (an area of the regulation of gene expression that is incompletely understood), the expression of an identical gene is dependent on whether the gene is inherited from the mother or father. For example, in Huntington disease, the clinical manifestations occur much earlier if the gene is inherited from the father rather than the mother. Modification of the genes by methylation of the DNA during development has been hypothesized as one explanation of the variability.

76. 46,XY,t(4:8)(p21; q22)—What does it all mean?

46	Normal number of chromosomes
XY	Genetic male
t(4:8)	The first set of parentheses refers to the chromosomes. The symbol in front indicates the change: *t* stands for reciprocal translocation, *del* for deletion, *dup* for duplication, and *inv* for inversion.
(p21; q22)	The second set of parentheses refers to the bands on the chromosomes. The short arm symbol is *p;* the long arm symbol is *q.*

In this case, a genetic male with a normal number of chromosomes has a reciprocal translocation between the short arm of chromosome 4 at band 21 and the long arm of chromosome 8 at band 22.

77. What are the features of the four most common sex chromosome abnormalities?

Characteristics of Sex Chromosome Disorders

	47,XXY (KLINEFELTER)	47,XYY	47,XXX	45,X (TURNER)
Frequency of live births	1/2000	1/2000	1/2000	1/8000
Maternal age association	Yes	No	Yes	No

(Table continued on next page.)

Characteristics of Sex Chromosome Disorders (Continued)

	47,XXY (KLINEFELTER)	47,XYY	47,XXX	45,X (TURNER)
Phenotype	Tall, eunuchoid habitus, under-developed sec-ondary sex characteristics, gynecomastia	Tall, severe acne, indistinguishable from normal males	Tall, indistinguish-able from normal females	Short stature, web neck, shield chest, pedal edema at birth, coarctation of aorta
IQ and behavior	80–100; behavioral problems	90–110; aggressive behavior	90–110; behavioral problems	Mildly deficient to normal IQ; spatial-perceptual difficulties
Reproductive function	Extremely rare	Common	Common	Extremely rare
Gonad	Hypoplastic testes, Leydig cell hyper-plasia, Sertoli cell hypoplasia, seminiferous tubule dysgenesis, few spermatogenic precursors	Normal size testes, normal testicular histology	Normal size ovaries, normal ovarian histology	Streak ovaries with deficient follicles

From Donnenfeld AE, Dunn LK: Common chromosome disorders detected prenatally. Postgrad Obstet Gynecol 6:5, 1986, with permission.

78. Is it possible to get identical twins of different sexes?

Yes. If anaphase lag (loss) of a Y chromosome occurs at the time of cell separation into twin embryos, a female fetus with karyotype 45,X (Turner syndrome) and a normal male fetus (46,XY) result.

79. Of the four most common types of sex chromosomal abnormalities, which is identifiable at birth?

Only infants with Turner syndrome have physical features easily identifiable at birth. Features include:

Dorsal hand and pedal edema	Broad chest with wide-spaced nipples
Low posterior hairline	Narrow, hyperconvex nails
Web neck (pterygium colli)	Prominent ears
Congenital elbow flexion (cubitus valgus)	Short fourth metacarpal or metatarsal

80. What causes the webbing of the neck in Turner syndrome?

Failure of canalization between the cervical and jugular lymphatic vessels causes trapped lymphatic fluid to accumulate progressively and to form large posterior nuchal cysts called cystic hygromas. Occasionally, resolution of fluid accumulation may occur during gestation with regression of the cystic hygroma, formation of nuchal webbing (called pterygium colli), nuchal skin redundancy, alteration in the zone of hair growth, protrusion of the lower auricles, and morphologic alterations of the fetal face. This is known as the jugular lymphatic obstruction sequence. It is hypothesized that if only a partial or temporary obstruction occurs, egress of lymphatic fluid may be possible, and the cystic hygroma will resolve with only redundant nuchal skin folds remaining. Therefore, the entire obstruction sequence will not develop. However, others believe that the pathogenesis of the web neck is not related to lymphatic obstruction but occurs as a primary developmental defect due to the chromosomal abnormality.

81. Describe the similarities and differences between Noonan syndrome and Turner syndrome.

Similarities: short stature, web neck, cardiac defects, low posterior hairline, broad chest, wide-spaced nipples, edema of the dorsum of the hands and feet, cubitus valgus

Differences:

Turner Syndrome	Noonan Syndrome
Females only	Both males and females
Chromosomal disorder (45,X)	Normal chromosomes (autosomal rec.)
Near-normal IQ	Mental deficiency
Coarctation most common cardiac defect	Pulmonary stenosis most common cardiac defect
Amenorrhea and sterility	Normal menstrual cycle in females

82. What is the most common inherited form of mental retardation?

Fragile X syndrome.

83. What is the nature of the mutation in fragile X syndrome?

When the lymphocytes of an affected male are grown in a folate-deficient medium and the chromosomes examined, a substantial number of X chromosomes demonstrate a break near the distal end of the long arm. This site, the fragile X mental retardation-1 gene (FMR-1), was identified and sequenced in 1991. At the center of the gene is a repeating trinucleotide sequence (CGG) that, in normal individuals, repeats 6–45 times. However, in carriers, the sequence expands to 50–200 times (called a premutation), and in fully affected individuals, it expands to 200–600 copies. These longer sequences cause malfunctioning of the gene. Expansion of trinucleotide repeat sequences are responsible for several other diseases including the neurodegenerative disorders myotonic dystrophy, spinocerebellar ataxia type 1, Kennedy disease, and Huntington disease.

84. What is in utero stem cell transplantation?

In utero stem cell transplantation is a potential alternative to postnatal stem cell transplantation for the treatment of selected congenital hematologic disorders that can be cured by bone marrow transplantation and can be diagnosed early in gestation.

Advances in prenatal diagnosis allow the diagnosis of congenital hematologic and genetic disorders by 10–12 weeks of gestation. In contrast to postnatal bone marrow transplantation, in utero stem cell transplantation aims to create a level of mixed chimerism adequate to ameliorate the clinical manifestations of the disease.

85. What are the in utero gene therapy techniques?

Successful gene therapy requires introduction of DNA into mammalian somatic cells to induce expression of a specific gene. Gene delivery to the host can be achieved through the use of two categories of vector systems: viral and nonviral delivery systems. The most promising are viral delivery systems comprising various recombinant viruses.

Recombinant viruses are composed of modified viral envelopes where the genes encoding for replication are deleted. The efficiency and biology of transduction differs between the specific wild-type viruses used to construct the vector. Some recombinant viral vectors infect only dividing cells; others can transduce nondividing cells. Unfortunately, immunogenicity acquired against the recombinant virus or against the transgene itself is the main factor limiting the duration of transgene expression.

Strategies for the treatment of each disease require specific vector design. In addition to the avoidance of an immune response, obstacles to overcome by vector design include safety issues, improving efficiency of ex vivo and in vivo gene delivery, and gene regulation post-cell transduction.

86. What are the potential advantages or rationales for performing in utero stem cell transplantation or in utero gene therapy?

1. The early gestational fetus is immunologically immature and uniquely tolerant to foreign antigens. The exposure to foreign antigens during this period of immunologic immaturity may allow the fetus to process the foreign antigens itself, obviating the need for immunosuppression. This donor-specific tolerance would permit readministrations of the stem cells or the viral vectors postnatally.

2. The maternal womb is the ideal sterile isolette.

3. Genetic disorders may result in irreversible damage to the fetus. In such cases, fetal gene therapy could preempt clinical manifestations of diseases.

4. The efficiency of transduction after fetal gene vector delivery may be increased because:
   - The proliferative fetal environment may allow more efficient transduction of cells by replication-dependent vectors.
   - There may be a greater expansion of the transduced cell population because of the competitive advantage of normal "transduced" cells over the host native cells.
   - There is an increased viral particle-to-cell ratio in the fetus.
   - There may be an increased volume of distribution of a viral vector in the fetal milieu.
   - The obstacles to gene delivery secondary to disease comorbidity (i.e., muscle destruction in muscular dystrophy) are absent in the fetus.

87. What disorders are potentially amenable to in utero stem cell transplantations?

1. Diseases that may benefit from in utero hematopoietic stem cell transplantation alone
   Rationale: Selective advantage for donor cells
   - Severe combined immunodeficiency disorder:
     X-linked
     ZAP 70
     Jac 3
     Adenosine deaminase deficiency
   - Wiskott-Aldrich syndrome
   - Chromosomal breakage syndromes:
     Fanconi anemia
     Bloom syndrome
   Rationale: Minimal engraftment requirement
   - Hyper IgM syndrome
   - Chronic granulomatous disease

2. Diseases that may benefit from in utero hematopoietic stem cell transplantation in combination with minimal ablative postnatal strategies
   Rationale: Successfully treated by mixed chimerism
   - Hemoglobinopathies: β-Thalassemia/? α-Thalassemia
   - Sickle cell disease
   Rationale: Prenatal tolerance induction; no matched sibling donor
   - Diseases that can be diagnosed early in gestation and successfully treated by postnatal stem cell transplantation

Diseases unlikely to benefit from in utero transplantation include hematologic disorders not cured by postnatal bone marrow transplantation, diseases that require a near-complete hematopoietic cellular replacement to effect a cure, and diseases that have CNS manifestations requiring large-scale CNS repopulation. Maturation of the blood-brain barrier restricts access to the CNS of transplanted cells.

88. What disorders are potentially amenable to in utero gene therapy?

Congenital malformations affect up to 3% of all newborns and cause as many as 20% of all infant deaths. Diseases that are potentially treatable by in utero gene therapy include:

- Hemophilia
- Tay-Sachs
- Lesch-Nyhan syndrome
- Leukodystrophies
- Generalized gangliosidosis

- Niemann-Pick disease
- Familial hypercholesterolemia
- Familial hyperbilirubinemia
  (Crigler-Najjar syndrome)
- Tyrosinemia type 1

- Cystic fibrosis
- Gaucher's disease
- Ornithine transcarba-
  mylase deficiency
- Muscular dystrophy

As with postnatal gene therapy, successful fetal gene therapy awaits the development of vectors with proven safety, efficacy, and long-term gene expression.

89. What are the potential risks of in utero gene therapy or stem cell transplantation for the fetus or the mother?

The risks of fetal therapy can be divided into procedural risks and biologic risks.

Procedural risks:

- The maternal risks include infection, hemorrhage, and possibly infertility. The risk of such complications should not be higher than that seen after similar obstetric procedures such as chorionic villous sampling, amniocentesis, or fetal transfusion. The risk of fetal loss is estimated between 1% and 3.5%.

Biologic risks:

- Similar to postnatal bone marrow transplantation, fetal or maternal graft-versus-host disease (GVHD) could develop.
- A major concern is the risk of germ cell line transduction with the possible transmission to future generations.
- Mutations occurring from random integration of the foreign gene into the host chromosome may lead to the development of neoplasms or other acquired diseases.
- Potential fetal toxicity can occur from the injected vectors or stem cells.
- Fetal organs or tissues may be damaged from the immune response to the viral vector or to the transgene.
- Transfer of viral vector, gene product, or donor stem cell to the mother through fetal-maternal microhemorrhages with possible untoward maternal effects.
- Fetal tolerance induction to a viral vector may have undesirable side effects, such as the inability to recognize a postnatal infection with the same virus. This theoretic situation could lead to silent organ or tissue damage with clinical manifestations developing after it is too late to intervene.

90. What are some of the ethical considerations of the fetus as a patient?

The fetus is considered to have "dependent" moral status. The previable fetus is thus totally dependent on the mother's autonomous decisions. Only she can present the fetus as a patient for treatment, and she has no moral obligation to present her fetus for experimentation. It is therefore essential to develop an ethical framework of nondirective counseling when discussing informed consent with the parents. The multidisciplinary team involved must ensure that the parents understand the available options, including postnatal treatment or termination of the pregnancy, and the possible outcomes of all the available treatments.

It is evident, however, that enormous ethical complexities with fetal gene therapy have only just begun to emerge. For example, if a disease does ultimately become treatable in utero with gene therapy, what does the physician do if the mother declines to have the fetus treated? If the disease under consideration is one that potentially leads to mental retardation and significant societal costs, what legislation should be developed to be sure that society is protected from the burden of life-long institutional care? In short, the discussions may be even more difficult to resolve than those of abortion.

91. Are there conditions under which there could be a competitive advantage of transplanted hematopoietic stem cells leading to a very high rate of engraftment?

High levels of donor cell engraftment can be expected when there is a competitive advantage for normal (transplanted) cells over deficient (host) cells. In the presence of a lineage deficiency, such as erythroid (anemia) or lymphoid (immunodeficiency), in utero hematopoietic stem cell transplantation can selectively reconstitute the defective lineage. A competitive advantage of transduced "normal" cells over deficient host cells may also exist in some circumstances after in utero gene delivery.

92. What are some of the barriers to engraftment of donor stem cells after in utero transplantation?

In utero stem cell transplantation differs from postnatal marrow transplantation in three major respects:

1. The myeloablative regimens and the irradiation used to permit engraftment following bone marrow transplantation alter the biology of the recipient hematopoietic microenvironment, which facilitates engraftment. This is not applicable to the fetal milieu. A limited number of receptive sites have been shown to represent one of the barriers to engraftment in fetal recipients.

2. After in utero transplantation, there is competition between the transplanted cells and the preexisting, vigorous, host hematopoietic compartment that is not present after myeloablation in postnatal bone marrow transplantation. Animal experiments have shown that it is primarily the ability of the host cells relative to the recipient cells to compete, rather than space, that determines ultimate engraftment.

3. The early gestational fetus is immunologically tolerant of foreign antigen. The fetal thymic microenvironment plays a major role in determination of self-recognition and repertoire of response to foreign antigen. Pre–T cells undergo positive and negative selection in the fetal thymus, the end result of which is the deletion of T-cell clones with high affinity for self antigen and preservation of T-cell repertoire against foreign antigens. However, immunorejection of transplanted cells may still occur from other mechanisms of rejection, including NK– or B-cell–mediated response. Experimental studies support the concept of fetal tolerance but suggest that it may be conditional and dependent on timing and appropriate presentation of antigen to the fetus.

93. What diseases have been successfully treated by in utero hematopoietic stem cell transplantation or in utero gene therapy?

Although there have been at least 26 human cases of in utero hematopoietic stem cell transplantation to date, the only clear successes have been in patients with severe combined immunodeficiency syndrome (SCID). Effective reconstitution of the immunodeficiency was achieved by CD34-enriched bone marrow transplantation to the fetus.

BIBLIOGRAPHY

 1. Burke WG, et al: Isolated single umbilical artery: The case for routine renal screening. Arch Dis Child 68:600–601, 1993.
 2. Chan CTJ, Clayton-Smith J, Cheng XJ, et al: Molecular mechanisms in Angelman syndrome: A survey of 93 patients. Am J Med Genet 30:895–902, 1993.
 3. Curry CJR: Pregnancy loss, stillbirth, and neonatal death. Pediatr Clin North Am 39:157–192, 1992.
 4. Deal CL: Parental genomic imprinting. Curr Opin Pediatr 7:445–458, 1995.
 5. DeBiasio P, Siccardi M, Volpe G, et al: First-trimester screening for Down syndrome using nuchal translucency measurement with free p-hCG and PAAP-A between 10 and 13 weeks of pregnancy: The combined test. Prenat Diagn 19:360–363, 1999.
 6. Dietz HC, Cutting GR, Pyeritz RE, et al: Marfan syndrome caused by a recurrent de novo missense mutation in the fibrillin gene. Nature 352:337–339, 1991.
 7. Enns G, Cox V, Goldstein, et al: Congenital diaphragmatic defects and associated syndromes, malformations, and chromosome anomalies: A retrospective study of 60 patients and literature review. Am J Med Genet 79:215–225, 1998.
 8. Flake A, Roncarolo MG, Puck J, et al: Treatment of X-linked severe combined immunodeficiency by in utero transplantation of paternal bone marrow. N Engl J Med 335:1806, 1996.
 9. Flake AW, Zanjani ED: In utero hematopoietic stem cell transplantation: Ontogenic opportunities and biologic barriers. Blood 94:2179–2191, 1999.
10. Geipel A, et al: Prenatal diagnosis of single umbilical artery: Determination of absent side, associated anomalies, Doppler findings, and perinatal outcome. Ultrasound Obstet Gynecol 15:114–117, 2000.

11. Haddew JE, et al: Prenatal screening for Down syndrome with use of maternal serum markers. N Engl J Med 327:588–593, 1992.
12. Hurst L, McVean G: Growth effects of uniparental disomies and the conflict theory of genomic imprinting. TIG 13:436–442, 1997.
13. James D: Diagnosis and management of fetal growth retardation. Arch Dis Child 65:390–394, 1990.
14. Johns DR: Mitochondrial DNA and disease. N Engl J Med 333:638–644, 1995.
15. Knoll JHM, Nicholls RD, Magenis RE, et al: Angelman and Prader-Willi syndromes have a chromosome 15 deletion but differ in parental origin of the deletion. Am J Med Genet 32:285–290, 1989.
16. Kohn DB, Parkman R: Gene therapy for the newborn. FASEB J 11:635–639, 1997.
17. Lam YH, Tang MH: Second-trimester maternal serum inhibin-A screening for fetal Down syndrome in Asian women. Prenat Diagn 19:463–467, 1999.
18. McCullough L, Chervenek F: Ethics in Obstetrics and Gynecology. New York, Oxford University Press, 1994.
19. Milunsky A (ed): Genetic Disorders and the Fetus: Diagnosis, Prevention, and Treatment, 3rd ed. Baltimore, Johns Hopkins University Press, 1998.
20. Rimion DL, Connor JM, Pyeritz RE (eds): Emery and Rimion's Principles and Practice of Medical Genetics, 3rd ed. New York, Churchill Livingstone, 1997.
21. Robinson WP, Bottani A, Xie YG, et al: Molecular, cytogenetic, and clinical investigations of Prader-Willi syndrome patients. Am J Hum Genet 49:1219–1234, 1991.
22. Romano G, Pacilio C, Giordano A: Gene transfer technology in therapy: Current applications and future goals. Stem Cells 17:191–202, 1999.
23. Shiang R, Thompson LM, Zhu YZ, et al: Mutations in the transmembrane domain of FGFR3 cause the most common genetic form of dwarfism, achondroplasia. Cell 78:335–342, 1994.
24. Stevenson RE, Hall J, Goodman R (eds): Human Malformations and Related Anomalies. Oxford Monographs on Medical Genetics, No. 27. New York, Oxford University Press, 1993.
25. Wald NJ, Watt HC, Hacksaw AK: Integrated screening for Down syndrome based on tests performed during the first and second trimesters. N Engl J Med 341:461–467, 1999.
26. Wilkie AO, Slaney SF, Oldridge M, et al: Apert syndrome results from localized mutations of FGFR2 and is allelic with Crouzon syndrome. Nature Gen 9:165–172, 1995.
27. Yang EY, Cass DL, Sylvester KG, et al: Fetal gene therapy: Efficacy, toxicity, and immunologic effects of early gestation recombinant adenovirus. J Pediatr Surg 34:235–241, 1999.
28. Zanjani ED, Anderson WF: Prospect for in utero human gene therapy. Science 285:2084–2088, 1999.

10. HEMATOLOGY

NORMAL RED BLOOD CELL INDICES AND
DIFFERENTIAL DIAGNOSIS OF ANEMIA

1. What are the normal values for hemoglobin level, mean cell volume (MCV), and reticulocyte count in preterm and term neonates on the first day of life?

Red Cell Values on First Postnatal Day

	GESTATIONAL AGE (WEEKS)							
	24–25	26–27	28–29	30–31	32–33	34–35	36–37	TERM
Hemoglobin (g/dl)	19.4 ± 1.5	19.0 ± 2.5	19.3 ± 1.8	19.1 ± 2.2	18.5 ± 2.0	19.6 ± 2.1	19.2 ± 1.7	19.3 ± 2.2
MCV (fl)	135 ± 0.2	132 ± 14.4	131 ± 13.5	127 ± 12.7	123 ± 15.7	122 ± 10.0	121 ± 12.5	119 ± 9.4
Reticulocyte (%)	6.0 ± 0.5	9.6 ± 3.2	7.5 ± 2.5	5.8 ± 2.0	5.0 ± 1.9	3.9 ± 1.6	4.2 ± 1.8	3.2 ± 1.4

Data derived from Zaizov R, Matoth Y: Red cell values on the first postnatal day during the last 16 weeks of gestation. Am J Hematol 1:276, 1976.

2. How does the site of blood sampling affect the hemoglobin and hematocrit?

Capillary samples obtained by heel stick shortly after birth have hemoglobin levels that are on average 3.6 g/dl higher than corresponding venous samples. The ratio of the capillary hematocrit to the venous hematocrit is 1.21 at 26–30 weeks' gestation and decreases to 1.12 in term infants and to 1.02 at 5 days of age in healthy infants. It is particularly important to remember that the differences between capillary and venous hemoglobins are most pronounced in sick, premature infants in whom anemia is most likely to be a clinical problem. Thus, unexpected changes in the hemoglobin level in such infants should prompt consideration of the site of sampling.

3. What is the normal red cell half-life in preterm and term infants?

As determined by chromium survival studies, the normal red cell half-life in preterm infants is 9–26 days (which corresponds to a red cell life span of 35–50 days) and in term infants is 13–35 days (which corresponds to a red cell life span of 60–70 days). In comparison, the normal red cell half-life in adults is 26–35 days, corresponding to a red cell life span of 65–70 days. In case you're wondering what happened to the concept of the 120-day life span of a normal red cell, remember that the values derived from chromium studies represent an average of all circulating red cells, not just those that are newly made and have a full 4 months of oxygen delivery ahead of them.

4. You are asked to evaluate a 10-week-old healthy infant who was born at term and found on a totally unnecessary but nonetheless complete blood count (CBC) to have a hemoglobin level of 9.8 g/dl. Your attending physician, after noting the red cell morphology to be normal, dismisses your twenty-four planned laboratory tests as unnecessary. Is he right, and, if so, why?

He's right. The mean hemoglobin level at 10 weeks for a term infant is 11.2 g/dl, and two standard deviations extend the lower limit of the normal range to 9.4 g/dl. In the absence of specific symptoms or signs of an underlying disorder, a work-up of a hemoglobin level of 9.8 g/dl is likely to be unrewarding.

5. What are the most common causes of anemia in the newborn?

As in children and adults, causes of neonatal anemia can be classified into three broad categories: decreased production, increased destruction, and blood loss. The most common causes of decreased red cell production include Diamond-Blackfan anemia, congenital leukemia, congenital infections, Down syndrome, osteopetrosis, and drug-induced red blood cell (RBC) suppression. In premature infants, the physiologic anemia begins early and may be confused with pathologic causes of decreased red cell production. Etiologies of increased red cell destruction include immune-mediated hemolysis (e.g., Rh, ABO, or minor blood group incompatibility, maternal autoimmune hemolytic anemia), membrane defects (e.g., spherocytosis, elliptocytosis, pyropoikilocytosis), enzyme defects (e.g., glucose-6-phosphate dehydrogenase [G6PD] or protein kinase [PK] deficiency), hemoglobinopathies (e.g., β-thalassemia syndromes), and acquired disorders (e.g., bacterial sepsis, congenital infections, disseminated intravascular coagulation [DIC], microangiopathic anemia). Blood loss is so common that it deserves its own question (see question 6).

6. Blood loss is the most common cause of anemia in the ill newborn; where can you find the lost blood?

In the laboratory where it has been sent for multiple tests.

7. What are the causes of blood loss in the infant other than phlebotomy?

Occult antenatal hemorrhage, obstetric accidents, placenta or umbilical cord malformations, and internal hemorrhage are the major categories of blood loss once excessive phlebotomy has been eliminated. Causes of antenatal hemorrhage include fetomaternal bleeding (e.g., abdominal trauma, traumatic amniocentesis, placental tumors) and twin-to-twin transfusions. Obstetric causes of blood loss include abruptio placentae, placental previa, incision of placenta during cesarean section, rupture of the umbilical cord or an anomalous vessel, and hematoma of the cord or placenta. Blood loss in the neonatal period may be due to intracranial hemorrhage, giant cephalohematoma, cephalohematoma, retroperitoneal, renal, or adrenal hemorrhage, a ruptured liver or spleen, or gastrointestinal (GI) bleeding.

When blood loss is acute, the neonate initially may have a surprisingly well-preserved hemoglobin level and unimpressive reticulocyte count despite signs of shock. In contrast, chronic blood loss is characterized by a low hemoglobin and increased reticulocyte count but, quite often, little evidence of distress.

8. Which hemoglobinopathies are clinically apparent at birth?

Because of the normal switch from gamma globin to beta globin that occurs in fetal and early neonatal development, different forms of thalassemia and other hemoglobinopathies may develop clinical manifestations at different times. For example, disorders of gamma globin production (γ-thalassemia) may cause a microcytic anemia in the fetus and newborn that subsequently resolves, whereas disorders of beta globin production (β-thalassemia) or beta globin structure (sickle cell disease) may be silent at birth but will reveal themselves at an older age. However, nature can play strange tricks. Although beta globin abnormalities are usually clinically silent at birth, circumstances resulting in excessive destruction or loss of fetal red cells, such as blood group incompatibility or intrauterine blood loss, may unmask a beta globin abnormality at a younger age by accelerating the production of red cells with adult hemoglobin.

Because alpha globin is made during most of fetal life as well as during infancy and adulthood, all forms of α-thalassemia, including α-thalassemia trait (two alpha gene deletions), hemoglobin H disease (three alpha gene deletions), and homozygous α-thalassemia with hydrops fetalis (four alpha gene deletions) may be apparent in the newborn period.

9. Can you diagnose hemoglobinopathies at birth, before symptoms appear?

You can and you should. Because beta globin production begins around 32 weeks gestation, hemoglobin S (Hb S) and other structural abnormalities of beta globin can be detected at term (or even earlier) by electrophoresis, high-pressure liquid chromatography, or other techniques. The presence of Hb S and the absence of Hb A at birth is diagnostic of sickle cell disease or sickle-beta zero thalassemia. The presence of only Hb F at term is indicative of homozygous β-thalassemia, and the presence of Hb H is indicative of Hb H disease or homozygous α-thalassemia.

10. What are the most useful initial laboratory studies in evaluating the anemic newborn?

When a hematologist asks you this question, the correct answer is always to look first at the peripheral smear. Microcytosis will point to iron deficiency or thalassemia, and excessive poly-chromasia or increased nucleated red cells will point to a destructive process or compensated blood loss. (Sure, the MCV and reticulocyte count can give you similar information, but real doctors want to see the smear.) Other abnormalities of red cell morphology may rapidly identify specific disorders. Spherocytes suggest spherocytosis or ABO incompatibility, blister cells suggest G6PD deficiency, and fragments suggest a microangiopathic anemia. The presence of blasts suggests leukemia. However, the interpretation of the peripheral blood smear of the newborn is not for the weak-hearted. Normal findings at this age, including target cells, spherocytes, variation in red cell size and shape, and occasional young, blast-looking lymphocytes, may resemble disease-related findings. Additional laboratory tests, such as a direct antiglobulin test (known to some as the direct Coombs' test) and the Kleihauer-Betke preparation are helpful in more conclusively identifying specific causes of anemia such as alloimmunization and fetomaternal bleeding.

11. Can you diagnose anemia in utero? If so, how can you treat it?

Percutaneous umbilical blood sampling allows the evaluation of fetal blood as early as 18 weeks' gestation, and anemia in the fetus may be treated with intrauterine transfusion. Blood is administered through the umbilical vein or into the peritoneal cavity. Fetal anemias that are sometimes managed with transfusions in utero include severe immune hemolysis, homozygous α-thalassemia, severe fetomaternal bleeding or twin-to-twin transfusion, and parvovirus B19 infection. Stem cell transplantation in utero is currently being evaluated for certain inherited hematologic diseases such as thalassemia and sickle cell anemia.

TRANSFUSION THERAPY

12. If the first blood sample drawn for type and crossmatch of an infant does not demonstrate the presence of maternally derived alloantibodies, when will another sample be required if there are ongoing transfusion requirements?

A sample for typing and crossmatching is required every 72 hours for older children and adults with ongoing RBC transfusion needs. Repeat samples are used to monitor the presence of new alloantibodies that have formed following exposure to RBC alloantigens. Infants < 4 months old are exempt from this requirement because of their inability to produce RBC alloantibodies upon exposure to allogeneic RBC. As a result, if a neonate's initial sample for type and cross-matching of RBC demonstrates no evidence of a maternally derived alloantibody, further pre-transfusing testing is not required until the child is > 4 months old.

13. Should infants receive O RhD-negative RBCs exclusively during the neonatal period?

Infants can be safely transfused with ABO/RH type-specific blood. O RhD-negative RBC is the so-called universal donor blood type and can therefore be safely transfused without establishing an infant's ABO/RH type. The practice of transfusing only O RhD-negative RBCs to infants unnecessarily depletes the availability of this resource, which is valuable in the context of emergency transfusion for infants, older children, and adults.

14. The storage of RBCs is associated with progressive leakage of K+ and hemoglobin out of the erythrocyte into the extracellular fluid. Under what circumstances is transfusion of stored RBCs associated with hyperkalemia that might be dangerous to the infant transfusion recipient?

The transfusion of RBCs that have been stored for > 1 week has resulted in hyperkalemia and death due to arrhythmia in the context or neonatal exchange transfusion or when large volumes of RBCs have been transfused rapidly to infants after open heart surgery. In these clinical situations, RBCs intended for transfusion should have been stored for < 1 week or, alternatively, can be washed to remove extracellular potassium.

15. Infants are among the most heavily transfused patient groups. Many premature infants require multiple small-volume RBC transfusions given as aliquots of 5–15 ml/kg body weight. The transfusions are given for a variety of indications, most commonly to treat the anemia of prematurity or to replace phlebotomy blood losses. What approach can be used to limit the number of donors to which an infant is exposed?

A premature infant, predicted to have a long hospital stay during which multiple transfusions would be required, can be assigned to receive RBCs from a single, dedicated unit of RBCs. Prospective studies have demonstrated that infants can safely receive small-volume transfusions of RBCs stored in either citrate-phosphate-dextrose-adenine-1 (CPDA-1) or additive solution until the unit expires. RBCs stored in additive solutions (AS) have a shelf-life of 42 days when stored at 3–5°C; those stored in CPDA-1 expire after 35 days of refrigerated storage.

16. In what clinical circumstances is the transfusion of fresh frozen plasma (FFP) indicated in an infant?

FFP contains 1 U/ml of the coagulation factors II, V, VII, VIII, IX, X, and XI. Indications for transfusion of plasma in neonates are relatively narrow. FFP is the appropriate therapy for the replacement of clotting factors in infants with bleeding due to deficiency of one clotting factor (e.g., factor X deficiency) or multiple clotting factors (as in DIC). When bleeding occurs in an infant with a specific factor deficiency for which a factor concentrate is commercially manufactured (as in hemophilia A or B), factor concentrates should be provided, if available. FFP is not indicated for replacement of intravascular volume (except in circumstances where coagulation factors need to be replaced).

17. What adverse reactions to transfusion are caused by the presence of passenger white blood cells (WBCs)?

Adverse reactions caused by passenger or contaminating WBC include:
  Sensitization to human leukocyte antigen (HLA)
  Febrile transfusion reactions
  Cytomegalovirus (CMV) transmission
  Transfusion-associated graft-versus-host disease (TA-GVHD)

Although HLA sensitization and febrile transfusion reactions are unusual in infants, transfusion-transmitted CMV and TA-GVHD are associated with serious, sometimes life-threatening outcomes. Although many physical methods for removing passenger WBCs exist, the most practical methods for leukoreduction utilize filters that remove WBCs by adhesion. Filtration is classified according to log reduction of WBCs in the component. Reducing the number of WBCs by 1–2 logs is usually effective in preventing febrile transfusion reactions, whereas HLA alloimmunization and prevention of transfusion-associated CMV requires a 3–4-log reduction per unit.

18. Can TA-GVHD be prevented by removing WBC (leukoreducing) cellular blood products?

TA-GVHD is caused by the transfusion of viable lymphocytes contained in cellular blood products to recipients unable to recognize the lymphocytes as foreign. Patients at risk for TA-GVHD fall into two categories: (1) those who are immunodeficient and (2) those who are otherwise healthy but receive cellular products from close biologic relatives. In either case, when the passenger lymphocytes engraft, they are capable of proliferation and attack the host, causing diarrhea, liver damage, and bone marrow failure. Because TA-GVHD is fatal in > 90% of cases, prevention is key. TA-GVHD is not effectively prevented by leukoreduction of cellular blood products but rather by gamma irradiation (dose = 2500 rads per component).

19. Which neonates are at a risk for transfusion-transmitted CMV disease and how can it be prevented?

Infants born to seronegative mothers with birth weights of < 1200 g are at highest risk for transfusion-transmitted CMV infection. Transmission can result in asymptomatic viruria, pneumonia, or sepsis. The risk of acquiring CMV from a transfusion correlates with the number of CMV-positive donors to which an infant is exposed. Between 40% and 90% of healthy blood donors have antibody to CMV.

Transfusion of cellular components from a donor negative for CMV antibody was until recently the best strategy for preventing CMV in those at risk. Because CMV resides in leukocytes, another approach to minimizing transmission of CMV through cellular blood products is leukoreduction (to a residual WBC of < 1×10^6 WBC/ml), usually by filtration. Leukoreduction results in a component with risk of transmitting CMV comparable to blood from donors who are CMV negative; i.e., both leukoreduced and CMV AB-negative components are considered CMV safe.

20. What is the difference between a random donor unit of platelets and a single donor unit? Aren't both types of platelets derived from one donor?

Both platelet products are taken from one volunteer donor. Random donor platelets (RDPs) are those separated from 1 unit of whole blood. One unit of RDPs contains at least 5.5×10^{10} platelets and is approximately 40 ml in volume. One dose of platelets for a thrombocytopenic infant can usually be supplied from a random donor unit. Single donor platelets (SDPs, also called platelets or apheresis) are derived from one donor and are harvested using hemapheresis technique, which allows for the collection of larger units containing at least 3×10^{11} platelets. SDPs are appropriate for the transfusion requirements of a thrombocytopenic adult.

21. When is an informed consent for the transfusion of blood components necessary? Are there any exceptions?

Obtaining informed consent prior to blood transfusion is a legal requirement in many states. A full informed consent allows discussion of the proposed transfusion, its risks and benefits, alternatives that may exist, and a prediction of what will happen if the transfusion does not proceed. The only circumstance under which transfusion can proceed without an informed consent is in the case of a true medical emergency.

22. Which neonates should receive irradiated blood?

All premature infants and infants < 1500 g should receive irradiated blood. Irradiation is used to prevent graft-versus-host (GVH) disease. In the very premature neonate, the WBC count may fall to a very low level at times, predisposing the neonate to population of WBCs from the donor transfusion. This may, in turn, set up a GVH reaction, because the population of white cells will recognize the native infant tissues as foreign.

23. How does phlebotomy in a premature infant compare with that in an adult?

Withdrawing 1 ml of blood from a 1000-g infant is equivalent to taking 70 ml of blood from an adult.

Blanchette VS, Ziporsky A: Assessment of anemia in newborn infants. Clin Perinatol 11:489–510, 1984.

DEVELOPMENTAL HEMATOPOIESIS

24. How does erythropoiesis develop in the fetus?

Hematopoiesis in the fetus starts in the yolk sac. By the 3rd postconceptional week, a "primitive" hematopoiesis is transferred to the liver. The primitive megaloblasts are thus replaced by non-nucleated erythrocytes. By the 20th week, hematopoiesis starts in the bone marrow; liver hematopoiesis progressively decreases and is fully terminated at birth.

25. How do the different cellular lines differentiate?

All cell lineages derive from the pluripotent **stem cells**. These are uncommitted and self-renewing. Under the influence of various cytokines, the pluripotent stem cells initially differentiate into colony-forming units (CFUs) that are capable of multiplication and maturation. There are three types: CFU-GM (granulocytes and monocytes), CFU-mega (megakaryocytes and platelets), and CFU-e (erythrocytes). The latter change to BFU-e (burst-forming units–erythrocytes), then to normoblasts, and ultimately, through the reticulocytes stage, into mature RBCs.

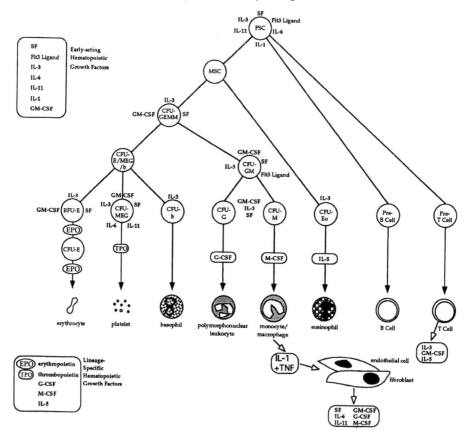

Major cytokine sources and actions. Cells of the bone marrow microenvironment such as macrophages (mP), endothelial cells (ec), and reticular fibroblastoid cells (fb) produce macrophage colony-stimulating factor (M-CSF), granulocyte macrophage colony-stimulating factor (GM-CSF), interleukin (IL-6), and probably Steel factor (SF: cellular sources not yet precisely determined) after induction with endotoxin (ma) or IL-1/TNF (ec, fb). T cells produce IL-3, GM-CSF, and IL-5 in response to antigenic and IL-1 stimulation. These cytokines have overlapping actions during hematopoietic differentiation, as indicated, and for all lineages optimal development requires a combination of early- and late acting factors. PSC = pluripotent stem cells; MSC = myeloid stem cells; TNF = tumor necrosis factor. (From Seiff CA, Nathan D, Clark SC: The anatomy and physiology of hematopoiesis. In Nathan DG, Orkin SH (eds): Nathan & Oski's Hematology of Infancy and Childhood, 5th ed. Philadelphia, W.B. Saunders, 1997, with permission.)

26. What types of hemoglobin are present in the fetus?

All types of hemoglobin are composed of two pairs of chains; adult erythrocytes contain two alpha (α) and two beta (β) chains. At the onset of primitive erythropoiesis, Hb Gower 1 ($\zeta_2\varepsilon_2$) is the prevalent hemoglobin. This is followed by Hb Gower 2 ($\alpha_2\varepsilon_2$) and Hb Portland ($\zeta_2\gamma_2$). These embryonic hemoglobins are rapidly replaced by fetal hemoglobin (Hb F–$\alpha_2\gamma_2$). Around the 30th week postconception, the synthesis of gamma chains decreases progressively and is replaced by the synthesis of beta chains, the characteristic chains of adult hemoglobin. By the time of birth, 50–70% of the hemoglobin is F. By 6 months, the level of Hb F is only 5–10%, and by 1 year, the adult level (< 1%) is reached.

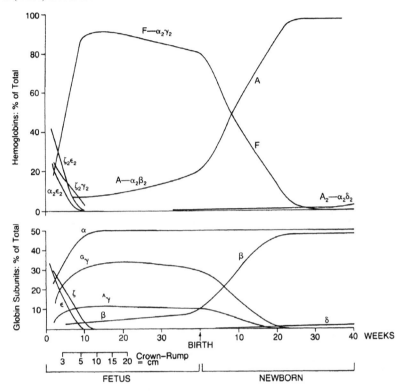

Changes in hemoglobin tetramers (*top*) and in globin subunits (*bottom*) during human development from embryo to early infancy. (From Bunn HF, Forget BG: Hemoglobin: Molecular, Genetic and Clinical Aspects. Philadelphia, W.B. Saunders, 1986.)

27. How do the red cells change during development?

The "primitive" megaloblast-like cells in the yolk sac are very large (~180 fl). By birth, however, the red cell size (MCV) decreases to 110–120 fl. By 1 year, the MCV reaches 82 fl.

28. What are the distinguishing characteristics of fetal red cells?

Fetal red cells are large (macrocytic, but not megaloblastic), have increased concentration of Hb F, express the i antigen (adult red cells express the I antigen), and have decreased levels of carbonic anhydrase. Cells with similar "fetal" characteristics are often produced during stress and in some congenital aplastic anemias (Fanconi anemia).

PHYSIOLOGIC ANEMIA

29. How do RBC indices change during the first months of life?

Changes in RBC indices are shown in the table (next page). The hemoglobin, hematocrit, MCV, and mean corpuscular hemoglobin (MCH) decrease gradually in the first 1–3 months of life, whereas the mean corpuscular hemoglobin concentration (MCHC) remains relatively unchanged.

Postnatal Changes in Red Blood Cell (RBC) Indices in Term Infants

RBC INDICES	DAYS			WEEKS			MONTHS					
	BIRTH (cord blood)	1	3	1	2	4	2	3	4	6	9	12
Hgb (g/dl)	16.5 (13.0)	18.5 (14.5)	18.6 (16.5)	17.5 (13.5)	16.6 (13.4)	13.9 (10.7)	11.2 (9.4)	11.5 (9.5)	12.2 (10.3)	12.6 (11.1)	12.7 (11.4)	12.7 (11.3)
Hct (%)	51 (42)	56 (45)	55	54 (42)	53 (41)	44 (33)	35 (28)	35 (29)	38 (32)	36 (31)	36 (32)	37 (33)
RBC ($\times 10^{12}$/L)	4.7 (3.9)	5.3 (4.0)	5.6	5.1 (3.9)	4.9 (3.9)	4.3 (3.3)	3.7 (3.1)	3.8 (3.1)	4.3 (3.5)	4.7 (3.9)	4.7 (4.0)	4.7 (4.1)
MCV (fl)	108 (98)	108 (95)	110 (104)	107 (88)	105 (88)	101 (91)	95 (84)	91 (74)	87 (76)	76 (68)	78 (70)	78 (71)
MCH (pg)	34 (31)	34 (31)	36.7	34 (28)	33.6 (30.0)	32.5 (29)	30.4 (27)	30 (25)	28.6 (25)	26.8 (24)	27.3 (25)	26.8 (24)
MCHC (g/dl)	33 (30)	33 (29)	33.1	33 (28)	31.4 (28.1)	31.8 (28.1)	31.8 (28.3)	33 (30)	32.7 (28.8)	35 (32.7)	34.9 (32.4)	34.3 (32.1)

Values represent mean (values in parentheses are –2 standard deviations). Data from Saarinen UM, Siimes MA: Developmental changes in red blood cell counts and indices of infants after exclusion of iron deficiency by laboratory criteria and continuous iron supplementation. J Pediatr 78:412–416, 1978; and Rudolph A (ed): Pediatrics, 16th ed. New York, Appleton-Century-Crofts, 1977. Reproduced from Ohls RK: Developmental erythropoiesis. In Polin RA, Fox WW (eds): Fetal and Neonatal Physiology. Philadelphia, W.B. Saunders, 1998, p 1767.

30. What happens to RBC production after birth?

Improved oxygenation after birth results in decreased red cell production in both term and preterm infants, reflecting a natural adaptation to the extrauterine environment. Erythropoiesis effectively stops as serum erythropoietin (EPO) concentrations decrease to 0–10 mU/ml. Reticulocyte (retic) counts drop from 6–10% at birth to < 1% by day 3–5.

31. What is the difference between physiologic anemia of the newborn and pathologic anemia of the newborn?

Anemia is defined as an inability of the circulating red cells to meet the oxygen demands of the tissues. The phrase "physiologic anemia of infancy" is actually a misnomer in that it describes the normal, nonpathologic drop in hemoglobin and hematocrit experienced by term and preterm infants. In healthy neonates, the hemoglobin concentration decreases over the first 2–3 months of life, reaches a nadir, and remains stable over the next several weeks, then slowly rises in the fourth to sixth month of life in response to increased EPO concentrations.

Pathologic anemia describes an abnormal condition in which the kinetics of erythropoiesis are altered, either through hemorrhagic or hemolytic blood loss or through decreased red cell production. Pathologic anemia in newborns is often discovered before a truly "anemic" state is achieved. In this sense, many of the pathologic conditions affecting newborn erythropoiesis represent early alterations from normal red cell indices and do not yet represent true anemia.

32. How does physiologic anemia in preterm infants differ from physiologic anemia in term infants?

The average decline in the hemoglobin of preterm infants is significantly different from that of term infants. Preterm infants reach a nadir of hemoglobin that averages 8g/dl at 4–8 weeks of age. Term infants reach a nadir of 11.5 g/dl at 6–10 weeks of age. Therefore, the physiologic anemia in preterm infants occurs sooner and to a greater degree than in term infants.

33. How does fetal hemoglobin differ from adult hemoglobin?

Fetal hemoglobin differs from adult hemoglobin primarily by its ability to bind oxygen. This is best illustrated by the hemoglobin-oxygen dissociation curve (see figure). The PO_2 at which

50% of hemoglobin is saturated is termed the **P_{50}**. The curve for fetal hemoglobin is said to be shifted to the left of the adult curve (a lower P_{50}), representing the greater affinity of fetal hemoglobin for oxygen at any given PO_2. This results in less of an ability of fetal hemoglobin to release oxygen to the tissues.

Factors that shift the hemoglobin oxygen curve to the right (and thereby increase oxygen delivery to tissues) include increased temperature, increased PCO_2, increased red cell 2,3-diphosphoglycerate (2,3-DPG) content, and increased hydrogen ion concentration (decreased pH).

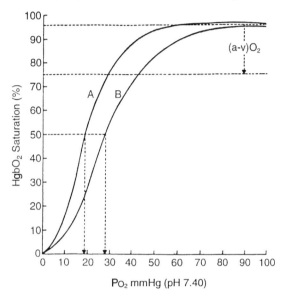

The oxyhemoglobin dissociation curve. Curve A represents the left-shifted fetal-neonatal relationship; P_{50} = 19 mmHg. Curve B represents the normal adult relationship; P_{50} = 27 mmHg. These curves can be shifted by changes in temperature, PCO_2, pH, and 2,3-DPG (2,3 diphosphoglycerate) level and percentages of HgB F and A. (From Sacks LM, Delivoria-Papadopoulos M: Hemoglobin-oxygen interactions. Semin Perinatol 8:169, 1987, with permission.)

ERYTHROPOIETIN

34. What is the source of EPO in the fetus?

Erythropoiesis in utero is controlled by erythroid growth factors produced solely by the fetus. EPO does not cross the placenta in humans; therefore, stimulation of maternal EPO production does not result in stimulation of fetal red cell production. In addition, suppression of maternal erythropoiesis by transfusion does not suppress fetal erythropoiesis. EPO is produced primarily by the fetal liver, although small amounts are produced by the fetal kidney during mid and late gestation. It is not known what factors regulate the switch of EPO production from the liver to the kidney around the time of birth. This switch may occur during the physiologic anemia of infancy.

35. How do the pharmacokinetics of EPO differ between preterm newborns and adults?

Pharmacokinetic studies in newborn humans and animals indicate that neonates have 2–4 times the volume of distribution and 3–4 times the clearance of EPO, necessitating the use of higher doses than required for adults. The half-life of EPO appears similar.

36. What is the best way to avoid transfusions in the first week of life in an otherwise healthy preterm very low birth weight (VLBW) infant?

KBIB (keep the blood inside the baby).

37. How is EPO administered to newborns?

EPO can be administered intravenously, subcutaneously, and (rarely) intramuscularly. EPO has been added to total parenteral nutrition (TPN) solutions and administered over 24 hours. Rapid IV injections result in serum EPO concentrations > 1000 mU/ml.

38. What laboratory tests should be ordered to determine if EPO is effective?

A reticulocyte (retic) count is the best measure of active erythropoiesis. In order to determine if EPO is effective, a comparison between a baseline retic count and one obtained 7–10 days following the start of EPO therapy will help determine if erythropoiesis has been stimulated. Reticulocyte counts can be presented as percentage of retics (uncorrected or corrected) or as absoluted reticulocyte counts (ARC). If reticulocytes are recorded as percentages, a corrected retic count can be obtained by multiplying the uncorrected percent retic by the hematocrit, then dividing by the expected hematocrit (this number varies with age and gestation of the infant).

The ARC can be calculated by multiplying the RBC count by the percent retic count. This number generally ranges from 30,000 cells/µl, reflecting inactive erythropoiesis, to greater than 500,000 cells/µl, reflecting active erythropoiesis. The ARC takes into account the number of red cells per volume of blood, and thus does not need to be corrected for anemia.

39. Does the use of EPO in the preterm infant decrease the transfusion requirement?

The use of EPO in the very low birth weight infant is controversial. Although it is accepted that EPO will decrease the need for RBC transfusions, it is uncertain if EPO also reduces donor exposures, because units of blood are generally separated into small aliquots. A conservative transfusion policy is clearly the most effective way to reduce the need for transfusion in the preterm infant.

NONIMMUNE HEMOLYTIC ANEMIAS

40. How do fetal red cell membranes differ from those in the older child and adult?

- The presence of i antigen in fetal erythrocytes and I antigen in adults
- Fetal membranes are more permeable to monovalent cations and contain less Na+, K+-adenosine triphosphatase (ATPase).
- Less phospholipid and cholesterol/cell
- The arrangement of membrane proteins may be slightly different, but the protein composition is qualitatively normal.
- Membrane fluidity is normal.

41. What causes congenital spherocytosis?

Hereditary spherocytosis (HS) is an inherited hemolytic anemia due to abnormalities in spectrin or proteins that anchor spectrin.

42. In which ethnic population is HS common, and how is the gene inherited?

- Northern European (affects 1/5000)
- Autosomal dominant
- Remember: In 20–25% of HS cases the mother and father are clinically normal, but exhibit subtle laboratory abnormalities consistent with a carrier state.

43. How is congenital spherocytosis classified?

Clinical Classification of Hereditary Spherocytosis

TRAIT	TRAIT	MILD SPHERO-CYTOSIS	MODERATE SPHERO-CYTOSIS	MODERATELY SEVERE SPHEROCYTOSIS*	SEVERE SPHEROCYTOSIS[†]
Hemoglobin (g/dl)	Normal	11–15	8–12	6–8	< 6
Reticulocytes (%)	1–3	3–8	≥ 8	≥ 10	≥ 10
Bilirubin (mg/dl)	0–1	1–2	≥ 2	2–3	≥ 3
Spectrin content (% of normal)[‡]	100	80–100	50–80	40–80[§]	20–50

(Table continued on next page.)

Clinical Classification of Hereditary Spherocytosis (Continued)

TRAIT	TRAIT	MILD SPHERO-CYTOSIS	MODERATE SPHERO-CYTOSIS	MODERATELY SEVERE SPHEROCYTOSIS*	SEVERE SPHEROCYTOSIS[†]
Peripheral smear	Normal	Mild spherocytosis	Spherocytosis	Spherocytosis	Spherocytosis and poikilocytosis
Osmotic fragility					
Fresh blood	Normal	Normal or slightly increased	Distinctly increased	Distinctly increased	Distinctly increased
Incubated blood	Slightly increased	Distinctly increased	Distinctly increased	Distinctly increased	Markedly increased

* Values in untransfused patients.
[†] By definition, patients with severe spherocytosis are transfusion dependent.
[‡] Normal ($\pm$ SD) = 245 $\pm$ 27 $\times$ 10^5 spectrin dimers per erythrocyte. In most patients ankyrin content is decreased to a comparable degree. A minority of HS patients lack band 3 or protein 4.2 and may have mild to moderate spherocytosis with normal amounts of spectrin and ankyrin.
[§] The spectrin content is variable in this group of patients, presumably reflecting heterogeneity of the underlying pathophysiology.
Adapted from Eber SW, Armbrust R, Schröter W: Variable clinical severity of hereditary spherocytosis: Relation to erythrocytic spectrin concentration, osmotic fragility and autohemolysis. J Pediatr 177:409, 1990; Pekrun A, Eber SW, et al: Combined ankyrin and spectrin deficiency in hereditary spherocytosis. Ann Hematol 67:89, 1993; and Lux SE, Palek J: Disorders of the red cell membrane. In Handin RI, Lux SE, Stossel TP (eds): Blood: Principles and Practice of Hematology. Philadelphia, J.B. Lippincott, 1995, pp 1701–1818. Reproduced from Gallagher PG, Forget BC, Lux S: Disorders of the erythrocyte membrane. In Nathan DG, Orkin SH (eds): Nathan & Oski's Hematology of Infancy and Childhood, 5th ed. Philadelphia, W.B. Saunders, 1998, with permission.

44. What are the laboratory abnormalities in HS?
- Spherocytes and microspherocytes on the peripheral smear
- Mild anemia
- MCHC is increased
- Abnormal osmotic fragility test (*Note:* About 25% of patients with HS will have a normal osmotic fragility test when freshly isolated cells are tested. However, incubation of the RBCs for 24 hours will bring out the abnormalities.)

45. Which condition in neonates is very difficult to differentiate from HS?
ABO incompatibility. Both conditions may have anemia, hyperbilirubinemia, microspherocytes, and an altered osmotic fragility test.

46. What is the role of G6PD in red blood cells?
- Generation of reduced nicotinamide adenine dinucleotide phosphate (NADPH). This intermediate helps keep glutathione (GSH) in a reduced state. GSH is important for maintenance of sulfhydril groups and prevention of oxidative damage.
- Mature RBCs are unable to synthesize G6PD.
- In normal cells, the half-life of G6PD is 60 days, and with severe deficiency, it may be 10 days or even less.

47. Does G6PD deficiency cause jaundice in newborn infants?
Neonatal jaundice is more common in infants with G6PD deficiency, but is not invariably observed. The increased incidence of hyperbilirubinemia does not correlate with the risk of anemia. Therefore, differences in hepatic metabolism (and not hemolysis) may account for the risk of hyperbilirubinemia.

IMMUNE HEMOLYTIC ANEMIAS

48. Who was the first person to describe hemolytic disease of the newborn?

Luoyse Bourgeois, a French midwife, described a set of twins with hemolytic disease of the newborn in 1609. The first twin was born hydropic and died shortly after birth, and the second twin died of kernicterus.

49. Who first suggested the term *erythroblastosis fetalis?*

Diamond and coworkers coined the term *erythroblastosis fetalis* in 1932 to describe infants with a hemolytic anemia, extramedullary hematopoiesis, hepatosplenomegaly, and an outpouring of immature erythroblasts. In addition, they showed that hydrops fetalis, icterus gravis, and kernicterus were different manifestations of the same disease.

50. What is erythroblastosis fetalis?

In this condition, antibody-mediated hemolysis in a fetus leads to severe anemia ultimately resulting in hydrops fetalis. Hydrops occurs due to a combination of extramedullary hematopoiesis leading to liver dysfunction and hypoalbuminemia, decreased plasma osmotic pressure, poor tissue oxygen delivery, capillary leak, and possibly a component of heart failure. In the classic scenario, an RhD-negative woman (15% of caucasians, 5% of African Americans, and < 1% of Asians) carrying an RhD-positive fetus is sensitized during pregnancy and produces anti-RhD antibodies, which, in subsequent pregnancies, cross the placenta and cause hemolysis in the fetus. Other Rh and minor blood group antigens occasionally cause isoimmunization and significant fetal hemolysis (see question 53). Prior to 1968, the incidence of erythroblastosis fetalis, or hemolytic disease of the newborn, was 6 per 1000 births, with a mortality as high as 25%.

51. What is the Rh blood system?

In the Rh blood group system, three pairs of antigens are present on the surface of the red blood cell (Cc, Ee, and Dd). The presence or absence of D signifies Rh positivity, and the d antigen does not exist. The antigens are inherited from each parent as a set of three. Cde and cDE are the most common genotypes. There are 43 other antigens in the Rh system, which are alleles of Cc, Ee, and D.

52. What is the significance of the D antigen?

The D^u antigen is an allele of D. The D^u antigen is weakly antigenic and is depressed by the presence of C on the opposite chromosome. Only rarely will the D^u antigen lead to isoimmunization.

53. What is RhoGAM and how effective is it at preventing Rh disease?

The introduction of RhoGAM (high-titer anti-D immune globulin) to prevent RhD isoimmunization in pregnancy dramatically decreased the incidence of erythroblastosis fetalis. RhoGAM is given as an intramuscular injection to RhD-negative women (unless the father is known to be RhD-negative as well) at 28 weeks' gestation, immediately after birth, and in situations in which there is a high risk of fetomaternal bleeding (including abortion, miscarriage, ectopic pregnancy, chorionic villous sampling, amniocentesis, percutaneous umbilical blood sampling, abdominal trauma, and placental abruption). The anti-D antibody binds to fetal RhD-positive red blood cells and decreases the load of foreign antigen presented to the maternal immune system. Since RhoGAM was introduced, the incidence of immune hemolytic disease of the newborn has declined to 6 per 10,000 births, and with advances in perinatal and neonatal care, the mortality has declined to less than 5%.

54. Since RhoGAM is so effective, why do women still get sensitized?

- An RhD-negative mother carrying an RhD-positive fetus receives no prenatal care
- Failure to recognize a clinical setting in which RhD sensitization may occur

• Inadequate dose of RhoGAM given
• Failure of the antibody to adequately block the maternal immune response

55. When an Rh-sensitized fetus is identified, what should be done?

A blood type and antibody screen are routinely performed on every woman in the first trimester of pregnancy. If the anti-D titer is greater than 1:8 or if the fetus shows signs of hydrops or polyhydramnios on ultrasound, amniocentesis or percutaneous umbilical cord blood sampling (PUBS) is performed. PUBS allows fetal RhD typing in cases in which the father is heterozygous (Dd), and measurement of fetal hematocrit, reticulocyte count, and Coombs' test. In cases in which the fetus is RhD-positive, amniotic fluid optical density (OD) analysis can be used to predict the severity of hemolysis. Bilirubin released into the amniotic fluid causes an increase in the OD at a wavelength of 450 nm. Using curves first developed in 1961 by Liley, the change in amniotic fluid OD_{450} over time may be plotted and used in conjunction with other tests such as ultrasonography to determine when intervention is required to prevent or treat hydrops fetalis. Intrauterine fetal blood transfusions are performed in cases of severe hemolytic anemia.

56. What is the most common cause of immune hemolytic anemia in the newborn?

Since RhoGAM became widely available, ABO incompatibility has become the most common cause of immune-mediated hemolysis in the newborn. An **ABO set-up** occurs when a woman who is blood type O delivers a baby who is blood type A, B, or AB. This occurs in about 15% of all pregnancies. Individuals with blood type O can produce a significant amount of IgG against A and B antigens. Unlike IgM, this IgG is actively transported across the placenta.

57. If 15% of all pregnancies have an ABO set-up, why do only 3% have ABO hemolytic disease?

• Maternal anti-A and anti-B antibodies may be IgG, IgM, or IgA, and the titer of IgG is variable.
• Red blood cells of newborns have less than a third the number of A and B antigens compared to adult red blood cells, and their sparse distribution contributes to low antibody binding.
• In contrast to Rh antigens, A and B antigens are found on many tissues besides red blood cells. Maternal antibody may be taken up in the placenta or in other tissues in the baby after birth.
• Anti-A and anti-B antibodies do not bind complement on neonatal cells and thus cause less severe hemolysis in neonates than in adults.

58. How would you manage a newborn whose mother is blood type O?

1. A general recommendation is to send cord blood for type and Coombs' test on all babies of blood type O mothers. The Coombs' test on cord blood is positive (often only weakly so) in about 30% of ABO-incompatible pregnancies. Blood drawn directly from the baby is less likely to be Coombs' positive, especially after the first day of life.
2. A serum bilirubin should be drawn on
   • All babies who appear jaundiced in the first 24 hours of life
   • Those who are Coombs' positive
   • Those who are ABO incompatible and are being discharged early (prior to day 3 of life)
   • Those in whom clinical assessment of jaundice may be difficult

Note: Even in the presence of a positive Coombs' test, only about 10% of newborns will require treatment for hyperbilirubinemia. On the other hand, a significant number of newborns with an ABO set-up who are Coombs' negative will also require phototherapy. If the direct Coombs' test is negative but hemolysis is suspected, a more sensitive assay may be done, which involves eluting RBC-bound antibodies and testing against a panel of cells of known antigen.

59. What clinical and laboratory features distinguish hemolytic disease due to Rh and ABO incompatibility?

Clinical and Laboratory Features of Rh and ABO Hemolysis in the Newborn

	Rh	ABO
Incidence	0.06% of pregnancies	3% of pregnancies
First pregnancy affected	Rare (< 5%)	Frequent (50%)
Subsequent pregnancies	Increasing severity	Not predictable
In utero hemolysis, hydrops	Common	Rare
Hepatomegaly	Moderate to severe	Mild or absent
Anemia at birth	Yes	No
Jaundice at birth	Possible	No
Jaundice by 24 hours	Yes	Yes
Direct Coombs' test	Strongly positive	Weakly positive
Reticulocytosis	Moderate to severe	Mild
Microspherocytosis	No	Yes
Need for exchange transfusion	50–70%	< 10%
Late anemia	Frequent	Uncommon

60. Which is worse, O-A or O-B incompatibility?

"B is Bad, but A is Awful." The A antigen is more antigenic than B and tends to cause more severe hemolysis.

61. What follow-up care is required for neonates with immune hemolytic disease?

Babies with significant hyperbilirubinemia should have a hearing screen performed prior to nursery discharge or within the first several months of life. In addition, a significant anemia may develop between 4 and 10 weeks of age (particularly in cases of Rh isoimmunization). Late anemia is generally well tolerated, and transfusion is rarely indicated unless signs of cardiorespiratory compromise are present. Early iron supplementation should be considered, except in babies who received intrauterine transfusions and have adequate iron stores.

62. What other antigens besides RhD and the ABO group may cause hemolytic disease of the newborn?

The majority of cases of minor blood group incompatibility are due to the antigens Kell, E, and c (which are about 1% as potent as the D antigen), and a small percentage of cases are caused by M or Duffy (less than 0.1% as potent as D). Hemolytic disease caused by the Kell antigen can be particularly severe ("Kell kills"). Management is the same as that for RhD disease.

HEMOGLOBINOPATHIES

63. Why isn't sickle cell disease symptomatic in the newborn infant?

The main hemoglobin at birth is fetal hemoglobin consisting of two α chains and two γ chains. Even in infants with homozygous sickle cell disease, the concentration of Hb S is only 20% at birth, which is not high enough to produce symptoms.

64. When does the chain switchover from γ to β occur during gestation?

32 weeks.

65. What are the manifestations of sickle cell disease in the newborn infant?

Jaundice   Respiratory distress
Fever   Abdominal distention
Pallor

66. When was sickle cell disease first described?

Herrick described sickle cell disease in a West Indian student in 1910. However, the mutation for sickle hemoglobin is believed to be at least 50,000 years old.

67. In infants with sickle cell disease, when does the risk of mortality from sepsis and sequestration increase?

At 2–3 months.

68. Is screening for sickle cell anemia in high-risk populations cost-effective?

Yes. Several studies have confirmed that neonatal diagnosis and follow-up can reduce mortality.

Powars D: Diagnosis at birth improves survival of children with sickle cell anemia. Pediatrics 83:830, 1989.

69. What are the complications of pregnancy in women with sickle cell disease?

- **Mother**—increase in severity and frequency of painful crises, increase in severity and frequency of chest syndrome, exaggeration of physiologic anemia of pregnancy, toxemia, and death (< 1%).
- **Fetus**—spontaneous abortion, prematurity, and intrauterine growth retardation (IUGR)

70. What are the effects of hemoglobin A and F on polymerization of Hgb S?

- Both Hb A and Hb F increase the delay time of polymerization of sickle hemoglobin and the solubility of Hgb S.
- Hb F is more potent than Hb A in both of those activities.

71. What are the varieties of thalassemia?

- **Silent carrier.** One out of four α-globin genes is inactivated. The MCV is somewhat lower in these infants, and levels of Bart's Hb (γ chain tetramer) are increased in cord blood.
- **α-Thalassemia trait.** Two out of four α-globin genes are inactivated. Levels of Bart's Hb are increased (4–6%) during the neonatal period. Affected infants develop a hypochromic microcytic hemolytic anemia.
- **Hemoglobin H disease.** Three out of four α-globin genes are inactivated. These infants exhibit a moderately severe hemolytic anemia, hypochromia, microcytosis, and increased levels of Hb H (a β chain tetramer—β_4).
- **Hydrops fetalis.** All four α-globin genes are inactivated. These infants are stillborn or die shortly after birth, and their blood contains only Hb Bart's (γ_4), Hb H (β_4), and small amounts of hemoglobin Portland ($\zeta_2\gamma_2$).

72. Why is it important to make the diagnosis of α-thalassemia trait at birth?

The diagnosis of α-thalassemia trait is easy to make at birth because of the presence of Bart's hemoglobin (γ_4) and microcytosis. As these babies grow, gamma chain production ceases, and the diagnosis becomes much more difficult. Importantly, infants with this disorder can be incorrectly diagnosed as iron deficient and erroneously placed on iron for long periods of time.

73. What is hemoglobin Constant Spring?

Some silent carriers of α-thalassemia produce small quantities of an unusual hemoglobin called **Constant Spring**. This hemoglobin was named after a small Jamaican town in which the first family known to carry the gene resided.

DIAMOND-BLACKFAN ANEMIA

74. What is Diamond-Blackfan anemia (DBA)?

DBA, also called congenital hypoplastic anemia or constitutional red cell aplasia, is a heterogeneous disorder involving the erythroid progenitor cells. This results in a progressive macrocytic anemia, which begins in infancy. The pathogenesis is unclear although the genetic abnormality has recently been found. There appears to be mutation in the gene that encodes the ribosomal protein S19 (located on chromosome 19q), which may play an important role in erythropoiesis and embryogenesis.

75. What are the clinical and laboratory features of DBA?

Affected children present most often in infancy with severe anemia. About a third of them have one or more congenital defects such as craniofacial dysmorphism, skeletal anomalies, congenital heart and urogenital defects, and mental retardation. There is usually growth retardation as well. Laboratory tests show a severe macrocytic anemia, with a normal white cell count and normal or increased platelet count. There is absolute reticulocytopenia. A bone marrow aspirate shows a decrease or absence of erythroid precursors.

76. How do you distinguish DBA from transient erythroblastopenia of childhood (TEC)?

	DBA	TEC
Etiology	Constitutional	Acquired
Genetics	19q13 mutation	—
Congenital malformations	30%	None
Short stature	Yes	No
MCV	Increased	Normal
Hb F	Increased	Normal
Adenosine deaminase	Increased	Normal
i antigen expression	Present	Absent
Role for steroids	yes	No
Recovery without treatment	15%	100%
Increased risk for tumors	Yes	No

77. What is the treatment of DBA?

The initial treatment of DBA should always be a trial of corticosteroids; 2 mg/kg/day of prednisone is a good start. Seventy-five percent of all patients will respond to this treatment, and steroids may then be tapered to a minimal alternate day dose to maintain adequate erythropoiesis, without the side effects of long-term corticosteroid therapy. In fact, some patients may remit spontaneously and be able to come off treatment. Oral or intravenous megadose pulse methylprednisolone has also been tried with some success. For those patients who do not respond to steroids, transfusions are the mainstay of treatment. This raises the obvious problem of transfusional iron overload, and chelation therapy with deferroxamine to prevent iron deposition and toxicity is required. Both bone marrow and peripheral or umbilical cord blood stem cell transplantation has been performed successfully in a small number of children with DBA. Recently hematopoietic growth factors such as EPO and interleukin-3 (IL-3) have been tried without sustained effect.

78. What is the prognosis of DBA?

The long-term prognosis remains uncertain. The average predicted survival of individuals with DBA is about 38 years. Causes of death include complications from iron overload in the transfused patients and sepsis or pneumonia in some of the others. There is an increased incidence of malignancies in these individuals, with leukemia being the most common. Osteogenic sarcoma, hepatocellular carcinoma, and gastric carcinoma are also reported.

METHEMOGLOBINEMIA

79. *Case 1.* **A 2-month-old infant living on a farm presents with unexplained cyanosis, vomiting, diarrhea, failure to thrive, a saturation of 90% on a pulse oximeter, but no respiratory distress.**

Case 2. **A 2-day-old infant with pulmonary hypertension on nitric oxide and FiO$_2$ of 60% drops his oxygen saturation to 85% on the pulse oximeter. The saturation does does not improve when the FiO$_2$ is increased to 100%.**

Case 3. **A 3-month-old former 27-week-gestation infant with bronchopulmonary dysplasia is undergoing bronchoscopy to rule out laryngotracheomalacia. The infant becomes bradycardic and cyanotic with oxygen saturation falling to 85%. The procedure is stopped, and the FiO$_2$ is increased to 100%, but there is only a minimal response in the infant's pulse oximeter oxygen saturation. A heparinized blood sample shows chocolate-brown blood that does not become bright red even when agitated with an air bubble.**

What presenting feature do these infants have in common? What would you do to investigate your suspicion as to the cause of the cyanosis? How would you confirm your diagnosis?

Each of the infants in these cases has methemoglobinemia. In the first case, exogenous exposure to inorganic nitrite compounds through drinking water is the cause of the constellation of toxic symptoms. In the second case, methemoglobinemia is a complication of inhaled nitric oxide therapy for pulmonary hypertension. In the third case, the use of a topical anesthetic agent resulted in methemoglobinemia. All three of the infants had a low functional SaO$_2$, manifested as persistently low oxygen saturation on the pulse oximeter. The third infant was also observed to have chocolate-colored blood that did not turn red upon mixing with ambient oxygen. The presence of chocolate-colored blood is indicative of methemoglobin (MetHb) and can be demonstrated by placing a drop of unclotted blood on filter paper. The color of this blood should be compared with that of a drop of blood from a normal control. Normal venous blood becomes bright red as it spreads into the filter paper; blood that does not brighten is characteristic of methemoglobinemia. The presence of methemoglobin can be confirmed by blood gas analysis using the cooximeter, which reads out separate values for MetHb and carboxyhemoglobin from the sample.

80. Why does the pulse oximeter give low readings when MetHb is present?

A pulse oximeter measures the functional SaO$_2$:

$$\text{Functional SaO}_2 = [O_2Hb/(O_2\,Hb + Hb)] \times 100$$

where Hb denotes reduced hemoglobin and O$_2$Hb, oxyhemoglobin. The pulse oximeter works on the principle of the Beer-Lambert law, which states that the concentration of an absorbing substance in solution can be determined from the intensity and wavelength of incident light, the transmission path, and the characteristic absorbence of the substance at that particular wavelength. The absorbence of the substance is dependent on its concentration in solution. In normal humans the solutes measured are oxygenated and reduced hemoglobin. The pulse oximeter measures red light at 660 nm and near infrared light at 940 nm. Reduced Hb absorbs incident light at 660 nm— ten times better than O$_2$Hb. At 940 nm, O$_2$HB has 10 times better absorbence than reduced Hb. Thus, functional SaO$_2$ can be calculated from the ratio of absorbencies at these wavelengths.

When methemoglobin is present, the ratio of absorbencies no longer reflects the ratio of oxygenated to total Hb. At 660 nm, MetHb has an absorbency similar to that of Hb, but at 940 nm, it has an absorbency like that of O$_2$Hb. Thus, the presence of MetHb will increase both numerator and denominator and drive the ratio [O$_2$Hb/Hb + O$_2$Hb)] toward one. This causes the calibrated saturation on the pulse oximeter to go toward 85%. In a nonhypoxic patient with methemoglobinemia, the saturation monitor underestimates the true oxygen saturation, whereas in a hypoxic patient, it overestimates the true oxygen saturation. The true fraction of methemoglobin can be calculated by the cooximeter using the following relationship:

$$\text{Fractional SaO}_2 = O_2Hb/(O_2Hb + Hb + COHb + MetHb) \times 100$$

Both carboxyhemoglobin (COHb) and MetHb can be measured using the in vitro wavelength cooximeter.

81. What is MetHb and how does the body deal with it?

MetHb is formed when the ferrous ion of the heme moiety is oxidized to the ferric form, destroying the oxygen-carrying capacity of heme. MetHb's presence also causes a shift in the oxygen dissociation curve to the left, reducing the transfer of oxygen to the tissues. In normal RBCs, a small amount of MetHb is constantly being formed, but the level remains low (< 1% of total Hb) because of the presence of two enzyme systems, the NADH-dependent cytochrome b_5 methemoglobin reductase system and NADH diaphorase. Cytochrome b_5 reductase uses NADH to reduce cytochrome b_5, which in turn reduces MetHb to Hb. A small amount of MetHb is reduced to hemoglobin by NADPH diaphorase. This mechanism is enhanced by methylene blue, the standard treatment for methemoglobinemia. Cellular antioxidants such as vitamin C and glutathione may reduce MetHb to Hb nonenzymatically.

82. What agents result in the production of MetHb?

MetHb production can be increased by **endogenous** oxidants, mainly nitric oxide (NO). Endogenous NO is produced during an inflammatory response (e.g., with sepsis or diarrheal diseases). Exposure to **exogenous** oxidants (e.g., drugs, food preservatives (sodium nitrite), and nitrites and nitrates in the water) has also been implicated. Typically, well water in farming communities is contaminated by nitrites and nitrates leached from minerals or from nitrogen-enriched fertilizers. Bacteria present in the water may degrade nitrates to nitrites. Current levels of safety for drinking water issued by the U.S. Environmental Protection Agency in 1991 are 1 mg/L of nitrites and 10 mg/L of nitrates. Drugs reported to cause methemoglobinemia include local anesthetics such as prilocaine (EMLA) and benzocaine, as well as dapsone, primiqine, amyl nitrite, isobutyl nitrite, and nitroglycerine. The single small dose of EMLA used for topical anesthesia in circumcision generally does not cause significant methemoglobinemia.

83. Why is methemoglobinemia more common in infants?

- In infants up to 6 months of age, there is a relative deficiency of NADPH diaphorase. This deficiency not only predisposes to methemoglobinemia, but also leads to a lack of response to methylene blue.
- Fetal hemoglobin is more sensitive to oxidation than adult hemoglobin.
- Congenital deficiencies of NADH diaphorase and methemoglobin reductase have been described.

84. Why are infants with G6PD deficiency at risk for methemoglobinemia?

G6PD deficiency is characterized by decreased production of NADPH, resulting in the hemolytic oxidation of RBCs and increased metHb levels in the presence of substances such as sulfa drugs. Decreased production of NADPH also leads to decreased reduction of methylene blue; thus, in patients with G6PD deficiency, methylene blue administration will cause hemolysis.

85. How do patients with methemoglobinemia usually present?

Acute or chronic presentations are possible. The hallmark of both is bluish or brownish cyanotic discoloration of lips and nail beds. In infants, irritability and excessive crying often occur with moderate levels of MetHb; drowsiness and lethargy develop as levels increase. Diarrhea can be one of the symptoms of acute toxicity. Chronic methemoglobinemia sometimes presents with vomiting and failure to gain weight.

Visible cyanosis occurs with as little as 1.5 g/dl of circulating methemoglobin; in contrast, at least 5 g/dl of reduced hemoglobin must be present before cyanosis is evident. Most patients whose MetHb level is less than 10% of total hemoglobin are clinically asymptomatic; however, cyanosis may be visible at MetHb < 6%. In otherwise healthy patients, MetHb > 30% may cause fatigue, headache, dyspnea, tachycardia, nausea, and weakness. MetHb > 55% is associated with lethargy and deteriorating consciousness. Cardiac arrhythmias and cardiovascular and neurologic depression may occur at higher levels. MetHb > 70% is usually fatal. Symptoms at any level may be worsened by anemia and cardiopulmonary disease.

86. How should infants with methemoglobinemia be treated?

- Identify possible etiologic agents and stop exposure.
- Provide 100% oxygen and airway and circulatory support as needed.
- Use gastric lavage or activated charcoal to treat exposure due to an ingested agent (e.g., adulterated food). The half-life of methemoglobin is 55 min and the MetHb level will usually fall quickly when the etiologic agent is cleared from the body.
- Asymptomatic patients with MetHb < 30% of total Hb should be closely observed but usually need no treatment.
- The MetHb levels found in patients with hereditary NADPH diaphorase deficiency rarely need treatment except for cosmetic reasons.
- Patients with MetHb > 30% should receive definitive treatment with methylene blue, used as a 1% solution in a dose of 1–2 mg/kg IV infused over 5–10 minutes. The dose can be repeated if the level of MetHb remains elevated an hour later or subsequently rises. The total dose of methylene blue should not exceed 7 mg/kg.
- If the MetHb level does not fall within an hour after treatment, consider exchange transfusion or hemodialysis. High doses of methylene blue may discolor the skin and interfere with pulse oximetry.
- Newborns and children of Afro-Caribbean, Asian, or Mediterranean descent should be screened for NADPH diaphorase deficiency and G6PD deficiency before treatment with methylene blue. If either of these conditions is present, methemoglobinemia should be treated with vitamin C, 300–1000 mg/day IV, divided into 3–4 doses and supplemented with oxygen and cardiopulmonary support.

FANCONI ANEMIA

87. What is Fanconi anemia?

Fanconi anemia is a congenital aplastic anemia that involves all bone marrow series erythrocytes, leukocytes, and platelets. It is often, but not always, associated with congenital malformations (usually bone anatomic abnormalities).

88. What is the pathogenesis of Fanconi anemia?

The syndrome results most likely from a failure of the DNA repair system. Cell complementation studies have shown several subtypes of Fanconi anemia. These are called complementation groups and are summarized in the table. Within each complementation group, different mutations may exhibit different degrees of severity.

Clinical Classification of Fanconi Anemia

GROUP	TRANSFUSIONS	ANDROGEN OR CYTOKINE TREATMENT	STATUS
1	Yes	No	Severe aplastic anemia; failed or never received androgens
2	Yes	Yes	Severe aplastic anemia; currently on but not responding to androgens
3	No	Yes	Previously severe or moderate aplasia; responding to androgens or cytokines
4	No	No	Severe or moderate aplastic anemia, needs treatment
5	No	No	Stable, with some sign of marrow failure (e.g., mild anemia, neutropenia, thrombocytopenia, high mean corpuscular volume, high Hb F)
6	No	No	Normal hematology ± normal Hb F

Hb F = hemoglobin F.
From Alter BP, Knobloch ME, Weinberg RS: Erythropoiesis in Fanconi's anemia. Blood 78:602, 1991. Reprinted in Alter BP, Young NS: The bone marrow failure syndromes. In Nathan DG, Orkin SH (eds): Nathan & Oski's Hematology of Infancy and Childhood, 5th ed. Philadelphia, W.B. Saunders, 1998.

89. What are the hematologic characteristics of Fanconi anemia?

Fanconi described the first family of three brothers with a "pernicious form" of macrocytic anemia in 1911. It was Naegeli in 1931 who first suggested the name "Fanconi's anemia" to describe the syndrome of familial aplastic anemia and congenital malformations. Affected individuals demonstrate evidence of "fetal" or "stress erythropoiesis." The red cells are large, display the i antigen, and have high levels of hemoglobin F. Patients are diagnosed with Fanconi anemia if they demonstrate chromosomal breaks when exposed to clastogenic agents.

90. What anomalies are seen in Fanconi anemia?

Skin
- Generalized hyperpigmentation on trunk, neck, and intertriginous areas: café-au-lait spots; hypopigmented areas; gray or bronze color; large freckles

Microsomia
- Short stature; delicate features; small size; underweight

Upper Limbs
- Thumbs: absent or hypoplastic; supernumerary, bifid, or duplicated; rudimentary or vestigial; short, low set, attached by a thread, triphalangeal, tubular, stiff, hyperextensible
- Radii: absent or hypoplastic (only with abnormal thumbs); absent or weak pulse
- Hands: clinodactyly; hypoplastic thenar eminence; six fingers; absent first metacarpal; enlarged, abnormal fingers; short fingers, transverse crease
- Ulnae: dysplastic

Gonads
- Males: hypogenitalia; undescended testes; hypospadias; abnormal genitalia; absent testis; atrophic testes; azoospermia; phimosis; abnormal urethra; micropenis; delayed development
- Females: hypogenitalia; bicornuate uterus; abnormal genitalia; aplasia of uterus and vagina; atresia of uterus, vagina, and ovary

Other Skeletal
- Head and face: microcephaly; hydrocephalus; micrognathia; peculiar face; bird face; flat head; frontal bossing; scaphocephaly; sloped forehead; choanal atresia
- Neck: Sprengel's deformity; short, low hair line; web
- Spine: spina bifida (thoracic, lumbar, cervical, occult sacral); scoliosis; abnormal ribs; sacrococcygeal sinus; sacral agenesis; Klippel Fell syndrome; vertebral anomalies; extra vertebrae

Eyes
- Small eyes; strabismus; epicanthal folds; hypertelorism; ptosis; slanting; cataracts; astigmatism; blindness; epiphora; nystagmus; proptosis; small iris; hypotelorism; anophthalmia

Ears
- Deafness (usually conductive); abnormal shape; atresia; dysplasia; low set, large, or small; infections; abnormal middle ear; absent drum; dimples; rotated; canal stenosis

Renal
- Kidneys ectopic or pelvic; abnormal, horseshoe, hypoplastic, or dysplastic; absent; hydronephrosis or hydroureter; infections; duplicated; rotated; reflux; hyperplasia; no function; abnormal artery

Gastrointestinal
- High arched palate; atresia (esophagus, duodenum, jejunum); imperforate anus, tracheoesophageal fistula, Meckel's diverticulum; umbilical hernia; hypoplastic uvula; abnormal biliary ducts; megacolon; abdominal diastasis; Budd-Chiari syndrome; anterior anus; persistent cloaca; annular pancreas

Lower Limbs
- Feet: toe syndactyly; abnormal toes; flat feet; short toes; club feet; six toes; supernumerary toe; abnormal
- Legs: congenital hip dislocation; Perthes' diseases; coxa vara; abnormal femur; thigh osteoma; abnormal legs

Cardiopulmonary
- Patent ductus arteriosus; ventricular septal defect; abnormal; peripheral pulmonic stenosis; aortic stenosis; coarctation; absent lung lobes; vascular malformation; aortic atheromas; atrial septal defect; tetralogy of Fallot; pseudotruncus; hypoplastic aorta; abnormal pulmonary drainage; double aortic arch; cardiac myopathy

Other
- Slow development; hyperreflexia; Bell's palsy; central nervous system arterial malformation; moyamoya syndrome; absent corpus callosum; stenosis of the internal carotid artery; small pituitary gland; accessory spleen; absent breast buds

91. How is Fanconi anemia diagnosed?

The diagnostic test consists of exposing a chromosomal preparation to agents such as DBO or mitomycin-C that induce over 15% of chromosomal breaks in affected individuals, but only a minor number of breaks in controls. This test is useful for prenatal detection of Fanconi syndrome and is positive in individuals who have the disease, even when hematologic parameters are normal.

92. Is Fanconi anemia always severe?

No. Degree of severity ranges from most severe to asymptomatic.

93. Is there an increased tendency to cancer in Fanconi anemia?

At least 20% of surviving patients develop cancer or leukemia. It appears that as the survival of the affected individuals improves, the probability of developing cancer increases. Cancer is a major cause of mortality in older patients.

94. Can Fanconi anemia be cured?

The only available cure is bone marrow transplantation, either from a histocompatible sibling or from cord blood. However, because of the underlying defect, cytotoxic drugs are not well tolerated, resulting in a higher probability of failure. When bone marrow transplant is not feasible, treatment with androgens (with or without corticosteroids) induces a slow, often incomplete remission of short duration.

95. What is the survival of Fanconi anemia patients?

Most patients succumb from infectious complications due to the profound agranulocytosis. Those who survive longer often die from leukemia (that rarely responds to therapy) or from other types of cancer. Patients treated with androgens have a high incidence of liver cancer.

TRANSIENT ERYTHROBLASTOPENIA OF CHILDHOOD

96. What is TEC?

Transient erythroblastopenia of childhood is a condition that affects otherwise healthy children between the ages of 6 months and 4 years. Temporary shut down of RBC production results in anemia and reticulocytopenia. The white cell and platelet counts are usually normal.

97. What is the etiology of TEC?

The precise etiology of this condition is unknown. It has been observed following viral infections such as parvovirus B19, herpesvirus type 6 variant B, and echovirus 11, but this is not a consistent finding. Only half the children affected report having a viral illness in the preceding 1–2 months. Other theories of pathogenesis include an autoimmune phenomenon; drugs such as aspirin, sulfonamides, and anticonvulsants; and a possible genetic predisposition.

98. How is the diagnosis of TEC made?

Clinically the patient is usually a well toddler with anemia. Symptoms such as lethargy and irritability may be present if anemia is profound. The CBC shows a moderate to severe normocytic anemia, with a reticulocyte count < 1%. A bone marrow exam is usually not indicated, but if done shows a decrease in the erythroid precursors and some increase in lymphocytes, but normal myeloid and megakaryocytic cell lines.

99. What other conditions may present with anemia in infancy?

By far the most common cause of anemia in infancy is iron deficiency. This microcytic anemia responds immediately to oral iron supplementation. Most inherited red cell abnormalities, such as thalassemia, sickle cell disease, spherocytosis, and enzyme deficiencies, may also present with anemia at this age. Differentiating these conditions from TEC is relatively easy because all will have elevated reticulocyte counts. The one condition that is difficult to distinguish from TEC is Diamond-Blackfan anemia or congenital hypoplastic anemia.

100. What is the treatment for TEC?

Expectant observation. As the name implies, TEC is always transient, and complete recovery is the rule. Transfusions are only indicated if the anemia is severe and symptomatic and there is evidence of cardiovascular compromise. Although steroids have been used, there is no evidence that they have any role in this condition. Most children recover within 1–2 months, but some may take as long as 4 months. Needless to say, the prognosis is excellent.

NEUTROPENIA

101. On the second day of life, a small-for-dates, but otherwise well preterm neonate who was delivered to a woman with pregnancy-induced hypertension is noted to have a blood neutrophil concentration of 700/µl. The differential count has a normal ratio of immature neutrophils to total neutrophils. What is the likely kinetic mechanism accounting for the neutropenia?

Neutrophils are produced by clonal maturation of progenitors in the bone marrow. The morphologically recognizable neutrophil precursors (myeloblasts, promyelocytes, and myelocytes) are capable of cell division and are collectively termed the **neutrophil proliferative pool** (NPP). The maturing neutrophils in the marrow that have lost mitotic capacity (metamyelocytes, band neutrophils, and segmented neutrophils) constitute a ready reserve, termed the **neutrophil storage pool** (NSP). Once neutrophils are released from the marrow into the blood, they become apportioned to one of two interchangeable pools, the **circulating** or the **marginated** pools. Together, these two blood pools of neutrophils are termed the **total blood neutrophil pool** (TBNP).

Neutropenia can be categorized kinetically as the result of
1. Diminished production of neutrophils in the marrow—decreased NPP, NSP, and TBNP
2. Accelerated neutrophil usage or destruction—increased NPP and decreased NSP and TBNP
3. Excessive neutrophil margination—normal NPP, NSP, and TBNP

During pregnancy-induced hypertension, fetal neutrophil production is reduced (diminished NPP), and this results in a small NSP and consequently a small TBNP. The neutropenia generally persists for less than 3 days but can last a week or more.

102. A neonate with early-onset sepsis and shock has a blood neutrophil concentration of 700/µl and a very high ratio of immature to total neutrophils (75% on the leukocyte differential cell count). What is the likely kinetic mechanism accounting for the neutropenia?

During a clinically significant bacterial infection, neutrophils exit the bone marrow and enter the blood at a more rapid rate than they do during steady-state. Likewise, neutrophils exit the blood and enter the infected tissues more rapidly than normal. In compensation, neutrophil production within the bone marrow increases (the NPP increases or remains stable). Neutropenia during sepsis is generally accompanied by a left shift, because of the egress of band neutrophils and metamyelocytes from the marrow. Thus, the NPP increases (or is normal) whereas the NSP and TBNP are low.

103. What is the kinetic mechanism accounting for neonatal alloimmune neutropenia?

Neonatal alloimmune neutropenia arises when a mother has IgG antibodies that cross the placenta and react with neutrophil antigens that are foreign to her but are expressed on fetal (and paternal) neutrophils. Immune destruction of fetal neutrophils, in the fetal bone marrow and blood, can lead to severe fetal and neonatal neutropenia. In compensation for the neutrophil destruction, neutrophil production within the marrow increases (NPP increases), while the NSP and TBNP decrease because of destruction of mature neutrophils.

104. What is the kinetic mechanism accounting for neutropenia immediately after experimental administration of bacterial endotoxin?

Endotoxemia causes excessive neutrophil margination. Thus, the NPP, NSP, and TBNP all remain normal, but the circulating neutrophil pool shifts to the marginated compartment.

105. What are the common hematologic findings among neonates delivered to women with pregnancy-induced hypertension?

Hyporegenerative neutropenia, hyporegenerative thrombocytopenia, reticulocytosis, elevated nucleated red blood cells, polycythemia.

106. An FDA indication exists for recombinant granulocyte-colony-stimulating factor (rG-CSF) in the treatment of "severe congenital neutropenia." Which of the following five varieties of neonatal neutropenia are severe congenital neutropenias?
  A. **Neutropenia accompanying early-onset sepsis**
  B. **Neutropenia accompanying pregnancy-induced hypertension**
  C. **Necrotizing enterocolitis**
  D. **Kostmann syndrome**
  E. **Shwachman-Diamond syndrome**

The varieties of neutropenia that accompany neonatal bacterial sepsis, PIH, and NEC are generally acute and short-lived. These varieties can be severe (< 500 neutrophils/μL), but seldom do they persist for more than a few days. In contrast, the neutropenia of Kostmann and Shwachman-Diamond syndromes are life-long problems. They are among the group termed "severe congenital neutropenia," and they generally respond to treatment with recombinant rG-CSF.

THROMBOCYTOPENIA

107. What is the normal platelet count for a newborn infant?

> 150,000/μl.

108. How well do "neonatal platelets" function?

Neonatal platelets appear to be functionally normal. However thrombocytopoiesis is not completely effective. Although healthy newborns have platelet counts similar to adults (150,000–450,000/ml), many apparently healthy newborns, particularly preterm ones, have platelet counts between 100,000 and 150,000/μl, without apparent cause. Moreover, in cases of infections, the platelet count of infants tends to drop precipitously. A marked rise in platelet count (up to 700,000/μl) is often seen between 2 weeks and 6 months of age. In the infant, as well as in older children, thrombocytosis is not associated with increased tendency to thrombosis, and thus it is not of clinical significance.

109. What physical findings suggest a specific etiology for thrombocytopenia in the neonate?
  • Blueberry rash (TORCH or viral infection)
  • Absence of radii (TAR syndrome)
  • Palpable flank mass and hematuria (renal vein thrombosis)
  • Hemangioma—often with bruit (Kasabach-Merritt syndrome)

- Abnormal thumbs (Fanconi syndrome, but it is unusual for affected infants to be thrombocytopenic at birth)
- Very small platelets (Wiskott-Aldrich syndrome)
- Markedly dysmorphic features (trisomy 13 or 18)

110. What is the most common mechanism for thrombocytopenia in the newborn infant?
Consumptive.

111. Why is thrombocytopenia difficult to diagnose and manage in babies?
1. The multitude of causes can make the differential diagnosis confusing and long.
2. It is difficult to obtain sufficient blood for evaluation (i.e., you can't get blood from a stone).

112. How common is neonatal thrombocytopenia in well term newborns and sick VLBW infants?
- Approximately 1 in 500–1000 infants born at term will have thrombocytopenia.
- Up to 20% of sick VLBW infants will demonstrate at least mild thrombocytopenia.

113. What are the etiologies of thrombocytopenia in sick premature infants?
Almost anything that will make the newborn sick will make them thrombocytopenic including bacterial and viral sepsis, NEC, consumptive coagulopathies, liver disease, hypersplenism, asphyxia, and renal vein thrombosis.

114. What is alloimmune thrombocytopenia (AIT)?
AIT is a platelet incompatibility between mother and fetus analogous to Rh disease. As with Rh disease, the mother makes antibody against "paternal" antigens (generally PL^{A1} or HPA-1). The antibody crosses the placenta and makes the fetus or neonate thrombocytopenic. In addition, the antibody can cause a qualitative defect in platelet aggregation.

115. When should one suspect AIT?
- The thrombocytopenia is unexplained.
- The mother has a normal platelet count and is well.
- The baby is not sick (other than purpura).
- The platelet count is very low ($\leq 50,000/\mu l$).
- There is a positive family history for thrombocytopenia (firstborn offspring are affected in about half the cases).
- Platelet counts stay low for an extended period of time (1–2 weeks).

116. If you suspect AIT, what should you do?
Call someone who knows what to do and follow the suggestions below.
- Bone marrow aspirates are not usually done because they are often uninformative
- Send blood specimens from the parents to the lab for:
  A. Platelet typing
  B. Platelet antibodies in the mother (paternal platelets are necessary for this test to see if the mother's antibody is directed against an antigen on the father's platelets)
  C. Determination of zygosity in the father. If the father is heterozygous, the risk in a subsequent pregnancy will be less.
  D. *Remember:* Just because the mother is PL^{A1}-negative doesn't mean she is making antibodies against a paternal antigen. Only 1 in 10 to 1 in 20 PL^{A1} women make antibody.
- Obtain a head ultrasound study. Intracranial hemorrhage occurs in 10–20% of cases. Physical examination is unreliable, and the presence of an intracranial hemorrhage will change the management.

- Speak to the mother about donating platelets. If her platelets are used, they must be washed to remove serum and irradiated to prevent graft-versus-host disease.
- If the platelet count is less than 30,000/µl, consider giving intravenous immunoglobulin (IVIG) at a dose of 1 gm/kg and methylprednisolone sodium succinate (Solu-Medrol; 2 mg/kg/day) until the platelet rises above 50,000.
- Consider giving random donor platelets (or even better PL^{A1}-negative platelets) and estimating platelet survival 1–2 hours and 12–16 hours after transfusion. Random donor platelets are not likely to be effective in small amounts because 98% of donors are PL^{A1} positive.

117. What are the clinical features of autoimmune thrombocytopenia?
- This diagnosis should be considered when both mother and infant have thrombocytopenia or when there is a history of thrombocytopenia in the mother. Note it is sometimes difficult to distinguish maternal idiopathic thrombocytopenic purpura (ITP) from the thrombocytopenia that occurs in pregnancy due to volume expansion (gestational thrombocytopenia).
- Autoimmune thrombocytopenia is milder in the newborn infant than AIT is.
- Platelet counts commonly fall after birth.
- The degree of maternal thrombocytopenia is a poor predictor of the degree of neonatal thrombocytopenia.

118. How is AIT treated?
If the baby's platelet count is < 50,000/µl, IVIG and Solu-Medrol therapy should be started.

119. What are the distinguishing characteristics of gestational thrombocytopenia?
- The platelet count is usually not less than 70,000/µl.
- No history of thrombocytopenia in the past (except at the time of a previous pregnancy).
- No history of bleeding symptoms.
- The platelet count goes back to normal after the pregnancy is completed.

120. When should platelets be administered to a sick infant with thrombocytopenia?
In a sick infant without bleeding manifestations, the platelet count should be kept above 25,000/µl. In an infant who is bleeding or after surgery, the platelet count should be kept $\geq$ 75,000/µl.

121. How long does the thrombocytopenia last in most infants with low platelet counts?
Assuming the cause of the thrombocytopenia has been eliminated, the platelet count generally rises to normal ranges by 1 week. In an occasional infant, it may actually overshoot.

POLYCYTHEMIA

122. A set of twins is born by cesarean section. Twin A is appropriate for gestational age (AGA), weighing 2.7 kg, and Twin B is small for gestational age (SGA), weighing 1805 g. Both have respiratory distress with tachypnea. Twin A requires an inspiratory oxygen concentration (FiO$_2$) of 80% to obtain a pulse oximetry value of 95%. Twin B requires an FiO$_2$ of 25%. Twin A has a chest x-ray that is normal, but Twin B's chest x-ray is mildly hazy, and there is some enlargement of the heart. A CBC is obtained on both twins. Twin A has a hematocrit of 71%, whereas Twin B has a hematocrit of 22%. What is the likely cause of the respiratory distress in these twins?

The classic signs of twin-to-twin transfusion are present in this case—disparate growth and hematocrit values. Twin A is polycythemic, and Twin B is anemic. There exists an inverse, linear correlation between hematocrit and pulmonary blood flow. Therefore, Twin A has very low pulmonary blood flow and increased pulmonary vascular resistance, accounting for the need for supplemental oxygen. Reduction of the hematocrit in Twin A will increase pulmonary blood flow and eliminate the need for oxygen. Twin B most likely has some fluid in his lungs or may have mild congestive heart failure secondary to anemia. A simple transfusion or partial exchange transfusion with packed red blood cells is indicated to increase the hematocrit.

123. An infant is born at term. Amniotic fluid volume had been normal during the pregnancy. At delivery there is a delay in the clamping of the cord. In the normal-newborn nursery, the infant is noted to be ruddy but has an otherwise normal examination. At 24 hours, the nurse notifies you that the infant has not voided. Investigation reveals that the infant is feeding well, and the physical examination remains normal. You elect to observe the infant. At 48 hours, the infant has only had a single void of 25 cc. How would you evaluate and treat this infant? Why is the urine output low?

Although it is prudent to evaluate the genitourinary system as a whole by obtaining a blood urea nitrogen (BUN), creatinine, and renal ultrasound study, it is unlikely to reveal a cause for significant oliguria in light of normal amniotic fluid volume and no perinatal asphyxia. A birth history of delayed cord clamping (a known cause of polycythemia) and the ruddy appearance of the infant make it likely that polycythemia exists. This is easily confirmed by measuring the infant's hematocrit. Whereas renal blood flow is unaffected by changes in hematocrit, the plasma fraction of the blood is reduced as the hematocrit increases. Therefore, renal plasma flow is reduced along with the creatinine clearance and urine production. A partial exchange transfusion will decrease the hematocrit, increase renal plasma flow, and restore normal renal function.

124. SGA infants, infants of diabetic mothers, and those born at a high altitude are at risk for polycythemia. What common factor is responsible for the increase in hematocrit in all three groups of babies?

In all three groups of infants, the oxygen content of fetal blood is reduced prior to birth. To compensate for the low PaO_2, the fetus increases its red cell mass by increasing erythropoietin production. In turn, this increases red cell mass until the oxygen content of the blood returns to a normal range.

125. You are called to see a large for gestational age (LGA) infant. The nursing staff reports that the "chemstrip" bedside glucose determinations have been low and a plasma glucose concentration was 20 mg/dl. An IV with 10% dextrose and water is begun at a rate of 80 cc/kg/day. Concerned about sepsis, you obtain a CBC and blood culture by arterial stick. The WBC and differential count are normal; however, the hematocrit is 72%. The plasma glucose remains in the hypoglycemic range despite increasing the rate of the IV and concentration of dextrose. How would you proceed?

Hypoglycemia is commonly seen in LGA infants. In addition, polycythemia is an independent risk factor for hypoglycemia. Hypoglycemia occurs in 10–40% of infants with polycythemia. An intravenous infusion of a dextrose solution will generally correct the hypoglycemia. In a number of the infants, however, the glucose will not normalize until the hematocrit is reduced by partial exchange transfusion. Two mechanisms for the hypoglycemia have been proposed. One thought is that the combination of a reduced plasma fraction (glucose primarily exists in the plasma fraction of blood) and reduced blood flow result in increased glucose extraction and hypoglycemia. A second suggested mechanism is decreased gluconeogenesis.

126. Should screening for polycythemia be done in every newborn infant?

In a healthy term newborn with a normal examination, there are no data to support the efficacy of obtaining a screening hematocrit. No etiologic link between polycythemia and neurologic injury has ever been established, and in population studies of asymptomatic polycythemic infants, all had normal long-term neurologic function.

127. A heel stick hematocrit was sent that was 76%. You are concerned about polycythemia and hyperviscosity. What should you do?

Obtain a central hematocrit.

128. What is the likelihood that a partial exchange transfusion will reduce the hematocrit and improve or protect the infant's long-term neurologic function?

Substantial data indicate that a partial exchange transfusion does not prevent neurologic injury. Polycythemia does reduce cerebral blood flow. However, the reduction in cerebral blood flow is not secondary to hyperviscosity, but is a physiologic response to the increase in arterial oxygen content resulting in normal cerebral oxygen delivery and metabolism. The decreased cerebral blood flow does not cause cerebral hypoxia. Therefore, it should not be surprising that studies have failed to show any benefit in long-term neurologic function by reducing the hematocrit. Lastly, several epidemiologic studies have suggested that it is the other events that occur in association with polycythemia such as asphyxia that cause the brain injury. Rather, polycythemia is a marker for fetal or perinatal distress and hypoxia.

HEREDITARY DISORDERS OF COAGULATION

129. What percentage of male infants with hemophilia who are circumcised in the neonatal period (before the diagnosis is established) will have unusual or excessive bleeding?

About 30–50%. The absence of bleeding at routine circumcision does not rule out the diagnosis of severe hemophilia.

130. At what age do boys with severe hemophilia typically begin to experience spontaneous hemarthrosis (joint bleeds)?

About 9–12 months, coincident with increased activity and ambulation. It is unusual for infants to have bleeding without specific trauma.

131. What fraction of infants born with hemophilia have factor VIII deficiency?

80–85% have hemophilia A, which is factor VIII deficiency, and 15–20% have hemophilia B, which is factor IX deficiency.

132. What is meant by "severe" hemophilia?

"Severe" refers to patients with a factor VIII or IX level less than 1% of the normal value. These patients will have frequent, spontaneous bleeding, such as hemarthrosis. A slightly higher baseline level (from 1–5%) is associated with a significantly milder phenotype in which bleeding typically occurs only with identifiable trauma.

133. How common is intracranial bleeding in infants with hemophilia?

Quite uncommon. Intracranial hemorrhage occurs in only 1–2% of severe cases, even with vaginal delivery.

134. Of hemophilia A and hemophilia B, which is X-linked?

Both are X linked. Both the factor VIII (hemophilia A) and factor IX (hemophilia B) genes are located on the long arm of the X chromosome.

135. Would cryoprecipitate be a good choice for empiric treatment in a newborn with an intracranial hemorrhage, an elevated PTT, and a family history of hemophilia before the factors levels are known?

No. Cryoprecipitate contains a higher concentration of factor VIII than FFP, but very little factor IX. Until the specific factor deficiency is known, FFP would be the best choice for factor replacement.

136. How can a male infant have hemophilia A if there is no family history of hemophilia on the mother's side? Why does this matter?

About a third of new cases of hemophilia A occur in families with no history of hemophilia. One possibility is that the family has female carriers but that, by random, no affected males have been previously born and identified. The other possibility is that a new mutation has occurred in one of the mother's factor VIII alleles. This gene is known to have a relatively high rate of new mutations. For the genetic counseling about future pregnancies, the risk of hemophilia in future male embryos depends on whether the mother and her sisters are carriers.

137. What is the risk of becoming infected with HIV from currently manufactured factor VIII and IX concentrate products?

Nearly nil. There are effective recombinant factor VIII and factor IX products available, and the plasma-derived, pooled products are all treated by solvent or detergent or heating processes that eliminate enveloped viruses. There have been no HIV transmissions from factors VIII and IX concentrates since before 1990.

138. What are the ways a female can "get" hemophilia?

There are several described mechanisms, all rare:
• She is the homozygous offspring of a hemophiliac male and a carrier female.
• She is a hemophilia carrier with extremely unfavorable "lyonization" such that most of her cells use the X chromosome with the defective gene.
• She has a chromosomal abnormality with only one X chromosome (XO) and that X chromosome has a hemophilia mutation.
• She has an extremely rare form of autosomally transmitted hemophilia.
• She is genetically normal and has an acquired inhibitor to factor VIII or IX.

139. What coagulation factor deficiencies result in an extremely prolonged partial thromboplastin time (PTT) but no bleeding diathesis?

Deficiencies of factor XII, prekallikrein, and high–molecular-weight kininogen. These factors are referred to as **contact factors** and are critical to initiating the activation of coagulation in the in vitro clotting assays, but do not contribute significantly to hemostasis in vivo.

140. How is von Willebrand disease inherited?

The most common and mildest forms are autosomal dominant. There are rare recessive variants. The disease is frequently so mild that the family history may be negative even when one of the parents is actually affected. Only the severe, autosomal recessive forms would be likely to present with bleeding manifestations in the newborn period.

141. How long after birth should one wait before screening an otherwise well newborn with a family history of hemophilia for factors VIII or IX deficiency?

Screening for factor VIII or factor IX levels can be done right away, even on cord blood. Neither factor VIII nor factor IX crosses the placenta. An infant with severe hemophilia and a factor VIII or IX level less than 1% should be reliably identified in the newborn period. However, the diagnosis of milder forms with higher endogenous factor levels, especially for factor IX, may be more difficult because the lower limit of normal range in a newborn is much lower than in adults.

142. Should the activated PTT (aPTT) be used to screen a newborn who is at risk for hemophilia because of a family history on the mother's side?

Probably not. The normal range for aPTT is wider in term newborns than older children and adults, and becomes even wider following a premature birth. An elevated aPTT does not distinguish between factor VIII and factor IX deficiency. The aPTT may also be within the normal range for a neonate with mild or moderate hemophilia. Therefore, it is better to order the definitive tests (factor VIII and factor IX levels).

143. What is a "PUP trial"?

The term refers to the design of a rigorous clinical trial of factor concentrate preparations in which the only eligible subjects are newborn hemophilia patients who have never received any other factor replacement therapy. Such patients are called **p**reviously **u**ntreated **p**atients (PUPs). PUP trials provide the cleanest estimates of rates of complications such as inhibitor formation and viral transmission. PUP trials are popular among the hemophilia families because the patients usually receive free factor while enrolled.

144. What coagulation factor deficiency is classically associated with delayed separation of the umbilical cord stump?

Factor XIII deficiency. Factor XIII stabilizes and crosslinks fibrin clots after they are formed. Factor XIII deficiency is a clinical bleeding disorder in which the screening tests, prothrombin time (PT), PTT, and platelet count are all normal.

DISSEMINATED INTRAVASCULAR COAGULATION

145. What is usually the earliest screening laboratory abnormality found during the course of DIC?

A low platelet count, related to consumption. With more advanced DIC, the PT typically becomes prolonged, and the PTT does as well.

146. What is the classic constellation of laboratory abnormalities seen in severe DIC?

Elevated PT, PTT, low platelet count, low fibrinogen, elevated fibrin split products (FSP).

147. What test can be used to distinguish DIC from liver (synthetic) failure?

Factor VIII level. This factor is thought to be synthesized in vascular endothelial cells, not in the hepatocyte. It is decreased in a state of consumption of coagulation factors, such as DIC, but remains normal in hepatic failure. Note that some factor VIII may be synthesized "in the liver" in endothelial cells rather than in hepatocytes.

148. What principles guide the approach to treating DIC?

1. **Identify** and treat the underlying disease process that is causing the DIC.

2. **Support** with blood products to replace the coagulation factors, platelets, and anticoagulant that are consumed in DIC. Platelet transfusions, FFP, and cryoprecipitate are typically given.

3. **Monitor** transfusion therapy with frequent coagulation tests to determine the dose and frequency of blood product administration.

4. **Consider heparin** therapy to interrupt the consumptive process. The value of this therapy is controversial.

149. How much cryoprecipitate should be given to treat DIC?

As much as it takes. Cryoprecipitate is typically used as a source of fibrinogen. The fibrinogen level should be monitored frequently—every 4–6 hours if possible. This information can be used to adjust the dose and frequency of cryoprecipitate transfusion to maintain the fibrinogen level above 100 mg/dl or at a sustainable level that prevents bleeding.

150. What are the first two things to do in response to a prolonged PTT in a term newborn?

1. Check to see that vitamin K was given after birth.

2. Repeat the PTT from a venipuncture to be sure the elevated PTT is real and not the result of a clotted specimen or heparin in a specimen drawn from a line.

151. What morphologic change may be seen in the red cells on the peripheral blood smear in severe DIC?

Schistocytes, or "microangiopathic" hemolytic anemia. These fragmented red cells, in a variety of shapes, are all smaller-than-normal, intact red cells. Schistocytes are thought to be formed when red cells must pass through small blood vessels that are partially occluded or distorted by excess fibrin deposited because of the DIC process.

152. Why do you need to collect the blood for FSPs into a special, separate tube?
Because the coagulation lab won't run the test if you don't. The biochemical reason is that fibrinogen interferes with the assay for FSPs, so it is necessary to remove all of the fibrinogen from the sample before measuring FSPs. The "special tube" contains a snake venom that completely converts the fibrinogen in the sample to insoluble fibrin, thereby removing the interference from the FSP assay.

CONGENITAL THROMBOTIC DISORDERS

153. What are the indications for thrombolytic therapy?
Thrombolytic therapy is used most commonly to treat arterial thrombi that are secondary to catheters placed in a peripheral artery, aorta, or femoral artery. The decision to use thrombolytic therapy is based on certain pieces of clinical information such as age and location of the thrombus and severity of the clinical symptoms. If there is potential loss of limb or critical organ function, thrombolytic therapy should be considered, provided there is no significant bleeding disorder, hemorrhage into the brain, hypertension, or other risk factors. In the presence of these complications, thrombolytic therapy might still be used if the baby's life is at risk. In the past, urokinase was the most commonly used thrombolytic agent in newborns, but it is in very short supply. Therefore, tissue plasminogen activator is now the drug of choice, and protocols are available. Heparin therapy is indicated either immediately following an infusion of a thrombolytic (provided the thrombolytic agent is infused for less than 12 hours) or during thrombolytic therapy (for infusions lasting more than 12 hours). Prolonged infusions of thrombolytic therapy (12–24 hours) will consume endogenous plasminogen (already physiologically decreased) and render the patient relatively resistant to thrombolytic therapy. Supplementation of plasminogen should be considered in these instances and can be achieved through the administration of FFP and cryoprecipitate.

154. What inherited disorders of coagulation proteins have been associated with a prothrombotic state?

Antithrombin III deficiency	Resistance to activated protein C due to
Protein C deficiency	the factor V Leiden mutation
Protein S deficiency	Dysfibrinogenemias

155. Can prothrombotic disorders be accurately diagnosed during the neonatal period?
Plasma concentrations of antithrombin III, protein C, and protein S are all physiologically decreased at birth with values that rapidly increase in the first days to week of life. Free protein S levels are similar to adults. Published reference ranges for healthy full-term and premature infants (30–40 weeks gestational age for the first 6 months of life) are available with reliable limits that encompass 95% of the population. Sick infants may have acquired deficiencies of these inhibitors that resolve with time. The evaluation of parents can be helpful in distinguishing an acquired from a congenital abnormality. Activated protein C ratios are decreased at birth, and adult reference ranges are not available. However, both factor V Leiden and prothrombin gene 20210A are DNA-based tests that are accurate in newborns.

Andrew M, Monagle P, Brooker L: Developmental hemostasis: Relevance to thromboembolic complications in pediatric patients. In Thromboembolic Complications During Infancy and Childhood. Hamilton, B.C. Decker, 2000, pp 5–46.

Andrew M, Paes B, Johnston M: Development of the hemostatic system in the neonate and young infant. Am J Pediatr Hematol Oncol 12:95–104, 1990.

156. How does one diagnose central venous line thrombosis in newborns?
Although ultrasound is the most commonly used diagnostic test, the sensitivity and specificity of ultrasound remains unknown. In children with thrombi in the upper venous system, ultrasound appears to be sensitive for clots in the jugular and axillary veins, but not in the inferior vena cava, subclavian, and innominate veins, where 80% of the thrombi are missed.

157. How should neonates with thrombi associated with central venous lines be treated?

In all situations, a determination must be made of how essential the line is for the infant. Additional options include supportive therapy, anticoagulation, and thrombolytic therapy. Local thrombolytic therapy with either urokinase or tissue plasminogen activator is commonly used and is very effective at restoring line patency. Systemic thrombolytic therapy is rarely indicated because the thrombi are usually old, occurring gradually over time with little likelihood of lysing. However, a new acute clot in the presence of an old clot may present with a relatively sudden superior vena cava syndrome. In this situation, thrombolytic therapy may be helpful in resolving the acute symptoms. Anticoagulation therapy with either unfractionated heparin or low–molecular-weight heparin can be very effective in preventing further progression of the thrombus.

158. How do infants with homozygous protein C or S deficiency present?

The classical clinical presentation of homozygous protein C or S deficiency consists of cerebral or ophthalmic damage that occurred in utero, purpura fulminans within days or hours of birth, and (on rare occasion) large vessel thrombosis. The skin lesions start as small ecchymotic sites that increase in size, develop bullae, and become necrotic. They occur mainly on the extremities, but can occur on the buttocks, abdomen, scrotum, and scalp. There is a severe diffuse DIC with secondary hemorrhagic complications and unmeasurable levels of protein C or S.

A second form of homozygous protein C or S deficiency presents with thromboembolic events during early childhood and then severe skin necrosis when placed on coumarin. Protein C or S levels in these patients are detectable and range from ~1–20% of normal. If coumarin is used to treat these patients, INR values must be maintained > 4, and there is a considerable risk of bleeding. An alternative approach is to use low–molecular-weight heparin.

159. How are infants with homozygous protein C or S disease managed?

FFP, 10 units/kg, three times a day until the skin lesions are healed.

NEOPLASMS

160. What biologic variables at the time of diagnosis distinguish congenital or infant leukemia from leukemia in an older child?

- Extreme leukocytosis
- Massive hepatosplenomegaly
- High incidence of CNS leukemia at diagnosis
- Hypogammaglobulinemia
- High incidence of coexpression of lymphoid and myeloid phenotypic markers
- Increased frequency of cytogenetic abnormalities
    Pseudodiploidy
    Hypodiploidy
    Translocations: t(4;11), 11q23 breakpoints involve MLL gene
- Five-year event free survival of 25%

161. On initial examination a full-term male infant is found to have an abdominal mass. A sonogram reveals a right suprarenal mass with calcification. What is the probable diagnosis and course of management?

The most likely diagnosis is a neuroblastoma. Neuroblastomas account for > 50% of the malignancies diagnosed in the neonatal period. However, their management remains controversial. Although small primary tumors without metastases may regress spontaneously without intervention, a biopsy to assess biologic markers is warranted. If no adverse parameters are found, observation only is acceptable. However, if unfavorable characteristics are identified or if respiratory compromise secondary to massive hepatic involvement is present, chemotherapy or radiotherapy should be instituted.

162. What prognostic variables in infants with neuroblastoma predict an unfavorable prognosis?

Unfavorable Prognostic Variable in Infants with Neuroblastoma

PROGNOSTIC VARIABLE	RESULT
Shimada histopathology	Unfavorable
N-myc amplication	> 10 copies
Catecholamines	Increased VMA, HVA
Serum ferritin	Elevated
Neuron-specific enolase	> 100 ng/ml
Stage	III, IV
Tumor cell ploidy	Hyperdiploidy
Karyotype	Terminal 1p deletions

163. On initial examination a full-term male infant is found to have an abdominal mass. A sonogram reveals a right renal mass. What is the probable diagnosis and course of management?

The most likely diagnosis is congenital mesoblastic nephroma (CMN), a monomorphous spindle-cell neoplasm that is a congener of Wilms tumor diagnosed early in life. Ninety percent of CMNs occur during the first 6 months of life. A meticulous, complete nephrectomy with clear surgical margins is required. Careful observation without additional therapy is curative.

164. A newborn infant with Down syndrome is found to have a white blood cell count of 150,000/mm³. What course of management would you recommend to the family?

Although children with Down syndrome have a 20-fold increased risk for developing acute leukemia as infants, they have a propensity for a "transient leukemia." The etiology of the myeloleukemoid reaction appears to arise from an intrinsic intracellular defect in the regulation of neutrophil proliferation and maturation within the bone marrow. Thus, it would be prudent to observe the patient and treat with supportive care measures. In the majority of patients with transient leukemia, the blood counts normalize in several weeks to months without treatment.

165. On exam a newborn male is noted to have bilateral leukocoria, or "cat's eye reflex" of the retina. An ophthalmologic exam confirms a diagnosis of retinoblastoma. What features characterize hereditary retinoblastoma?

- Bilateral presentation
- Diagnosis established at an early age
- May be present in newborns
- Occurs in 20–30% of newly diagnosed cases of retinoblastoma
- Ocular tumors are multifocal
- Arise from a mutation in a germinal cell
- Presence of chromosome 13q14 deletion
- Loss of two retinoblastoma gene alleles
- Offspring may be affected
- Increased risk of second malignant neoplasms, particularly sarcomas

166. A female infant presents with constipation and is found to have a sacrococcygeal mass. What is the most likely diagnosis?

Germ cell tumor. Approximately 70% of sacrococcygeal germ cell tumors occur in females, and 50% are diagnosed in the neonatal period. At diagnosis, 50% are benign, 30% are malignant, and 20% have immature embryonic elements and although not frankly malignant have malignant potential. Clinically sacrococcygeal masses may be classified in order of frequency as follows:

Type I—predominantly external with minimal presacral component

Type II—external with significant intrapelvic component

Type III—external with predominant pelvic mass extending into the abdomen

Type IV—entirely presacral without an external component

167. Describe the clinical presentation and management of an infant with familial ery-throphagocytic lymphohistiocytosis (FEL).

FEL is a rare, poorly understood disease that has an autosomal recessive pattern of inheritance. It is characterized by a positive family history, hemophagocytosis, and defective cellular and humoral immunity. Infants present with irritability, fever, wasting, hepatosplenomegaly, hyperlipidemia, and a coagulopathy. Treatment consists of an exchange transfusion, chemotherapy, and an experimental allogeneic bone marrow transplant. The prognosis is poor.

168. What are the clinical manifestations of Langerhans histiocytosis (LH)?

The clinical presentation of infants and children with LH is varied. The spectrum of symptoms ranges from mild discomfort secondary to lytic bone lesions, diabetes insipidus, seborrhea, and chronic otitis media to generalized symptoms of fever, failure to thrive, hepatosplenomegaly, pulmonary compromise, and bone marrow failure. The diagnosis is confirmed by the presence of Birbeck granules and CD1 expression in lesional cells.

BIBLIOGRAPHY

Normal Red Blood Cell Indices and Differential Diagnosis of Anemia
1. Brugnara C, Platt OS: The neonatal erythrocyte and its disorders. In Nathan DG, Orkin SH (eds): Hematology of Infancy and Childhood, 5th ed. Philadelphia, W.B. Saunders, 1998, pp 19–52.
2. Cloherty JP, Stark AR: Manual of Neonatal Care, 3rd ed. Boston, Little, Brown, 1991.
3. Flake AW, Zanjani ED: In utero transplantation for thalassemia. Ann N Y Acad Sci 850:300–311, 1998.

Tranfusion Therapy
4. Blanchette VS, Gray E, Hardie MJ, et al: Hyperkalemia following exchange transfusion: Risk eliminated by washing red cell concentrates. J Pediatr 105:321, 1984.
5. Goodstein MH, Locke RG, Wlodarczyk D, et al: Comparison of two preservative solutions for erythrocyte transfusions in newborn infants. J Pediatr 123:783–788, 1993.
6. Manno CS: What's new in transfusion medicine? Pediatr Clin North Am 43:793–808, 1996.

Developmental Hematopoiesis
7. Bunn HF, Forget BG: Hemoglobin: Molecular, Genetic, and Clinical Aspects. Philadelphia, W.B. Saunders, 1986.
8. Seiff CA, Nathan D, Clark SC: The anatomy and physiology of hematopoiesis. In Nathan DG, Orkin SH (eds): Hematology of Infancy and Childhood, 5th ed. Philadelphia, W.B. Saunders, 1998.

Physiologic Anemia
9. Alverson DC: The physiologic impact of anemia in the neonate. Clin Perinatol 22:609–626, 1995.
10. Oski FA: The erythrocyte and its disorders. In Nathan DG, Orkin SH (eds): Hematology of Infancy and Childhood, 4th ed. Philadelphia, W.B. Saunders, 1993, pp 18–43.

Erythropoietin
11. Ohls RK, Veerman MW, Christensen RD: Pharmacokinetics and effectiveness of recombinant erythropoietin administered to preterm infants by continuous infusion in parenteral nutrition solution. J Pediatr 128:518–523, 1996.
12. Ohls RK: Erythropoietin to prevent and treat the anemia of prematurity. Curr Opin Pediatr 11:108–114, 1999.
13. Oski FA: The erythrocyte and its disorders. In Nathan DG, Orkin SH (eds): Hematology of Infancy and Childhood, 4th ed. Philadelphia, W.B. Saunders, 1993, pp 18–43.
14. Zipursky A: Erythropoietin for premature infants: Cost without benefit. Pediatr Res 48:136, 2000.

Nonimmune Hemolytic Anemias
15. Gallagher PG, Forget BC, Lux S: Disorders of the erythrocyte membrane. In Nathan DG, Orkin SH (eds): Hematology of Infancy and Childhood, 5th ed. Philadelphia, W.B. Saunders, 1998.

Immune Hemolytic Anemias
16. Bowman JM: Immune hemolytic disease. In Nathan DG, Orkin SH (eds): Hematology of Infancy and Childhood, 5th ed. Philadelphia, W.B. Saunders, 1998, pp 53–78.
17. Gollin YG, Copel JA: Management of the Rh-sensitized mother. Clin Perinatol 22:545–560, 1995.
18. Peterec SM: Management of neonatal Rh disease. Clin Perinatol 22:561–592, 1995.

Diamond-Blackfan Anemia
19. Alter BP: Bone marrow transplant in Diamond-Blackfan anemia. Bone Marrow Transpl 21:965–966, 1988.
20. Glader BE: Diagnosis and management of red cell aplasia in children. Hematol Oncol Clin North Am 1:341–347, 1987.
21. Willig TN, Ball SE, Tehernia G: Current concepts and issues in Diamond-Blackfan anemia. Curr Opin Hematol 5:109–115, 1998.
22. Young NS, Alter BP: Aplastic Anemia: Acquired and Inherited. Philadelphia, W.B. Saunders, 1994.

Methemoglobinemia
23. Avery AA: Infantile methemoglobinemia: Reexamining the role of drinking water nitrates. Environm Health Persp 107:583–586, 1999.
24. Coleman MD, Coleman NA: Drug-induced methemoglobinemia. Treatment issues. Drug Safety 14:394–405, 1996.
25. Fran AM, Steinberg VE: Health implications of nitrate and nitrite in drinking wter: An update on methemoglobinemia occurrence and reproductive and developmental toxicity. Regul Toxicol Pharmacol 23:35–43, 1996.
26. Griffin JP: Methaemoglobinaemia. Adv Drug Reactions Toxicol Rev 16:45–63, 1997.
27. Higasa K, Manabe JI, Yubisui T, et al: Molecular basis of hereditary methemoglobinemia types I and II: Two novel mutations in the NADH-cytochrome b5 reductase gene. Br J Haematol 103:922–930, 1998.
28. Plotkin JS, Buell JF, Njoku MJ, et al: Methemoglobinemia associated with dapsone treatment in solid organ transplant recipients: A two-case report and review. Liver Transplant Surg 3:149–152, 1997.
29. Sinex JE: Pulse oximetry: Principles and limitations. Am J Emerg Med 17:59–67, 1999.
30. Taddio A, Ohlsson A, Einarson TR, et al: A systematic review of lidocaine-prilocaine cream (EMLA) in the treatment of acute pain in neonates. Pediatrics 101:E1, 1998.

Franconi Anemia
31. Alter BP, Young NS: The bone marrow failure syndromes. In Nathan DG, Orkin SH (eds): Hematology of Infancy and Childhood, 5th ed. Philadelphia, W.B. Saunders, 1998.

Neutropenia
32. Al-Mulla Z, Christensen RD: Neutropenia in the neonate. Clin Perinatol 22:711–739, 1995.
33. Calhoun D, Christensen RD: Recent advances in the pathogenesis and treatment of nonimmune neutropenias in the neonate. Curr Opin Hematol 5:37–41, 1998.
34. Calhoun, Christensen RD: The role of hematopoietic growth factors in neonatal neutropenia and infection. Semin Neonatol 4:17–26, 1999.
35. Papoff P, Christensen RD: New therapies for neonatal sepsis. Curr Top Neonatal 3:200–231, 1999.
36. Schibler KR: Leukocyte development and disorders during the neonatal period. In Christensen RD (ed): Hematologic Problems of the Neonate. Philadelphia, W.B. Saunders, 1999, pp 311–342.

Polycythemia
37. Lindermann R, Haga P: Evaluation and treatment of polycythemia in the neonate. In Christensen RD (ed): Hematologic Problems of the Neonate. Philadelphia, W.B. Saunders, 2000, pp 171–183.
38. Rosenkrantz TS, Oh W: Cerebral blood flow velocity in infants with polycythemia and hyperviscosity: Effects of partial exchange transfusion with Plasmanate. J Pediatr 101:94–98, 1982.
39. Rosenkrantz TS, Stonestreet BS, Hansen NB, et al: Cerebral blood flow in the newborn lamb with polycythemia and hyperviscosity. J Pediatr 104:276–280, 1984.
40. Rosenkrantz TS, Philipps AF, Skrzypczak PS, Raye JR: Cerebral metabolism in the newborn lamb with polycythemia. Pediatr Res 23:329–333, 1988.
41. Rosenkrantz TS: Polycythemia. In Burg FD, Ingelfinger JR, Wald ER, Polin RA (eds): Current Pediatric Therapy, 16th ed. Philadelphia, W.B. Saunders, 1999, pp 318–320.
42. Rosenkrantz TS: Polycythemia. In Sunshine P, Stevenson DK (eds): Fetal and Neonatal Brain Injury: Mechanisms, Management, and the Risks of Practice, 2nd ed. New York, Oxford University Press, 1997, pp 532–538.

Hereditary Disorders of Coagulation
43. Coleman RW, Hirsh J, Marder V, Salzman EW (eds): Hemostasis and Thrombosis: Basic Principles and Clinical Practice, 3rd ed. Philadelphia, J.B. Lippincott, 1994.
44. Lane DA, Grant PJ: Role of hemostatic gene polymorphisms in venous and arterial thrombotic disease. Blood 95:1532, 2000.

Disseminated Intravascular Coagulation
45. Rivlin KA, Bussell JB: Thrombosis and hemostasis. In Spitzer AR (ed): Intensive Care of the Fetus and Newborn. St. Louis, Mosby, 1996, pp 1098–1111.

Congenital Thrombotic Disorders
46. Andrew M, deVeber G: Pediatric Thromboembolism and Stroke Protocols. Hamilton, Canada, B.C. Decker, 1999.
47. Monagle P, Andrew M, Halton J, et al: Homozygous protein C deficiency: Description of a new mutation and successful treatment with low-molecular-wight heparin. Thromb Haemostas 79:756-761, 1998.

Neoplasms
48. Link MP (ed): Pediatric Oncology. Pediatric Clinics of North America, vol. 44. Philadelphia, W.B. Saunders, 1997.
49. Pizzo PA, Poplack DG (eds): Principles and Practice of Pediatric Oncology, 3rd ed. Philadelphia, Lippincott-Raven, 1997.

11. INFECTION AND IMMUNITY

DEVELOPMENTAL IMMUNOLOGY

1. What is the maternal contribution of IgG to the fetus and newborn infant and how quickly does it disappear postnatally?

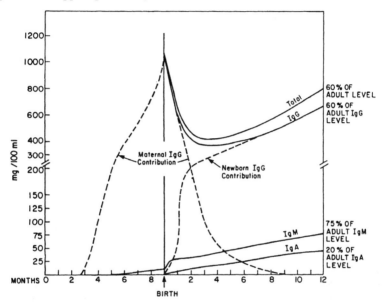

From Wilson CB, Lewis DB, Penix LA: The physiologic immunodeficiency of immaturity. In Stiehm ER (ed): Immunologic Disorders in Infants and Children, 4th ed. Philadelphia, W.B. Saunders, 1996, p 267, with permission.

The IgG of the fetus and newborn infant is entirely maternal in origin. Levels of all classes of IgG fall rapidly after birth, and the respective concentrations derived from the maternal placental transfer and active production by the young infant are approximately equal by 2 months postnatal age. By 10–12 months of age, catabolism of passively acquired IgG is complete, and all circulating IgG is infant in origin.

2. What are the principal types of IgA in the newborn infant?

Because IgA does not cross the placenta, all the IgA in neonatal serum and secretions is derived from the baby. The two principal types are IgA_1 and IgA_2. Some of their properties are summarized in the table.

	IgA_1	IgA_2
IgA Subunits	Monomer	Dimer
J-piece and secretory component	Absent	Present
Major site	Serum	Secretions
Presence at birth	Yes	No
Adult levels attained	16 yr–adult	6–8 yr

261

Despite the presence of circulating IgA_1 at birth, the respiratory and gastrointestinal (GI) tracts remain vulnerable to the entry of infectious organisms in the absence of secretory IgA_2.

3. What are the levels of serum complement at birth relative to the adult?

Complement components are synthesized as early as 6–14 weeks of gestation. However, levels of virtually all components of both the classic and alternative pathways are reduced at birth in both term and preterm newborn infants, with greater deficits noted in the latter.

Summary of Published Complement Levels in Neonates

COMPLEMENT COMPONENT	MEAN % OF ADULT LEVELS	
	TERM NEONATE (NO. OF STUDIES)	PRETERM NEONATE (NO. OF STUDIES)
CH_{50}	56–90 (4)	45–71 (3)
AP_{50}	49–65 (3)	40–51 (2)
C1q	65–90 (3)	27–58 (2)
C4	60–100 (4)	42–91 (3)
C2	76–100 (2)	96 (1)
C3	60–100 (5)	39–78 (4)
C5	75 (1)	—
C6	47 (1)	—
C7	67 (1)	—
C8	~ 20 (1)	
C9	< 20 (2)	—
B	35–59 (8)	36–50 (3)
P	33–71 (5)	13–65 (2)
H	61 (1)	—
C3bi	55 (1)	—

Data derived from Johnston RB, Stroud RM: Complement and host defense against infection. J Pediatr 90:169–179, 1977; Notarangelo LD, Chirico G, Chiara A, et al: Activity of classical and alternative pathways of complement in preterm and small for gestational age infants. Pediatr Res 18:281–285, 1984; David CA, Vallota EH, Forristal J: Serum complement levels in infancy: Age related changes. Pediatr Res 13:1043–1046, 1979; and Lassiter HA, Watson SW, Seifring ML, Tanner JE: Complement factor 9 deficiency in serum of human neonates. J Infect Dis 166:53–57, 1992. Adapted from Lewis DB, Wilson CB: Developmental immunology and role of host defenses in fetal and neonatal susceptibility to infection. In Remington JS, Klein JO (eds): Infectious Diseases of the Fetus and Newborn Infant, 4th ed. Philadelphia, W.B. Saunders, 2001, p 88.

Overall activity ad components of the alternative pathway are more consistently decreased than those of the classical pathway. This finding is especially problematic for neonates who are exposed to organisms with polysaccharide capsules such as *Escherichia coli* K1 and group B *Streptococcus* and cannot rely on classical pathway activation due to the lack of specific antibodies. In addition to differences in concentration, functional differences in C3 have also been described resulting in deficits of opsonization.

4. What phenomena are responsible for "depletion" or "exhaustion" neutropenia in the neonate?

The precursors of neutrophils, the colony-forming unit–granulocyte macrophage (CFU_{GM}), appear to proliferate at or near the maximal rate in neonates under baseline conditions. Consequently, these cells may not be able to increase their number in response to infection. In addition, the postmitotic storage pool in the bone marrow is small relative to the circulating pool in neonates (approximately 2–3:1) compared to adults (approximately 10–15:1).

As shown in the figure, the neutrophil storage pool compartment expands during development. Although the data in humans are not as precise, evidence suggests similar patterns with relatively small pools expanding into large ones with advancing age. Thus the small neonatal storage pools are rapidly released from the bone marrow in response to infection and cannot be

readily replaced by the early neutrophilic precursors that are already in a state of maximal proliferation. As a result, rather than develop neutrophilia as might occur in the adult, the neonate will
rapidly develop neutropenia due to "exhaustion" or "depletion" of his/her storage pools.

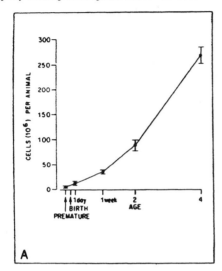
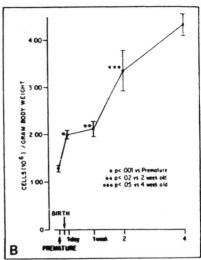

Neutrophil storage data in an animal model. (From Erdman SH, Christensen RD, Bradley PP, Rothstein G:
Supply and release of storage neutrophils: A developmental study. Biol Neonate 41:132–137, 1982, with
permission.)

5. When do thymocytes first appear during fetal life and what are their stages of development?

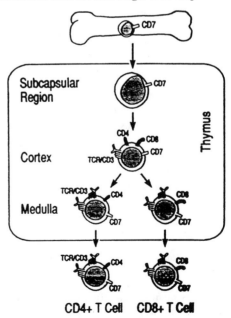

Cell Type	Major Developmental Events
Prothymocyte	Migration into thymus from bone marrow
Type I thymocyte	Proliferation, TCR gene rearrangement
Type II thymocyte	Selection of the αβ-TCR repertoire
Type III thymocyte	Emigration to periphery
Peripheral CD4+ and CD8+ T cells	

From Lewis DB, Wilson CB: Developmental immunology and role of host defenses in fetal and neonatal susceptibility to infection. In Remington JS, Klein JO (eds): Infectious Diseases of the Fetus and Newborn
Infant, 4th ed. Philadelphia, W.B. Saunders, 2001, p 38, with permission.

Prothymocytes bearing the CD7 and CD34 surface antigens enter the thymus at approximately 8.5 weeks' gestation. As the separation between the thymic cortex and medulla becomes apparent after 12 weeks, thymocytes localize according to their stage of maturation. Subcapsular thymocytes (type I) are negative for CD3, a molecule whose interaction with T-cell receptors is critical for the function of the latter, as well as negative for CD4 and CD8. Cortical thymocytes (type II) are positive for expression of CD3, CD4, and CD8. During this stage, the process of "positive" and "negative" selection occurs, resulting in selective survival of cells with specificities for a particular repertoire of antigens. Type III thymocytes located in the medulla are CD3-positive and express either CD4 *or* CD8. This latter cell type is the immediate precursor to the peripheral T lymphocyte.

6. When does cell-mediated immunity mature in the fetus?

By the 12th week of gestation, lymphocytes obtained from the human thymus respond to mitogens and foreign histocompatibility antigens. Furthermore, fetal cells stimulated with alloantigens exhibit normal antigen-specific cytotoxicity. In contrast, the phenotypic appearance and proportion of circulating cells are diminished, and the production of some cytokines is reduced in the neonate. The most significant defect appears to be a deficiency of memory T cells, which may be responsible for the deficient production of interferon-γ in the neonate.

7. How do neutrophils in the neonate differ functionally from the adult?

Despite the conflicting data in the literature, there is enough information to demonstrate that neonatal neutrophils are deficient in adherence, deformability, and chemotaxis. These properties would result in a relatively slow influx of neutrophils into sites of microbial invasions, resulting in rapidly progressive infections.

CHARACTERISTIC	NEONATE FUNCTION VS. ADULT
Neutrophils in circulation	↑
Neutrophil storage pool	↓
Adherence	↓
Adhesion content and regulation	Abnormal
Deformability	↓
Locomotion	
Random migration	Normal
Chemotaxis	↓
Binding of chemotactic factors	Normal
Signal transduction	Some elements abnormal
Phagocytosis	Normal
Degranulation	Normal
Lactoferrin content	↓
Bactericidal capacity	Normal (↓ during stress)
Respiratory burst	
O_2^-, H_2O_2	Normal or ↑
·OH, chemiluminescence	Normal or ↓

Note: some functions have not been studied thoroughly, and the biochemical basis for most defects is not understood.

Adapted from Speer CP, Johnson RB: Neutrophil function in newborn infants. In Polin RA, Fox WW (eds): Fetal and Neonatal Physiology, 2nd ed. Philadelphia, W.B. Saunders, 1998, p 1958.

8. Why do newborn infants respond poorly to polysaccharide vaccines or encapsulated bacteria such as group B streptococci?

The ability of the B lymphocytes to respond to specific antigens develops chronologically and in a manner that depends on whether the response requires T lymphocyte "help." In humans and in mice, the antigens can be divided into three groups based on the nature of the immune response: (1) thymus dependent (TD) antigens, which include most protein antigens, (2) thymus independent type 1 (TI-1) antigens, which bind directly to B lymphocytes and do not require T cells at all for antibody production, and (3) thymus independent type 2 (TI-2) antigens, which are mostly polysaccharides composed of multiple identical subunits and require small numbers of T lymphocytes for antibody production to occur. The response to TI-2 antigens appears last chronologically at approximately 6 months of age, accounting for the poor neonatal response to polysaccharide vaccines and to infection with encapsulated organisms such as group B streptococcus. Interestingly, although the *Haemophilus influenzae* type B PRP vaccine is poorly immunogenic in neonates, the coupling of *Haemophilus influenzae* polysaccharide to carrier proteins renders it immunogenic by converting it from a TI-2 antigen to a TD antigen, for which responsiveness is already present at birth.

9. Why are neonates particularly susceptible to infection with viruses such as herpes simplex?
The defenses against viral infections involve numerous mechanisms including antibody neutralization of extracellular virus, direct cytolysis of infected cells by natural killer (NK) cells, and antibody-dependent cellular cytotoxicity (ADCC) as well as specific cell-mediated cytotoxicity through T lymphocytes. The neonatal patient has deficits in virtually all of these components. Infants infected at the time of parturition depend on the presence of passively acquired maternal antibody, which will not be present in large quantity in mothers with primary infection, the setting in which the most severe neonatal infection occurs. Insofar as NK cells are concerned, they appear early in gestation and reach normal numbers by mid to late gestation. However, even at term, they are largely immature in phenotype, consisting of 50% CD56-negative cells. These cells are deficient in their ability to kill virus-infected cells and in the ability to produce critical cytokines such as interferon-γ. Furthermore, virus-specific T-cell–mediated immunity is also diminished or delayed in the human neonate with decreased T cell killing and production of interferon-γ. Consequently, infection with herpes simplex virus in the neonate can result in a rapidly progressive, fulminant, and often fatal infection.

10. In a young infant with prolonged retention of the umbilical cord and recurrent severe infections, what diagnosis should be considered?
Leukocyte adhesion deficiency (LAD) type I. This disorder is caused by a mutation in the CD18 gene, whose product is required for the expression of the β_2 integrins on the membranes of leukocytes. This group of surface molecules consists of MAC-1, leukocyte function-associated antigen 1 (LFA-1) and p 150,95, which are heterodimers of CD11a, CD11b, and CD11c, respectively, and CD18, and are essential to the ability of neutrophils to adhere to and migrate within sites of inflammation. As a result, patients with this disorder will demonstrate virtual absence of neutrophils in inflammatory exudates despite marked elevations of peripheral blood leukocyte counts. Patients with LAD type I are highly susceptible to life-threatening infections of the skin, mucous membranes, and GI tract with the degree of severity varying with the degree of expression of the β_2 integrins. For example, patients with moderately severe disease who express these molecules at 2.5–6.0% of normal values have been described. Delayed separation of the cord, which normally occurs on the average at 15.0 ± 7.2 (standard deviations [SD]) days, has been described in some of the most severe patients. Diagnosis can be made through use of specific immunophenotyping reagents to demonstrate the severe reduction in expression of the β_2 integrins.

EARLY ONSET NEONATAL SEPSIS: EPIDEMIOLOGY

11. How has the use of maternal intrapartum antibiotics altered the incidence of early onset neonatal sepsis?
Since consensus guidelines were developed in 1996, the incidence of early onset group B streptococcal (GBS) infections has declined by 65% overall with a 75% decline in black infants. During the same time period, however, intrapartum antibiotic administration has been associated with drug-resistant neonatal sepsis (particularly ampicillin).

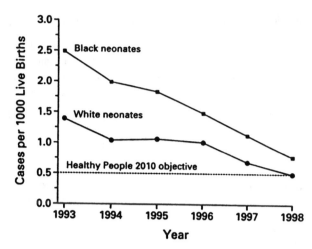

Incidence of early-onset invasive group B streptococcal disease in black neonates and white neonates in four active surveillance areas (California, Georgia, Tennessee, and Maryland), 1993 through 1998. The Healthy People 2010 objectives, released by the U.S. Department of Health and Human Services, constitute a national prevention strategy for substantially improving the health of people in the United States. Live births for 1998 were approximated on the basis of 1997 data. (From Schrag SJ, Phil D, Zywicki S, et al: Group B streptococcal disease in the era of intrapartum antibiotic prophylaxis. N Engl J Med 342:17, 2000, with permission.)

12. Which maternal and neonatal factors increase the infant's risk of early-onset disease?

Several obstetric and neonatal factors have been identified that may be associated with an increased risk of neonatal infection. The presence of any of these factors alone is not an indication for a complete sepsis workup and antibiotic therapy; however, combinations of risk factors are clearly additive and should greatly enhance the suspicion of sepsis.

Risk Factors for Perinatally Acquired Neonatal Bacterial Infection

MATERNAL	NEONATAL
Prolonged rupture of membranes > 18–24 hr	Prematurity
Premature rupture of membranes (< 37 wk)	Low birth weight (< 2500 g)
Maternal fever ≥ 100.4°F	Male gender
Intra-amniotic infection	5-minute Apgar < 6
Maternal colonization with GBS	Multiple gestation (?)
GBS bacteriuria	
Previous infant with invasive GBS disease	
Maternal urinary tract infection at delivery	

Adapted from Eichenwald EC: Perinatally transmitted neonatal bacterial infections. Inf Dis Clin North Am 11:226, 1997.

13. How does the epidemiology of early-onset sepsis differ in the very low birth weight (VLBW) infant (< 1500 g)?

Among VLBW infants, the incidence of early-onset sepsis increases with decreasing gestational age (19 cases/1000 live births vs. 2.5 cases/1000 live births in term infants). Whereas most VLBW infants become infected with microorganisms colonizing the maternal genital tract (e.g., *E. coli* or GSB), in rare circumstances early-onset infections can be caused by pathogens commonly associated with nosocomial sepsis (coagulase-negative staphylococci). These infections reflect the relative immaturity of the immune system in the VLBW infant and the need for invasive monitoring and procedures.

14. What is very-early-onset neonatal sepsis?

Whereas early-onset disease usually presents in the first few days of life with multisystem involvement, a third category of "very-early-onset" sepsis has been suggested. The major difference with early-onset disease is the age of onset, suggesting an in utero origin for very-early-onset infections. These infants are often symptomatic before birth with abnormalities of fetal heart rate. The onset of symptoms is within the first few hours after birth (see table).

Characteristics of Neonatal Bacteremia

CHARACTERISTICS	VERY EARLY ONSET	EARLY ONSET
Age of onset	< 12 hr	> 24 hr and < 3 days
Presence of maternal risk factors	Almost always	Frequently
Source of microorganisms	Maternal genital tract	Maternal genital tract
Clinical presentation	Fulminant multisystem involvement; pneumonia; shock	Wide spectrum: multisystem involvement to asymptomatic bacteremia
Mortality rate (%)	< 10	15–50

Adapted from Kaftan H, Kinney JS: Early onset neonatal bacterial infections. Semin Perinatol 22(1):17, 1998.

NOSOCOMIAL SEPSIS

15. What are nosocomial infections?

Nosocomial infections are hospital-acquired infections and, therefore, are potentially preventable by nursery infection control practices.

16. What percentage of VLBW infants develop a nosocomial infection?

Approximately 25% of VLBW infants will develop one or more episodes of blood culture–proven late-onset sepsis.

17. What are the most common nosocomial pathogens isolated from preterm VLBW infants?

In recent years, coagulase-negative staphylococci have emerged as the most frequently isolated pathogens responsible for late onset sepsis. Other pathogens associated with late-onset sepsis include *Staphylococcus aureus*, *Enterococcus*, *Klebsiella* species, *Enterobacter*, *Pseudomonas aeruginosa*, and fungi (especially *Candida albicans*).

18. What are the adverse consequences of late-onset neonatal infections among VLBW infants?

- Prolonged length of mechanical ventilation
- Prolonged need for parenteral nutrition (TPN), and need for indwelling catheters
- Prolonged length of hospitalization
- Increased cost of care
- Increased risk of death

19. What factors distinguish early-onset infections from late- and late, late-onset infections?

Characteristics of Early- and Later-Onset Infections

CHARACTERISTIC	EARLY-ONSET	LATE-ONSET	LATE, LATE-ONSET
Age at onset	Birth–7 days	7–30 days	> 30 days
Maternal OB complications	Common	Uncommon	Varies
Prematurity	Frequent	Varies	Usual, especially < 1000 g
Source of organism	Maternal genital tract	Maternal genital tract or environment	Environment/community
Clinical presentation	Multisystem	Multisystem or focal	Multisystem or focal
Mortality rate	10–20%	5–10%	< 5%

Adapted from Baker CJ: Group B streptococcal infections. Clin Perinatol 24:59–70, 1997.

20. What are the major risk factors for late-onset neonatal sepsis?

Risk Factors for Late-Onset Neonatal Sepsis

RISK FACTOR	COMMENTS
Prematurity/low birth weight	Risk of infection is inversely related to gestational age and birth weight.
Intravascular catheters	Intravascular catheters provide a portal of entry for infectious organisms, and risk of infection is directly related to number of catheter days.
Parenteral nutrition	TPN requires vascular access, which increases risk; intralipids enhance the growth of lipophilic organisms, particularly coagulase-negative staphylococci and malassezia fur fur.
Enteral nutrition	Human milk decreases and formula feeding increases risk.
Intubation/ventilation	Endotracheal intubation provides a portal of entry for colonization and infection with potential pathogens.
Invasive procedures	Provide portal of entry for organisms by breaking the skin and mucous membrane barriers.
Medications	Dexamethasone and H_2 blocker use increase risk of infection; widespread and prolonged use of broad-spectrum antibiotics may predispose to infections caused by resistant organisms and/or fungi.
Duration of hospitalization	Prolonged length of stay increases risk of exposure to hospital pathogens.
Overcrowding/understaffing	Increases the likelihood of poor infection control practices (especially poor handwashing), which increase the risk of infection.

DIAGNOSIS OF NEONATAL SEPSIS

21. What are the major risk factors for a neonate to develop perinatally acquired sepsis?

- Prolonged rupture of membranes (> 18 hours)
- Maternal fever
- Premature prolonged rupture of membranes
- Maternal colonization with GBS
- Maternal urinary tract infection (UTI) or GBS bacteriuria
- Sepsis in a sibling of a multiple birth
- Previous sibling with GBS sepsis
- Premature birth

22. What is the attack rate for neonatal sepsis if these sepsis risk factors are present?

As a general rule of thumb, presence of a major risk factor (such as premature rupture of fetal membranes [PROM] or maternal GBS colonization) leads to a sepsis attack rate of about 1% for proven sepsis or 2% for proven or highly suspected sepsis. If a second risk factor is present, the attack rate rises to 4–6% for proven and 10% for proven or highly suspected sepsis. Further risk factors are additive; the presence of three risk factors raises the sepsis risk 25-fold over baseline with no risk factors.

23. What is the significance of maternal fever (defined as $\geq 100.4°F$)?

If the fever is one of a constellation of symptoms for the diagnosis of chorioamnionitis (fever + 2 or more other abnormalities including fetal tachycardia, uterine tenderness, foul vaginal discharge, or maternal leukocytosis), there is a significant sepsis risk for the neonate, with reported attack rates ranging from 6% to 20%. However, if the fever is isolated, the sepsis attack rate is low. This issue is further compounded by the use of epidural anesthesia, which is associated with maternal fever without raising the neonatal sepsis rate. If the maternal fever is > 101°F, there is a risk of other adverse outcomes for the neonate, including seizures.

Lieberman E, Lang J, Richardson DK, et al: Intrapartum maternal fever and neonatal outcome. Pediatrics 105:8–13, 2000.

24. What are the possible presenting signs and symptoms of neonatal sepsis?

The signs and symptoms of neonatal sepsis are protean and nonspecific. Almost any symptom in the neonate may be an indication of sepsis, but there is extensive overlap with other conditions and with normal newborn transitional findings. The points to consider include respiratory distress, lethargy, hypotonia, "not looking well," grunting, vomiting, abdominal distention, unexplained jaundice, fever, hypothermia, hypoglycemia, apnea, seizures, shock, petechiae, and purpura.

25. With all of these possible signs of sepsis, how does one differentiate sepsis from other conditions, particularly after antibiotics have been started and decisions need to be made regarding duration of treatment?

Laboratory data are important in this regard, including cultures and sepsis screen strategies. With regard to what constitutes symptomatic sepsis, it is important to remember that sepsis usually presents with a constellation of signs and symptoms, the symptoms usually persist for more than 12 hours even when treated, and symptomatic sepsis can receive a low priority on the differential diagnosis if one makes a firm diagnosis of a noninfectious condition such as transient tachypnea of the newborn (TTN) or transitional hypoglycemia.

26. How reliable is the blood culture in the diagnosis of neonatal sepsis?

Unfortunately, the sensitivity of the blood culture is not very high in this condition. In patients with well-defined clinical GBS sepsis, only 50% may have positive blood cultures. In studies of neonates who died, the postmortem diagnosis of sepsis was confirmed by premortem blood cultures in only 80% of cases. The current extensive use of maternal antibiotic administration further confounds the reliability of the blood culture.

27. When should lumbar puncture (LP) be performed?

In retrospective studies, early-onset meningitis was detected in 1–2% of LPs performed. However, if there are no symptoms of meningitis and the sepsis evaluation is done for nonspecific reasons or for respiratory distress, the incidence of meningitis is either 0% or < 1%. On the other hand, Wiswell reported that 37% of cases of meningitis would be missed if one relied on symptoms or positive blood cultures and that at least 15% of proven meningitis occurs with a negative blood culture. Because neonatal meningitis is a low-incidence disease (0.25/1000 live births), an informal meta-analysis of published reports shows that one would need to do at least 1000 LPs to diagnose one case that would be missed by lack of symptoms or a negative blood culture.

One rational approach is to perform an LP if there are symptoms of meningitis *or* if sepsis is the leading diagnosis. One would not perform the LP if respiratory distress or nonspecific symptoms have led to a sepsis evaluation, but sepsis is a secondary consideration.

Wiswell TE, Baumgart S, Gannon CM, Spitzer AR: No lumbar puncture in the evaluation for early neonatal sepsis: Will meningitis be missed? Pediatrics 95:803–806, 1995.

28. Which characteristics of laboratory tests (sensitivity, specificity, positive predictive accuracy, and negative predictive accuracy) are most important for the diagnosis of neonatal sepsis?

The ideal laboratory test is one in which sensitivity, specificity, positive predictive accuracy, and negative predictive accuracy are all high. Unfortunately, no tests for sepsis fulfill that criterion. Specificity and positive predictive accuracy are less important because the treatment of neonatal sepsis is relatively benign and unlikely to result in serious medical consequences. Tests with a high negative predictive accuracy are particularly useful because the purpose of laboratory testing is to exclude "disease" in uninfected babies who do not require antibiotics or in whom antibiotics can be discontinued at the earliest possible time.

29. What is the relevance of C-reactive protein (CRP) in the diagnosis of neonatal sepsis?

Serum CRP is an acute phase reactant, which becomes elevated in the face of inflammation or infection, with a response time of 6–8 hours. The normal value in the neonate is < 1.0 mg/dl. An elevated CRP at 12–24 hours after onset of possible sepsis has a positive predictive value of only 7–43%, but a negative predictive value of 97–99.5%; thus, CRP is quite useful in ruling out sepsis. A marked elevation of CRP (> 5.0 mg/dl) has a positive predictive value for sepsis of 10%.

> Gerdes JS: Clinicopathologic approach to the diagnosis of neonatal sepsis. Perinatol 18:361–381, 1991.
>
> Benitz WE, Han MY, Madan A, Ramachandra P: Serial serum C-reactive protein levels in the diagnosis of neonatal infection. Pediatrics 102:E41, 1998.

30. Can a normal white blood cell (WBC) count, immature-to-total (I:T) neutrophil ratio, neutrophil count, or CRP be used to rule out sepsis on admission?

Unfortunately not. Neither these nor any other tests can be used to reliably rule out infection in the neonate. The usefulness of the tests improves markedly with serial measurements, because there have been many cases of sepsis described in which the WBC or CRP became abnormal 12–24 hours after the onset of the disease. Furthermore, these tests can be combined in a sepsis screen in which several parameters are used to improve the diagnostic accuracy.

31. What clinical factors affect neutrophil counts?

COMPLICATIONS	TOTAL NEUTROPHILS		TOTAL IMMATURE INCREASE	INCREASED I:T RATIO	APPROXIMATE DURATION
	DECREASE	INCREASE			
Maternal hypertension	++++	0	+	+	72 hr
Maternal fever, neonate healthy	0	++	+++	++++	24 hr
≥ 6 hr intrapartum oxytocin	0	++	++	++++	120 hr
Stressful labor	0	+++	++++	++++	24 hr
Asphyxia (5 min Apgar ≤ 5)	+	++	++	+++	24–60 hr
Meconium aspiration syndrome	0	++++	+++	++	72 hr
Pneumothorax with uncompli- cated hyaline membrane disease	0	++++	++++	++++	24 hr
Periventricular hemorrhage, no seizures	+++	+	++	++++	120 hr
Seizures—no hypoglycemia, asphyxia, or central nervous system hemorrhage	0	+++	+++	++++	24 hr
Prolonged (≥ 4 min) crying	0	++++	++++	++++	1 hr
Asymptomatic blood sugar ≤ 30	0	++	+++	+++	24 hr
Hemolytic disease	++	++	+++	++	7–28 days
Surgery	0	++++	++++	+++	24 hr
High altitude	0	++++	++++	0	6 hr

Adapted from Powell K, Marcy M: Laboratory aids in the diagnosis of neonatal sepsis. In Remington JS, Klein JO (eds): Infectious Diseases of the Fetus and Newborn Infant. Philadelphia, W.B. Saunders, 1995.

32. When evaluating an infant for possible sepsis, when is the best time to obtain a WBC count and differential count?

Counts obtained immediately after birth are frequently normal because there has not been sufficient time for inflammatory mediators to disturb neutrophil indices. Counts obtained 12–24 hours following birth are more likely to be abnormal in infants with sepsis. In the symptomatic infant (term or preterm), delaying the WBC for 12–24 hours should pose no problem because most symptomatic infants are treated with antibiotics empirically. In these infants, the main issue is whether antibiotics can be discontinued before a full course of treatment is given. In asymptomatic infants an "early" WBC or differential count should only be obtained if it will influence the decision to begin antibiotics.

33. What parameters are useful in creating a sepsis screen strategy?

A combination of diagnostic tests improves the predictive values over use of a single test. In this strategy, negative serial sepsis screens substantially reduce the likelihood that the infant has sepsis. One suggested sepsis screen is as follows:

TEST	POINT VALUE
Absolute neutrophil count < 1750/mm^3	1 point
Total WBC < 7500 or > 40,000/mm^3	1 point
I:T neutrophil ratio $\geq$ 0.2	1 point
I:T neutrophil ratio $\geq$ 0.4	2 points
CRP+ ($\geq$ 1.0 mg/dl)	1 point
CRP+ ($\geq$ 5.0 mg/dl)	2 points

The screen is considered positive if 2 or more points are present. It is important to recognize that no sepsis screen is perfect, and one should err on the side of caution with neonatal sepsis.

34. Are cytokine determinations helpful in the diagnosis of neonatal sepsis?

A number of inflammatory mediators are now being investigated as possible diagnostic tests for neonatal sepsis. Interleukin-6 (IL-6) has been studied extensively, and the following results have been observed.

- IL-6 is an early mediator of inflammation that is partly responsible for the increase in acute phase reactants.
- IL-6 is elevated in most infants with systemic infection (> 90% sensitivity)
- During the course of sepsis, levels of IL-6 fall quickly to normal.
- IL-6 is more likely than CRP to be elevated (especially when a sample is taken early in the course of sepsis).

Inflammatory mediators may, therefore, add to our information base when considering a diagnosis of sepsis.

ANTIMICROBIAL THERAPY

35. Ampicillin is used in conjunction with gentamicin as empiric therapy for early-onset sepsis. Why is ampicillin used?

Ampicillin is the antimicrobial of choice for treatment of GBS, *Listeria monocytogenes*, and most enterococci. Other beta-lactam antibiotics have acceptable activity against GBS, but only ampicillin provides good coverage for *Listeria* and enterococci.

36. Is cefotaxime an acceptable alternative to gentamicin?

The third-generation cephalosporins (such as cefotaxime and ceftazidime) have excellent activity against group B streptococci and gram-negative organisms. Some data, however, indicate that resistance of gram-negative organisms developed rapidly when cefotaxime was used for presumptive therapy. Therefore it is prudent to restrict their usage to infants with meningitis due to susceptible gram-negative organisms.

37. What are the theoretical advantages of third-generation cephalosporins?

- Low toxicity
- Measurement of serum levels is unnecessary

Note: cefotaxime is the third-generation cephalosporin of choice because it is not excreted in the bile and has been used extensively in neonates.

38. What are the advantages of once-a-day gentamicin dosing for all neonates?

- Higher peak concentrations may enhance bacterial killing.

- There is a postantibiotic effect especially when used in conjunction with a beta-lactam antibiotic.
- There may be less nephrotoxicity.

39. Is once-daily dosing of gentamicin appropriate for all neonates?

No. Certain groups of infants require dosing intervals more often than every 24 hours including
   Infants > 38 weeks
   Asphyxiated infants
   Infants with patent ductus arteriosus (PDA)
   Infants receiving indomethacin
Suggested doses and dosing intervals are shown in the table.

GESTATIONAL AGE (weeks)	DOSE (mg/kg/dose)	INTERVAL (hours)
≤ 29*	5	48
30–33	4.5	48
34–37	4	36
≥ 38	4	24

* or significant asphyxia, or significant PDA, or treatment with indomethacin.
Adapted from Young TE, Magnum B (eds): Neofax, 13th ed. Battle Creek, MI, Acorn Publishing, 2000.

40. Why shouldn't ceftriaxone be used in neonates?

Ceftriaxone can displace bilirubin from albumin and may increase the risk of kernicterus in a jaundiced infant.

41. How long should proven bacterial sepsis be treated?

There are as many answers to this question as there are neonatologists in the world. The following are commonly accepted guidelines:
   Bacterial sepsis with minimal or absent focal infection: 7–10 days
   Meningitis: 21 days

42. What is acceptable empiric therapy for late-onset sepsis?

Because *Staphylococcus epidermidis* is the most common cause of nosocomial sepsis in neonates, empiric therapy should include vancomycin. This antibiotic is generally paired with an aminoglycoside antibiotic to cover gram-negative organisms.

43. The laboratory calls you with peak and trough gentamicin serum concentrations of 10 μg/ml and 4 μg/ml, respectively. What adjustments should you make in dosing?

The trough level is elevated. Trough levels are determined to assess the potential for nephrotoxicity and ototoxicity. The dosing interval should be lengthened. This can be done empirically or can be accomplished by measuring serial trough levels until the serum concentration is within an acceptable range. That interval can then be used to administer subsequent doses.

44. What are the major adverse reactions to antimicrobials commonly used in neonates?

ANTIBIOTIC	ADVERSE EFFECTS
Ampicillin	Rare hypersensitivity reactions*
Amphotericin B	Hypokalemia Reversible nephrotoxicity due to reduced glomerular filtration rate
Acyclovir	Reversible renal dysfunction secondary to the formation of acyclovir crystals in renal tubules[†]
Cefotaxime	Rare, occasional leukopenia

(Table continued on next page.)

ANTIBIOTIC	ADVERSE EFFECTS
Ceftriaxone	Displaces bilirubin from albumin, resulting in higher bilirubin concentrations Gallbladder sludging
Gentamicin	Irreversible ototoxicity and reversible nephrotoxicity
Vancomycin	Rare, nephrotoxicity, enhanced by combination with an aminoglycoside. Red man syndrome (rash and hypotension)[‡]

[*] Hypersensitivity reactions are not commonly seen in the neonatal period.
[†] Adequate hydration helps to prevent this complication.
[‡] Appears rapidly and resolves within minutes and hours. Lengthening infusion time usually eliminates risk for subsequent doses.

GROUP B STREPTOCOCCAL INFECTIONS

45. Early-onset GBS disease is a consequence of maternal GBS colonization. Are there other adverse outcomes of pregnancy associated with maternal GBS colonization?

Higher titer colonization is associated with:

Early fetal loss	Low birth weight
Premature rupture of membranes	Maternal sepsis
Preterm labor	Maternal chorioamnionitis

46. Are special methods needed to isolate group B streptococci?

The majority of studies using selective broth media containing antibiotics (e.g., nalidixic acid, gentamicin, colistin) demonstrate at least a twofold yield of positive cultures from genital and rectal sites of adults in comparison to nonselective methods. This is because of the suppression of overgrowth by co-colonizing bacteria.

On the other hand, standard laboratory methods for isolation of GBS from blood and spinal fluid are fully adequate. In addition, nonselective (standard trypticase-soy agar [TSA] blood agar plates) media give higher yield of positive surface cultures of newborns during the first 24–48 hours of life (because the antibiotics in selective media are slightly inhibitory to GBS and most GBS surface isolates are pure cultures in the first 2 days of life).

47. Is GBS sexually transmissible?

Yes. Several studies in the 1970s demonstrated increased efficacy in antepartum treatment to eradicate GBS colonization by concurrent treatment of sexual partners of colonized women, supporting the speculation that these organisms can be sexually transmitted. A definitive study from Japan published in 1999 demonstrated sexual transmission and reinfection during pregnancy in longitudinal studies of couples with 92% serotype concurrence among infected couples.

Although it is apparent that GBS is sexually transmissible, epidemiologic data for GBS colonization are significantly different from those of classic sexually transmissible diseases (STDs), such as gonorrhea and *Chlamydia trachomatis*. GBS colonization is most common in women of higher age, lower parity, and limited sexual activity based on number of sexual partners/lifetime, and age at onset of sexual activity.

48. How many serotypes of GBS have been identified? What is the clinical and immunologic significance of the serotypes?

Seven serotypes have been identified: Ia, II, III, IV, V, VI, and VIII. Early studies of GBS disease in North America demonstrated a predominance of type III, thought also to be the most virulent serotype. It remains the most commonly isolated serotype to cause meningitis in this country. Since the 1970s there has been a progressive change in predominance of serotypes with Ia now the leading cause of early-onset infection. During the last decade, several new serotypes have been identified.

Serotype V, initially isolated from nonpregnant HIV-positive adults in the U.S., has become a common colonizing serotype among healthy pregnant women.

Serotype IV is more commonly isolated in Europe, and serotypes VI and VIII predominate in Asia.

From an immunologic and public health perspective, the recognition of multiple new serotypes has confounded the efforts of investigators to develop an effective multivalent vaccine to prevent this disease in newborns.

49. What are the major distinguishing characteristics of early- and late-onset GBS disease?

	EARLY-ONSET DISEASE	LATE-ONSET DISEASE
Age at onset*	First 7 days of life	Beyond day 7
Symptoms	Respiratory distress, apnea, PPHN, hypotension	Irritability, fever, poor feeding
Serotypes	All	All
Mode of transmission	Vertical transmission from mother to infant	Nosocomial acquisition
CDC IAP†	50–65% reduction in attack rate	No effect

* Ages at onset were once (classically) defined as early onset occurring during the first 5 days of life and late onset occurring beyond day 10. Recent surveillance studies have redefined early onset as < day 7 and late onset as > day 7.

† Centers for Disease Control and Prevention (CDC) recommendations for intrapartum antibiotic prophylaxis (IAP) to prevent GBS disease.

50. What are the CDC recommendations for IAP to prevent early-onset GBS disease?

The 1996 CDC consensus strategies recommended use of an antepartum screening strategy *or* a risk factor–based strategy on which to formulate intrapartum treatment guidelines.

Antepartum screening strategy. Originally, antepartum screening at 22–23 weeks and 35–37 weeks using a combined vaginal-rectal swab processed in selective media was advocated as the screening strategy. Most recent revisions of the screening strategy recommend screening only at 35–37 weeks. Antepartum treatment was not recommended. At the time of admission for delivery, antibiotic treatment should be given during labor if the mother:

- Is colonized with group B streptococcus and has one or more of the risk factors listed below *or*
- Chooses to have IAP in the absence of risk factors

Risk factor–based strategy. Patients presenting for delivery with any of the risk factors listed below will be treated in labor:

- Delivery prior to 37 weeks
- Membrane rupture prior to 37 weeks
- Duration of membrane rupture > 18 hours
- Maternal temperature in labor > 100.4°F
- History of a sibling with early-onset GBS disease
- Urine culture positive for GBS during this pregnancy

Intrapartum management of parturients. Patients identified by either of the above strategies will be treated with antibiotics:

- Penicillin G, 5 million units loading IV, followed by 2.5 million units every 4 hours until delivery *or*
- Ampicillin, 2 g IV loading dose, followed by 1 g every 4 hours until deliver

In cases of penicillin allergies:

- Clindamycin, 900 mg IV, every 8 hours until delivery *or*
- Erythromycin, 500 g IV, every 6 hours until delivery

51. What are the pros and cons of intrapartum antibiotic prophylaxis?

Pro: IAP has resulted in a dramatic reduction in incidence of early-onset disease. The figure illustrates the decline in incidence of early-onset GBS disease over the past decade as IAP programs were implemented. The graph is based on composite data from CDC surveillance centers, a National Institute of Child Health and Development (NICHD) multicenter study reviewing disease rates from 1992 to 1997, and ongoing surveillance at the author's center. The incidences of disease from 1990 to 1993 represent the pre-IAP era, whereas data from 1993 to 1996 followed the American College of Obstetrics and Gynecology (ACOG) and American Academy of Pediatrics (AAP) recommendations published in 1993. The third data set reflects the impact of the CDC recommendations published in 1996.

Cons:
- Risk of maternal anaphylaxis
- IAP not 100% effective; 25% of infants with positive blood cultures are born to treated mothers
- Risk factor–based strategy identifies only maximum of 75% of affected infants' mothers
- Screening-based strategy identifies only maximum of 85–90% of affected infants' mothers
- Emergence of infections in mothers and infants by resistant organisms (e.g., *E. coli*, *Enterococcus* species)
- Increasing resistance of GBS to clindamycin and erythromycin
- Does not address other adverse outcomes of pregnancy, e.g., early fetal loss, preterm labor, PROM

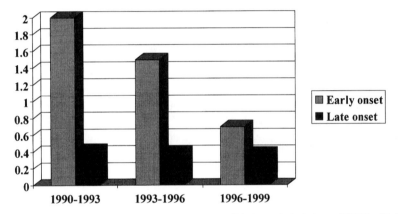

Group B streptococcal disease in the era of intrapartum antibiotic prophylaxis (cases/1000 live births).

52. What is the natural history of nosocomial acquisition of GBS in late-onset disease?

The majority of infants who present with late-onset disease acquire the organism outside the hospital. These infants' mothers have no history of genital colonization with GBS during pregnancy. The most common group of infants who develop late-onset disease comprises VLBW infants who acquire colonization during prolonged neonatal intensive care unit (NICU) hospitalizations.

53. How does late-onset disease due to GBS presenting as cellulitis differ from the majority of cases of late-onset sepsis?

Late-onset sepsis associated with cellulitis may be due to transient bacteremia during delivery with later presentation of infection. Other distinguishing characteristics include:

Male infant predominance	Overrepresentation of preterm infants
Serotype III predominance	Maternal history of colonization
History of earlier treatment with antibiotics	during pregnancy

54. How does osteomyelitis due to GBS differ in presentation compared with neonatal osteomyelitis due to other organism in the newborn period (usually *Staphylococcus aureus*)?

- Indolent onset
- Better prognosis

- Presenting symptoms: decreased movement and pain with manipulation; swelling and erythema rare
- Site is proximal humerus in 55% of cases
- Single bone involvement

STAPHYLOCOCCUS EPIDERMIDIS

55. Should vancomycin prophylaxis be used to prevent neonatal nosocomial coagulase-negative *Staphylococcus* (CONS) sepsis?

The answer is controversial. Selective use of vancomycin may prevent CONS bacteremia, but the risks of usage are high. Risks include emergence of fungal or gram-negative infections in vancomycin-treated infants and the more general problem of emergence of vancomycin-resistant strains of CONS or enterococci in NICUs as a whole. Because coagulase-negative staphylococci are generally organisms of low virulence, one wonders about the risk/benefit ratio of such prevention strategies.

56. What are the risk factors for bloodstream infections with coagulase-negative staphylococci?

Prematurity
Central venous catheters
Lipid emulsions
Mechanical ventilation

57. Does the I:T neutrophil ratio predict neonatal CONS infection?

The I:T neutrophil ratio is sensitive for the detection of nosocomial infection in infants. However, I:T neutrophil ratios may be normal in the presence of CONS disease, perhaps because of the relative avirulence of this organism.

58. Name the focal complications of persistent bacteremia with CONS.

Infective endocarditis
Necrotizing enterocolitis (NEC)
Pneumonia
Meningitis

59. What is the recommended therapy for CONS infection?

The initial recommended therapy is vancomycin, which may be modified if the organism is sensitive to oxacillin and an aminoglycoside. In cases of persistent bacteremia, a combination of vancomycin and rifampin may be the best therapeutic regimen. In cases of an infected indwelling catheter, antibiotic therapy through the catheter is mandatory, and removal of the catheter may be necessary if the culture remains positive. The same is true for meningitis secondary to an infected cerebrospinal fluid (CSF) shunt.

CANDIDA

60. What are the most important risk factors for neonatal systemic candidiasis?

Several predisposing factors for systemic candidiasis have been identified:
- Long-term use of broad-spectrum antibiotics suppresses normal GI flora and allows candidal overgrowth.
- Prematurity and host immunosuppression are associated with abnormal skin barriers, humoral and cellular immune deficits, neutrophil dysfunction, and complement deficiencies.
- Central intravenous catheterization and parenteral hyperalimentation allow a portal of entry for the organism into the bloodstream.
- Prolonged steroid use may impair neutrophil function.

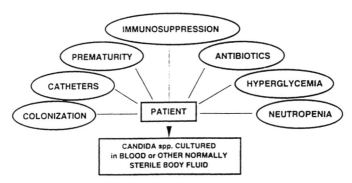

Risk factors for infection with *Candida* species. (From Hostetter MK: Infections with *Candida* species. In Long SS, Pickering LK, Prober CG (eds): Principles and Practice of Pediatric Infectious Diseases. New York, Churchill Livingstone, 1997, with permission.)

61. Describe the spectrum of candidal disease in neonates.

Vertical transmission of *C. albicans* occurs in approximately 10% of term and 30% of preterm infants. Most commonly, acquisition leads to neonatal thrush or a perineal diaper rash with little associated morbidity. The more serious illnesses associated with candida are shown in the table. Early-onset candidal disease, or **congenital candidiasis**, arises following exposure of the infant to organisms colonizing the maternal genital tract. Cutaneous findings are the hallmark of the disease, but the association with pulmonary disease conveys a grave prognosis despite systemic antifungal therapy. **Catheter-associated fungemia** generally arises from organisms within the GI tract. Affected infants have resolution of fungemia with prompt removal of the catheter and parenteral amphotericin therapy for 10–14 days. In contrast, infants with **disseminated candidiasis** have involvement of distant organs, including heart, kidney, bone, eyes, lungs, and meninges. Long-term therapy is recommended, and prognosis is guarded in these cases.

CLINICAL FEATURES	CONGENITAL CANDIDIASIS	CATHETER-RELATED FUNGEMIA	SYSTEMIC CANDIDIASIS
Age at onset	Birth	> 7 days	> 7 days
Risk factors	None	Necessary	Necessary
Skin involvement	Hallmark	None	None
Respiratory involvement	Occasionally	Never	Frequent
Positive blood culture	No	Yes	Yes
Multiorgan involvement	Never	Rare	Frequent
Treatment	Topical antifungals*	Catheter removal *and* parenteral amphotericin B	Parenteral amphotericin B
Prognosis	Excellent	Good	Fair-poor

* Death may occur in premature infants with pulmonary involvement, and parenteral amphotericin B should be used in these infants.
Adapted from Bendel CM, Hostetter MK: Semin Pediatr Infect Dis 5:34–41, 1994.

62. Has late-onset candidal disease been described?

Recently, the recurrence of candidal disease has been described in 4 immunocompetent infants following a prolonged period of latency (up to 1 year). All of the infants presented with candidal arthritis and osteomyelitis, were born prematurely, had received parenteral nutrition through indwelling catheters, and had a history of systemic candidiasis during the newborn period. The pathogenesis of these latent infections is unknown.

Harris MC, Pereira GR, Myers MD, et al: Candidal arthritis in infants previously treated for systemic candidiasis during the newborn period. Pediatr Emerg Care 16:249–251, 2000.

63. Is there an association between *Candida* sepsis and retinopathy of prematurity (ROP)?

One study has suggested an association between *Candida* sepsis and ROP in extremely low birth weight (ELBW) infants. The study found increased severity of ROP and need for laser therapy following candidal infection. Although the mechanism is unknown, endothelial injury by the organism, elaboration of proinflammatory cytokines, and production of angiogenic substances may be involved.

Mittal M, Dhannireddy R, Higgins RD: Candida sepsis and association with retinopathy of prematurity. Pediatrics 101:654–657, 1998.

64. How can systemic candidal disease be prevented?

Attempts to prevent candidal disease have not been very successful given the increased survival of VLBW premature infants requiring complex medical therapies. Limitation of the use of broad-spectrum antibiotics may prevent fungal colonization of the GI tract in susceptible neonates. Alternatively, early introduction of enteral feedings may lessen the duration of parenteral nutrition and need for intravenous catheters. The efficacy of prophylactic antifungal therapies in preventing disseminated candidiasis in high-risk patients has not been demonstrated.

65. What is the recommended treatment of neonatal systemic candidal infection?

There is currently no consensus regarding the best approach to the treatment of systemic candidal infections in neonates, because large, controlled studies of treatment strategies have not yet been performed. Amphotericin B remains the mainstay of therapy. It is a polyene macrolide antibiotic, which binds to the fungal cell membrane, causing leakage of cellular contents and cell death. The dose is 1 mg/kg/day administered for 14 days (catheter associated fungemia: total dose 10–15 mg/kg) to 6 weeks (disseminated disease: total dose 25–30 mg/kg), depending on disease severity and site. Although side effects include nephrotoxicity, hypokalemia, hepatotoxicity, and bone marrow suppression, the drug appears to be well tolerated in neonates.

Amphotericin B lipid complex, which is incorporated into unilamellar liposomes, was developed to eliminate the severe adverse effects of conventional amphotericin with good CNS penetration. To date, randomized, clinical trials have not been performed to compare its efficacy to that of conventional amphotericin B, but several smaller studies have shown safety. 5-Flucytosine is a nucleoside analogue that inhibits DNA replication in candida. It may be used as adjunctive synergistic therapy for candidal meningitis or persistent fungemia because amphotericin B penetrates the spinal fluid poorly. Others have recommended combination therapy for all patients as optimal therapy. Fluconazole, another alternative agent, binds to fungal cytochrome P450 and affects fungal membrane integrity. There have been no controlled trials of this agent in neonatal candidiasis, so it is not recommended as first-line therapy in neonates. An additional therapeutic concern is the emergence of relative resistance of non-albicans species to conventional treatment with amphotericin B, necessitating susceptibility testing in cases refractory to therapy.

WHITE CELL FUNCTIONAL DISORDERS

66. What factors diminish the capacity of neutrophils derived from preterm infants to kill bacterial pathogens?

Respiratory distress syndrome and sepsis decrease bactericidal activity of neutrophils isolated from preterm infants. A low neutrophil-to-bacterial ratio (1:100) is also associated with decreased bacterial killing. Certain bacterial strains (*E. coli*, *S. aureus*, and group B streptococcus) are more readily killed by neutrophils isolated from well term neonates and adult subjects than those from preterm infants.

67. What neutrophil defect causes chronic granulomatous disease?

Dysfunction of the neutrophil cell membrane reduced nicotinamide adenine dinucleotide phosphate (NADPH) oxidase results in inadequate generation of superoxide anion and other reactive oxygen intermediates. Deficiency of these reactive oxygen intermediates results in poor bactericidal activity and recurrent infections. Treatment includes prophylactic antibiotics, aggressive antibiotic treatment of infections, steroids, and interferon-γ. Bone marrow transplantation has been successful.

68. What is the most common neutrophil defect observed in neonates treated with high doses of glucocorticoids?

The anti-inflammatory effects of glucocorticoids primarily affect granulocyte trafficking. Neutrophils demonstrate diminished adhesion to vascular endothelium. This may be due in part to diminished endothelial and leukocyte expression of adhesion molecules as a result of decreased macrophage production of proinflammatory mediators (cytokines, arachidonic acid metabolites, and platelet activating factor).

69. Which of the following components of neonatal host defense constitutes the primary barrier to invasive infections?
A. **Neutrophils**
B. **Macrophages**
C. **Skin and mucous membranes**
D. **Natural killer (NK) cells**

Skin and mucous membranes are the primary defense against invading microbes. Neutrophils, macrophages, and NK cells attempt to eradicate those organisms that manage to bypass the primary defense barrier. The high incidence of nosocomial infections in preterm neonates may not be effectively diminished until new strategies that augment skin and mucous membrane defense mechanisms are discovered.

IMMUNOTHERAPY

70. What nutrient is believed to decrease the risk of nosocomial sepsis in the very low birth weight infant?

In a randomized, double-blind study (n = 68 subjects), enteral **glutamine** supplementation during the first 30 days of life in infants born at 24–32 weeks improved tolerance to oral feedings and decreased the incidence of hospital-acquired sepsis.

Neu J, Roig JC, Meetze WH, et al: Enteral glutamine supplementation for very low birth weight infants decreases morbidity. J Pediatr 131:691–699, 1997.

71. What are the clinically beneficial effects of pentoxifylline administration to premature infants with culture-proven sepsis?

Pentoxifylline has been shown to inhibit cytokine production. In a randomized, double-blind, placebo-controlled study, intravenous administration of 5 mg/kg/day of pentoxifylline to premature (n = 78 patients) infants with culture-proven sepsis resulted in a significant decrease in mortality, metabolic acidosis, oliguria/anuria, disseminated intravascular coagulation (DIC), hypotension, and NEC. Pentoxifylline (a methyl xanthine) has principally been used in Europe. At this time its use should be considered experimental.

Lauterbach R, Pawlik D, Kowalczyk D, et al: Effect of the immunomodulating agent, pentoxifylline, in the treatment of sepsis in prematurely delivered infants: A placebo-controlled, double-blind trial. Crit Care Med 27:807–814, 1999.

72. What is the single most important determinant of efficacy when treating septic neonates with granulocyte transfusions?

The primary determinant of efficacy is the dose of granulocytes transfused. Infusion of $> 0.5 \times 10^9$ cells/kg to septic neonates produced an 18-fold increase in the odds of survival. However, this survival benefit did not reach statistical significance when a meta-analysis of published studies was restricted to the results of randomized, controlled trials because of the limited number of patients enrolled. Therefore, white cell transfusions to augment the host defense of septic neonates remain experimental.

73. In what clinical setting does administration of intravenous immunoglobulin (IVIG) appear to be beneficial in augmenting neonatal host defense?

IVIG has minimal benefit in prophylaxis of late-onset sepsis in neonates. However, in septic neonates, IVIG administration confers at least a six-fold decrease in mortality rate according to the authors of a recent meta-analysis of all the relevant published studies.

Jensen HB, Pollock BH: The role of intravenous immunoglobulin for the prevention and treatment of neonatal sepsis. Semin Perinatol 22:6–13, 1998.

74. Which of the following statements is correct with regard to growth factor immunotherapy?
   A. Prophylactic administration of granulocyte-macrophage colony-stimulating factor (GM-CSF) has been reported to prevent early-onset neonatal sepsis and is recommended for preterm infants.
   B. Intrapartum administration of granulocyte colony-stimulating factor (G-CSF) to women in preterm labor results in an increase in the circulating absolute neutrophil count in exposed newborn infants.
   C. When studied in a randomized, placebo-controlled fashion, G-CSF administration to newborn infants with neutropenia and clinical signs of sepsis failed to increase circulating absolute neutrophil counts or ameliorate severity of illness, morbidity, or mortality.

C. Although GM-CSF prophylaxis has been reported to abolish neutropenia in most well and sick premature infants, significant benefit in preventing sepsis (early or late onset) has not yet been reported because of limited numbers of enrolled patients in randomized, controlled trials. Intravenous intrapartum G-CSF administration results in an increase in the absolute neutrophil count of the treated mothers but not in their infants.

NEONATAL MENINGITIS

75. What are the normal values for cells, protein, and glucose in the CSF of healthy term and preterm infants?

	WBC	PMN	PROTEIN	GLUCOSE
Term	7* ± 13	0.8* ± 6.2	64* ± 24	51* ± 13
	4[†]	0[†]		
Preterm (< 1000 g)	4* ± 3	6 ± 15%	160 ± 56	61 ± 34
	6[†]			

WBC = white blood cell; PMN = polymorphonuclear neutrophil
* mean ± standard deviation; [†] median
Term infant data from Ahmed A, Hickey SM, Ehrett S, et al: Cerebrospinal fluid values in the term infant. Pediatr Infect Dis J 15:298–303, 1996. Preterm infant data from Rodriguez AF, Kaplan SL, Mason EO: Cerebrospinal fluid values in the very low birth weight infant. J Pediatr 116:971–974, 1990.

76. Should a lumbar puncture be done on an asymptomatic infant who is born to a mother with risk factors for infection?

The answer to this question is controversial. Meningitis occurs in 10–20% of neonates with positive blood cultures. With increased use of intrapartum antibiotics, a postnatal blood culture is no longer a reliable way to determine if an infant was bacteremic. In a retrospective study by Wiswell et al. of infants with proven meningitis (n = 43), there were 7 infants with meningitis who were totally asymptomatic (i.e., they had no signs or symptoms consistent with meningitis). Four of these 7 infants also had a negative blood culture. However, in other recent retrospective studies of infants who were being evaluated for possible sepsis, meningitis only occurred in infants who were symptomatic. Therefore, in an asymptomatic "high-risk" infant, it seems appropriate to do a lumbar puncture only in situations where laboratory testing or history strongly suggests the infant is bacteremic. All other babies should be closely observed.

Wiswell TE, et al: No lumbar puncture in the evaluation for early neonatal sepsis: Will meningitis be missed? Pediatrics 95:803–806, 1995.

77. What are the mechanisms of brain injury in meningitis?
- Vascular infarcts (vasospasm/thrombosis)
- Reactive oxygen species
- Excitotoxic amino acids
- Alterations in cerebral blood flow

78. What factors influence antibiotic concentrations in CSF?

VARIABLE	EFFECT ON CNS PENETRATION	EXAMPLE
High degree of protein binding	Reduced	Ceftriaxone
Lipid solubility	Enhanced	Rifampin
High degree of ionization	Reduced	Beta lactams
Active transport system	Enhanced	Penicillin
Meningeal inflammation	Enhanced*	Beta lactams, vancomycin

* Meningeal inflammation only influences penetration of hydrophilic antibiotics.

79. What are the recommendations for initial empiric therapy of meningitis in the neonate?
- A regimen of ampicillin and cefotaxime or a combination of a penicillin (e.g., ampicillin) and an aminoglycoside is recommended for initial empiric therapy.
- Ceftazidime is probably as efficacious as cefotaxime, but should be reserved for *P. aeruginosa* infections.

80. How should gram-positive and gram-negative meningitis be treated during the neonatal period?

Treatment of meningitis caused by enteric organisms. There are no data demonstrating the superiority of cefotaxime or ceftriaxone over ampicillin plus an aminoglycoside. However, for gram-negative meningitis, cefotaxime is preferred and is often paired with an aminoglycoside. Gram-negative meningitis should be treated for at least 3 weeks.

Treatment of meningitis due to gram-positive organisms. Because there is synergism between ampicillin and aminoglycosides for most GBS, *Listeria monocytogenes*, and enterococci, combination therapy is recommended until the CSF is sterilized. If the GBS disease is shown to be tolerant to ampicillin (MBC/MIC $\geq$ 30/1), combination therapy should be used for the duration of treatment (~ 14 days).

81. Are cytokine determinations of CSF helpful in deciding whether an infant has aseptic or bacterial meningitis?
- Both proinflammatory cytokines (tumor necrosing factor-α [TNF-α], IL-1, and IL-6) and anti-inflammatory cytokines (IL-10, IL-ra, tumor growth factor-β [TGF-β]) are found in the CSF of children with meningitis.
- CXC and CC chemokines are found in both bacterial and aseptic meningitis.
- High levels of TNF-α, Il-1, and IL-8 are found in bacterial meningitis (sensitivity ~ 80%; specificity ~ 95%).
- At this time, it is not clear that cytokine determinations are superior to standard ways of differentiating bacterial from aseptic meningitis (e.g., CSF count, differential count, protein, and glucose).

INFECTION CONTROL

82. What is the difference between incidence rate and prevalence rate?

Incidence rate is the ratio of the number of new occurrences of a disease in a given period to the number of persons at risk (e.g., number of cases of bacteremia per 1000 catheter-days). Prevalence rate is the ratio of persons with a disease entity in a defined population at a specific time without regard to when the disease began.

83. What is the difference between endemic and epidemic nosocomial infections?

Sporadic (endemic) infections represent the bulk of nosocomial infections and are the usual level of infection expected during a given period for a given population. Epidemic infections are marked by an unusual increase in the incidence of disease entity. A knowledge of the endemic levels of a disease is needed to make this assessment.

84. Which kinds of patients need to be isolated in negative-pressure rooms?

Patients **suspected** of having tuberculosis, chickenpox, or measles need to be placed on respiratory isolation in negative-pressure rooms to prevent aerosol spread of their infection. It is important to assess the family members of such patients for infection or immune status as well.

85. A nurse tells you that she has just been exposed to chickenpox and she never had it as a child. What do you tell her about the period of isolation?

Patients (or nonimmune staff or visitors) need to be isolated from day 10 to day 21 after documented exposure to a person with active varicella zoster virus infection. If a patient has received varicella zoster immune globulin (VZIG), the incubation period is extended to 28 days.

86. What is contact isolation?

Contact isolation is a category of isolation for infectious entities that can be spread through direct contact with infectious secretions or fomites contaminated with infectious secretions. Patients on contact isolation should be placed in a single room (when available), and health care workers should wash hands upon entering and leaving the room and wear gowns and gloves for contact with the patient or the patient's environment.

87. Which diseases require contact isolation?

Clostridium difficile	Croup
Rotavirus	Herpes simplex
Respiratory syncytial virus	

88. What are droplet precautions?

Droplet precautions are used to prevent transmission of diseases that are spread through large, aerosolized droplets containing infectious particles. Such particles are spread through sneezing and coughing and rapidly settle on horizontal surfaces within a few feet of the source patient. Examples include adenovirus, *Parvovirus*, rubella, and meningitis caused by *Haemophilus influenzae* or *Neisseria meningitidis*.

89. What is the best way to determine if patient-to-patient transmission of a pathogen has occurred?

This possibility should be investigated in two ways:

1. Epidemiologic investigation to determine if there is a known epidemiologic link between the patients (e.g., sharing a hospital room or common health care workers).

2. Further confirmation by molecular epidemiology (analysis of the DNA of the bacteria or fungus) to assess clonality of the patient's organisms.

90. What are the most frequently cited reasons that nursery personnel do not wash their hands?

- Handwashing takes too much time
- Lack of soap (54%) and lack of towels (65%)
- One thorough wash/day is sufficient (26%)
- Gloves can substitute for handwashing (25%—including 50% of physicians)
- Handwashing is not important if an infant is receiving antibiotics (10%)

Wharton KN, Karlowicz MG: Barriers to full compliance with handwashing in a neonatal intensive care unit. Pediatr Res 43:254A, 1998.

91. What are the current recommendations for perinatal care handwashing?
- Removal of all rings; no nail polish or false nails
- Initial 3-minute scrub to the elbow
- A 10-second scrub before and after handling each infant

92. Do careful handwashing practices reduce the incidence of nosocomial infection?
Six of seven hospital-based studies (including two in NICUs) have demonstrated that improved handwashing techniques will reduce infection rates.

Larson E: Skin hygiene and infection prevention: More of the same or different approaches? Clin Infect Dis 29:1287–1294, 1999.

93. Is washing with soap and water an effective way to "de-germ" hands?
Handwashing with soap and water does not reliably prevent microbial transmission and may actually increase it by dispersing bacterial colonies.

94. What is the disadvantage of frequent handwashing?
Frequent handwashing may actually transmit more bacteria by affecting skin health and raising pH.

Ojajarvi J, Makela P, Rantasalo I: Failure of hand disinfection with frequent handwashing: A need for prolonged field studies. J Hyg (Lond) 79:107–119, 1977.

95. What is the value of skin emollients?
Skin emollients decrease the dispersal of bacteria. In two small studies, topical emollients without antibiotics have been shown to decrease the frequency of nosocomial infection in neonates. *Note:* alcohol-based formulations (with appropriate emollients) are equivalent or superior to antiseptic detergents. In addition, they require no washing or drying, thereby reducing damage to the skin.

Abstracts, fifteenth annual educational conference, Association for Practitioners in Infection Control. May 1–6, 1988, Dallas. Am J Infect Control 16:73–92, 1988.

Nopper AJ, Horji KA, Sookdeo-Drost S, et al: Topical ointment therapy benefits premature infants. J Pediatr 128:660–669, 1996.

96. Does gowning prevent infections in the NICU?
There are very limited data to support the efficacy of gowning and much data to say that it is ineffective. The risk of transmitting infection through clothing is 2/10,000 encounters.

97. Does gowning serve as a reminder for personnel to wash their hands?
No!

Donowitz LG: Failure of the overgown to prevent nosocomial infection in a pediatric intensive care unit. Pediatrics 77:35–38, 1986.

98. For which kinds of infants in the nursery should nursery personnel wear gown and gloves?
- Infants colonized with a resistant microorganism or a bacterium known to cause infection in the nursery.
- Infants requiring contact isolation because of colonization with *Clostridium difficile*, rotavirus, respiratory syncytial virus, or herpes simplex virus.

CONJUNCTIVITIS

99. What are the common causes of neonatal conjunctivitis and when do they present?

ETIOLOGY	USUAL TIME OF ONSET AFTER BIRTH
Chemical (with silver nitrate prophylaxis)	6–24 hours
C. trachomatis	5–14 days

(Table continued on next page.)

ETIOLOGY	USUAL TIME OF ONSET AFTER BIRTH
N. gonorrhea	2–5 days
Other bacterial etiology:	> 5 days
Staphylococcus aureus	
Haemophilus species	
Streptococcus pneumoniae	
Enterococcus species	
Herpes simplex	5–14 days

The times of onset for infections caused by these organisms may overlap, particularly in the presence of prolonged rupture of membranes. In 10–46% of babies who present with conjunctivitis in the first month of life, *C. trachomatis* is the cause. The incidence of chlamydial conjunctivitis will probably decrease because pregnant women are now being screened and treated for chlamydia. *Haemophilus influenzae* and *S. pneumoniae* are frequently isolated in babies with lacrimal duct obstruction. Viral causes of conjunctivitis are rare during the first month; however, 70% of cases with viral etiology are due to herpes simplex, which may also cause severe systemic disease. *Pseudomonas* is a rare cause of bacterial conjunctivitis in healthy term newborns, but the organism deserves mention because it is sometimes responsible for epidemic conjunctivitis in premature babies. *Pseudomonas* can be a dangerously virulent organism, and pseudomonas conjunctivitis requires systemic as well as local (even subconjunctival) antibiotic therapy.

100. A 5-day-old full-term baby presents in the emergency room with pus coming from one eye. What work-up should you do? What treatment should be given?
You must do a Gram stain first. If the Gram stain shows gram-negative intracellular diplococci with abutting flattened sides, *N. gonorrhea* should be assumed to be the cause of the eye discharge, and the baby should be admitted for systemic treatment. A bacterial culture should be sent, along with a specific gonorrhea culture, to confirm the diagnosis. Note that the eye discharge seen in gonococcal ophthalmia is often thick, copious, and golden yellow in color. If the Gram stain is negative for intracellular diplococci, a culture for *C. trachomatis* and a rapid test for chlamydia (such as DFA, EIA, or DNA probe) should be performed in addition to bacterial cultures. A combined DNA probe for detection of both *N. gonorrhea* and *C. trachomatis* is commercially available. The chlamydia tests need to be done on conjunctival scrapings, because *Chlamydia* organisms are obligate intracellular organisms. If herpes conjunctivitis is suspected, a rapid test for herpes simplex and culture should be sent to the lab.

Conjunctivitis caused by gonorrhea should be treated with ceftriaxone at a dose of 50 mg/kg administered intravenously or intramuscularly once a day for 7 days. Additional topical therapy is not needed when ceftriaxone is used, but the infant's eyes should be irrigated with normal saline frequently until the discharge is gone.

If gonococcal ophthalmia is not suspected, 0.5% erythromycin ointment can be applied to each eye four times a day for 7 days. If the chlamydia test comes back positive, oral erythromycin (50 mg/kg/day divided into four equal doses) should be given for 14 days. Azithromycin is still undergoing clinical testing for newborns, but this drug at an oral dose of 20 mg/kg given once a day for 3 days may become the treatment of choice. After systemic antibiotics are started, topical treatment of the eye may be discontinued.

Herpes conjunctivitis is rare and is almost always accompanied by other systemic manifestations of neonatal herpes. The treatment for neonatal herpes conjunctivitis is acyclovir, 10 mg/kg IV every 8 hours for 10 days, plus topical therapy with 1% Trifluridine solution applied to the eye every 2 hours for 7 days or until cornea has reepithelialized.

101. Why doesn't conjunctivitis caused by *C. trachomatis* cause blindness in neonates when it causes so many cases of blindness in third world countries?
The visual loss from trachoma is caused by irreversible corneal damage from chronic folliculitis due to repeated chronic infection. Because of their immature immune system, newborns

lack the requisite lymphoid tissue in their conjunctiva to mount such a response. The length of infection also makes a difference. Even older children do not develop folliculitis until the infection has been present for at least 1–2 months; newborn conjunctivitis caused by *C. trachomatis* usually clears by 2 months even without antibiotic treatment, so no permanent scarring occurs. Another important factor may be that the serotypes of *C. trachomatis* that cause endocervical infections in women and conjunctivitis in neonates (types D–K) differ from the serotypes that cause blinding trachoma (types A–C).

102. Does the use of antibiotic eye prophylaxis at birth decrease the incidence of neonatal conjunctivitis secondary to *C. trachomatis*?

No. Topical silver nitrate, tetracycline, and erythromycin given at birth are equally effective in preventing gonococcal ophthalmia neonatorum, but none of these agents significantly decreases the incidence of chlamydial conjunctivitis.

CHLAMYDIA INFECTIONS

103. What is the risk of chlamydial infection in infants born to mothers whose endocervical culture is positive for *Chlamydia trachomatis*?

Neonatal acquisition usually occurs at the time of birth. In the absence of treatment during pregnancy, 50–75% of infants born to mothers with endocervical cultures positive for *C. trachomatis* become infected in at least one of the following anatomic sites: nasopharynx, conjunctiva, rectum, or vagina. Twenty to fifty percent develop conjunctivitis at 5–14 days of age that is generally not prevented by antibiotic eye prophylaxis at birth. Ten to twenty percent develop pneumonia between 4 and 12 weeks of life. The remaining infants develop an apparently asymptomatic colonization of the nasopharynx, rectum, or vagina. These infants can remain colonized for up to 3 years, although most clear even without treatment by 1 year of age.

Note that successful treatment of the mother during pregnancy with oral erythromycin or azithromycin prevents most cases of vertical transmission (see question 105).

104. What procedures are used to diagnose *C. trachomatis* infection in infants?

Chlamydia culture of the conjunctiva (for conjunctivitis) or nasopharynx (for pneumonia) is considered the gold standard for diagnosis, but there are disadvantages to this method. Culture specimens require special handling, which can make transport to the laboratory difficult. The fact that cultures generally require 3–7 days to process may delay treatment.

Since the mid-1980s, several commercial rapid tests have been developed. Direct fluorescent antibody (DFA) tests and enzyme immunoassays (EIA) have been approved by the U.S. Food and Drug Administration (FDA) for detection of *C. trachomatis* in infants with conjunctivitis or pneumonia; these tests have a sensitivity of 93–100% and specificity of 94–97% compared with culture. Results are usually available in less than 24 hours. A DNA probe was marketed more recently. DNA probes have a detection sensitivity and specificity similar to that of the EIA test and, in the commercial version, have the additional advantage of being combined with a DNA probe for *N. gonorrhea*. This test has received clearance by the FDA for use with conjunctival specimens but not for use with nasopharyngeal specimens. Newly developed amplified DNA tests based on polymerase chain reaction (PCR) and ligase chain reaction (LCR) appear to be even more sensitive than culture for chlamydia detection, but these are expensive. These tests are not yet FDA approved for infant conjunctival or nasopharyngeal specimens but may become the diagnostic test of choice when a very sensitive test is needed.

Remember that *C. trachomatis* is an obligate intracellular organism, so the collection swab must be scraped across the conjunctiva or nasopharynx to ensure that there are adequate cells for detection. In the eye, the pus should be wiped away before the conjunctival scrapings are obtained.

105. What is the proper treatment for *C. trachomatis* infections?

Mothers with positive endocervical cultures should be treated during pregnancy. Maternal treatment consists of erythromycin base, 500 mg orally 4 times a day for 7 days. Treatment for *C.*

trachomatis is hampered by its long growth cycle and requires prolonged therapeutic levels of antibiotics. Compliance can be a problem with this erythromycin course. Azythromycin is a macrolide antibiotic that has a lower incidence of side effects and a much longer half-life, so once-a-day dosing for shorter periods is possible. Post-treatment follow-up cultures should be preformed to determine whether or not treatment has been successful; if not, a second course of treatment may be indicated. Sexual partners of positive women must be treated as well. Chlamydia infection in both male and female genital tracts can be asymptomatic, which is why routine screening, especially in pregnancy, is warranted.

Until recently, the American Academy of Pediatrics (AAP) *Red Book* recommended that babies born to mothers with untreated chlamydial cervical infections receive oral erythromycin (50 mg/kg per day in four divided doses) for 14 days, starting on the first day of life. However, the efficacy of prophylactic treatment is unknown; moreover, reports of an association between the pro- phylactic use of oral erythromycin for pertussis and infantile hypertrophic pyloric stenosis have ap- peared. The AAP now recommends that treatment be reserved for infants with actual infection.

Neonates with chlamydial conjunctivitis should receive oral erythromycin, 50 mg/kg/day in four divided doses, for 14 days. Additional topical therapy is not needed. Erythromycin with the same dose given for 2–3 weeks is the treatment of choice for chlamydial pneumonia. Treatment failure requiring a second course of erythromycin occurs in about 20% of cases.

Azithromycin may soon be approved for use in neonates. Its shorter treatment course and less severe GI side effects should improve treatment compliance. Preliminary data indicate that azithromycin, in a dose of 20 mg/kg once a day for 3 days, successfully treats conjunctivitis caused by *C. trachomatis.*

106. What are the characteristics of *C. trachomatis* pneumonia?

The onset of *C. trachomatis* pneumonia is usually between 4 and 12 weeks of age (a few cases present as early as 2 weeks, but none has been reported beyond 4 months). Most infants have a prodrome of about 1 week's duration of a stuffy nose without fever and a persistent parox- ysmal staccato cough that can lead to breathlessness. They may present with tachypnea and in- spiratory rales. Expiratory wheezing occurs in less than 25% of infants with the disease; 60% have abnormal eardrum findings. Although a severe illness is relatively rare, they appear irritable, eat poorly, and cough often. The chest x-ray shows hyperinflation with bilateral diffuse nonspe- cific infiltrates. Lab values are significant for eosinophilia (> 300 to 400/mm^3), an elevated total serum IgG (> 500 mg/dl) and an elevated total IgM (> 110 mg/dl). Without treatment, symptoms last an average of 6 weeks. Treatment of any previous conjunctivitis with oral erythromycin seems to prevent this pneumonia, although there are case reports of treatment failures. Half of the infants with chlamydial pneumonia do not have a history of previous conjunctivitis.

107. Does *C. pneumoniae* cause disease in newborns?

C. pneumoniae, a recently discovered species of the genus *Chlamydia*, has not been iso- lated in any children under the age of 2 years. It is a common cause of pneumonia, bronchitis, and upper respiratory tract infections in older children between the ages of 5 and 15 years.

108. Does *C. trachomatis* infection in pregnant women cause complications other than neonatal infection?

Although studies are conflicting, *C. trachomatis* infection in pregnancy is weakly linked to premature rupture of membranes and premature delivery. Ten to thirty percent of women with chlamydial infections who undergo induced abortions develop late endometritis. Chronic salpin- gitis caused by *C. trachomatis* can lead to infertility and an increased risk for ectopic pregnancy.

OSTEOMYELITIS AND SEPTIC ARTHRITIS

109. What pathogens cause neonatal osteomyelitis?

• *Staphylococcus aureus*
• Group B streptococcus

- Gram-negative enteric bacilli (e.g., *E. coli*, *Klebsiella* spp., *Pseudomonas* spp.)
- *Candida* species
- *Mycoplasma hominis*
- *T. pallidum*

110. What is the incidence of osteomyelitis in the neonate?

The overall rate of nosocomial bone and joint infections is 1–2/1000 admissions.

111. What is the pathogenesis of osteomyelitis in the newborn?

Hematogenous dissemination is responsible for most infections; however, skeletal infections can also result from:
- Extension from infection in surrounding tissues
- Direct inoculation
- Transplacental infection leading to fetal sepsis (syphilis)

112. What distinct anatomic and physiologic features place the newborn at risk for osteomyelitis and septic arthritis?

The metaphysis is usually the site of seeding caused by sluggish flow in the metaphyseal vessels (also referred to as sinusoidal vessels) and decreased phagocytic activity. In the newborn period, these transphyseal vessels form a conduit between the metaphysis and the epiphysis. Additionally, the relatively thin cortex and loosely applied periosteum are poor barriers against spread of infection. The hip, shoulder, and knee can easily become infected because the epiphyseal-metaphyseal junction is entirely within the joint capsule.

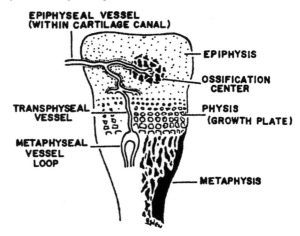

Schematic depiction of blood supply in the neonatal epiphysis. Normally in children, there are two separate circulatory systems: (1) the metaphyseal loops, derived from the diaphyseal nutrient artery, and (2) the epiphyseal vessels, which course through the epiphyseal cartilage within structures termed cartilage canals. In the neonatal period, sinusoidal vessels, termed the transphyseal vessels, connect these two systems. With ensuing skeletal maturation, these vessels disappear, and the epiphyseal and metaphyseal systems become totally separated. (From Ogden JA, Lister G: The pathology of neonatal osteomyelitis. Pediatrics 55:474–478, 1975, with permission.)

113. What are the manifestations of osteomyelitis in the neonate?

- Systemic signs are usually absent in neonatal osteomyelitis, but occasionally are present.
- In most infants, the earliest presenting signs are pain (with pseudoparalysis), limitation of motion, and swelling. Discoloration and increased warmth may accompany the swelling.
- Feeding and weight gain are usually undisturbed.
- The distribution of bone involvement is as follows:

Femur (39%)	Ulna (3%)
Humerus (18%)	Clavicle (2%)
Tibia (14%)	Tarsal bones (2%)
Radius (5%)	Ribs (2%)
Maxilla (4%)	Vertebrae (1%)

Remington JS, Klein JO (eds): Infectious Diseases of the fetus and Newborn Infant. Philadelphia, W.B. Saunders, 1995.

114. How often are bacterial cultures positive in neonatal osteomyelitis?
- 60% of blood cultures are positive
- 70% of bone aspirates are positive

115. Is the erythrocyte sedimentation rate (ESR) or C-reactive protein (CRP) more helpful in the management of osteomyelitis?

In most studies, the ESR was significantly elevated on days 2–5. ESR values slowly returned to normal within 3 weeks of therapy. In contrast, CRP rises within 6–12 hours of a triggering stimulus and returns to normal within a week of therapy. A secondary rise in either ESR or CRP could be a sign of recrudescence.

116. How common is fungal septic arthritis?

Candida species cause 17% of septic arthritis in premature infants.

117. What are the unique features of *Candida* bone infections?
- Unlike bacterial infections, there is no inflammatory sign other than edema of the extremity.
- Fungal infections on x-ray are "punched out" metaphyseal lucencies that appear less aggressive than staphylococcal osteomyelitis.
- Affected babies often have a history of central line–related fungemia.
- Fungal septic arthritis can appear as late as 1 year after a treated fungal infection.
- Fluconazole may be a good alternative to amphotericin B because of good joint penetration.

118. What is the first line of management for a suspected septic arthritis in a newborn infant?

Joint aspiration with incision and drainage whenever there is significant collection of pus in the soft tissues. Often surgical drainage is indicated for relief of intra-articular pressure when the hip or shoulder is affected.

119. What radiologic studies are helpful in the diagnosis of osteomyelitis?

TEST	PROS	CONS
Skeletal x-rays	Eventually bony changes will be seen (i.e., punched out lytic lesions, osseous lucencies, and periosteal elevation). Multiple sites of involvement can eventually be seen. Trauma (i.e., fracture) as a cause of swelling or pseudoparalysis can be ruled out.	X-ray changes do not occur for 7–12 days. Conventional radiographs are insensitive to destruction of < 30% of the bone matrix.
^{99m}Technetium (Tc)	Osteomyelitis can be detected earlier than on traditional skeletal surveys. With the higher resolution gamma cameras used today, multiple sites of infection are often noted.	Patient is exposed to radiation. False-negative studies have been reported. False-positive results occur from increased metabolic bone activity.
Gallium bone scan	In equivocal ^{99m}Tc bone scans, gallium might be useful.	The radiation dose is significantly higher than in ^{99m}Tc bone scan.
Sonography	Most useful as a tool for finding or guiding needle aspiration of fluid collections in joints or adjacent to bone. It is inexpensive. There is no radiation exposure.	An experienced sonographer is required. Accuracy is variable in the neonate.
Magnetic resonance imaging (MRI)	MRI detects inflammatory or destructive intramedullary disease in older children or adults.	Not helpful in neonates because the marrow compartment is rarely involved.

120. What is the presentation of maxillary osteomyelitis?

1. Early edema and redness of the cheeks
2. Unilateral nasal discharge
3. Swelling of the eyelid with conjunctivitis

121. What are the initial antibiotics used for the treatment of osteomyelitis?

Optimal coverage is provided by a penicillinase-resistant penicillin coupled with an amino-glycoside until an organism is identified and antibiotic sensitivities have been determined. Therapy should be continued for a minimum of 4–6 weeks. In the neonatal age group, orally administered antibiotics are not used because there are insufficient data regarding their absorption and efficacy.

PYELONEPHRITIS AND URINARY TRACT INFECTION

122. A 10-day-old male infant presents with a 2-day history of fever, vomiting, lethargy, and jaundice. Examination reveals a temperature of 39°C; blood pressure, 65/40; and pulse 170/min; there are no focal abnormal physical findings. Laboratory data include bilirubin, 7 mg/dl (direct 2 mg/dl); creatinine, 0.2 mg/dl; WBC count, 20,000 cells/mm³; and urinalysis 60 WBCs per high-power field. What is the most likely diagnosis?

The signs and symptoms indicate an acute infectious process. The urinalysis suggests a diagnosis of acute pyelonephritis. Symptomatic urinary tract infections (UTIs) occur in 1.4/1000 newborns.

123. What is the incidence of asymptomatic bacteriuria in the neonate?

Asymptomatic bacteriuria occurs in 2% of healthy full-term neonates and up to 10% of premature infants. Males are affected more often than females in the neonatal period, and uncircumcised males are even more susceptible.

124. What is the pathogenesis of UTI in the neonate?

Unlike older infants, hematogenous spread of infection is more common than ascending infection. For this reason, some neonates may have associated meningitis and septicemia. Therefore, in addition to urinalysis and urine culture, neonates more than 3 days of age should have blood and CSF cultures drawn prior to initiation of antibiotics. The yield of urine culture in neonates less than 3 days of age is poor. Unlike the distinction of cystitis and pyelonephritis in older infants and children, infection of the urinary tract in the neonate often includes that of the kidney.

125. What are the signs and symptoms of UTI in the neonate?

The symptoms of UTI are often nonspecific and include vomiting, diarrhea, failure to thrive, fever, lethargy, and jaundice, which is unconjugated if the UTI occurs in the first week of life and conjugated if UTI occurs later.

126. How is the diagnosis of a UTI in the neonate made?

The definitive diagnosis is by positive culture of urine that is obtained using sterile precautions. Urinalysis is not very helpful; up to 25 leukocytes/mm³ in males and up to 50 leukocytes/mm³ in clean-catch specimens are considered normal. Absence of pyuria does not rule out UTI.

127. What are the common organisms responsible for UTI in newborn infants?

The most common organism causing UTI in neonates is *E. coli*, which accounts for 91% of community-acquired infection in children less than 8 weeks of age. Other organisms include *Proteus, Pseudomonas, Klebsiella, Enterococcus,* and *Staphylococcus aureus,* which may be associated with suppurative lesions in the testis, epididymis, or kidneys. With prolonged hospitalization, coagulase-negative *Staphylococcus* and *Candida* can also cause UTI. Predisposing factors for *Candida* UTI include prematurity, intravascular catheters, parenteral nutrition, cutaneous fungal infection, and use of broad-spectrum antibiotics. Candidiasis can be associated with fungal balls in the kidney and renal pelvis, which can lead to obstruction.

128. How should pyelonephritis be treated?

Treatment of pyelonephritis is similar to that of bacterial UTI and consists of parenteral antibiotics, usually a combination of a penicillin and an aminoglycoside, or, in older infants, a third-generation cephalosporin. For suspected staphylococcal infection, a penicillinase-resistant penicillin could be used. Amphotericin is used for candida infection, and in premature neonates, liposomal amphotericin can be used to reduce nephrotoxicity. The duration of therapy is 10–14 days, and it is advisable to repeat a urine culture after 48 hours to ensure clearance of the organisms from the urinary tract. Antibiotic prophylaxis is indicated for structural anomalies of the urinary tract or vesicoureteric reflux. Prophylaxis is used until spontaneous resolution or surgical correction of the underlying lesion has occurred.

129. In addition to urinalysis and urine culture, what other tests are indicated in the treatment of an infant with possible UTI?

In addition to diagnosing UTI, it is also important to evaluate the urinary tract for underlying structural or functional abnormalities that may predispose to recurrent UTIs. Urinary tract anomalies have been detected in 30–55% of infants with UTI younger than 2 months of age, but rarely occur in the early neonatal period.

Abdominal ultrasound is a safe and noninvasive method of evaluating structural abnormalities of the urinary tract and is the initial imaging test of choice. Plain x-ray of the abdomen does not allow adequate visualization of the kidneys. **Intravenous pyelography** can be useful in assessing the function of the kidneys. **Radionuclide scans** such as DMSA scans can be used to evaluate function and structural abnormalities, specifically renal scars following UTI. **Vesicoureterography** to evaluate the presence or absence of vesicoureteric reflux should be performed after completion of treatment of the UTI, because transient vesicoureteral reflux commonly occurs with the acute infection.

IMPETIGO

130. What are the two types of impetigo in the neonate?

1. **Nonbullous (traditional, classic) impetigo:**
   - Accounts for 70% of cases.
   - Typically, lesions appear initially on areas of the skin of the face or extremities that have been traumatized (e.g., insect bites, varicella, abrasions, lacerations, and burns).
   - Initially, a tiny vesicle or pustule forms and rapidly develops into a honey-colored crusted plaque, generally < 2 cm in diameter.
   - Infection causes an exudate with spongiosis, vesiculation, and the accumulation of neutrophils, often in pustules. The exudation on the cutaneous surface results in formation of the typical golden crusts of impetigo.
   - Lesions are associated with little to no pain and minimal or no surrounding erythema.
   - Constitutional symptoms are generally absent.
   - The courses of most cases are indolent and resolve without scarring within approximately 2 weeks.
2. **Bullous impetigo:**
   - Less common than the nonbullous form and affects younger children, mainly infants and young children. May occur among neonates in nursery epidemics.
   - Lesions appear most commonly on the skin of the face, buttocks, trunk, perineum, and extremities.
   - Neonatal bullous impetigo can begin in the diaper area.
   - Characterized by flaccid, transparent bullae 1–2 cm in diameter arising from normal intact skin.

- Rupture of the bullae occurs easily, leaving a narrow rim of scale at the edge of a shallow, moist erosion.
- Surrounding erythema and regional adenopathy are generally absent.
- Lesions result from the subcorneal epidermal cleft caused by the staphylococcal toxin exfoliatin.
- Infants are sensitive to the exfoliative action, and infection can result in extensive epidermal dyshesion, namely staphylococcal scalded skin syndrome.

131. What bacterial etiologic agents are linked to impetigo?

Nonbullous impetigo is predominantly caused by *Staphylococcus aureus* (not phage group 2) and group A beta-hemolytic streptococci (GABHS). Bullous impetigo is always caused by coagulase-positive *Staphylococcus aureus*, approximately 80% from phage group 2 (60% of those in phage group 2 are type 71; most of the remainder are types 3A, 3B, 3C, and 55).

132. What are the complications of impetigo?

The infectious agents causing impetigo can occasionally disseminate, causing osteomyelitis, septic arthritis, pneumonia, sepsis, or meningitis. Cellulitis is observed in 10% of infants with nonbullous impetigo. Bullous impetigo may occasionally progress to staphylococcal scalded skin syndrome (SSSS). In SSSS, intact bullae are consistently sterile, unlike those of bullous impetigo. Infections with nephritogenic strains may result in glomerulonephritis.

133. What is the noninfectious differential diagnosis of bullous impetigo?

Thermal burns	Dermatitis herpetiformis
Mast cell disease	Epidermolysis bullosa, congenital porphyria
Histiocytosis X	Stevens-Johnson syndrome
Acrodermatitis enteropathica	

134. How should infants with impetigo be treated?

Impetigo is commonly treated with topical antibiotics (e.g., mupirocin [Bactroban]) for 7–10 days. The use of parenteral antibiotics is controversial. Systemic antimicrobial therapy should probably be administered to all infants who do not respond to conventional treatment and who have extensive involvement or signs consistent with sepsis.

OMPHALITIS

135. What are the presenting signs of omphalitis in the neonate?

- Foul-smelling discharge
- Periumbilical erythematous streaking, induration, and tenderness to palpation
- Purulent or serosanguinous discharge
- On rare occasions, signs of a systemic infection

136. What is the incidence of omphalitis?

In hospitalized infants the incidence is ~ 2%. In infants delivered at home the incidence may be as high as 21%.

137. What are the predisposing factors for omphalitis?

Prematurity	Improper severing of the umbilical cord
Complicated delivery	Poor hygienic practices during the neonatal period

138. Which bacteria cause omphalitis?

- *Staphylococcus aureus*
- *Streptococcus pyogenes* (infections with group A, beta-hemolytic streptococci may result in a wet malodorous stump with only mild evidence of inflammation
- Gram-negative organisms (e.g., *E. coli*, *Klebsiella* sp.)

139. What are the noninfectious causes of increased umbilical drainage?

Serosanguinous drainage may be seen with a patent urachus or omphalomesenteric duct.

140. What are the major complications of omphalitis?

- Septic umbilical arteritis
- Suppurative thrombophlebitis of the umbilical or portal veins (resulting in portal vein thrombosis and portal hypertension)
- Liver abscess
- Endocarditis
- Abdominal wall necrotizing fasciitis
- Peritonitis

141. How should infants with omphalitis be treated?

Infants with omphalitis should receive a penicillinase-resistant penicillin and an aminoglycoside antibiotic. Local therapy should be used to eliminate surface colonization.

142. What syndrome can be associated with chronic omphalitis or delayed separation of the umbilical cord?

Leukocyte adhesion deficiency (LAD) is a life-threatening, autosomal-recessive inherited deficiency of cell adhesion molecules associated with chronic omphalitis or delayed separation of the umbilical cord. The hallmark of LAD is the absence of granulocytes at the site of infection.

143. You are informed during sign-out rounds that a newborn is suspected to have funisitis. Where should you look for that infection?

Funisitis is no fun for the baby or the attending physician caring for the child! Funisitis is an inflammation of the umbilical cord vessels and Wharton's jelly and has been described as either an acute exudative or subacute necrotizing process accompanying chorioamnionitis. The predominant organisms identified as etiologic agents are gram-negative bacteria, including *E. coli*, *Klebsiella*, and *Pseudomonas*. Gram-positive organisms (e.g., streptococci, staphylococci) and candidal species are less commonly responsible.

LISTERIOSIS

144. Is *Listeria monocytogenes* still a significant pathogen to consider when evaluating sepsis in neonates?

Yes. Although it is an uncommon infection in the United States (7.4 cases per million population according to the CDC), an estimated 1850 cases per year result in 425 deaths. The largest affected groups are neonates and adults older than 60 years of age. Pregnant women account for about 27% of cases and have an increased tendency to develop listeriosis during the third trimester, often resulting in septic abortion. Vertical transmission from the colonized mother is the only human-to-human acquisition of the organism.

145. How do mothers acquire *Listeria monocytogenes*?

L. monocytogenes is acquired by susceptible adults (those with lower cellular immunity) through eating contaminated food. Surprisingly, the incidence of *L. monocytogenes* infection is low considering that food contamination is relatively common. The CDC sampled all refrigerator foods, 11% of which yielded the organism. *L. monocytogenes* loves refrigerator temperatures (4–10°C), which facilitates its growth. Additionally, it resists killing by routine pasteurization. Therefore, soft cheese products are the most common sources, along with delicatessen meats, fish, and poultry products. However, any undercooked food source is likely to contain this common organism (prevalent also in all soil and raw vegetable matter). One recent outbreak occurred with gravad-treated (cold-smoked) rainbow trout.

146. What are the signs and symptoms of clinical infection in the pregnant mother?

Following ingestion of the microorganism, mothers may incubate *L. monocytogenes* for 11–70 days (mean 31 days). Invasion of the intestinal mucosal barrier ensues with bacteremia resulting in a flu-like illness with fever, chills, myalgias, arthralgias, headache, and backache. Symptoms may be mild and manifest most commonly between 26 and 30 weeks' gestation. Often the placenta becomes a reservoir for bacterial proliferation resulting in amnionitis with persistence of symptoms until abortion or delivery occurs, with a 22% occurrence of either stillbirth or neonatal death. If cultured and recognized, the mother may be treated effectively, preserving the pregnancy.

147. How do *Listeria* infections present in the neonate?

Neonate infection may manifest at birth as disseminated listeriosis termed *granulomatosis infantiseptica*, with microabscesses throughout the body, but particularly the liver and spleen. This entity may be accompanied by hemorrhagic amnionitis presenting as "chocolate syrup" meconium. Death usually occurs with a few hours. Vertical transmission from the mother may occur shortly before or at birth, resulting in either early-onset neonatal sepsis with pneumonia before 2 weeks of life (from organisms inhaled with amniotic fluid) or late-onset sepsis with meningitis within the first month. Papular rash (pinpoint, evanescent) and conjunctivitis are reported but are not specific for listeriosis. As with any virulent bacterial infection, DIC and multiple organ system involvement are common. Mortality reports vary from 50% to 100%, with the highest death rates occurring in early-onset infections in the premature infant.

Clinical and Laboratory Features of Early-onset Listeriosis

FEATURE	BANCROFT. ET AL. (1971)	ALBRITTON ET AL. (1976)	AHLFORS ET AL. (1977)	LENNON ET AL. (1984)	EVANS ET AL. (1985)	% (TOTAL)	
Age at onset (days)	< 1	< 1	< 1	< 1	< 1		
Sex (M/F)	9M/4F	12M/7F	5M/0F	9M/5F	7M/8F	64 M	(42/24)
Preterm infants[a]	8/13	14/19	3/5	11/22	12/15	63	(38/60)
Mortality (of live-born infants)	1/13	6/18	1/5	1/14	3/11	15	(7/48)
Features in infants							
Meconium stain	8/13	NA	5/5	NA	7/11	69	(20/29)
Pneumonia	10/13	NA	3/5	NA	5/11	62	(18/29)
Anemia[b]	NA[c]	NA	4/5	NA	6/11	62	(10/16)
Thrombocytopenia[d]	—	NA	3/5	2/10	4/11	35	(9/26)
Meningitis[e]	3/13	NA	1/5	NA	2/11	21	(6/29)
Source of isolate							
Blood	7/8	13/18	5/5	8/14	8/11	73	(41/56)
Maternal features							
Flu-like illness[f]	5/13	NA	2/5	NA	8/15	45	(15/33)
Blood isolate[g]	NA	NA	NA	4/15	3/5	35	(7/20)

[a] Preterm infants: gestation age < 35 weeks or, if gestation not indicated, birth weight < 2500 g.

[b] Anemia defined as hemoglobin < 14 and/or hematocrit < 45.

[c] NA = not available.

[d] Thrombocytopenia: author's criteria.

[e] Meningitis based on compatible clinical or autopsy findings or observation of organism on Gram stain of cerebrospinal fluid. Isolation of organism was not sufficient criteria as blood contamination of cerebrospinal fluid is frequent.

[f] Flu-like illness defined as presence of respiratory symptoms, myalgia, fever occurring from 3 days to 1 month prior to delivery.

[g] Isolates of *L. monocytogenes* from blood of mother at any time before delivery of infant.

Adapted from Bortolussi R, Schlech WF: Listeriosis. In Remington JS, Klein JO (eds): Infectious Diseases of the Fetus and Newborn Infant. Philadelphia, W.B. Saunders, 1995.

Clinical and Laboratory Features of Late-onset Listeriosis

FEATURE	ALBRITTON ET AL. (1976)	VISINTINE ET AL. (1977)	FILICE ET AL. (1978)	KESSLER AND DAJANI (1990)	% (TOTAL)	
Mean age (days)	14.7	—	12.1	19.7		
Sex (M/F)	14M/7F	18M/7F	4M/3F	11M/6F	67 M (47/23)	
Signs at presentation						
Fever	NA	25/26	7/7	15/17	94	(47/50)
Irritability	NA	18/25	5/7	14/17	75	(37/49)
Diarrhea	NA	NA	4/7	NA		—
Isolates						
CSF	19/21	25/26	6/7	17/17	94	(67/71)
Blood	2/21	7/25	1/7	2/17	17	(12/70)
Lab Features*						
WBC (blood)	NA	18,000	13,600	20,400		—
WBC (CSF)	NA	2750	3874	3792		—

* Mean cells per mm^3; WBC = white blood cell count.
Adapted from Bortolussi R, Schlech WF: Listeriosis. In Remington JS, Klein JO (eds): Infectious Diseases of the Fetus and Newborn Infant. Philadelphia, W.B. Saunders, 1995.

148. What is the pathogenesis of *L. monocytogenes* infection, and why does insufficiency of cellular immunity in particular contribute to the development of disease?

L. monocytogenes is a small gram-positive rod sometimes mistaken as a diptheroid or culture contaminant. The organism is an intracellular, facultative anaerobic parasite. Once phagocytized, *L. monocytogenes* replicates rapidly within the cytosol, but repels phagosome killing through its major virulence factor, listeriolysin O (characteristic of only this species of *Listeria*). Using the cell's own cytoskeletal actin polymerization mechanism, *L. monocytogenes* pushes outward on the host cell's membrane forming filopods, which are then injected into neighboring cells. Cell-to-cell transmission spreads rapidly without exposure to circulating humoral antibodies or neutrophils. T-lymphocytes, therefore, provide the only natural recognition and immunity toward *L. monocytogenes*, although macrophage killing (probably using nitric oxide) may also occur. Because cellular immunity is suppressed during pregnancy and is naturally deficient during early neonatal life, *L. monocytogenes* enjoys an advantage during these host-vulnerable periods. In the cellular immune competent host, significant infection is rare and self-limited.

149. How is the diagnosis of listeriosis made?

L. monocytogenes growth on cultures of blood, cerebral spinal fluid, meconium, and amniotic fluid may be selectively cold enhanced; however, specific media are now preferred and used routinely in clinical laboratories for rapid confirmation of the diagnosis. *L. monocytogenes* should be suspected in any neonatal sepsis work-up, particularly if gram-positive rods are present on Gram stain of placental membranes, meconium, or amniotic fluid. Serology via a peptide limited to detect the aminoterminal end of listeriolysin O has recently shown promise for early identification of *L. monocytogenes* in endemic outbreaks.

150. How should listeriosis be treated in the neonate?

L. monocytogenes remains sensitive to ampicillin, and gentamicin may augment antimicrobial killing. Because of the organism's tendency to hide in tissue reservoirs, higher doses of ampicillin (200 mg/kg/day) are usually recommended for extended durations (2 weeks for bacteremia, 3 weeks for meningitis). Trimethoprim-sulfamethoxazole (TMP-SMX) is the best alternative for mothers who are penicillin sensitive, although erythromycin has been used in case reports (not currently recommended). Iron therapy for anemia should be withheld during treatment of listeriosis, because iron enhances the organism's growth in vitro and is therefore a virulence factor contributing to host susceptibility to infection.

SYPHILIS

151. In 1987, the reported rate of congenital syphilis was 10.5 cases/100,000 live births. By 1991, this had risen to 107 cases/100,000 births. What factors account for these changes?
- New surveillance case definition
- Substantial under-reporting of actual disease
- Coinfection with HIV
- Insufficient public health resources
- Promiscuity, failure to implement safer sexual practices, drug use, particularly among adolescents and young adults

The last several years, however, have seen a reversal of this trend, perhaps because of public awareness, wider screening practices, and community-based prevention programs.

152. What are the recommendations for syphilis screening in pregnancy?
All women should have a VDRL (Venereal Disease Research Laboratory test for syphilis) performed at the first prenatal visit, with a second screen during the third trimester. If the nontreponemal test is positive, treponemal serology should be obtained. The CDC currently recommends that no infant be discharged from the hospital without a determination of maternal serology for syphilis.

153. What are the effects of maternal coinfection with HIV on fetal infection with *Treponema pallidum*?
Although the effects of maternal HIV infection on the transmission of syphilis are incompletely understood, the cellular immune abnormalities associated with HIV may allow greater treponemal proliferation and higher fetal infection. In addition, HIV-infected women may not respond adequately to benzathine penicillin, rendering their fetuses more susceptible to disease.

154. What is the relationship between maternal drug use and congenital syphilis?
Recent studies have found an increased risk of congenital syphilis among neonates following maternal illicit drug use, particularly cocaine. Reasons suggested include poor prenatal care among pregnant drug addicts and predisposing sexual behaviors in this population.

155. Which infants should be evaluated for congenital syphilis?
Asymptomatic infants born to successfully treated mothers do not need evaluation. Infants born to seropositive mothers (nontreponemal test confirmed by treponemal test) should be evaluated if mothers:
- Have untreated syphilis
- Were treated for syphilis < 1 month before delivery
- Were treated for syphilis with a nonpenicillin regimen
- Did not have the expected decrease in nontreponemal antibody titers after treatment
- Were treated but had insufficient follow-up during pregnancy

156. What is pneumonia alba?
The pneumonia alba of congenital syphilis is characterized by yellow-white, heavy, grossly enlarged lungs. There is a marked increase in the amount of connective tissue in the interalveolar septa and interstitium histologically, with loss of alveolar spaces and obliterative fibrosis.

157. What is Hutchinson's triad?
The findings of Hutchinson's teeth, interstitial keratitis, and eighth nerve deafness comprise Hutchinson's triad and are virtually pathognomonic for late congenital syphilis. The stigmata represent scars induced by the lesions of early congenital syphilis or reactions to persistent inflammation.

158. How useful are treponemal antibody tests in the diagnosis of congenital syphilis?

Not very. Both treponemal and nontreponemal tests currently available detect maternal IgG antibody. Moreover, although treponemal antibody tests are more specific and sensitive for diagnosis, they remain reactive indefinitely, so active versus past infection cannot be distinguished. Therefore, treponemal antibody tests are not recommended screens for newborn infants.

159. Which infants should be treated for congenital syphilis?

Even if the evaluation is normal, all infants born to mothers who are untreated or who have evidence of relapse or reinfection should be assumed to be infected and treated.

Infants should be treated if they have:
- Any evidence of active disease (physical examination findings or x-ray)
- A reactive CSF VDRL
- An abnormal CSF finding, regardless of serology
- Quantitative nontreponemal antibody titers that are 4 times greater than maternal titers

160. What is the derivation of the word *syphilis*?

Syphilis is derived from the name of the shepherd Syphilus, the hero of a poem written by Frascatorius in 1530. Syphilis was afflicted with this disease as punishment for cursing the gods.

HUMAN IMMUNODEFICIENCY VIRUS

161. What is the relative seroprevalence of HIV infection among pregnant women?

It depends on location. Worldwide, the rate varies markedly. In the United States, the overall prevalence is estimated at 1.5/1000 women, with much higher rates reported from urban areas. In Philadelphia, the rate is about 7.5/1000, whereas in New York City, the prevalence is around 25/1000 (or 1 in 40). These numbers pale in comparison to those found in sub–Saharan Africa where rates as high as 25–33% (250–330/1000 pregnant women) are reported from several prenatal care centers.

162. What is the risk of transmission of HIV infection to newborns?

Untreated, the rate varies worldwide, from a high of 30–40% in Africa (confounded by breast-feeding and poor nutritional status) to 20–25% in the United States, and 13–15% in Europe. With the use of perinatal zidovudine (AZT, ZDV) the rate of infant infection drops to 8%. When perinatal zidovudine is combined with elective cesarean section, the rate of infant infection is less than 5%. When pregnant women are treated with two to three drugs in combination therapy and maintain a low viral load, the risk to the infant is less than 3–4%.

163. What risk factors are associated with increased risk of perinatal transmission of HIV infection?

Maternal AIDs diagnosis	Breast-feeding
CD4 count < 200/mm³	Preterm delivery
High viral load	Chorioamnionitis
Prolonged rupture of membranes	Vaginal delivery
Vitamin A deficiency (?)	Untreated STDs (?)

164. When during the perinatal period is HIV transmitted?

HIV infection may be transmitted in utero, intrapartum, or after birth through breast-feeding. In the absence of breast-feeding, it is believed that approximately 20–30% of perinatal infections occur in utero, with the remaining 70–80% occurring during the intrapartum period. In the event an infant escapes infection in utero and during delivery but is then breast-fed, the risk is approximately 15% when breast-feeding is continued for at least 6 months.

165. Which pregnant women should be offered HIV testing?

All. Because risk factor assessments fail to detect more than 40% of HIV-infected pregnant women, the AAP and ACOG both recommend routine HIV counseling to all pregnant women, with voluntary HIV testing. This is all the more important in light of major advances in perinatal treatment strategies to reduce the incidence of HIV transmission to newborns.

166. What percentage of HIV-exposed neonates will be positive by the enzyme-linked immunosorbent assay (ELISA) HIV antibody screening test?

Virtually all. The ELISA measures IgG anti-HIV antibodies, which readily cross the placenta in the third trimester; hence, all infants born to antibody-positive women will be antibody-positive themselves. These maternal antibodies will remain detectable in the infants' bloodstream until 12–18 months of age.

167. What is the best diagnostic test for defining HIV infections in infants, and when should it be ordered?

All HIV-exposed infants should have an HIV PCR DNA assay (or HIV blood culture) performed at birth, at 1 month of age, and at 3–4 months of age. Any positive test should be repeated immediately. If the tests at 1 month and 4 months of age are negative, the infant is considered HIV uninfected. Currently, quantitative RNA measurements (termed *viral load*) are not recommended for diagnostic purposes. In addition, the p24 antigen test is no longer used for diagnosis.

168. What tests are used to monitor immune dysfunction related to HIV infection, and how do the normal values differ from those in adults?

The CD4 percentage and the absolute CD4 count are used to monitor immunogenic function in HIV infection. It should be remembered that normal CD4 counts for infants and children are much higher than those found in adults (normal infant CD4 count is $2500–3500/ml^3$, and normal adult values are $700–1000/ml^3$).

169. What therapies are recommended for pregnant HIV-infected women?

Close prenatal monitoring, attention to nutritional issues, antiretroviral therapy (at a minimum, prenatal and intrapartum AZT followed by 6 weeks of AZT to the neonate) and elective cesarean section are now all part of recommended care for infected pregnant women.

170. What are the major HIV-related complications seen in HIV-infected infants?

Pneumocystis carinii pneumonia (PCP) is the most common serious HIV-related infection in infancy. The peak age of onset is 3–9 months, and it carries a 50% mortality rate. Fortunately, PCP can be prevented by thrice weekly TMP-SMX as prophylaxis. All exposed infants should be placed on PCP prophylaxis at 6 weeks of age and continued on the medicine until HIV infection is definitively ruled out (two negative HIV PCR DNA tests, both after 1 month of age). Growth failure (FTT) and a progressive encephalopathy are also common serious complications of HIV infection in the first year of life.

CYTOMEGALOVIRUS

171. What is the most common congenital viral infection in the United States?

Congenital cytomegalovirus infection, occurring in 1–2% of all live births.

172. What are the most common manifestations of congenital cytomegalovirus infection in neonates?

Petechiae	Hepatosplenomegaly
Small for gestational age (SGA) birth weight	Jaundice at birth

Istas AS, Demmler GJ, Dobbins JG, Stewart JA: Surveillance for congenital cytomegalovirus disease: A report from the National Congenital Cytomegalovirus Disease Registry. J Infect Dis 20:665–670, 1995.

173. What are the most reliable methods for diagnosing congenital cytomegalovirus infection?

Isolation of cytomegalovirus from urine during the first 3 weeks of life is the most reliable method for diagnosing congenital infection. Specimens must be obtained at that time because neonates who acquire cytomegalovirus at the time of birth can start to shed virus as early as 3 weeks of age. Detection of IgM antibodies to cytomegalovirus in serum obtained within the first few days after birth is highly suggestive of congenital infection. False-positive results may be reported by laboratories that do not use appropriate methods for detecting IgM antibodies to cytomegalovirus.

174. How can neonates acquire cytomegalovirus infection other than by maternal-fetal transmission?

Cytomegalovirus can be transmitted to neonates through blood transfusion.

175. What methods are available to prevent transmission of cytomegalovirus to neonates through blood products?

Transmission of cytomegalovirus to neonates by blood transfusion can be prevented by use of blood obtained from seronegative donors, frozen in glycerol, or depleted of white blood cells.

176. What is the frequency of hearing loss in infants with congenital cytomegalovirus infection?

HEARING LOSS		
TYPE	SEVERITY*	% AFFECTED
Bilateral		11
	Mild	5
	Moderate to profound	6
Unilateral		8
	Mild	4
	Moderate to profound	4

Data from Hanshaw J et al. (1976), Stagno S et al. (1983), Saigal S et al. (1982), and Kumar M et al. (1984).
* Mild hearing loss, 22–55 dB; moderate to profound ≥ 55 dB.
Adapted from Volpe JJ (ed): Neurology of the Newborn, 3rd ed. Philadelphia, W.B. Saunders, 1995.

177. What is the relationship between neonatal clinical signs and neurologic outcome in congenital cytomegalovirus infection?

		NEUROLOGIC SEQUELAE*		
NEONATAL SIGNS	NORMAL	MAJOR	MINOR	DEATH
Neurologic				
Microcephaly, intracranial calcifications, chorioretinitis	7	79	0	14
Other	40	50	0	10
Systemic				
Jaundice, hepatosplenomegaly, or purpura, but no neurologic signs	48	12	36	4
No neurologic or systemic signs	81	3	16	0

Data from MacDonald and Tobin and based on 80 infants.
* Expressed as percentage of those with designated neonatal clinical signs.
Adapted from Volpe JJ (ed): Neurology of the Newborn, 3rd ed. Philadelphia, W.B. Saunders, 1995.

HERPES SIMPLEX VIRUS

178. What diagnostic approaches should be taken when a baby develops skin vesicles in the neonatal period?

Newborn babies with skin vesicles should be rapidly worked up for the possibility of neonatal herpes simplex virus (HSV) infection, which is considered at least a semiemergency. The most useful test for rapid diagnosis of HSV is a smear of material obtained from a skin vesicle that is fixed and stained with monoclonal antibodies to HSV, which are commercially available. This test is simple to perform and highly sensitive and accurate; results can be available within an hour and will indicate if the virus is type 1 or type 2. Cultures for virus should also be performed, but this will often take as long as 48 hours to be completed. PCR, if available, can also be useful for diagnosis.

Babies in whom the diagnosis is established or who are strongly suspected of having neonatal HSV should be further tested for the possibility of disseminated infection and involvement of the central nervous system (CNS). Usually this means performing liver function tests, an ophthalmologic examination, lumbar puncture, and magnetic resonance imaging (MRI) or computed tomography (CT) scan. These tests usually need to be repeated after 1–2 weeks, with the first battery of tests often serving as a base-line.

179. How should women with a past history of genital herpes be screened during pregnancy?

Until fairly recently, it was thought that women with frequent reactivation episodes of genital HSV were at greatest risk to deliver an infected infant and that they should, therefore, be screened for HSV infection during pregnancy. Prospective studies, however, indicate that the infant at greatest risk to develop neonatal HSV is born to a woman with primary asymptomatic genital HSV at term. The risk of infection of the infant is only about 2% in mothers with recurrent HSV but 50% in those with primary HSV at term. Therefore, the women who should be screened at term are those who have no history of past HSV and who feel well. Unfortunately, however, there is still no good screening test for these women. Obtaining viral cultures on so many women is impractical and expensive. PCR does not necessarily indicate the presence of infectious HSV and in any case is not widely available. It is now possible to determine whether a woman has been infected with HSV type 2 in the past by a special antibody test. Women lacking antibodies to the glycoprotein G of HSV 2 are considered susceptible and are at risk to develop primary infection with this virus. However, the best screening test for prevention of severe neonatal HSV is a high index of suspicion when an infant develops vesicular skin lesions. There is no real need to screen women with a past history of genital HSV because these women are at very little risk to deliver an infected baby.

180. How is neonatal HSV classified, and what is the importance of the classification with regard to prognosis?

Clinically, the infection is divided into three categories: (1) skin, eye, or mouth (SEM) involvement; (2) disseminated infection that has extended to the viscera, especially the liver and lungs; and (3) CNS involvement. Even with appropriate antiviral therapy, the prognosis for infants with disseminated HSV and CNS disease is much poorer with regard to morbidity and mortality than infants who have infection confined to the SEM. It is believed that early therapy with acyclovir (ACV) to infants with SEM disease can prevent much of disseminated and CNS disease. Therefore, it is recommended that all infants with skin lesions due to HSV, even if they are otherwise well, be treated with ACV.

Typing of the infecting virus is also important because type 1 infections have a better prognosis than type 2 infections. Most infants with encephalitis due to type 1 HSV have a good long-term prognosis, whereas those with HSV 2 encephalitis do not.

181. What is the differential diagnosis for an infant with clinical signs of meningitis and sepsis whose cultures for bacteria are negative?

Two viral infections need to be considered. The first is **disseminated HSV with CNS involvement**. One helpful diagnostic clue is the development of skin vesicles, which can also be used as a source from which to isolate virus for diagnosis. However, about 20% of babies with this form of HSV never develop skin vesicles. Other sources of virus for culture include respiratory secretions, blood, and CSF. The CSF should be cultured for virus although it is rare to isolate HSV from this source. If infection with HSV is strongly suspected, therapy with ACV can begin while viral cultures and other tests remain pending.

The other viral infection associated with such a severe neonatal syndrome is **enteroviral infection**, usually due to coxsackie virus or enteric cytopathic human orphan (ECHO) virus. Because both HSV and enterovirus infections of the neonate are related to maternal infection, it is important to obtain a history from the mother, examine her, and perform viral cultures on her throat, rectum, and genitalia. Acute and convalescent antibody titers for HSV and enteroviruses may also be useful, particularly if an enterovirus is isolated from her stool. At present there is no therapy for enterovirus infections of the newborn, but because antiviral drugs are now being developed, it is important to be aware of this infection.

182. What is the usual pathogenesis of HSV infections that present in the newborn?

Most often, the virus multiplies on the mucosa of the maternal genital tract, and the baby is infected during the vaginal delivery. In only about 5% of infections does it appear that the virus crossed the placenta and caused congenital rather than neonatal infection. If the diagnosis of maternal primary HSV is known at delivery and the membranes are not ruptured, infections in infants can be prevented by performing a cesarean section. The chances of infection of the infant are increased if the skin is broken for any reason (e.g., from a scalp monitor).

Infants also can be infected with HSV type 1 if a mother has primary active HSV 1 infection, usually in the throat and mouth, at delivery. Presumably in this case, infection of the infant occurs from close maternal contact, such as kissing the baby, and aerosols.

Once the virus has infected the infant, it is thought to multiply locally and then disseminate by viremia.

183. What is the treatment for neonatal HSV?

The treatment is administration of intravenous ACV to all infants in whom the diagnosis of neonatal HSV is either established or pending diagnostic results. ACV is an antiviral drug that interferes with the replication of HSV DNA by acting as a chain terminator and interfering with the action of DNA polymerase. Because its action occurs mainly in infected cells, it is very well tolerated. Early therapy with ACV has decreased mortality and morbidity from serious HSV infections by 30–50%. Even more importantly, although it is difficult to quantitate, treatment of babies with minimal involvement (SEM) prevents dissemination of the virus and severe infections from developing. ACV is usually administered at a dosage of 30 mg/kg/day IV for 14–21 days, depending on the condition of the infant.

184. How should infants with neonatal HSV be followed after treatment?

Follow-up is best individualized. Most asymptomatic infants should have a CT or MRI scan at some point following completion of therapy and discharge, usually after 4–6 weeks. Infants with symptoms such as recurrent skin vesicles, developmental delay, or seizures may have scans performed after a shorter interval. Infants who develop new or recurring symptoms should have a lumbar puncture for examination of the CSF. Those with CSF abnormalities or in whom the PCR remains positive should probably receive another course of intravenous ACV and be followed up closely again after the second discharge. Infants suspected of having continued low-grade replication of HSV in the CNS may be given oral ACV on a long-term basis.

185. How safe is long-term therapy with acyclovir for an infant?

This therapy is considered an off-label use of ACV, and it needs to be discussed carefully with the parents. Long-term therapy is used by some physicians who suspect that low-grade multiplication of HSV in the CNS is ongoing. This form of therapy is not of proven use, but intuitively it makes sense. The dose is 300 mg/m^2, three times a day, orally. Monitoring for toxicity, particularly on the bone marrow, is important and should be performed every 1–2 weeks while the medication is being administered. The usual duration of long-term therapy is several months. Although short-term safety seems not to be a problem (dosage can be lowered if toxicity occurs), long-term safety is unknown.

186. How should infants born to women with active recurrent genital HSV infection be managed?

This remains somewhat controversial. Some obstetricians perform a cesarean section on any woman at term known to have active genital HSV. Others no longer recommend cesarean section in women with known recurrent HSV because the risk of infection to the infant is very low—about 2%.

187. Are antibody titers useful for diagnosis of HSV, and what are their limitations?

Antibody titers are of little use for diagnosis of HSV because it takes at least several days after infection for antibodies to rise. Therefore, it is preferable to demonstrate the presence of virus or viral antigens or DNA in tissues for diagnosis. In instances when no virus can be demonstrated, antibody titers may be useful. Ideally, acute and convalescent sera (10–14 days apart) from mother and baby should be obtained. In addition to examining these sera for antibodies to HSV, antibodies to other congenital and neonatal pathogens such as toxoplasmosis and cytomegalovirus can be measured. Practically speaking, however, by the time it becomes clear that antibody titers might be useful, the acute serum samples have already been discarded.

It is now possible to identify women who have not been infected with HSV 2 previously by measuring antibodies to a HSV antigen that is not shared between type 1 and type 2 (glycoprotein G). Commercial availability of this assay is gradually increasing.

VARICELLA-ZOSTER VIRUS

188. What is the congenital varicella syndrome?

This congenital syndrome is usually associated with maternal varicella between 8 and 20 weeks of pregnancy. Transmission of varicella-zoster virus (VZV) from mother to infant occurs in 25–50% of cases of infected mothers. Fortunately, however, the syndrome is much less common than fetal infection. The syndrome in the infant occurs in only about 2% of cases of maternal chickenpox. Common manifestations of the syndrome include skin scarring (either generalized or localized in a dermatomal distribution), limb deformities (such as hypoplasia or missing digits), eye involvement (such as chorioretinitis, cataract, nystagmus, and hypoplasia), low birth weight, and mental retardation. Reactivation of VZV acquired in utero is a common event. Thus, zoster develops in about 20% of infants with the congenital syndrome in the first few years of life. The presence of antibodies to virus VZV in a baby over 8 months old would distinguish between actual infection of the infant with VZV and presence of transplacental antibodies. However, the presence of these antibodies indicates infection but not necessarily the syndrome. It is hoped that as the rubella vaccine has nearly eliminated congenital rubella, the varicella vaccine will make the congenital varicella syndrome even more rare.

189. What is the appropriate management of an infant born to a woman with varicella at term delivery?

Infants whose mothers have the onset of the rash of varicella within 4 days prior to delivery and within 2 days postpartum have about a 50% chance of also developing varicella. In as many as 30% of infants who are untreated, the varicella may be disseminated and even fatal. This form of varicella resembles that seen in highly immunocompromised patients such as children with leukemia receiving chemotherapy. It is possible to prevent this severe form of infant varicella by administering varicella-zoster immune globulin (VZIG) to the baby as soon as possible after birth. Rarely, VZIG may be ineffective in infants, so babies given this prophylaxis warrant close follow-up. Many will develop a mild form of clinical varicella with less than 100 skin vesicles despite VZIG. Indications for adding antiviral therapy (acyclovir) are extensive skin lesions and development of pneumonia, which suggests severe varicella. It is thought that an important element of risk to the infant is VZV infection across the placenta during the time of maternal viremia. Therefore, infants whose mothers develop varicella more than 2 days postpartum are at significantly less risk from varicella and do not require VZIG, although some physicians may elect to administer it. In this case, infection of the infant would not be from exposure to VZV in utero, but from postpartum exposure. Infants whose mothers had the onset of varicella more than 5 days prior to delivery do not need to receive VZIG because they will have developed sufficient transplacental VZV antibodies by this time (as if nature provided them with a dose of VZIG). With regard to isolation of infants perinatally exposed to VZV, there are two points to consider:

    1. The incubation period can be as short as 10 days and is counted from the time of onset of maternal rash.

    2. Infants are contagious only around the time when rash is expected to occur.

190. What is the appropriate management of an infant born to a woman with zoster at term?

There is almost no chance that such an infant will develop varicella, and no special management is required. Women with zoster have high antibody titers to VZV, and their infants are well protected from the virus by transplacental antibodies.

191. When is it appropriate to administer acyclovir to a pregnant woman with chickenpox?

There is no question that varicella in adults tends to be more severe than in children. Although the data are far from conclusive, most experts believe that varicella in pregnant women is likely to be more severe than in nonpregnant women, especially in the third trimester of pregnancy. Therefore, pregnant women with varicella should be closely observed, particularly for development of primary pneumonia. Pneumonia usually presents with fever, cough, dyspnea, and bilateral fluffy interstitial infiltrates on chest x-ray. Pregnant women with varicella pneumonia or even suspected varicella pneumonia should be treated with intravenous ACV (30 mg/kg/day, divided into three doses). Usually treatment is continued for 7 days. Maternal ACV therapy has not been associated with fetal malformations; nevertheless, it is advisable to avoid its use if possible. Orally administered ACV is not well absorbed and has demonstrated only modest success against varicella in clinical trials. Therefore, it is preferable to monitor pregnant women with varicella closely and to intervene if necessary with intravenous ACV, which is known to be effective if given early in the course of illness.

192. Should children be immunized against varicella when their mother, who has never had varicella, is pregnant?

Each instance is best individualized, weighing the potential risks and benefits to the mother. For example, in a family with several young, varicella-susceptible children who attend school or day care, there is a very high likelihood (estimated at 9% per child) that they will introduce chickenpox into the household while their mother is pregnant. In such a situation, it is preferable to immunize the children against chickenpox. Only about 5% of immunized children develop rash following immunization, and the infectivity of these children to others is extremely low. Should the vaccine virus nevertheless infect the mother, the illness is predicted to be mild, and no cases of the congenital varicella syndrome have been associated with vaccine-type VZV. In contrast, the wild-type VZV is highly contagious, so, if the children bring this virus home, maternal infection is inevitable, may be severe, and is known to be associated with a congenital syndrome. On the other hand, in the family in which there is only one child who is cared for at home and who has few visitors, it may be preferable to immunize the child after the mother is delivered. There would be no known risk to the newborn if the sibling developed a vaccine-associated rash.

CONGENITAL TOXOPLASMOSIS

193. You are scheduled to see a 3-month-old infant whose family recently moved to your community. The child is thriving with a normal birth history. This is the mother's second pregnancy. Both parents are healthy. During the third trimester of this pregnancy, the infant's mother reported having a systemic febrile illness associated with a swollen right cervical lymph node that was severe enough to prompt a visit to her family doctor. The enlarged

lymph node resolved over a 4-week interval. Mother is an avid gardener. They own no pets. The physical examination is normal except for a mild left eye strabismus, which is intermittent. You refer the patient to an ophthalmologist. He calls you a week later. On exam he sees pigmented macular lesions, left greater than right. He is concerned about toxoplasmosis. *Toxoplasma gondii*-specific IgG antibodies were detected in the infant's serum. What further evaluation is needed to establish the diagnosis of congenital toxoplasmosis?

Suggested Evaluation of the Infant Suspected of Having Congenital Toxoplasmosis

TESTS	RATIONALE/FINDING
Nonspecific tests	
Head circumference	Microcephaly
Ophthalmologic evaluation	Chorioretinitis?
	Cataract?
Neurologic evaluation	Psychomotor retardation?
Brain CT scan	Intracranial calcifications?
	Hydrocephalus?
Blood tests:	
CBC with differential and platelet counts	Anemia
	Eosinophilia
Serum total IgM, IgG, IgA, and albumin	To establish specific antibody load (see question 197)
Serum alanine aminotransferase, total and direct bilirubin	Jaundice
CSF cell count, glucose protein, and total IgG	Pleocytosis or elevated protein as newborn?
T. Gondii*-specific tests	
Infant/newborn serum tests:[†]	
Sabin-Feldman dye test	Detection of IgG antibodies
IgM ISAGA (immunosorbent agglutination assay)	Increased sensitivity for detection of IgM antibodies (best for newborns and infants < 6 months)
IgA EIA (enzyme immunoassay)	Useful to confirm IgM assays in pre-and postnatal diagnosis
IgE EIA/ISAGA	IgE antibodies generally indicate a more acute phase than IgM or IgA antibodies; useful in diagnosis of acute infection
Newborn blood (if prenatal suspicion) for inoculation into mice	This method is more sensitive than tissue culture but is slow (up to 6 weeks)
Lumbar puncture:[‡]	
Sabin-Feldman dye test	Detection of specific IgG antibodies in the CSF
IgM EIA	Same as above except IgM is detected
PCR (1 ml frozen and shipped dry ice)	Detection of *T. gondii* DNA in the CSF
Placental tissue (100 g in saline not frozen in cold packs)	Inoculation into mice as above
Maternal serum tests:	
Sabin-Feldman dye test	As above
IgM EIA	The EIA is used in adults versus ISAGA test above
IgA EIA	As above
IgE EIA/ISAGA	As above
AC/HS (differential agglutination)	Detects IgG antibodies. Helpful to differentiate acute from nonacute infection in adults.

* Recommend sending the Toxo Panel–Adult on the mother and Toxo Panel–Infants to Research Institute, Palo Alto Foundation, 860 Bryant Street, Palo Alto, CA 94301; Telephone: 650-853-4820; Fax 650-614-3292; Email: toxolab@pamfri.org

[†] Newborn serum 0.5–1 ml.

[‡] CSF, 1 ml for PCR testing shipped on dry ice by overnight courier.

194. How is the infection acquired in the mother?

Toxoplasma gondii is a protozoan parasite that exists in three developmental stages: tachyzoite, tissue cyst, and oocyst. Once infected with the tachyzoite, the organism may encyst commonly in the skeletal muscles. Ingestion of the oocyst, probably the most common route of infection, is found only in the intestinal tract of cats and other felines. Oocysts must mature or sporulate in the soil (at least 24 hours) before they are infectious.

Therefore, toxoplasma infection is acquired through ingestion of undercooked or raw meat containing tissue cysts or if water or other foods become contaminated by oocysts that have been excreted in the feces of infected cats. In the case above, the history reveals that the child's mother is an avid gardener and may have become infected through exposure to soil contaminated with cat feces.

The incidence of acute toxoplasmosis during pregnancy based on seroprevalence among women of child-bearing years is estimated at 0.2–1%. Transmission rates to the fetus depend on the stage of the pregnancy and treatment during pregnancy (see table).

	WITHOUT MATERNAL TREATMENT	WITH MATERNAL TREATMENT
1st trimester	10–15%	5%
2nd trimester	30%	17%
3rd trimester	60%	29%

Treatment during pregnancy consists of spiramycin throughout the remainder of the pregnancy. Pyrimethamine-sulfadiazine is alternated with spiramycin if fetal infection was confirmed by prenatal testing.

Wong SY, Remington JS: Toxoplasmosis in pregnancy. Clin Infect Dis 18:853–862, 1994.

195. If the newborn is infected, what are the signs and symptoms and the prognosis in congenital toxoplasmosis?

Congenital toxoplasmosis affects approximately 3500 newborns in the United States each year. Most infected newborns are born asymptomatic, and only on thorough evaluation can infection be suspected. The clinical manifestations of congenital toxoplasmosis include:

Intrauterine growth retardation	Strabismus
Developmental delay	Myocarditis
Encephalitis	Hydrops fetalis
Hydrocephalus	Thrombocytopenia
Intracranial calcifications	Eosinophilia
CSF pleocytosis	Nephrotic syndrome
Seizures	Hepatomegaly with calcification and jaundice
Deafness	Metaphyseal bone lucencies
Blindness	Interstitial pneumonia
Cataracts	Petechial purpura
Chorioretinal scars or chorioretinitis	Maculopapular rash
Nystagmus	

196. What is the treatment for neonates?

MEDICATION	DOSAGE
Sulfadiazine	100 mg/ml; half of the infant's weight (kg) equals number of milliliters given in A.M. and P.M.
Pyrimethamine	2 mg/ml; half of the infant's weight (kg) equals number of milliliters e given once daily.
Sulfadiazine	100 mg/ml; 10 mg (2 tablets) on Monday, Wednesday, and Friday. Crush and give with formula or apple juice.

The treatment is continued for approximately 12–14 months (consult infectious diseases expert). The dosage should be adjusted weekly. In addition, a CBC with differential should be done by finger stick twice weekly to measure the absolute neutrophil count. Remember pyrimethamine is a folic acid antagonist and therefore may cause thrombocytopenia, granulocytopenia, and anemia secondary to bone marrow suppression. The use of folinic acid can counteract this side effect.

197. If maternal infection is suspected but full evaluation for toxoplasmosis in the newborn is negative except for *T. gondii*-specific IgG antibodies, what is the best management plan?

In this case, transfer of maternal antibodies may be suspected if all other evaluations are negative. A monthly Sabin-Feldman dye test should be obtained from the infant to observe a fall in antibody titers over time (50% per month). One may calculate toxoplasma antibody load with the following formula:

Toxoplasma antibody load = (dye test titer × dye test sensitivity)/quantitative IgG

Here is an example of the expected fall in antibody titers in an infant without infection and transfer of maternal antibody only:

AGE (DAYS)	DYE TEST TITER	TEST SENSITIVITY*	QUANTITATIVE IMMUNOGLOBULINS (mg/dl)	ANTIBODY LOAD
10	1–16,000	0.2	886	3.61
28	1–8000	0.2	518	3.09
43	1–4096	0.2	427	1.92
67	1–2048	0.2	285	1.08
102	1–1024	0.2	255	.80
132	1–256	0.2	119	.43
189	1–64	0.2	209	.06

* Value obtained from Research Institute, Palo Alto Foundation

UREAPLASMA UREALYTICUM

198. What is the carriage rate of *Ureaplasma urealyticum* in the female lower genital tract?

Seventy percent, with a range of 40–80%. Colonization in adults is related to the number of sexual exposures but occurs in 50% of men and 70% of women with three or more partners.

199. What is the rate of vertical transmission for *U. urealyticum*, and what factors influence that rate?

The vertical transmission rate ranges from 25–60%. Transmission occurs in utero by ascending infection or during delivery through an infected birth canal. Preterm and VLBW infants are more likely to acquire *U. urealyticum* in their lower respiratory tract. The mode of delivery does not influence the rate of transmission, but it is increased in the presence of clinical intraamniotic infection and histologic chorioamnionitis and may be increased in the presence of prolonged rupture of membranes.

200. What are the clinical manifestations of *U. urealyticum* infection?

- It is the most common agent isolated when there is chorioamnionitis and is the most frequent isolate from placentas following preterm delivery.
- Several case reports and studies looking at radiographic changes and neutrophils in endotracheal aspirates suggest that *U. urealyticum* causes pneumonia in the newborn.
- Surfactant-deficient respiratory distress syndrome (RDS) is twice as frequent in premature infants < 34 weeks' gestation who have *U. urealyticum* isolated from the endotracheal aspirate. However, there is no association with superficial colonization.

- In two meta-analyses, *U. urealyticum* colonization was associated with a relative risk (RR) of chronic lung disease (CLD) of approximately 1.8. This increased RR has been borne out in the post-surfactant era. It is hypothesized that infection causes a subacute pneumonia and chronic damage. This is supported by the finding of increased levels of cytokines, IL-1-β and TNF-α in colonized VLBW infants.
- *U. urealyticum* has been isolated from CSF frequently. In the preterm population, it may be associated with hydrocephalus. There may not be a pleocytosis, and it may persist for weeks. Several case reports describe a clinical response to treatment.

201. How is *U. urealyticum* diagnosed?

Although usually limited to research settings, it is appropriate to sample endotracheal aspirates, blood, and CSF from the premature neonate, if available. The organism is fastidious and should be transported to the laboratory in special transport media and refrigerated if transport is not immediately possible.

- Culture is done in solid and liquid media.
- Polymerase chain reaction (PCR) using different nucleotide sequences has been done on neonatal specimens and is at least as sensitive as culture.
- Serologic diagnosis remains a research tool.

202. Does treatment of *U. urealyticum* prevent CLD?

Although numerous studies have demonstrated the association of colonization of the lower respiratory tract and CLD, several randomized, controlled trials have not demonstrated any decrease in the incidence of CLD after treating infants colonized with *U. urealyticum* with erythromycin.

TUBERCULOSIS

203. How do the fetus and newborn infant become infected with *Mycobacterium tuberculosis*?

The most common route of infection is hematogenously through the umbilical vessels from a focus in the placenta. Because the umbilical vessels transmit the *M. tuberculosis*, the primary complex is formed in the fetal liver and periportal lymph nodes. Other routes are aspiration or ingestion of infected amniotic fluid and by direct contact with infected cervix. The former usually presents with multiple primary focus in the gut, lungs, and middle ear. In the early postnatal period, the newborn also can be infected by the airborne route, which can be confused with true congenital tuberculosis. This route of infection is typical of what is seen in all other age groups with a primary focus in the lungs.

204. What are the criteria for diagnosing congenital tuberculosis?

Before antitubercular treatments were developed, Beitzke outlined strict criteria to diagnose congenital tuberculosis.

1. Tuberculosis in the child must be established firmly
2. There must be a primary complex in the liver, confirmation of which often requires autopsy
3. If the primary complex in the liver is undocumented or lacking, the tubercular lesions must be only a few days old and extrauterine infection must be excluded with certainty.

Recently Cantwell et al. proposed a new set of criteria for the diagnosis of congenital tuberculosis. The newborn should have proven tuberculous lesion along with at least one of the following:

1. Lesions in first week of life
2. A primary hepatic complex or caseating hepatic granuloma
3. Tuberculous infection of the placenta or maternal genital tract
4. Exclusion of the possibility of postnatal transmission by thorough investigation of contacts of the child

205. What is the difference among tubercular exposure, infection, and disease?

Exposure is contact with the person with suspected or confirmed contagious pulmonary tuberculosis. Some of these patients develop positive PPD subsequently. Tubercular **infection** is defined as positive PPD test with x-ray that either is normal or reveals only granulomas or calcification in the lung or regional lymph nodes. **Disease** is defined as those patients with infection in whom signs and symptoms or x-ray manifestations of tuberculosis are apparent.

206. How does tuberculosis present in the newborn?

Congenital tuberculosis most commonly presents as hepatosplenomegaly and respiratory distress. These signs can be associated with nonspecific constitutional symptoms. Twenty percent may present with ear discharge. The disease should be suspected if the mother has tuberculosis or has symptoms that point toward tuberculosis. Postnatally acquired tuberculosis presents mainly with constitutional symptoms of fever, lethargy, weight loss, anorexia along with involvement of respiratory system. If untreated, the majority of newborns will progress to a severe form of disease such as meningitis or miliary tuberculosis within the first 2 years of life.

207. What is the approach to diagnose and treat a newborn whose mother has positive PPD?

The approach suggested by the Committee on Infectious Disease of the AAP follows:

MOTHER WITH POSITIVE PPD BUT THE FOLLOWING CONDITION	SEPARATION	MATERNAL TREATMENT	NEWBORN TREATMENT	HOUSEHOLD CONTACTS
Negative x-ray	No	Treat infection	No evaluation	PPD testing
Abnormal x-ray but no active disease	Yes, until mother is fully evaluated	Treat infection	Follow-up care	PPD testing
Abnormal x-ray but active disease	Yes, until mother is fully evaluated and receiving treatment until deemed non-contagious	Treat disease	Evaluation for congenital infection and HIV. If positive, treated and followed by PPD	Reporting to public health department, thorough investigations including PPD

208. What is the yield of *M. tuberculosis* from different specimens in children with perinatal tuberculosis?

SPECIMEN/PROCEDURE	YIELD*
Gastric aspirate	10/12 (83%)[†]
Liver biopsy	10/10 (100%)
Nodal biopsy	3/3 (100%)
Spinal fluid	2/7 (28%)
Aural discharge	1/2 (50%)
Tracheal aspirate	2/2 (100%)
Bone marrow	2/4 (50%)
Urine	1/2 (50%)
Nasopharyngeal secretions	1/1 (100%)

* Yield = number of positive results/total number.
† One specimen had only a positive smear.
Data from Hageman J, Shulman S, Schreiber M, et al: Congenital tuberculosis: Critical reappraisal of clinical findings and diagnostic procedures. Pediatrics 66:980, 1980.
From Smith MHD, Teele DW: Tuberculosis. In Remington JS, Klein JO (eds): Infectious Diseases of the Fetus and Newborn Infant. Philadelphia, W.B. Saunders, 1995, with permission.

209. How should tuberculosis be treated in the neonate?

Regimens include:

- A 2-month regimen of isoniazid (INH), rifampin, and pyrazinamide followed by INH and rifampin for 4 months
- A 9-month regimen of INH and rifampin

If drug resistance is suspected, at least one other agent (pyrazinamide, ethambutol, or streptomycin) should be included.

Suggested Dosages of Antituberculosis Drugs* for Neonates

DRUG	SIZES OF AVAILABLE PREPARATIONS	SINGLE DAILY DOSE (mg/kg)
INH tablets[†]	50, 100, 300	10–15
Rifampin capsules[‡]	150–300	10–20
Pyrazinamide tablets	500	20–30[§]
Ethambutol tablets	100, 400	15–25
Ethionamide tablets	250	15–20
Streptomycin for intramuscular use only	1- and 5-g vials	20–30

* Antituberculosis drugs are available without cost from most health departments once the physician has officially reported the case.
[†] Available for parenteral use and supplied in 10-ml vials containing 100 mg/ml.
[‡] Available for parenteral use in the United States. Consult Dow Chemical Co.
[§] This is the usually recommended dose; however, some clinicians who frequently use this drug for infants recommend a dose of 30–40 mg/kg to a maximal daily dose of 1.5 g.
From Smith MHD, Teele DW: Tuberculosis. In Remington JS, Klein JO (eds): Infectious Diseases of the Fetus and Newborn Infant. Philadelphia, W.B. Saunders, 1995, with permission.

210. How should tuberculosis be treated during pregnancy?

Both INH and ethambutol cross the placenta and are not teratogenic. Rifampin crosses the placenta, but it inhibits DNA-dependent RNA polymerase. Therefore, it has the potential to be teratogenic; however, no malformations have been observed. Streptomycin is ototoxic to the fetus. Treatment regimens for pregnant women generally consist of isoniazid, rifampin, and ethambutol for 1–2 months followed by rifampin and INH for 9 months. An alternative regimen is ethambutol and isoniazid for 18 months.

INFECTIOUS HEPATITIS

211. What are the common causes of infectious hepatitis in the neonate?

Several infectious agents can cause hepatitis of neonates and infants and include the TORCH pathogens: *Toxoplasma gondii*, **o**ther infectious etiologies (syphilis, hepatitis B, C, and D, and rarely hepatitis A virus [HAV]), **r**ubella, **c**ytomegalovirus (CMV), and **h**erpes simples I and II. Additional etiologies in this age group include generalized viral infections with adenovirus, coxsackievirus, enterovirus, Epstein-Barr virus (EBV), HIV, and varicella.

212. How is hepatitis B virus (HBV) transmitted?

HBV is transmitted by percutaneous or mucosal exposure to infectious body fluids, sexual contact, or perinatal transmission from an infected mother to her newborn. Women who are HBeAg-positive are more likely to transmit hepatitis (70–90% to their infants than women who are hepatitis B surface antigen (HBsAg)-positive only (5–20%).

213. What are the most helpful serologic assays to diagnose HBV?

Serologic tests can distinguish between acute and chronic infection and time of onset of infection with HBV (see table, next page). Hepatitis B early antigen (HBeAg) is present during acute infection, cleared during convalescence, and variably present in chronic disease. HBV DNA is best used to monitor response to treatment of chronic infection.

Interpretation of Hepatitis B Virus Serologic Test Results

HBsAG	IGM ANTI-HBc	TOTAL ANTI-HBc	ANTI-HBs	INTERPRETATION
+	–	–	–	Early HBV infection prior to anti-HB core response
+	+	+	–	Early HBV infection, onset within 6 mo
–	+	+	+ or –	Recent HBV infection, within 4–6 mo with resolution
+	–	+	–	HBV infection, onset ≥ 6 mo, probable chronic infection
–	–	–	+	HBV vaccine response
–	–	+	+	Past HBV infection, recovered

HBsAg = hepatitis B surface antigen; HBc = hepatitis B core antigen.
Adapted from Mahoney FJ: Update on diagnosis, management, and prevention of hepatitis B virus infection. Clin Microbiol Rev 12:351–366, 1999.

214. What are the best ways to prevent transmission of HBV from an infected mother to a newborn?

- Screening all pregnant women for hepatitis B
- Providing active immunization with hepatitis B vaccine and passive immunization with hepatitis B immunoglobulin (HBIG) within 12–24 hours of birth. Breast-feeding is not associated with increased risk.
- Routine immunization of all infants
- Vaccination of all 11–12-year-olds and high-risk adolescents

215. What are the complications of HBV?

Hepatic complications of hepatitis B include chronic active hepatitis and cirrhosis that can progress to liver failure and hepatocellular carcinoma. The risk of chronic infection is inversely related to age; as many as 90% of newborns, 30% of children 1–5 years of age, and 5–10% of older children may have persistence of HBsAg.

216. How is hepatitis C virus (HCV) transmitted, and how are the clinical manifestations different from hepatitis A and B?

Hepatitis C is transmitted by parenteral exposure to blood and blood products from a hepatitis C–infected person. Sexual transmission is less common. Approximately 5% of infected women transmit HCV to their neonates. Only 25% of patients are jaundiced, and liver function abnormalities are frequently less severe than those seen with HBV. However, 85% of persons infected with HCV develop persistent infection, and as many as 70% develop chronic hepatitis, 20% develop cirrhosis, and some may progress to hepatocellular carcinoma.

PARVOVIRUS

217. What percentage of women of child-bearing age are immune to parvovirus B19 infection?

Approximately 50%. This means that B19 infection in pregnancy is only a concern for about 50% of pregnant women, because previous infection confers immunity. Immunity can be assessed by screening for parvovirus B19 IgG antibody. If exposure to *Parvovirus* or clinical signs or symptoms suggestive of B19 infection occur during pregnancy in a woman with unknown B19 status, both IgG and IgM anti-B19 antibodies should be measured to determine whether recent infection has occurred.

218. If B19 infection occurs during pregnancy, what is the risk for an adverse fetal outcome (i.e., nonimmune hydrops fetalis or fetal demise)?

Less than 10%. When intrauterine B19 infection associated with hydrops was first described, a high risk for fetal complications following maternal infection was emphasized. With prospective follow-up of a large number of women with B19 infection in pregnancy, adverse fetal outcome appears to be the exception, not the rule. Harger et al. reported no fetal or neonatal deaths attributable to B19 infection in 52 IgM-positive women, and the calculated frequency of hydrops and death from B19 infection is 0–8.6% (95% CI). These data are similar to data from other prospective studies.

Obstetric follow-up of women with B19 infection usually relies on frequent ultrasound examinations in the weeks following infection. Based on the low risk for adverse outcomes, Harger et al. suggest brief "screening" ultrasound to detect fetal ascites or other early signs of nonimmune hydrops with full exams only if abnormalities are detected.

Harger JH, Adler SP, Koch WC, Harger GF: Prospective evaluation of 618 pregnant women exposed to parvovirus B19: Risks and symptoms. Obstet Gynecol 91:413–420, 1998.

219. You get a call from a worried mother of a 2-year-old patient. The family puppy was just diagnosed with parvovirus hemorrhagic colitis. She is concerned about possible transmission to her toddler or herself (she is 3 months pregnant). What advice do you give?

Not to worry. Canine parvovirus is not a human pathogen!

220. Parvovirus B19 is the cause of erythema infectiosum (EI). How often do children or adults infected with B19 develop classic EI?

Classic EI with "slapped cheeks" appearance followed by a characteristic lacy or reticular rash on the trunk and limbs is fairly easy to diagnose clinically. Unfortunately, most individuals infected with B19 do not develop classic EI. A nondiagnostic exanthem may be present in approximately one-third to one-half of infections. In the study by Harger et al., 38% of B19-infected women manifested rash; none were clinically diagnosed as EI. In adults, especially women, joint symptoms occur in 60–80% of cases and may be helpful diagnostically. The clinical illness in adults, with fever, rash, and joint symptoms, mimics rubella.

221. Why does B19 infection cause aplastic anemia in patients with hemolytic anemia?

Parvoviruses require actively dividing cells to replicate, and B19 preferentially infects RBC precursors. In patients with hemolytic anemia and a high RBC turnover, the viral cytopathic effect destroys bone marrow RBC precursors, resulting in reticulocytopenia. The transient arrest of erythrocyte production results in profound anemia in individuals with a shortened RBC survival, such as patients with hemolytic anemia. In fetuses, shortened RBC survival (60–80 days vs. 110–120 days in adults) also contributes to the severity of anemia in some cases.

BIBLIOGRAPHY

Developmental Immunology
1. Erdman SH, Christensen RD, Bradley PP, Rothstein GJ: Supply and release of storage neutrophils: A developmental study. Biol Neonate 41:132–137, 1982.
2. Speer CP, Johnston RB: Neutrophil function in newborn infants. In Polin RA, Fox WW (eds): Fetal and Neonatal Physiology, 2nd ed. Philadelphia, W.B. Saunders, 1998, p 1958.
3. Stiehm ER (ed): Immunologic Disorders in Infants and Children, 3rd ed. Philadelphia, W.B. Saunders, 1989.
4. Yoder MC, Polin RA: Developmental immunology. In Fanaroff AA, Martin RJ (eds): Neonatal-Perinatal Medicine, 6th ed. St. Louis, Mosby, 1997, pp 685–717.

Early-Onset Neonatal Sepsis
5. Eichenwald EC: Perinatally transmitted neonatal bacterial infections. Infect Dis Clin North Am 11:223–239, 1997.
6. Hickman ME, Rench MA, Ferrieri P, Baker CJ: Changing epidemiology of group B streptococcal colonization. Pediatrics 104:203–209, 1999.
7. Kaftan H, Kinney JS: Early onset neonatal bacterial infections. Semin Perinatol 22:17, 1998.
8. Stoll BJ, Gordon T, Korones SB, et al: Early-onset sepsis in very low birth weight neonates: A report from the National Institute of Child Health and Human Development Neonatal Research Network. J Pediatr 129:72–80, 1996.

Nosocomial Sepsis
9. Schuchat A, Zywicki SS, Dinsmoor MJ, et al: Risk factors and opportunities for prevention of early-onset neonatal sepsis: A multicenter case-control study. Pediatrics 105:21–26, 2000.

10. Stoll BJ, Gordon T, Korones S, et al: Late-onset sepsis in very low birth weight neonates: A report from the NICHD Neonatal Research Network. J Pediatr 129:63–71, 1996.

11. Stoll BJ, Holman RC, Schuchat A, et al: Decline in sepsis-associated neonatal and infant deaths in the United States, 1979 through 1994. Pediatrics 102:E18, 1994.

12. Stoll BJ, Temprosa M, Tyson JE, et al: Dexamethasone therapy increases infection in very low birth weight infants. Pediatircs 104:E63, 1999.

Diagnosis of Neonatal Sepsis

13. Benitz WE, Han MY, Madan A, Ramachandra P: Serial serum C-reactive protein levels in the diagnosis of neonatal infection. Pediatrics 102:E41, 1998.

14. Gerdes JS: Clinicopathologic approach to the diagnosis of neonatal sepsis. Clin Perinatol 18:361–381, 1991.

15. Lieberman E, Lang J, Richardson DK, et al: Intrapartum maternal fever and neonatal outcome. Pediatrics 105:8–13, 2000.

16. Powell K, Marcy M: Laboratory aids in the diagnosis of neonatal sepsis. In Remington JS, Klein JO (eds): Infectious Diseases of the Fetus and Newborn Infant, 4th ed. Philadelphia, W.B. Saunders, 1995.

Antimicrobial Therapy

17. Edwards MS, Baker CJ: Nosocomial infections in the newborn. In Long SS, Pickering LK, Prober CG (eds): Principles and Practice of Pediatric Infectious Diseases. New York, Churchill Livingstone, 1997, pp 619–625.

18. Klein JO, Marcy SM: Bacterial sepsis and meningitis. In Remington JS, Klein JO (eds): Infectious Diseases of the Fetus and Newborn Infant, 4th ed. Philadelphia, W.B. Saunders, 1995, pp 835–890.

19. Young TE, Magnum OB (eds): Neofax: A Manual of Drugs Used in Neonatal Care, 12th ed. Raleigh, NC, Acorn Publishing, 1999.

Group B Streptococcal Infections

20. Lim K, Clemens J, Azimi P, et al: Capsular polysaccharide types of group B streptococcal isolates from neonates with early-onset systemic infection. J Infect Dis 177:790–792, 1998.

21. Schrag SJ, Zywicki S, Farley MM, et al: Group B streptococcal disease in the era of intrapartum antibiotic prophylaxis. N Engl J Med 342:15–20, 2000.

22. Schuchat A: Epidemiology of group B streptococcal disease in the United States: Shifting paradigms. Clin Microbiol Rev 11:497–513, 1998.

Staphylococcus epidermidis

23. Baier RJ, Bocchini JA, Brown EG: Selective use of vancomycin to prevent coagulase-negative staphylococcal nosocomial bacteremia in high-risk very low birth weight infants. Pediatr Infect Dis J 17:179–183, 1998.

24. Baltimore RS: Neonatal nosocomial infections. Semin Perinatol 22:25–32, 1998.

Candida

25. Butler KM, Baker CJ: *Candida:* An increasingly important pathogen in the nursery. Pediatr Clin North Am 35:543–563, 1988.

26. Harris MC, Bell LM, Pereira GR, et al: Candidal arthritis in infants previously treated for systemic candidiasis during the newborn period: Report of three cases. Pediatr Emerg Care 16:249–251, 2000.

27. Hughes WT, Flynn PM: Candidiasis. In Feigin RD, Cherry JD (eds): Textbook of Pediatric Infectious Diseases, 4th ed. Philadelphia, W.B. Saunders, 1998, pp 2303–2313.

28. Mittal M, Dhanireddy R, Higgins RD: Candida sepsis and association with retinopathy of prematurity. Pediatrics 101:654–657, 1998.

White Cell Functional Disorders

29. Johnston RB: Function and cell biology of neutrophils and mononuclear phagocytes in the newborn infant. Vaccine 16:1363–1368, 1998.

30. Speer C, Johnston RB: Neutrophil function in newborn infants. In Polin RA, Fox WW (eds): Fetal and Neonatal Physiology, 2nd ed. Philadelphia, W.B. Saunders, 1997, pp 1954–1998.

Immunotherapy

31. Jenson HB, Pollock BH: The role of intravenous immunoglobulin for the prevention and treatment of neonatal sepsis. Semin Perinatol 22:6–13, 1998.

32. Lauterbach R, Pawlik D, Kowalczyk D, et al: Effect of immunomodulating agent, pentoxifylline, in the treatment of sepsis in prematurely delivered infants: A placebo-controlled, double-blind trial. Crit Care Med 27:807–814, 1999.

33. Neu J, Roig JC, Meetze WH, et al: Enteral glutamine supplementation for very low birth weight infants decreases morbidity. J Pediatr 131:691–699, 1997.

Neonatal Meningitis

34. Wiswell TE, Baumgart S, Gannon CM, Spitzer AR: No lumbar puncture in the evaluation for early neonatal sepsis: Will meningitis be missed? Pediatrics 95:803–806, 1995.

Infection Control
35. American Academy of Pediatrics: 1997 Red Book: Report of the Committee on Infectious Diseases, 24th ed. Elk Grove Village, IL, AAP, 1997.
36. Bennett JV, Brachman PS: Hospital Infections. Boston, Little, Brown, 1992.
37. Mayhall CG: Hospital Epidemiology and Infection Control. Baltimore, Williams & Wilkins, 1996.

Conjunctivitis
38. de Toledo AR, Chandler JW: Conjunctivitis of the newborn. Infect Dis Clin North Am 6:807–813, 1992.
39. Hammerschlag MR: Neonatal conjunctivitis. Pediatr Ann 22:346–351, 1993.
40. Hammerschlag MR, Cummings C, Roblin PM, et al: Efficacy of neonatal ocular prophylaxis for the prevention of chlamydial and gonococcal conjunctivitis. N Engl J Med 320:769–772, 1989.

Chlamydia Infections
41. American Academy of Pediatrics: Chlamydial infections. In Pickering LK (ed): 2000 Red Book: Report of the Committee on Infectious Diseases, 24th ed. Elk Grove Village, IL, AAP, 2000, pp 205–212.
42. Hammerschlag MR: *Chlamydia trachomatis* in children. Pediatr Ann 23:349–353, 1994.
43. Hammerschlag MR, Gelling M, Roblin PM, et al: Treatment of neonatal chlamydial conjunctivitis with azithromycin. Pediatr Infect Dis J 17:1049–1050, 1998.
44. Hammerschlag MR, Rawstron SA: Sexually transmitted infection. In Jenson HB, Baltimore RS (eds): Pediatric Infectious Diseases: Principles and Practice. Norwalk, CT, Appleton & Lange, 1995, pp 1249–1276 .
45. Normann E, Gnarpe J, Gnarpe H, Wettergren B: *Chlamydia pneumoniae* in children with acute respiratory tract infections. Acta Paediatr 87:23–27, 1998.

Osteomyelitis and Septic Arthritis
46. Asmar BI: Osteomyelitis in the neonate. Infect Dis Clin North Am 6:124–125, 1992.
47. Jaramillo D, Treves ST, Kasser JR, et al: Osteomyelitis and septic arthritis in children: Appropriate use of imaging to guide treatment. AJR Am J Roentgenol 165:399–403, 1995.
48. Ogden J, Lister G: The pathology of neonatal osteomyelitis. Pediatrics 55:474–478, 1975.
49. Swanson H, Hughes P, Messer SA, et al: *Candida albicans* arthritis one year after successful treatment of fungemia in a healthy infant. J Pediatr 129:688–694, 1996.
50. Trujillo M, Nelson JD: Suppurative and reactive arthritis in children. Semin Pediatr Infect Dis 8:242–249, 1997.
51. Unkila-Kallio L, Kallio MJ, Eskola J, Peltola H: Serum C-reactive protein: Erythrocyte sedimentation rate and white blood cell count in acute hematogenous osteomyelitis of children. Pediatrics 93:59–61, 1994.
52. Wong M, Isaacs D, Howman-Giles R, Uren R: Clinical and diagnostic features of osteomyelitis occurring in the first three months of life. Pediatr Infect Dis J 14:1047–1053, 1995.

Pyelonephritis and Urinary Tract Infection
53. Jakobsson B, Berg U, Svensson L: Renal scarring after acute pyelonephritis. Arch Dis Child 70:111–115, 1994.
54. Klein JO, Long SS: Bacterial infections of the urinary tract. In Remington JS, Klein JO (eds): Infectious Diseases of the Fetus and Newborn Infant, 4th ed. Philadelphia, W.B. Saunders, 1995, pp 925–934.

Impetigo
55. Darmstadt GL, Lane A: Cutaneous bacterial infections. In Behrman RE, Kliegman RM, Arvin AM, Nelson WE (eds): Nelson Textbook of Pediatrics, 15th ed. Philadelphia, W.B. Saunders, 1996, pp 1889–1891.
56. Darmstadt GL: Oral antibiotic therapy for uncomplicated bacterial skin infections in children. Pediatr Infect Dis J 16:227–240, 1997.
57. Feingold DS: Staphylococcal and streptococcal pyodermas. Semin Dermatol 12:331–335, 1993.
58. Freij BJ, McCracken GH: Acute infections. In Avery GB, Fletcher MA, MacDonald MG (eds): Neonatology: Pathophysiology and Management of the Newborn, 5th ed. Philadelphia, Lippincott Williams & Wilkins, 1999, pp 1212–1213.
59. Marcy SM, Klein JO: Focal bacterial infections. In Remington JS, Klein JO (eds): Infectious Diseases of the Fetus and Newborn Infant, 3rd ed. Philadelphia, W.B. Saunders, 1990, pp 722–728.
60. Margileth AM: Dermatologic conditions. In Avery GB, Fletcher MA, MacDonald MG (eds): Neonatology: Pathophysiology and Management of the Newborn, 5th ed. Philadelphia, Lippincott Williams & Wilkins, 1999, pp 1345–1347.
61. Melish ME, Bertuch AA: Bacterial skin infections. In Feigin RD, Cherry JD (eds): Textbook of Pediatric Infectious Diseases, 4th ed. Philadelphia, W.B. Saunders, 1998, pp 741–745.
62. Saiez-Llorens X, McCracken GH: Perinatal bacterial diseases. In Feigin RD, Cherry JD (eds): Textbook of Pediatric Infectious Diseases, 4th ed. Philadelphia, W.B. Saunders, 1998, p 917.
63. Sam EE, Esterly NB: The skin. In Fanaroff AA, Martin RJ (eds): Neonatal-Perinatal Medicine: Diseases of the Fetus and Infant, 6th ed. St. Louis, Mosby, 1997, pp 1648–1649.

64. Shinefeld HR: Staphylococcal infections. In Remington JS, Klein JO (eds): Infectious Diseases of the Fetus and Newborn Infant, 4th ed. Philadelphia, W.B. Saunders, 1995, pp 878–879.
65. Siegfried EC, Shah PY: Skin care practices in the neonatal nursery: A clinical survey. J Perinatol 19:31–39, 1999.
66. Tunnessen WW: Bacterial infections of the skin: Symposium on pediatric dermatology. Pediatr Clin North Am 30:515–532, 1983.
67. Tunnessen WW: Practical aspects of bacterial skin infections in children. Pediatr Dermatol 2:255–265, 1985.

Omphalitis
68. Brook I: Microbiology of necrotizing fasciitis associated with omphalitis in the newborn infant. J Perinatol 18:28–30, 1998.
69. Cushing AH: Omphalitis: A review. Pediatr Infect Dis 4:282–285, 1985.
70. Faridi MMA, Rattan A, Ahmed SH: Omphalitis neonatorum. J Ind Med Assoc 91:283–285, 1993.
71. Guvenc H, Aygun AD, Uysar P, et al: Omphalitis in term and preterm appropriate for gestational age and small for gestational age infants. J Trop Pediatr 43:368–372, 1997.
72. Hartman GE, Boyajian MJ, Choi SS, et al: General surgery. In Avery GB, Fletcher MA, MacDonald MG (eds): Neonatology: Pathophysiology and Management of the Newborn, 5th ed. Philadelphia, Lippincott Williams & Wilkins, 1999, pp 1036–1037.
73. Mason WH, Andrews R, Ross LA, Wright HT: Omphalitis in the newborn infant. Pediatr Infect Dis J 8:521–525, 1989.
74. Meberg A, Schoyen R: Hydrophobic material in routine umbilical cord care and prevention of infections in newborn infants. Scand J Infect Dis 22:729–733, 1990.
75. Monu JUV, Okola AA: Diffuse abdominal wall cellulitis in ascending omphalitis: A lethal association in neonatal necrotizing fasciitis. J Natl Med Assoc 85:457–459, 1993.
76. Nezelof C: Chronic omphalitis in a 4-month-old girl. Path Res Pract 187:334–337, 1991.
77. Oudesluys-Murphy AM, Eilers GAM, deGroot CJ: The time of separation of the umbilical cord. Eur J Pediatr 146:387–389, 1987.
78. Samuel M, Freeman NV, Vaishnav A, et al: Necrotizing fasciitis: A serious complication of omphalitis in neonates. J Pediatr Surg 29:1414–1416, 1994.
79. Sawin RS, Schaller RT, Tapper D, et al: Early recognition of neonatal abdominal wall necrotizing fasciitis. Am J Surg 167:481–484, 1994.

Listeriosis
80. Bortolussi R, Schlech WF: Listeriosis. In Remington JS, Klein JO (eds): Infectious Diseases of the Fetus and Newborn Infant, 4th ed. Philadelphia, W.B. Saunders, 1995.

Syphilis
81. American Academy of Pediatrics: 1997 Red Book: Report of the Committee on Infectious Diseases, 24th ed. Elk Grove Village, IL, AAP, 1997.
82. Sanchez PJ, Wendel GD: Syphilis in pregnancy. Clin Perinatol 24:71–90, 1997.
83. Sison CG, Ostrea EM, Reyes MP, Salari V: The resurgency of congenital syphilis: A cocaine-related problem. J Pediatr 130:289–292, 1997.

Human Immunodeficiency Virus
84. American Academy of Pediatrics Committee on Pediatric AIDS: Evaluation and medical treatment of the HIV-exposed infant. Pediatrics 99:909–917, 1997.
85. Centers for Disease Control and Prevention: Public Health Service Task Force recommendations for the use of antiretroviral drugs in pregnant women infected with HIV-1 for maternal health and for reducing perinatal HIV-1 transmission in the United States. MMWR 47:RR2, 1998.
86. Centers for Disease Control and Prevention: U.S. Public Health Service Recommendations for Human Immunodeficiency Virus Counseling and Voluntary Testing for Pregnant Women. Atlanta, CDC.
87. Centers for Disease Control and Prevention: Working Group on Antiretroviral Therapy and Medical Management of HIV-Infected Children: Guidelines for the use of antiretroviral agents in pediatric HIV infection. MMWR 47:1–43, 1998.

Cytomegalovirus
88. Volpe JJ (ed): Neurology of the Newborn, 4th ed. Philadelphia, W.B. Saunders, 1995.

Herpes Simplex Virus
89. Annunziato PW, Gershon A: Herpes simplex virus infections. Pediatr Rev 17:415–423, 1996.
90. Brown Z, Selke S, Zeh J, et al: The acquisition of herpes simplex during pregnancy. N Engl J Med 337:509–515, 1997.
91. Prober CG, Arvin AM: Perinatal herpes: Current status and obstetric management strategies: The pediatric perspective. Pediatr Infect Dis J 10:832–835, 1995.

Varicella-Zoster Virus
92. Enders G, Miller E, Cradock-Watson J, et al: Consequences of varicella and herpes zoster in pregnancy: Prospective study of 1739 cases. Lancet 343:1548–1551, 1994.
93. Gershon A: Chickenpox, measles, and mumps. In Remington JS, Klein JO (eds): Infectious Diseases of the Fetus and Newborn Infant, 4th ed. Philadelphia, W.B. Saunders, 1995.

Congenital Toxoplasmosis
94. Wong SY, Remington JS: Toxoplasmosis in pregnancy. Clin Inect Dis 18:853-862, 1994.

Ureaplasma urealyticum
95. Wang EE, Matlow AG, Ohlsson A, Nelson SC: *Ureaplasma urealyticum* infections in the perinatal period. Clin Perinatol 24:91–105, 1997.

Tuberculosis
96. Smith MHD, Teele DW: Tuberculosis. In Remington JS, Klein JO (eds): Infectious Diseases of the Fetus and Newborn Infant, 4th ed. Philadelphia, W.B. Saunders, 1995.
97. Starke JR: Tuberculosis: An old disease but a new threat to the mother, fetus, and neonate. Clin Perinatol 24:107, 1998.

Infectious Hepatitis
98. Fishman LN, Jonas MM, Lavine JE: Update on viral hepatitis in children. Pediatr Clin North Am 43:57-74, 1996.
99. Mahoney FJ: Hepatitis B virus. In Long SS, Pickering LK, Prober CG (eds): Principles and Practice of Pediatric Infectious Diseases. New York, Churchill Livingstone, 1997, pp 1194-1205.
100. Mahoney FJ: Update on diagnosis, management, and prevention of hepatitis B virus infection. Clin Microbiol Rev 12:351-366, 1999.
101. Snyder JD: Acute hepatitis. In Long SS, Pickering LK, Prober CG (eds): Principles and Practice of Pediatric Infectious Diseases. New York, Churchill Livingstone, 1997, pp 448-453.

Parvovirus
102. Harger JH, Adler SP, Koch WC, Harger GF: Prospective evaluation of 618 pregnant women exposed to parvovirus B19: Risks and symptoms. Obstet Gynecol 91:413–420, 1998.

12. NEUROLOGY

NEUROLOGIC EXAMINATION OF THE NEWBORN INFANT

1. What are the basic elements of the neonatal neurologic examination?

The neonatal neurologic exam in concept differs little from the examination of a child or an adult. The examiner desires to know how well the individual is able to function in his or her environment. The following are therefore tested:

- Mental status (level of alertness)
- Cranial nerves
- Motor and sensory function
- Primitive reflexes

Primitive reflexes are the one aspect that makes the neonate unique, because these are only seen during the newborn period.

2. What is the gestational age examination?

External physical and neurologic characteristics of the newborn are used to assess the newborn infant's gestational age. This examination is accurate to within 1–2 weeks of gestational age. The modified Ballard score is an example. One performs an examination and categorizes all the findings shown. The total score is then added to derive the approximate gestational age. These exams become slightly less accurate at the lower limits of viability, although recent modifications have attempted to address this problem.

3. What is the Ballard score?

The Ballard score, recently modified, is a simplified method of assessing neonatal maturity, based on characteristics found on the physical examination (see figure, next page).

4. What neonatal reflexes compete with the plantar reflex?

- **Contact avoidance** results in extension of the toes when the dorsum of the foot is stroked.
- **Nociceptive withdrawal** results in extension of the toes with flexion of the hip, knee, and ankle.
- **Plantar grasp** results in flexion of the toes with pressure on the distal aspect of the ball of the foot.
- **Positive supporting reaction** results in flexion of the toes to pressure on the plantar surface of the foot.

5. Is ankle clonus normal in the newborn infant?

Bilateral ankle clonus of 5–10 beats may be a normal finding, especially in infants who are crying, hungry, or jittery. This is particularly true if the clonus is unaccompanied by other signs of upper motor neuron dysfunction.

6. What is the size of mature newborn breast tissue?

Mature newborn breast tissue is > 1 cm on one or both sides. The less mature the infant is, the smaller the amount of breast tissue. Before 28 weeks' gestation, the breast bud is barely perceptible. In caring for premature infants, however, one should not forget that the breast tissue is present and that injury to the breast bud may cause problems later. Most commonly, the insertion of a chest tube to treat a tension pneumothorax in a female infant may cause a permanent deformity if the tube is inserted into this area. Because the areola may not be visible before 32 weeks' gestational age, care should be taken to avoid this easily preventable complication by not inserting tubes or needles in this region of the thorax.

Neuromuscular Maturity

	-1	0	1	2	3	4	5
Posture							
Square window (wrist)	> 90°	90°	60°	45°	30°	0°	
Arm recoil		180°	140°–180°	110° 140°	90°–110°	< 90°	
Popliteal angle	180°	160°	140°	120°	100°	90°	< 90°
Scarf sign							
Heel to ear							

Physical Maturity

								Maturity Rating	
Skin	Sticky, friable, transparent	Gelatinous, red, translucent	Smooth pink, visible veins	Superficial peeling &/or rash, few veins	Cracking, pale areas, rare veins	Parchment, deep cracking, no vessels	Leathery, cracked, wrinkled	**Score**	**Weeks**
Lanugo	None	Sparse	Abundant	Thinning	Bald areas	Mostly bald		-10	20
								-5	22
Plantar surface	Heel-toe 40–50 mm: -1 < 40 mm: -2	> 50 mm no crease	Faint red marks	Anterior transverse crease only	Creases ant. 2/3	Creases over entire sole		0	24
								5	26
Breast	Imperceptible	Barely perceptible	Flat areola, no bud	Stippled areola, 1–2 mm bud	Raised areola, 3–4 mm bud	Full areola, 5–10 mm bud		10	28
								15	30
Eye/ear	Lids fused loosely: -1 tightly: -2	Lids open pinna flat stays folded	Sl. curved pinna; soft; slow recoil	Well-curved pinna; soft but ready recoil	Formed & firm, instant recoil	Thick cartilage, ear stiff		20	32
								25	34
Genitals male	Scrotum flat, smooth	Scrotum empty, faint rugae	Testes in upper canal, rare rugae	Testes descending, few rugae	Testes down, good rugae	Testes pendulous, deep rugae		30	36
								35	38
Genitals female	Clitoris prominent, labia flat	Prominent clitoris, small labia minora	Prominent clitoris, enlarging minora	Majora & minora equally prominent	Majora large, minora small	Majora cover clitoris & minora		40	40
								45	42
								50	44

The Ballard scoring system. (From Ballard JL, Khoury JC, Wedig K, et al: New Ballard Score, expanded to include extremely premature infants. J Pediatr 119:417–423, 1991, with permission.)

7. What characteristic of the pinna of the ear is associated with immaturity?

Flexibility. The immature pinna is soft, flat, shapeless, and easily folded and does not recoil because of insufficient cartilage. The amount of cartilage present in the ear increases as gestational age increases.

8. At what gestational age are the testes usually descended into the scrotum and the scrotum covered with rugae?

By 38–40 weeks' gestational age, the testes should be well into the scrotum, and the scrotum should have rugae present. Many infants, however, particularly those in cold environments, will not have easily palpable testes, because they readily retract back into the inguinal canal. Careful milking of the testes along the route of the inguinal canal should enable the examiner to easily bring the testis back to the base of the scrotum.

9. Are there any simple confirmatory tests of gestational age that do not use a complex scoring system?

Examination of the vascularity of the anterior capsule of the lens by direct ophthalmoscopy is very simple and accurate. With increasing maturation, the vascularity of the anterior capsule decreases (see figure). This can be used to confirm the gestational age exam.

Grade 4	Grade 3	Grade 2	Grade 1
27 to 28 weeks	29 to 30 weeks	31 to 32 weeks	33 to 34 weeks

From Hittner H, Hirsch NJ, Rudolph AJ: Assessment of gestational age by examination of the anterior capsule of the lens. J Pediatr 91:455–458, 1977, with permission.

10. When does olfactory discrimination develop?

By 29–32 weeks of gestation, the majority of infants appear to demonstrate sucking or arousal/withdrawal to an olfactory stimulant.

11. What are the major etiologies of deafness in the newborn?

Parents often become aware of hearing loss in their child before it is apparent to the physician. Early intervention can be critical and assists in the development of speech and improved learning. It is, therefore, helpful for the neonatologist to screen any infants in the following groups on a routine basis:

- Low birth weight
- Congenital infections (rubella, toxoplasmosis, cytomegalovirus, syphilis, herpes)
- Toxins (including ototoxic antibiotics)
- Hyperbilirubinemia
- Hypoxic-ischemic encephalopathy
- Craniofacial anomalies
- Familial

12. What is the estimate of visual acuity of a full-term infant, and when does color vision develop?

Many parents ask this basic question. There appears to be an innate desire of mothers and fathers to have their infant recognize them as soon as possible. At birth, the newborn has at least 20/150 vision, and color vision develops at 2 months of age.

13. What is the difference between dysconjugate gaze and skew gaze?

Dysconjugate gaze is an abnormality in the horizontal plane, whereas skew gaze is an abnormality in the vertical plane. A small degree of dysconjugate gaze may be seen in a normal newborn infant, particularly after the child first awakens from sleeping. Dysconjugate gaze should disappear no later than 6 months of age. Persistence beyond this age, or evidence of dysconjugate gaze for longer periods during the day, should be referred to a pediatric ophthalmologist for evaluation.

14. Do newborns prefer to turn their heads to the right or left?

Healthy neonates prefer to turn their heads to the right, which may reflect the normal asymmetry of cerebral function at this age. This preference has been observed as early as 28 weeks' gestation. By 39 weeks' gestation, 90% of newborn infants spend about 80% of the time with the head turned to the right side.

15. When does the Moro reflex appear and disappear?

The Moro reflex is one of the most fascinating of the primitive reflexes. It is thought to be an evolutionary remnant that relates to the way that man's ancestors carried their infants. Monkeys and apes carry their young in front, and the young animal typically wraps its arms and legs around the mother. With movement, the young animal extends the arms and legs and tightens its grasp around the mother. In man, the Moro reflex begins to appear at about 30 weeks' post-conceptional age, is strongly present at birth in a full-term infant, begins to extinguish at around 3 months of life, and disappears by 6 months of age.

16. What is craniosynostosis? What are the different variations of this problem?

Craniosynostosis occurs when there is premature closure of a cranial suture resulting in the arrest of growth perpendicular to the affected suture.

Types of craniosynostosis and their appearance are:
- **Dolichocephaly**—sagittal synostosis (long, narrow head)
- **Brachycephaly**—coronal synostosis (wide head)
- **Acrocephaly**—coronal, sagittal, and lambdoidal synostosis (tower head)
- **Trigonocephaly**—metopic synostosis (pointed front of the head)

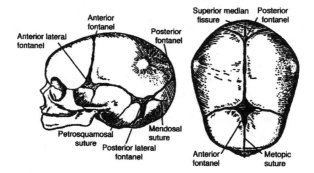

Normal cranial sutures. (From Silverman FN, Kuhn JP (eds): Caffey's Pediatric X-ray Diagnosis, 9th ed. St. Louis, Mosby, 1993, p 5, with permission.)

 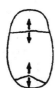

Normocephaly Dolichocephaly Trigonocephaly Plagiocephaly Plagiocephaly Brachycephaly

From Gorlin RJ: Craniofacial defects. In Oski FA, et al (eds): Principles and Practice of Pediatrics, 2nd ed. Philadelphia, J.B. Lippincott, 1994, p 508, with permission.

17. What are the normal cerebrospinal fluid (CSF) values for healthy neonates?

In the CSF examination of a group of high-risk neonates who did not have infection, the values (mean and range) were:

	TERM	PRETERM
WBC count (cells/mm^3)	8.2 (0–32)	9.0 (0–29)
Protein (mg/dl)	90 (20–170)	115 (65–150)
Glucose (mg/dl)	52 (34–119)	50 (24–63)
CSF/blood glucose (%)	81 (44–248)	74 (55–105)

18. When examining the sensory system, what clinical signs can be observed for painful stimuli in a neonate?

In response to painful stimuli, an infant can demonstrate changes in heart rate, blood pressure, respiration, motor phenomena (including withdrawal of the limb and facial grimacing), cry, and hormonal and metabolic changes. During surgery, these signs may be very important in assessing the adequacy of anesthesia for the procedure.

19. In newborns with facial paralysis, how is peripheral nerve involvement distinguished from central nerve involvement?

Peripheral injury usually results from compression of the peripheral portion of the nerve by prolonged pressure from the maternal sacral promontory. The use of forceps alone is not thought to be an important causative factor. Peripheral paralysis is unilateral. The forehead is smooth on the affected side, and the eye is persistently open.

Central nerve injury often results from contralateral CNS injury (temporal bone fracture or posterior fossa hemorrhage or tissue destruction). It involves only the lower half or two-thirds of the face. The forehead and eyelids are not affected.

In both forms of paralysis, the mouth is drawn to the normal side when crying, and the nasolabial fold is obliterated on the affected side.

THE SPINE

20. What are the presenting signs of cervical spinal cord injury in a neonate?

Spinal cord injury is fortunately an uncommon occurrence in neonates. It can occur, however, when excessive traction is applied to the neck during a difficult delivery, especially if there is shoulder dystocia. The presentation in a newborn consists of flaccid weakness of all four extremities with sparing of the face and cranial nerves.

21. When should an occult spinal dysraphism be suspected?

Occult spinal dysraphism should be suspected in children who have the following dorsal midline features:

• An abnormal collection of hair
• Cutaneous abnormalities (e.g., hemangioma or pigmented nevi)
• Cutaneous dimples or tracts or a subcutaneous mass on the lower back

In 80–90% of cases, there is an associated vertebral abnormality. The diagnosis should also be suspected in patients with symptoms of progressive lower extremity weakness or sensory loss, gait abnormalities, foot deformities, or neurogenic bowel and bladder problems.

EXTERNAL HEMORRHAGE

22. Following a difficult delivery, what three major forms of extracranial hemorrhage can occur?

Caput succedaneum, cephalohematoma, and subgaleal hemorrhage.

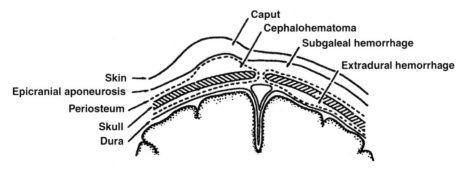

Types of traumatic external hemorrhage. (Adapted from Volpe JJ (ed): Neurology of the Newborn, 3rd ed. Philadelphia, W.B. Saunders, 1995, p 770, with permission.)

Major Varieties of Traumatic External Hemorrhage

LESION	FEATURES OF EXTERNAL SWELLING	INCREASES AFTER BIRTH	CROSSES SUTURE LINES	MARKED BLOOD LOSS
Caput succedaneum	Soft, pitting	No	Yes	No
Subgaleal hemorrhage	Firm, fluctuant	Yes	Yes	Yes
Cephalohematoma	Firm, tense (may calcify and later liquefy)	Yes	No	No

From Volpe JJ (ed): Neurology of the Newborn, 3rd ed. Philadelphia, W.B. Saunders, 1995, p 770, with permission.

23. If a cephalohematoma is suspected, should a skull x-ray be done to evaluate for fracture?
Cephalohematomas occur in up to 2.5% of live births. The incidence of associated fractures ranges from 5% to 25% in studies. These fractures are almost always linear and nondepressed and do not require treatment. Thus, in an asymptomatic infant with a cephalohematoma over the convexity of the skull and without suspicion of a depressed fracture, an x-ray is not necessary. If the exam suggests cranial depression or if neurologic signs are present, radiographic imaging is warranted.

INTRACRANIAL HEMORRHAGE

24. What are the major types of intracranial hemorrhage and their typical pathogenesis?
Subdural hemorrhage is usually caused by trauma, with more occurring in term than premature infants. Subdural bleeding is usually seen more commonly with forceps or vacuum extractions, compared with spontaneous vaginal deliveries or cesarean section births.

Intraventricular hemorrhage is usually the result of hypoxemic-ischemic events, most often seen in the premature baby and not in the term infant.

Intraparenchymal hemorrhage is usually the result of hypoxemic-ischemic events, most often seen in the premature baby and not in the term infant. These bleeds may be observed in term infants with intrauterine infarcts of the brain and neonatal stroke syndrome.

Subarachnoid hemorrhage is typically the result of hypoxemic-ischemic events. It is usually seen in the premature baby but occasionally can occur in association with trauma or aneurysm in the term infant.

Intracerebellar hemorrhage is often the result of hypoxemic-ischemic events, usually seen in the premature baby. It also may be seen with external compression of the occiput in premature infants. In term infants, this type of bleeding is uncommon but may result from traumatic birth injury.

25. How does the presentation of a congenital cerebral arterial aneurysm differ from that of an arteriovenous malformation?
The aneurysm presents with signs of acute increased intracranial pressure due to massive subarachnoid hemorrhage, often with sudden neurologic deterioration. There are often focal seizures and focal neurologic findings.

The most common arteriovenous malformation in the newborn is the vein of Galen malformation, which typically presents as congestive heart failure. Arteriovenous malformations that do not involve the vein of Galen typically present with signs of intracranial hemorrhage such as seizures, hydrocephalus, or brain stem signs.

26. What causes subarachnoid hemorrhage (SAH) in the newborn?
SAH in the neonate is believed to result from traumatic or hypoxic events that increase traction on or flow through small fragile vascular channels, which are the remnants of anastomoses present between the leptomeningeal arteries during brain development.

27. What are the three clinical presentations of SAH?

1. **Asymptomatic.** In most cases, only small amounts of hemorrhage have occurred and minimal or no clinical signs are present.

2. **Well baby with seizures.** In patients without significant hypoxic-ischemic encephalopathy, seizures secondary to SAH have their onset on the second day of life. In the interictal period, these babies appear well. They usually continue to appear well even after their seizure. These events usually leave little to no residual deficits.

3. **Catastrophic deterioration.** In rare instances, newborn infants with large SAHs follow a rapidly fatal course characterized by coma, respiratory disturbance, seizures, loss of brain stem reflexes, and flaccidity.

28. What is the site of origin of the intraventricular hemorrhage in the preterm infant?

Most neonatal intraventricular hemorrhage comes from the subependymal germinal matrix, a highly cellular region at the level of the head of the caudate nucleus, adjacent to the ventrolateral aspect of the lateral ventricles. This region is prominent in the developing fetus (23 weeks) and involutes by about 36 weeks of gestation. It is an area of the brain that is highly vascular and poorly supported by connective tissue, so bleeding readily occurs in the premature infant.

29. What is the procedure of choice for the diagnosis of germinal matrix–intraventricular hemorrhage and why?

Cranial ultrasound is a reliable, portable, safe, and cost-effective method for evaluating infants for intraventricular hemorrhage. Because it can be performed at the bedside with minimal disturbance of the infant, it has emerged as the study of choice since it was introduced in the 1980s.

30. What variables contribute to the development of intraventricular hemorrhage in the premature newborn?

Many of the following factors are simultaneously active and can lead to intraventricular hemorrhage in the premature neonate:

- Increased cerebral venous pressure associated with labor and delivery and altered or abnormal cardiorespiratory dysfunction
- Increased cerebral blood flow associated with systemic hypertension, volume expansion, and hypercarbia
- Fluctuating cerebral blood flow due to mechanical ventilation, hypotension with reperfusion, or presence of a patent ductus arteriosus (PDA)
- Coagulopathy due to thrombocytopenia and platelet dysfunction
- The immature, friable, and highly metabolic microvascular network in the germinal matrix

31. What are the major courses of progression of posthemorrhagic ventricular dilatation and their rates of occurrence?

Slowly progressive ventricular dilatation with spontaneous arrest (< 4 weeks)—65%
Persistent slowly progressive ventricular dilatation (> 4 weeks)—30%
Rapidly progressive—5%

Of the persistent slowly progressive group, about 67% will have arrest of progression whereas 33% will continue to progress. Of the spontaneous arrested groups, about 5% will have late progressive ventricular dilatation.

32. What are some of the various treatment options for intraventricular hemorrhage?

Close observation is the initial step in managing these conditions. Attention should be paid to the infant's clinical condition and the rate of head growth. Head growth greater than 1 cm/week is abnormal and deserves further investigation. Serial ultrasonography is used to monitor changes in ventricular size.

Serial LP is an effective treatment for posthemorrhagic hydrocephalus in some cases. This management approach can be used when there is communication between the lateral ventricles and the lumbar subarachnoid space. Typically, 10–15 ml/kg of CSF are removed with each therapeutic LP. This procedure should be monitored with cranial ultrasonography after each "tap" and carried out until there is absence of recurrence (typically, daily for about 2–3 weeks).

Carbonic anhydrase inhibitors can be used to reduce CSF production. Acetazolamide (100 mg/kg/day) has been shown to decrease CSF production by 50%. This treatment can be combined with furosemide (1–2 mg/kg/day) to control the progression of posthemorrhagic hydrocephalus. Careful attention must be paid to electrolytes and acid-base balance with these drugs to avoid significant metabolic disturbances.

Ultimately, **ventricular drainage** and **shunting** are required for these infants who do not respond to the therapies described above. Ventricular drains are temporizing measures whereas shunts are definitive therapy. Shunts often become infected or obstructed in premature infants, although many babies will become shunt independent over time.

33. Can serial lumbar punctures (LPs) prevent posthemorrhagic hydrocephalus?

Although LPs are useful in lowering increased intracranial pressure and in treating hydrocephalus once it has developed, they appear to be of little benefit in preventing the onset. Infants with slowly progressive ventricular dilatation and increasing head circumference who do not show signs of spontaneous arrest and improvement within 4 weeks should undergo a trial of serial LPs. Their effectiveness should be assessed with ultrasound. If there is no benefit, the placement of a ventriculoperitoneal shunt is necessary.

34. Which ventricular region is most readily affected by the ventricular dilatation? When does ventricular dilatation occur in relation to intraventricular hemorrhage?

The posterior horns of the lateral ventricles dilate before and to a greater degree than the anterior horns. Ventricular dilatation typically follows intraventricular hemorrhage by 1–3 weeks. Ventricular dilatation often does not produce rapid head growth for 1–2 weeks after the ventricular enlargement begins to appear.

35. What is the incidence of long-term neurologic sequelae in infants with germinal matrix–intraventricular hemorrhage?

The incidence of long-term neurologic sequelae is related to the severity of the germinal matrix–intraventricular hemorrhage. Mild intraventricular hemorrhage (grade I) has a 5% incidence of neurologic sequelae compared with 15% in grade II, 35% in grade III, and 90% in severe cases with periventricular infarction (grade IV).

36. Which areas of the central nervous system (CNS) are injured by hypoxia and ischemia?

In full-term infants, hypoxia and ischemia produce injuries in the peripheral and dorsal aspects of the cerebral cortex. Lesions involve gyri at the depths of the sulci and the neuronal nuclei of the basal ganglia. In premature infants, injury is localized to the germinal matrix and the periventricular region, while the cortex is relatively spared.

The reason for the different sites of injury has much to do with the significant differences in the brain of the very premature infant compared to the term baby. In particular, there is a deficiency of glial cells in the supporting regions of the germinal matrix in the preterm infant. When coupled with the extraordinary friability of the vasculature in this region, the possibilities for hemorrhage in the periventricular region are substantial. As the vasculature further develops during gestation, however, the term infant becomes more susceptible to injury in watershed areas of the brain that are prone to ischemic injury.

37. What are the five major neuropathologic varieties of neonatal hypoxic-ischemic encephalopathy?

1. **Selective neuronal necrosis:** usually occurs in a characteristic, although possibly widespread region.

2. **Status marmoratus:** following neuronal loss, the development of gliosis and hypermyelination, often in the basal ganglia and thalamus

3. **Parasagittal cerebral injury:** "watershed infarcts" due to ischemia

4. **Periventricular leukomalacia:** loss of white matter in characteristic patterns due to ischemia, particularly in premature infants

5. **Focal and multifocal ischemic brain necrosis:** infarction due to ischemia, with large areas of necrosis in the distribution of major vessels

PERIVENTRICULAR LEUKOMALACIA

38. What is periventricular leukomalacia (PVL)?

PVL is a condition manifesting as necrosis of the white matter dorsal and ventral to the lateral ventricles (particularly around the anterior horns and the trigones). Scarring or gliosis of neural tissue in these regions of the brain leads to an alteration of neuronal migration. Ultrasonographically, it is often seen as cystic dilatation in this area of the brain. There is a significant correlation between PVL and subsequent development of cerebral palsy.

39. What are the major etiologic factors involved in the development of PVL?

The exact etiology of PVL is not entirely understood. It does appear, however, that the key factors in its etiology are (1) the increasing survival of very premature infants (to at least 6 days of age) and (2) some degree of hypoxic-ischemic injury to the brain. In addition, recent evidence has suggested that neonatal infection may have an important role in the development of PVL. PVL is known to occur in utero, at the time of birth, or after birth. It is not necessary for an intraventricular hemorrhage to be present for a baby to develop PVL.

The regions involved in this condition are located in the arterial border zones' "watershed areas" of the deep penetrating vessels of the middle, anterior, and posterior cerebral, lenticulostriate, and choroidal arteries. These regions are at particular risk at times of decreased cerebral blood flow. The vessels in this region are also noted to continue their development through the last few months of gestation. The immature vasculature of this developing region has impaired autoregulation capabilities and is described as "pressure passive circulation." Finally, other factors include the relatively high metabolic activity of the cerebral white matter and the susceptibility of the region to local cytotoxic substrates. Under conditions of extreme prematurity and neonatal lung disease, all of these factors may be altered, ultimately leading to PVL.

The role of infection is somewhat less clear in the development of PVL. It is thought, however, that proinflammatory cytokines may be critical to the pathogenesis of this neurologic injury. Prolonged tocolysis has also been implicated in the etiology of this lesion, again suggesting that elevated levels of cytokines may be a triggering mechanism.

40. Can hemorrhage be an associated factor with PVL?

Yes, a common and serious complication of PVL is hemorrhage. Intraventricular hemorrhage may also be associated with PVL, but it is not a cause of PVL. The same factors that result in PVL are probably operative in the etiology of intraventricular hemorrhage, hence the relationship between the two.

41. How early can PVL be noted on cranial ultrasonography?

Within 1–3 weeks after the hypoxic-ischemic insult, cystic changes can be detected on head ultrasound. Part of the difficulty with PVL comes from the fact that the timing of the hypoxic-ischemic insult is usually difficult to determine. The role of sepsis in this process is also unclear at present and may be more important than was previously believed.

42. What are the common neurologic sequelae of PVL?

The long-term sequelae of PVL are still being established through follow-up studies. The principle sequelae, however, at this time appear to include spastic diplegia and visual and cognitive deficits.

43. Name the primary visual deficits related to PVL.
Poor visual acuity
Delayed visual maturation
Strabismus
Supranuclear disorders of eye movement

CEREBRAL PALSY

44. What is the definition of cerebral palsy (CP)?
Cerebral palsy is a term used to describe the condition in a child with damage to the brain that occurs early in life (typically before age 3 years) that is nonprogressive and results in a disability of motor function.

45. How is CP classified?
Clinical classification is based on the nature of the movement disorder, muscle tone, and anatomic distribution. A single patient may have more than one type.

CLASSIFICATION	DISTRIBUTION	CHARACTERISTICS
Spastic	65%	Characterized by neurologic signs of upper motor neuron damage with increased "clasp knife" muscle tone, increased deep tendon reflexes, pathologic reflexes, and spastic weakness
Hemiplegia	30%	Primarily unilateral involvement, arm usually more than leg
Quadriplegia	5%	All limbs involved, with legs often more involved than arms
Diplegia	30%	Legs much more involved than arms, which may show no or only minimal impairment
Dyskinetic	20%	Characterized by prominent involuntary movements or fluctuating muscle tone with choreoathetosis the most common subtype. Distribution is usually symmetric along the four limbs.
Ataxic	15%	

Adapted from Palmer FB, Hoon AN: Cerebral palsy. In Parker S, Zuckerman B (eds): Behavioral and Developmental Pediatrics. Boston, Little, Brown, 1995, pp 88–94, with permission.

46. Which newborns are at greatest risk for CP?
Premature infants are at the highest risk. The lower the birth weight and gestational age, the greater the chance for the child to develop CP.

BIRTH WEIGHT	INCIDENCE OF CEREBRAL PALSY/1000 LIVE BIRTHS
> 2500 g	2/1000 (0.2%)
< 1500 g	50/1000 (5%)
< 1000 g	120/1000 (12%)

47. Why is CP difficult to diagnose clinically in the first year of life?
• Hypotonia is more common than hypertonia and spasticity in the first year, making prediction of CP difficult.
• Early abundance of primitive reflexes (with variable persistence) may confuse the clinical picture.
• Infants have a limited variety of volitional movements for evaluation.
• Substantial myelination takes months to evolve and may delay the clinical picture of abnormal tone and increased deep tendon reflexes.
• Most infants who develop CP do not have identifiable risk factors. Most cases are not related to labor and delivery events.

48. What problems are commonly associated with CP?

- Mental retardation. Two-thirds of all patients experience this. It is most commonly observed in children with spastic quadriplegia.
- Learning disabilities
- Ophthalmologic abnormalities (strabismus, amblyopia, nystagmus, refractive errors)
- Hearing deficits
- Communication disorders
- Seizures. One-third of all patients have seizures. They are most commonly observed in children with spastic hemiplegia
- Failure to thrive
- Feeding problems
- Gastroesophageal reflux
- Behavioral and emotional problems (especially attention deficit hyperactivity disorder, depression)

Eicher PS, Batshaw ML: Cerebral palsy. Pediatric Clin North Am 40:537–551, 1993.

49. What is the most common ultrasonographic abnormality of the brain in infants who ultimately go on to have CP?

Large (> 3 mm in diameter) periventricular cysts indicate permanent damage to the white matter of the corticospinal tracts. The neuronal cells in that region, which migrate and populate other areas, essentially have died and are replaced by fluid initially, then scar tissue. These are cells that have gone through apoptosis (programmed cell death) and are no longer capable of further development. As a result, the child is left with permanent injury. The cysts are part of the process of PVL when examined pathologically.

50. What are the chances that a child with an Apgar score of ≤ 3 for 15–20 minutes will have CP?

Only 10–15%. Although a low Apgar score is a risk factor for CP, 55% of children with CP that developed at a later time in life had Apgar scores of 7–10 at 1 minute, and 73% had scores of 7–10 at 5 minutes.

51. What is the correlation between abnormalities on electronic fetal monitoring and subsequent CP?

There is a very poor correlation between abnormal fetal heart rate tracings and CP. Late decelerations and decreased beat-to-beat variability are associated with an increased risk of CP. However, 99.8% of infants with these abnormalities on monitoring do not develop CP, and 75% of children with CP do not have any abnormalities on electronic monitoring.

52. How do electronic fetal monitoring and prompt cesarean section for "fetal distress" affect the incidence of CP?

They don't. Children delivered by cesarean section have the same rate of CP as those delivered vaginally. Historically, as the rate of cesarean section deliveries has increased, the incidence of CP has remained unchanged and more recently has actually risen. It is unclear whether this rise represents the increased survival of extremely low birth weight babies or whether other factors are the cause.

53. How does maternal infection affect the incidence of CP in term children of normal birth weight?

Maternal fever above 38°C (100.4°F) during labor or a clinical diagnosis of chorioamnionitis is associated with a marked (nine-fold) increased risk of CP, especially spastic quadriplegic CP (19-fold increase).

54. How has the prevalence of CP changed since the advent of neonatal intensive care in the 1960s?

The prevalence has risen approximately 20% from the early 1960s to the late 1980s, almost entirely because of increased survival of low and very low birth weight infants. One of the most disconcerting aspects of newborn intensive care has been the fact that, as smaller and more critically ill infants survive, the incidence of CP has risen. Such outcome data are most discouraging.

The fact is, however, there are now many completely intact infants who previously would have died but now survive to become normal children.

55. What percentage of cases of CP are caused by intrapartum asphyxia?

Although obstetricians are frequently made to feel that they are responsible for all cases of CP, the fact is that spastic CP is the result of intrapartum asphyxia in only about 10% of children. Because so many children with spastic CP often have no definable etiology for their problem, recent attention has focused on the possibility that in utero infection may be more important than previously thought in the etiology of CP.

56. What is the evidence to suggest that inflammatory cytokines have been found to be associated with prematurity and with development of CP?

The levels of interleukin-1 (IL-1), IL-8, IL-9, and tumor necrosis factor-α (TNF-α) in dried neonatal blood have been found to be significantly higher in infants who subsequently were diagnosed with CP than in controls. These markers have also been associated with prematurity. Other factors found in higher-than-normal concentrations in children who went on to have CP include antiphospholipid antibody, antibodies to antithrombin 3, and antibodies to protein C and S. These data suggest that coagulation defects may also play a role in fetal brain injury and pregnancy wastage.

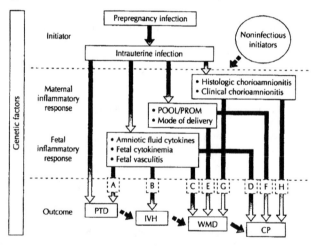

Some presumed pathways from initiators to inflammatory responses in mother and fetus and links (labeled A through H) between some of these and the adverse outcomes preterm delivery (PTD), intraventricular hemorrhage (IVH), white matter damage (WMD), and cerebral palsy (CP). (From Dammann O, Leviton A: Role of the fetus in perinatal infection and neonatal brain damage. Curr Opin Pediatr 12:100, 2000, with permission.)

57. What features in an infant suggest a progressive CNS disorder rather than CP as the cause of a motor deficit?

- Abnormally increasing head circumference (possible hydrocephalus, tumor)
- Eye anomalies such as cataracts, retinal pigmentary degeneration, optic atrophy (possible neurodegenerative disease)
- Skin abnormalities such as vitiligo, café-au-lait spots, nevus flammeus (possible Sturge-Weber disease, neurofibromatosis)
- Hepatomegaly or splenomegaly (possible storage disease)
- Decreased or absent deep tendon reflexes
- Sensory abnormalities (loss of diminished sense of pain, position, vibration, or light touch)

NEONATAL SEIZURES

58. Name four reasons why it is important to recognize, diagnose, and treat neonatal seizures.

1. Seizures are the most common clinical sign of a neonatal neurologic disorder.

2. Neonatal seizures are usually caused by a significant illness that may be systemic or purely neurologic. Some of these conditions (e.g., hypoglycemia, meningitis) will continue to cause brain damage until they are recognized and treated.

3. Neonatal seizures may interfere with the physician's ability to provide general medical care such as oral alimentation and assisted ventilation.

4. Some clinical and experimental data suggest that neonatal seizures are not just an innocent symptom of neurologic disease but may themselves contribute to the ultimate extent of brain injury (controversial).

59. Are neonatal seizures more likely to be symptomatic of an acute illness or idiopathic?

It is sometimes said that the term *idiopathic* means that we doctors are "idiots" for not being able to figure out the "pathology." Seizures occurring during the neonatal period are more likely to be symptomatic of an acute illness than idiopathic. The reported incidence of neonatal seizures varies with the population studied, gestational age, and risk status. It also depends on whether subclinical seizures (seizures only seen on the electroencephalogram [EEG] without any visible clinical signs) are included. The reported clinical incidence of neonatal seizures varies from 0.5% to 3.0%. There are two broad categories of seizures in the neonatal period. The first is the "well child" with seizures. These may be due to early epilepsy, simple hypocalcemia, small stroke, mild subarachnoid hemorrhage, or cerebral dysgenesis. The other group is the "sick child" with seizures and an acute neonatal encephalopathy due to hypoxia-ischemia, shock, sepsis, meningitis, inborn errors of metabolism, and other potentially serious conditions.

60. In premature and full-term infants, how do the causes of seizures vary in relative frequency and time of onset?

Variance in Relative Frequency and Time of Onset of Causes of Seizures

ETIOLOGY	POSTNATAL TIME OF ONSET		RELATIVE FREQUENCY	
	0–3 DAYS	> 3 DAYS	PREMATURE	FULL-TERM
Hypoxic-ischemic	+		+++	+++
Intracranial hemorrhage	+	+	++	+
Hypoglycemia	+		+	+
Hypocalcemia	+	+	+	+
Intracranial infection	+	+	++	+
Developmental defects	+	+	++	++
Drug withdrawal	+	+	+	+

From Volpe JJ (ed): Neurology of the Newborn, 3rd ed. Philadelphia, W.B. Saunders, 1995, p 184, with permission.

61. How are seizures classified in the newborn infant?

Seizures are, in general, defined as sudden paroxysmal alterations in neurologic function (behavior, motor, autonomic function) due to abnormal, excessive discharges on the EEG. In other words, the clinical seizure is caused by an electrical seizure of the brain, demonstrated as an ictal EEG. Neonatal seizures are usually clinically classified as clonic, tonic, myoclonic, and subtle seizures.

Clonic seizures are sustained, repetitive, rhythmic jerking movements of a muscle. Holding or repositioning the involved body part does not stop them. Clonic seizures may be focal (e.g., involving just the face, arm, or leg) or multifocal (involving several body parts, often in a migrating fashion). They may be seen with a focal structural abnormality (e.g., a stroke or bleed) or with diffuse conditions such as metabolic encephalopathies. Most clonic seizures are accompanied by EEG seizure activity (electrographic seizures).

Tonic seizures are abrupt changes in muscle tone that produce sustained changes in muscle posture. Focal tonic seizures involve just an arm or leg or the extraocular muscles (producing sustained deviation of both eyes to one side). Generalized tonic seizures produce an abnormal posture of the whole body (head, neck, trunk, and limbs). Thus, they resemble "decerebrate" posturing or opisthotonus. Generalized posturing is often associated with severe intracranial hemorrhage but usually is not epileptic (i.e., the simultaneous EEG is negative for electrographic seizure activity).

Myoclonic seizures are rapid shock-like jerks of the muscle occurring as single or repetitive jolts of the affected muscles. The jerks are faster than clonic seizures and not rhythmic. Myoclonic seizures may be focal, multifocal, or generalized. They occur primarily in the flexor muscle groups. These abnormal-appearing movements are usually not triggered. Focal myoclonic seizures usually are not associated with electrographic seizures.

Subtle seizures are frequently overlooked and may be difficult to diagnose. They are repetitive, paroxysmal stereotyped alterations in motor activity or neonatal behavior. Examples of subtle seizure are swimming movements in the arms, chewing, tongue thrusting, bicycling movements of the legs, autonomic changes, and apnea. Subtle seizures are more common in premature than full-term infants and usually not linked to ictal EEG activity.

Volpe J: Neonatal seizures: Current concepts and revised classifications. Pediatrics 84:422–428, 1989.

62. After an asphyxial event, how long should feeding be delayed?

During an asphyxial event, vasoconstriction of the mesenteric vessels can result in intestinal ischemia. Because of the relationship between ischemia and the incidence of necrotizing enterocolitis, feedings should be delayed for 2–3 days to allow for repair of the intestinal mucosa.

63. What is the study of choice to diagnose neonatal strokes?

In any sick infant with seizures or a clinical neurologic abnormality, the suspicion for an underlying structural lesion should be high. Although the head ultrasound examination is easy and noninvasive, it is not very sensitive in detecting strokes. Computed tomography (CT) is superior to ultrasound in the acute setting, but lacks the detail of magnetic resonance imaging (MRI) and exposes the infant to radiation. MRI is the diagnostic test of choice. A relatively new magnetic pulse sequence called diffusion-weighted imaging (DWI) can detect very recent strokes if performed within a week of the insult. Traditional MRI is adequate for older strokes. DWI is therefore important for detection of early stroke and can help time the insult.

Cowan FM, et al: Early detection of cerebral infarction and hypoxic ischemic encephalopathy in neonates using diffusion-weighted magnetic resonance imaging. Neuropediatrics 25:172–175, 1994.

64. How are neonatal strokes treated, and what are their outcomes?

Once a neonatal stroke is diagnosed, an etiologic work-up should be undertaken. A magnetic resonance angiogram (MRA) helps visualize the cerebral arteries. The work-up also should include an echocardiogram to rule out a cardiac source of emboli and coagulation studies for an acquired or inherited prothrombotic condition. Initial management includes general medical support and administration of antiepileptic medications if the child is seizing.

The use of thrombolytic agents (tissue plasminogen activator [TPA] and urokinase) during acute strokes has not been evaluated in neonates. In rare prothrombotic conditions, heparin, warfarin (Coumadin), aspirin, or other anticoagulants may be needed to prevent further strokes. The outcome from focal strokes in neonates is variable, but "size does matter," and children with a large hemispheric injury are likely to develop at least a hemiparesis. Like real estate, "location, location, location" is the key! Small strokes in noneloquent cortex may not produce any long-term adverse effects. Nevertheless, longitudinal, comprehensive, neurologic follow-up is important to screen for developmental delays and learning disabilities and to institute therapy early if needed.

Mercuri E, et al: Early prognostic indicators of outcome in infants with neonatal cerebral infarction: A clinical, electroencephalogram, and magnetic resonance imaging study. Pediatrics 103:39–46, 1999.

MALFORMATIONS OF THE CENTRAL NERVOUS SYSTEM

65. What is the risk of seizure activity in an anencephalic infant?

None! Anencephalic infants lack a cerebral cortex and therefore exhibit no cortical function. Seizure activity is a dysfunction of the cerebral cortex. Although it is believed that subcortical seizures may occasionally occur in neonates, the disorganization of the anencephalic brain is so significant that seizure activity simply does not occur.

66. Polyhydramnios is seen in approximately 50% of patients with anencephaly. What is the mechanism accounting for polyhydramnios in fetal neurologic disease?

Neurologically impaired fetuses often lack normal swallowing activity, resulting in an abnormal accumulation of amniotic fluid. Polyhydramnios most commonly occurs for idiopathic reasons, but swallowing dysfunction or high intestinal obstruction may result in polyhydramnios.

67. What fetal conditions are associated with an elevated alpha-fetoprotein in maternal serum?

Elevated alpha-fetoprotein (defined as > 2.5 ml) is seen in open neural tube defects, abdominal wall defects, esophageal or duodenal atresia, congenital nephrosis, and fetal demise. Alpha-fetoprotein is synthesized by the fetal liver and excreted by the kidney, normally peaking at 10–13 weeks estimated gestational age. The level may vary with gestational age, number of fetuses, and maternal weight and race.

68. What is the difference between an Arnold-Chiari type I malformation and an Arnold-Chiari type II malformation?

An Arnold-Chiari type I malformation is defined as elongation of the cerebellar tonsils and displacement of the inferior lobes of cerebellum into the cervical spinal canal. It is thought to be an acquired malformation. The elements of an Arnold-Chiari type II malformation include cerebellar dysplasia; elongation of the fourth ventricle; and caudal displacement of the vermis, cerebellar tonsils, pons, and medulla oblongata into the upper cervical canal. It is associated with the presence of myelomeningocele and hydrocephalus. The etiology is felt to be secondary to defective rhombogenesis, a primary rather than acquired brain malformation.

69. What is the difference among meningocele, myelomeningocele, and spina bifida occulta? What is the incidence of myelomeningocele?

A meningocele is a protrusion of meninges only through a bony defect in the vertebral column. A myelomeningocele is a protrusion of meninges and spinal cord through a bony defect in the vertebral column. Spina bifida occulta is a vertebral defect in the absence of spinal cord or meningeal herniation. The incidence of myelomeningocele is 0.5–1/1000 live births.

70. What dietary deficiency plays a role in the etiology of a myelomeningocele?

An estimated 60% of cases of myelomeningocele are due to inadequate intake of folic acid in pregnant women. Current recommendations are that all women of child-bearing age consume at least 0.4 mg of folic acid per day. The recommendation for women who have already delivered a child affected with myelomeningocele is 4 mg of folic acid per day starting at least 4 weeks prior to conception and continuing through the first 3 months of pregnancy.

71. What is the full anatomic expression of a myelomeningocele?

Children with myelomeningocele have a complex, multifaceted, congenital disorder of structure, which represents a dysraphic state (a defective closure of the embryonic neural groove). In its full expression, it is typified anatomically by:

- The presence of unfused or excessively separated vertebral arches of the bony spine (spina bifida)
- Cystic dilation of the meninges that surround the spinal cord (meningocele)

• Cystic dilation of the spinal cord itself (myelocele)
• Hydrocephalus and spectrum of congenital cerebral abnormalities

72. If the diagnosis of myelomeningocele is made prenatally, should delivery be done by cesarean section?

In one study, infants delivered by cesarean section prior to the onset of labor had significantly less paralysis at age 2 years than did infants with comparable lesions who were delivered vaginally following a period of labor.

Luthy DA, Wardinsky T, Shurtleff DB, et al: Cesarean section before the onset of labor and subsequent motor function in infants with meningocele diagnosed antenatally. N Engl J Med 324:662–666, 1991.

73. Which congenital cerebral disorders are associated with myelomeningocele?

1. A **type II Arnold-Chiari malformation** may occur in which the hindbrain is abnormal and enclosed in a small posterior fossa. The medulla oblongata and the "tonsils" of the cerebellum are displaced or herniated downward to occupy the normal position of the upper cervical cord. The impaired egress of CSF caused by aqueductal stenosis commonly results in hydrocephalus. Arnold-Chiari malformations sometimes coexist with other abnormalities of the cerebral cortex.

2. **More severe cerebral malformations** may occur in the maximal expression of the dysraphic state. Incomplete closure of the cranial bones results in cranium bifidum. Protrusion of abnormal brain tissue through the defective skull bone results in an encephalocele. Gross failure of neural groove fusion results in craniorachischisis or, in its maximal form, anencephaly.

3. **Hydrocephalus** is seen in 95% of children with thoracic or high lumbar myelomeningocele. The incidence decreases progressively with more caudal spinal defects to a minimum of 60% if the myelomeningocele is located in the sacrum.

74. What is the usual cause of stridor in a child with myelomeningocele?

Stridor is usually due to dysfunction of the vagus nerve, which innervates the muscles of the vocal cords. In their resting position, the edges of the cords meet in the midline; in speech, they move apart. Hence, in bilateral vagal nerve palsies, the free edges of the vocal cords are closely opposed and obstruct air flow, resulting in stridor. In symptomatic patients the motor nucleus of the vagus nerve may be congenitally hypoplastic or aplastic. More commonly, the vagal dysfunction is believed to arise from a mechanical traction injury secondary to hydrocephalus, which produces progressive herniation and inferior displacement of the abnormal hindbrain. Shunting the hydrocephalus may alleviate the traction and improve the stridor. Sometimes, the later recurrence of stridor indicates reaccumulation of hydrocephalus due to ventriculoperitoneal shunt failure.

Children with myelomeningocele may have a variety of forms of apnea and bradycardia because of this defect. In addition to vagal dysfunction as described, these children may have central apnea from brain stem compression or structural abnormality. It is occasionally helpful to monitor such patients at home.

75. How frequently is myelomeningocele associated with mental retardation?

Only 15–20% of patients have associated mental retardation. Hydrocephalus per se does not cause the mental retardation associated with this syndrome. (Recall that children with appropriately treated congenital hydrocephalus due to simple aqueductal stenosis usually have normal psychomotor development.) Lower intellectual function is more commonly seen in patients with higher cord lesions, hydrocephalus, ventriculoperitoneal shunts, and a history of intracranial bleeding or infections. Mental retardation is usually attributed to acquired secondary CNS infection or subtle microscopic anomalies of neuronal migration and differentiation, which may coexist with the macroscopically visible malformation of the hindbrain.

Infection is particularly problematic for patients with shunts. Many children with recurring infections who initially appear to be developmentally normal may have significant subsequent developmental problems as shunts are replaced, and infection and shunt obstruction become chronic care issues.

76. In an infant born with myelomeningocele, how does the initial evaluation predict long-term ambulation potential?

- **Thoracic.** No hip flexion is noted. Almost no younger children will ambulate, and only about a third of adolescents will ambulate with the aid of extensive braces and crutches.
- **High lumbar (L1, L2).** Infant is able to flex hips but no has no knee extension. About a third of children and adolescents will ambulate, but only with extensive assistive devices.
- **Mid lumbar (L3).** Infant is able to flex hips and extend knee. The percentage of ambulators is midway between those with high and low lumbar lesions.
- **Low lumbar (L4, L5).** Infant is able to flex knee and dorsiflex ankle. Nearly half of younger children and all adolescents will ambulate with varying degrees of crutches or braces.
- **Sacral (S1–S4).** Infant can plantar flex ankles and move toes. Nearly all children and adolescents will ambulate with minimal or no assistive devices.

77. What is a tethered cord? How is it diagnosed?

A tethered cord is the prolongation of the conus and thickening of the filum terminale, producing limited mobility of the caudal end of the cord and resulting in injury to the cord. The signs present on physical examination in the neonatal period are limited to dermal defects such as hair tufts and sacral dimples. Ultrasound of the distal cord is diagnostic. If left untreated, potential long-term sequelae include incontinence, delayed ambulation, or loss of ambulation.

78. Name the three types of holoprosencephaly. What is the difference between holoprosencephaly and hydranencephaly?

The three types of holoprosencephaly are **alobar**, **semilobar**, and **lobar**. Holoprosencephaly is a primary brain malformation resulting from failure of cleavage of the cerebral hemispheres. Hydranencephaly is a disruption, probably secondary to bilateral infarction of the internal carotid arteries.

79. What is the most common type of fetal hydrocephalus? What is the most common cause of fetal hydrocephalus?

The most common type of fetal hydrocephalus is obstructive noncommunicating; this refers to an increase in the volume of CSF within the skull secondary to an obstruction that is intrinsic to the ventricular system. The most common cause of fetal hydrocephalus is myelomeningocele accompanied by an Arnold-Chiari type II malformation.

80. What is hydrocephalus ex vacuo?

Hydrocephalus ex vacuo is the presence of enlarged ventricles secondary to a lack of brain growth. It most commonly occurs after some form of cerebral injury, either before or after birth. Critically ill neonates with chronic or recurring hypoxemic-ischemic disease may demonstrate ventriculomegaly or hydrocephalus ex vacuo as a result of ongoing neuronal loss.

81. How does hydrocephalus occur in premature neonates?

In **communicating hydrocephalus**, the baby appears to develop ventriculomegaly from obstruction of CSF reabsorption in the arachnoid villi. The onset of hydrocephalus usually occurs several weeks after the original hemorrhage and is slowly progressive. Infants with head circumference growth in excess of 1 cm/week should have a head sonogram to see if hydrocephalus is present. Occasionally, this form of hydrocephalus will respond to repeat LPs with or without the use of acetazolamide. The repeat taps simply allow sufficient time for the reabsorption of the fibrin deposits that are thought to be obstructing the reabsorption of CSF. In approximately 60% of cases, a ventriculoperitoneal shunt is needed.

In **noncommunicating or obstructive hydrocephalus,** a clot or fibrin organization has become lodged in the ventricular system, most commonly at the aqueduct of Sylvius. Spinal fluid flow is blocked, and head growth proceeds rapidly in most instances. A shunt is virtually always needed, although many infants will outgrow their need for a shunt at a later time.

82. Name the components of the Dandy-Walker malformation.

The components of the Dandy-Walker malformation are dilatation of the fourth ventricle, partial or complete agenesis of the cerebellar vermis, and enlargement of the posterior fossa. The Dandy-Walker malformation may occur in isolation or as part of a multiple malformation complex.

ADDICTION IN THE NEONATE

83. When does withdrawal occur in infants of narcotic-addicted mothers?

Most withdrawal occurs within 72 hours after birth; the range is from shortly after birth to as late as 2 weeks after delivery. In general, the closer to delivery the mother has used the drug, the greater the delay in onset of signs.

84. Should heroin-exposed infants with perinatal depression receive a narcotic antagonist?

No. The administration of narcotic antagonists may precipitate seizures in the infant.

85. What special diagnostic studies should be ordered at birth for well-appearing infants born to cocaine-addicted mothers?

None. Although there are reports of perinatal brain infarctions, CNS hemorrhage, genitourinary malformations, cardiac abnormalities, and an increase in sudden infant death syndrome (SIDS) in infants with in utero cocaine exposure, there are no recommendations for studies of any sort, unless dictated by abnormal clinical condition or history.

Hurt H: Substance use during pregnancy. In Spitzer AR (ed): Intensive Care of the Fetus and Neonate. Philadelphia, Mosby, 1996.

86. Of cocaine, heroin, alcohol, marijuana, and cigarettes, which is considered usually compatible with breast-feeding by the American Academy of Pediatrics (AAP)?

Alcohol. The AAP states that maternal alcohol use is usually compatible with breast-feeding; some recent literature, however, suggests that infants with chronic alcohol exposure may have lower scores on the Psychomotor Index of the Bayley Scales of Infant Development.

Committee on Drugs: The transfer of drugs and other chemicals into human milk. Pediatrics 93:137–150, 1994.

87. Do most children with in utero cocaine exposure demonstrate significant neurologic damage?

No. Although controversy exists regarding long-term neurodevelopmental outcome of cocaine-exposed children, as a group, these children have not demonstrated the severe irreparable brain damage first predicted. The terms *crack kid* and *cocaine-addicted baby* are considered pejorative and unfounded.

88. If maternal drug abuse is suspected, which specimen from the infant is most accurate in detecting exposure?

Although urine has traditionally been tested when maternal drug abuse is a possibility, meconium has a greater sensitivity than urine and positive findings that persist longer. It may contain metabolites gathered over multiple weeks, compared with urine, which represents more recent exposure. Of note, maternal self-reporting is notoriously inaccurate as an indicator of drug use. In an informal, anonymous study conducted at a major hospital in Philadelphia, approximately 20% of inner city mothers and 15% of suburban mothers screened around the time of birth were positive for cocaine and other illicit drugs. One must always be suspicious about maternal drug use if an infant's problems are not easily explained. It should be noted, however, that in some states informed maternal consent must be given prior to drug screening of the neonate, which can hinder diagnosis and surveillance.

Ostrea EM Jr, Brady M, Gause S, et al: Drug screening of newborns by meconium analysis: A large-scale, prospective, epidemiologic study. Pediatrics 89:107–113, 1992.

89. What are the manifestations of drug withdrawal in the neonate?

The signs and symptoms of drug withdrawal in the neonate can be remembered by using the mnemonic **WITHDRAWAL.**

W   Wakefulness
I   Irritability
T   Tremulousness, temperature variation, tachypnea
H   Hyperactivity, high-pitched persistent cry, hyperacusis, hyperreflexia, hypertonus
D   Diarrhea, diaphoresis, disorganized suck
R   Rub marks, respiratory distress rhinorrhea
A   Apneic attacks, autonomic dysfunction
W   Weight loss or failure to gain weight
A   Alkalosis (respiratory)
L   Lacrimation

NEUROCUTANEOUS SYNDROMES

90. What are the three most common neurocutaneous syndromes?
1. Neurofibromatosis
2. Tuberous sclerosis
3. Sturge-Weber syndrome

91. Describe the inheritance patterns of the various neurocutaneous syndromes.

SYNDROME	INHERITANCE PATTERN
Neurofibromatosis	Autosomal dominant
Tuberous sclerosis	Autosomal dominant
Von Hippel-Lindau syndrome	Autosomal dominant
Incontinentia pigmenti	X-linked dominant
Sturge-Weber syndrome	Sporadic
Klippel-Trenaunay-Weber syndrome	Sporadic

92. What is the derivation of the term *phakomatosis?*

The term *phakomatosis* is derived from the Greek *phakos*, meaning "spot," and refers to patchy, circumscribed dermatologic lesions that are the hallmark of this group of disorders. In addition to dermatologic features, these syndromes have hamartomatous involvement of multiple tissues, especially the CNS and eye. More commonly, the term *neurocutaneous syndrome* is used.

93. How common are café-au-lait spots at birth? How common is a positive family history in cases of neurofibromatosis?

Up to 2% of black infants will have three café-au-lait spots at birth, and only one café-au-lait spot occurs in 0.3% of white infants. White infants with multiple café-au-lait spots at birth are more likely than black infants to develop neurofibromatosis. In older children, a single café-au-lait spot > 5 mm can be found in 10% of white and 25% of black children. Because of the high spontaneous mutation rate for this autosomal dominant disease, only about 50% of newly diagnosed cases are associated with a positive family history. (See figure, top of next page.)

Hurwitz S: Neurofibromatosis. In Clinical Pediatric Dermatology, 2nd ed. Philadelphia, W.B. Saunders, 1993, pp 624–629.

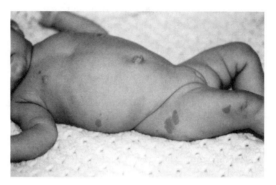

Multiple café-au-lait macules of > 5 mm diameter in an infant. (From Halbert AR: Neurocutaneous disorders. In Fitzpatrick JE, Aeling JL (eds): Dermatology Secrets. Philadelphia, Hanley & Belfus, 1996, pp 28–34, with permission.)

94. What are the primary clinical diagnostic features of tuberous sclerosis in the neonatal period?
- Subependymal nodules or giant cell astrocytomas (histologic confirmation)
- Multiple calcified subependymal nodules protruding into the ventricle (radiographic confirmation)
- Multiple retinal astrocytomas
- Cardiac hamartomas
- Skin lesions are uncommon in the neonate, although hypopigmented macules are seen, as are occasional café-au-lait spots

95. Which types of facial port-wine stains are most strongly associated with ophthalmic or CNS complications?
Port-wine stains can occur as isolated cutaneous birthmarks or, particularly in the areas of underlying the birthmark, in association with structural abnormalities in (1) choroidal vessels of the eye leading to glaucoma, (2) leptomeningeal vessels in the brain leading to seizures (Sturge-Weber syndrome), and (3) hemangiomas in the spinal cord (Cobb syndrome). In a study by Tallman et al., glaucoma or seizures were most associated with port-wine stains in children demonstrating:
- Involvement of the eyelids
- Bilateral distribution of the birthmark
- Unilateral involvement of all three branches (V1, V2, V3) of the trigeminal nerve

Ophthalmologic assessment of radiologic studies (CT or MRI) are indicated for children exhibiting these findings.

Tallman B, Tan OT, Morelli JG, et al: Location of port-wine stains and the likelihood of ophthalmic and/or central nervous system complications. Pediatrics 87:323–327, 1991.

96. What are the three stages of incontinentia pigmenti?
Incontinentia pigmenti is an X-linked dominant disorder associated with seizures and mental retardation. The condition is presumed lethal to males in utero because nearly 100% of cases are female:
- Stage 1 (vesicular stage)—Lines of blisters on the trunk and extremities in the newborn that disappear in weeks or months. They may resemble herpetic vesicles. Microscopic examination of the vesicular fluid demonstrates eosinophils.
- Stage 2 (verrucous stage)—Lesions develop around age 3–7 months that are brown and hyperkeratotic, resembling warts. These disappear over 1–2 years.
- Stage 3 (pigmented stage)—Whorled, swirling (marble cake-like) macular hyperpigmented lines develop. These may fade over time, leaving only remnant hypopigmentation in late adolescence or adulthood (which is sometimes considered a fourth stage).

NEUROMUSCULAR DISORDERS

97. How does electromyography (EMG) help differentiate myopathic and neurogenic disorders?

EMG measures the electrical activity of resting and voluntary muscle activity. Normally, the action potentials are of standardized duration and amplitude with 2–4 distinguishable phases. In myopathic conditions, the durations and amplitudes are shorter than expected. In neuropathies, they are longer. In both conditions, extra phases (i.e., polyphasic units) are usually noted.

98. What is the differential diagnosis of hypotonia?

Hypotonia is a common but nonspecific sign in neonates and young infants. Because of the fundamental nature of the central nervous system in the developing infant, many different categories of problems can alter the muscle tone of the child. These changes can include:

1. Acute serious generalized medical illness, such as infection, shock, dehydration, or hypoglycemia

2. Chromosomal abnormalities and various syndromes (without definable chromosomal changes) may have accompanying hypotonia

3. Connective tissue alterations may produce excessive joint laxity and decreased tone

4. Metabolic disorders with encephalopathy, such as hypothyroidism, Lowe syndrome, or Canavan disease

5. CNS disorders, such as cerebellar dysfunction, acute spinal cord disease, neuromuscular disorder, hypotonic cerebral palsy, or benign congenital hypotonia.

6. Birth trauma and birth asphyxia may have accompanying hypotonia, either on a temporary or permanent basis

In the absence of an acute encephalopathy, the differential diagnosis of hypotonia is best approached by asking the question: Does the patient have normal strength despite the hypotonia, or is the patient weak and hypotonic? The combination of weakness and hypotonia usually points to an abnormality of the anterior horn cell or the peripheral neuromuscular apparatus, whereas hypotonia with normal strength is more characteristic of brain or spinal cord disturbances.

99. In a newborn with weakness and hypotonia, what obstetric and delivery features suggest a diagnosis of myotonic dystrophy?

A history of spontaneous abortions, polyhydramnios, decreased fetal movements, delays in second-stage labor, retained placenta, and postpartum hemorrhage all raise the concern for congenital myotonic dystrophy. Because the mother is nearly always affected in congenital myotonic dystrophy, a careful clinical and EMG evaluation of the mother is essential in such cases.

100. Why is myotonic dystrophy an example of the phenomenon of "anticipation"?

Genetic studies have shown that the defect in myotonic dystrophy is an expansion of a trinucleotide (CTG) in a gene on the long arm of chromosome 19 that codes for a protein kinase. In successive generations, this repeating sequence has a tendency to increase, sometimes into the thousands (normal is < 40 CTG repeats), and the extent of repetition correlates with the severity of the disease. Thus, each succeeding generation is likely to get more extensive manifestations and earlier presentations of the disease (i.e., the phenomenon of "anticipation").

101. How does the pathophysiology of infant botulism differ from that of food-borne botulism?

Infant botulism results from the ingestion of *Clostridium botulinum* spores that germinate, multiply, and produce toxin in the infant's intestine. The source of the spores is often unknown, but is has been linked to honey in some cases, and spores have been found in corn syrups. Therefore, these foods are not advised for infants < 1 year of age. In food-borne botulism, preformed toxin is already present in the food. Improper canning and anaerobic storage permits spore germination, growth, and toxin formation, which results in symptoms if the toxin is not destroyed by proper heating. Wound botulism, which is rare, occurs if spores enter a deep wound and germinate.

102. What is the earliest indication for intubation in an infant with botulism?

Loss of protective airway reflexes. This occurs before respiratory compromise or failure because diaphragmatic function is not impaired until 90–95% of the synaptic receptors are occupied. Indeed, an infant with hypercarbia or hypoxia is at very high risk for imminent respiratory failure.

103. Why are antibiotics and antitoxins not used in cases of infant botulism?

- By the time the diagnosis is made, most patients are usually stable or improving.
- Antibiotics may result in bacterial death with the potential release of additional toxin (hypothetical).
- Aminoglycoside antibiotics may also interfere with neuromuscular transmission and can precipitate respiratory failure.
- They pose the risk of serum sickness and anaphylaxis.
- Circulating unbound toxin is not found in ongoing disease.
- Previously bound toxin is irreversibly bound (recovery based on growth of new nerve sprouts).
- There is excellent prognosis with aggressive supportive care alone.

104. In an infant with severe weakness and suspected botulism, why is the use of aminoglycosides relatively contraindicated?

The botulism toxin acts by irreversibly blocking acetylcholine release from the presynaptic nerve terminals. Aminoglycosides, as well as tetracyclines, clindamycin, and trimethoprim, also interfere with acetylcholine release. Therefore, they have the potential to act synergistically with the botulinum toxin to worsen or prolong neuromuscular paralysis.

105. How is neonatal myasthenia gravis differentiated from infant botulism?

Very few cases of botulism have been reported in neonates. Symptoms have always occurred after discharge from the neonatal nursery. Botulism is usually heralded by constipation followed by early facial and pharyngeal weakness, ptosis, and dilated, sluggishly reactive pupils with diminished deep tendon reflexes. The injection of edrophonium does not improve muscle strength. EMG examination demonstrates distinctive abnormalities such as brief small-amplitude polyphasic potentials (BSAPS) and an incremental response in the amplitude of evoked muscle potentials to repetitive nerve stimulation. Stool cultures may be positive for the toxin or clostridia.

Transient neonatal myasthenia gravis usually presents at birth or within the first few days of life. There may be a family history of myasthenia in the mother or siblings. The distribution of weakness depends on the specific subtype of myasthenia, but pupils and deep tendon reflexes are spared. The EMG examination shows a distinctive progressive decline in the amplitude of compound motor action potentials with repetitive stimulation of the nerve. Edrophonium temporarily improves the patient's clinical strength and abolishes the pathologic EMG response to repetitive stimulation.

106. What are the risks to a neonate born to a mother with myasthenia gravis?

Passively acquired neonatal myasthenia develops in about 10% of infants born to myasthenic mothers because of the transplacental transfer of antibody directed against acetylcholine receptors (AChR) in striated muscle. Signs and symptoms of weakness typically arise within the first hours or days of life. Pathologic muscle fatigability commonly causes feeding difficulty, generalized weakness, hypotonia, and respiratory depression. Ptosis and impaired eye movements occur in only 15% of cases. The weakness virtually always resolves as the body burden of anti-AChr immunoglobulin diminishes. Symptoms typically persist about 2 weeks but may require several months to disappear entirely. General supportive treatment is usually adequate, but oral or intramuscular neostigmine may help to diminish symptoms.

107. How does the pathophysiology differ in permanent congenital myasthenia versus transient neonatal myasthenia gravis?

Permanent (also referred to as juvenile and adult) myasthenia gravis is caused by circulating antibodies to the AChR of the postsynaptic neuromuscular junction. Transient neonatal myasthenia gravis does not have an autoimmune basis. It is caused by morphologic or physiologic features affecting the pre- and postsynaptic junctions, including defects in ACh synthesis, endplate acetylcholinesterase deficiency, and endplate AChR deficiency.

108. How is the edrophonium (Tensilon) test done?

Edrophonium is a rapid-acting anticholinesterase drug of short duration that improves symptoms of myasthenia gravis by inhibiting the breakdown of ACh and increasing its concentration in the neuromuscular junction. A test dose of 0.15 mg/kg is given intravenously, and if tolerated, the full dose of 0.15 mg/kg (up to 10 mg) is given. If measurable improvement in ocular muscle or extremity strength occurs, myasthenia gravis is likely. Because edrophonium may precipitate a cholinergic crisis (e.g., bradycardia, hypotension, vomiting, bronchospasm), atropine and resuscitation equipment should be available.

109. What are the four characteristic features of damage to the anterior horn cells?
1. Weakness
2. Fasciculations
3. Atrophy
4. Hyporeflexia

110. What processes can damage the anterior horn cells?
- **Degenerative** (spinal muscular atrophy): Werdnig-Hoffmann disease, Kugelberg-Welander, Pena-Shokeir, and Manden-Walker syndromes
- **Metabolic:** Tay-Sachs disease (hexosaminidase deficiency), Pompe disease, Batten disease (ceroid-lipofuscinosis), hyperglycinemia, neonatal adrenoleukodystrophy
- **Infections:** poliovirus, coxsackievirus, enteric cytopathic human orphan (ECHO) viruses

RETINOPATHY OF PREMATURITY

111. What infants require ophthalmologic evaluation for retinopathy of prematurity (ROP)? When should the examination be performed?

The AAP recommends that an individual experienced in neonatal ophthalmology and indirect ophthalmoscopy examine the retinae of all premature neonates (i.e., those who are delivered at < 35 weeks' gestation or who weigh < 1800 g) who require supplemental oxygen. Infants who are less mature at birth (i.e., < 30 weeks' gestation or < 1300 g) should be examined regardless of oxygen exposure. The original recommendation was that the examination is best done prior to discharge or at 4–7 weeks of age if the infant is still hospitalized. Recent data, however, suggest that the extremely low birth weight infant may be at added risk and should be examined earlier, to prevent a certain percentage of these babies from being examined for the first time when they already have prethreshold or threshold ROP.

Subhani MT, et al: Screening guidelines for retinopathy of prematurity (ROP): The need for revision in extremely low birth weight infants. Pediatrics [in press].

112. What are the stages of ROP?

Stage I:	Line of demarcation separates vascular and avascular retina
Stage II:	Ridging of line of demarcation secondary to scar formation
Stage III:	Extraretinal fibrovascular proliferation present (In addition, in stages II and III, the term *plus disease* refers to active inflammation, as manifested by tortuosity of retinal vessels, which increases the risk of progression of ROP)
Stage IV:	Subtotal retinal detachment
Stage V:	Complete retinal detachment

113. What are the indications for cryotherapy or laser therapy in ROP?

In a multicenter trial by the Cryotherapy for ROP Cooperative Group, **threshold disease**, defined as a level of severity at which the risk of blindness approaches 50%, was chosen for treatment. This diagnosis required the presence of at least five contiguous or eight cumulative 30° sectors (clock hours) of stage III ROP (in zone 1 or 2) and the presence of plus disease.

114. How is vitamin E used in the prevention and treatment of ROP?

Recent trials of vitamin E therapy have not shown it to be effective in preventing ROP. However, because of its activity as an antioxidant, vitamin E treatment may lessen the severity of ROP. Serum vitamin E levels should be maintained at 1–2 mg/dl. Higher levels may be associated with toxicity (necrotizing enterocolitis or sepsis).

115. A baby has developed stage II ROP in the nursery. One of the attending neonatologists wants to restrict the use of oxygen in this infant, even though the child has significant apnea and bradycardia. Another attending believes that keeping the oxygen at consistently higher levels is better for the baby. Who is correct?

One of the debates that has raged in neonatology for many years is what oxygen levels are responsible for the development of ROP. Since the first observation by Campbell in the early 1950s associating oxygen with ROP, neonatologists have worried that unrestricted use of oxygen may lead to deterioration in eye disease in this condition. Furthermore, in the early 1970s, many malpractice judgments were awarded to babies who developed ROP in which there was only one arterial $paO_2 > 100$ mmHg during the entire hospitalization! Fortunately, those days have ended. Nevertheless, the optimal arterial levels of oxygen in the clinical circumstances outlined above have remained controversial.

Recently, the STOP-ROP Study trial group showed that there was no deterioration in retinopathy with the use of supplemental oxygen. In fact, there was a suggestion that babies with prethreshold disease might actually do somewhat better with oxygen saturation levels kept between 96% and 99%, although the results were not quite statistically significant. However, supplemental oxygen should be used with caution. Infants in the high saturation group in the STOP-ROP study exhibited more adverse pulmonary events.

STOP-ROP Multicenter Study Group: Supplemental therapeutic oxygen for prethreshold retinopathy of prematurity (STOP-ROP): A randomized, controlled trial. I: Primary ouctomes. Pediatrics 105: 294–310, 2000.

NEURORADIOLOGY

116. Two skilled and experienced observers have performed cerebral ultrasound scans on an infant born at 25 weeks' gestation who is now some weeks old. How likely are they to agree on their findings, and how likely are they to agree with the intracranial findings of the pathologist if the child died suddenly later that day?

There are surprisingly few data available on the interobserver variability of cerebral ultrasonography. However, both interobserver variability and prediction of pathologic appearances seem to depend on the type of lesion. Agreement is good with hemorrhagic lesions, such as germinal layer hemorrhage, intraventricular hemorrhage, and hemorrhagic parenchymal infarction. However, agreement between observers and with pathologic assessment for ischemic lesions and diffuse white matter disease rarely occurs. Diffuse echogenicity is an ultrasound diagnosis that is rarely agreed on among independent observers and should be treated with caution. If you don't believe this, try it for yourself with your colleagues.

117. How useful is an MRI scan for determining prognosis after neonatal encephalopathy?

Remarkably good if used properly. Certain features of MRI scans have poor interobserver agreement and predict tissue damage and outcome poorly. However, if interpretation is confined to observation of certain features, it is very good. Abnormal signal in the posterior limb of the internal capsule has a positive predictive value for bad outcome of nearly 100%, as long as the infant is more than 36 week's gestation and 3 days after birth. Other features can be useful but are less reliable for the formal assignation of prognosis.

BIBLIOGRAPHY

Neurologic Examination of the Newborn Infant
1. Ballard JL, Khoury JC, Wedig K, et al: New Ballard Score, expanded to include extremely premature infants. J Pediatr 119:417–423, 1991.
2. Ballard JL, Novak KK, Driver M: A simplified score for assessment of fetal maturation of newly born infants. J Pediatr 95:769–774, 1979.
3. Hittner H, Hirsch NJ, Rudolph AJ: Assessment of gestational age by examination of the anterior capsule of thelens. J Pediatr 91:455–458, 1977.

External Hemorrhage
4. Volpe JJ (ed): Neurology of the Newborn, 3rd ed. Philadelphia, W.B. Saunders, 1995, p 770.

Intracranial Hemorrhage
5. Paneth N, Rudelli R, Monte W, et al: White matter necrosis in very low birth weight infants: Neuropathologic and ultrasonographic findings in infants surviving six days or longer. J Pediatr 116:975–984, 1990.
6. Volpe JJ: Intraventricular hemorrhage and brain injury in the premature infant: Neuropathology and pathogenesis. Clin Perinatol 16:361–386, 1989.
7. Volpe JJ: Intraventricular hemorrhage and brain injury in the premature infant: Diagnosis, prognosis, and prevention. Clin Perinatol 16:387–411, 1989.

Periventricular Leukomalacia
8. Miller SP, Shevell MI, Patenaude Y, O'Gorman AM: Neuromotor spectrum of periventricular leukomalacia in children born at term. Pediatr Neurol 23:155–159, 2000.
9. Nwaesi CG, Pape KE, Martin DJ, et al: Periventricular infarction diagnosed by ultrasound: A postmortem correlation. J Pediatr 105:106–110, 1984.

Cerebral Palsy
10. Eicher PS, Batshaw ML: Cerebral palsy. Pediatr Clin North Am 40:537-551, 1993.
11. Grether JK, Nelson KB: Maternal infection and cerebral palsy in infants of normal birth weight. JAMA 278:207–211, 1997.
12. Nelson KB, Dambrosia JM, Grether JK, Philips TM: Neonatal cytokines and coagulation factors in children with cerebral palsy. Ann Neurol 44:665–675, 1998.
13. Palmer FB, Hoon AN: Cerebral palsy. In Parker S, Zuckerman B (eds): Behavioral and Developmental Pediatrics. Boston, Little, Brown, 1995, pp 88–94.
14. Shapiro BK, Capute AJ: Cerebral palsy. In Oski FA (ed): Principles and Practice of Pediatrics, 2nd ed. Philadelphia, Lippincott Williams & Wilkins, 1994, pp 679–686.
15. Taft LT: Cerebral palsy. Pediatr Rev 6:41, 1984.
16. Wu YW, Colford JM Jr: Chorioamnionitis as a risk factor for cerebral palsy: A meta-analysis. JAMA 234:1417–1424, 2000.

Neonatal Seizures
17. Cowan FM, Pennock JM, Hanrahan JD, et al: Early detection of cerebral infarction and hypoxic ischemic encephalopathy in neonates using diffusion-weighted magnetic resonance imaging. Neuropediatrics 25:172-175, 1994.
18. Mercuri E, Rutherford M, Cowan F, et al: Early prognostic indicators of outcome in infants with neonatal cerebral infarction: A clinical, electroencephalogram, and magnetic resonance imaging study. Pediatrics 103:39–46, 1999.
19. Volpe JJ: Neonatal seizures: Current concepts and revised classifications. Pediatrics 84:422–428, 1989.

Malformations of the Central Nervous System
20. Halamek LP: Malformations of the central nervous system. In Spitzer AR (ed): Intensive Care of the Fetus and Neonate. St. Louis, Mosby, 1996, pp 42–59.
21. Luthy DA, Wardinsky T, Shurtleff DB, et al: Cesarean section before the onset of labor and subsequent motor function in infants with meningomyelocele diagnosed antenatally. N Engl J Med 324:662–666, 1991.

Addiction in the Neonate
22. American Academy of Pediatrics Committee on Drugs: The transfer of drugs and other chemicals into human milk. Pediatrics 93:137–150, 1994.
23. Hurt H: Substance use during pregnancy. In Spitzer AR (ed): Intensive Care of the Fetus and Neonate. St. Louis, Mosby, 1996.
24. Hurt H, Brodsky NJ, Braitman LE, Giannetta J: Natal status of infants of cocaine-users and control subjects: A prospective comparison. J Perinatol 15:297–304, 1995.
25. Hurt H, Brodsky NJ, Betancourt L, et al: Cocaine-exposed children: Follow-up through 30 months. J Dev Behav Pediatr 16:29–35, 1995.

26. Mayes LC, Granger RH, Bornstein MH, Zuckerman B: The problem of prenatal cocaine exposure: A rush to judgment. JAMA 267:406–408, 1992.
27. Ostrea EM, Brady M, Gause S, et al: Drug screening of newborns by meconium analysis: A large-scale, prospective, epidemiologic study. Pediatrics 89:107–113, 1992.

Neurocutaneous Syndromes
28. Hurwitz S: Neurofibromatosis. In Hurwitz S (ed): Clinical Pediatric Dermatology: A Textbook of Skin Disorders of Childhood and Adolescence, 2nd ed. Philadelphia, W.B. Saunders, 1993, pp 624–629.
29. Tallman B, Tan OT, Morelli JG, et al: Location of port-wine stains and the likelihood of ophthalmic and/or central nervous system complications. Pediatrics 87:323–327, 1991.

Neuromuscular Disorders
30. Finegold SM, Arnon SS: Clostridial intoxication and infection. In Feigin RD, Cherry ID (eds): Textbook of Pediatric Infectious Diseases, 2nd ed. Philadelphia, W.B. Saunders, 1987.
31. Schreiner MS, Field E, Ruddy R: Infant botulism: A review of 12 years' experience at the Children's Hospital of Philadelphia. Pediatrics 87:159–165, 1991.

Retinopathy of Prematurity
32. Fierson WM, Palmer EA, Biglan AW, et al: Retinopathy of prematurity guidelines. Pediatrics 101:1093, 1998.
33. Wright K, Anderson ME, Walker E, Lorch V: Should fewer premature infants be screened for retinopathy of prematurity in the managed care era? Pediatrics 102:31–34, 1998.

13. ORTHOPAEDICS AND NEONATAL PAIN MANAGEMENT

1. How does Erb palsy differ from Klumpke palsy?

ERB PALSY	KLUMPKE PALSY
Involves upper plexus (C5, C6, and in 50% of cases, C7	Involves lower plexus (C8, T1)
Arm held adducted, internally rotated, and pronated with wrist and fingers flexed ("waiter's tip")	Small muscles of hand and wrist affected ("claw hand")
Biceps reflex absent, Moro reflex with hand movement but no shoulder abduction, palmar grasp present	Up to one-third have associated Horner syndrome
5% have ipsilateral diaphragmatic involvement	

2. What factors place the fetus and neonate at greater risk for brachial plexus palsy?

Birth brachial plexus palsy is a traumatic injury caused by stretching one or more components of the brachial plexus. It occurs in 0.4–2.5 per 1000 live births. Risk factors include high birth weight, prolonged labor, breech presentation, and shoulder dystocia. It is classified according to the severity of damage (mild, moderate, severe) and according to the components of the plexus that are injured. The palsy may involve the upper arm (the paralysis of Erb-Duchenne [C5, C6]), the lower arm (the paralysis of Klumpke [C8, T1]), or the entire arm.

3. What are the child's chances for recovery?

Recovery depends on the circumstances of delivery and the degree of paralysis noted. In most cases of Erb or Klumpke injury, there is a high likelihood of recovery, because the brachial plexus is not severed completely, but stretched and injured. With a paralysis of the entire arm, recovery is less likely, because the injury is more extensive.

4. What findings are helpful in the diagnosis of brachial plexus palsy?

On physical examination, close observation of spontaneous movement is important. In brachial plexus palsy, the affected arm lies motionless at the side with the elbow in extension. There is no motion in response to painful stimuli. The Moro reflex is absent on the affected side. One may also see an ipsilateral Horner syndrome or a phrenic nerve palsy. Radiographs of the upper extremity that include the clavicle should be taken to rule out a fracture.

5. How is brachial plexus injury treated?

Therapy must be aimed at preventing contractures. For the first 7–10 days, the arm is gently immobilized against the abdomen to minimize further hemorrhage and swelling. Following this initial period, passive range of motion exercises at the shoulder, elbow, wrist, and hand are performed. In addition, wrist splints to help stabilize the fingers and avoid contractures should be used.

6. What is the outcome of neonatal brachial plexus palsy?

Approximately 90% of patients have normal examinations by 12 months of age. Onset of recovery occurs within 2 weeks, and involvement of only the proximal upper extremity is a favorable prognostic sign.

7. What should be included in the differential diagnosis of birth brachial plexus palsy?

1. Birth fractures with pseudoparalysis of the upper extremity, including separation of the proximal humeral epiphysis, fracture of the clavicle, and fracture of the humeral shaft

2. Septic arthritis of the shoulder joint
3. Osteomyelitis of the humerus

8. A newborn infant is noted to have external rotation of the lower extremities at rest, with little spontaneous movement and bilateral foot deformities. What radiographs should be ordered?

Both spine and pelvis radiographs. The abnormalities described can be due to anomalies of the spine or the lower extremities.

9. A premature newborn infant on ventilator support in the neonatal intensive care unit (NICU) has decreased movement in the right lower extremity. What diagnostic tests may be appropriate?

Baseline laboratory testing should be considered (complete blood count [CBC], C-reactive protein, sedimentation rate) as part of the evaluation for possible joint infections, which are not uncommon in this setting. These tests may not be rewarding because infants may develop infection without abnormalities in their laboratory values. Plain radiographs of the entire extremity should be obtained to help detect subtle fracture that may not be apparent on clinical examination. Radiographs are often normal in the early phases of bone and joint infection. In this setting, bone and joint infections most often involve more than one site. Therefore, careful clinical assessment to detect subtle joint effusions or swelling over long bones is indicated. Often an ultrasound is helpful in confirming a joint effusion in the hip, because overlying muscle may mask the usual clinical findings. A technetium-99 (Tc-99) bone scan is very useful in detecting other sites of multicentric infection.

10. Initial evaluation of a first-born infant reveals multiple stiff joints in both the upper and lower extremities and thin, tapered, and "shiny" fingers. What is the main diagnostic consideration?

Arthrogryposis multiplex congenita (AMC) is a clinical syndrome characterized by poor development of the joints in utero leading to multiple contractures. This does not appear to be a hereditary condition, and there is no increased risk in siblings of the same family. Many mothers report decreased fetal movement in utero. On clinical examination, the limbs are usually symmetrical. Joints may have either flexion or extension contractures. There is decreased active and passive motion of the affected joints. The normal skin creases are usually absent, and the skin is taut and glossy. Dimpling at the joints may be present. There is atrophy of the limbs. Often the hips are dislocated, and clubfoot (talipes equinovarus) or congenital vertical talus affects the feet. The upper extremities are usually internally rotated at the shoulder, with elbow flexion or extension contractures. There are often radial head dislocations. The forearms are pronated with adduction deformity of the thumbs. Delivery may be difficult as a consequence of the stiff elbow and knee joints. This may result in birth fractures of the humerus and the femur. General health is not affected by this syndrome, although patients often exhibit minor respiratory difficulties and failure to thrive as newborns.

11. What congenital spine malformation is associated with maternal insulin-dependent diabetes?

Lumbosacral agenesis is more common in women with insulin-dependent diabetes. It is characterized by an absence of variable amounts of the sacrum and lumbar spine and the associated neural elements. There may also be concomitant anomalies of the genitourinary and gastrointestinal (GI) tracts. The level of the lesion may vary, and this will influence the clinical picture. These lesions are classified into four types according to the Renshaw classification.

• Type I is either partial or total sacral agenesis.
• Type II, the most common, is partial sacral agenesis with a symmetrical defect but a stable sacroiliac joint.

• Type III is variable lumbar agenesis with total sacral agenesis. The ilia articulate with the lowest lumbar vertebra that is present.

• Type IV is similar to type III but with the endplate of the most caudal vertebra resting on a fused ilia.

Depending on the severity of the agenesis, the patient may have variable foot deformities and abnormalities of the hips and knees.

12. A newborn child is suspected of having a genetic skeletal dysplasia. What is the most critical orthopaedic radiographic examination?

The most important radiograph is the lateral cervical spine. More than 150 distinct osteochondrodysplasias have been identified. Each has distinctive features, but many also have similar radiographic findings. One of the most common is agenesis or hypoplasia of the upper cervical spine elements. This can lead to instability and places the child at great risk of spinal cord injury during ordinary handling. Detection of cervical instability is mandatory to allow proper stabilization and protection.

13. Why has the term *developmental dysplasia of the hips* (DDH) replaced the term *congenital hip dislocation?*

DDH is now preferred over CHD to reflect the evolutionary nature of hip problems in infants in the first months of life. About 2.5–6.5 infants per 1000 live births develop problems, and a significant percentage of these problems are not present on neonatal screening examinations. Clearly, the overt pathologic process may not be present at birth, and periodic examination of the infant's hip is recommended at each routine well-baby exam until the age of 1 year.

14. What signs are indicative of DDH in the newborn?

The most reliable clinical methods of detection remain the **Ortolani reduction** and the **Barlow provocative maneuvers**. The infant should be lying quietly supine. The examiner then flexes the hip and thigh to 90°. The Ortolani test is done by lifting the greater trochanter toward the acetabulum as the leg is abducted in an attempt to palpate and reduce a dislocated femoral head. The Barlow test is an effort to dislocate the hip by adduction of the thigh and gentle downward pressure.

15. What is the significance of a "hip click" in a newborn?

A hip click is the high-pitched sensation felt at the very end of abduction when testing for developmental dysplasia of the hip with Barlow and Ortolani maneuvers. It occurs in up to 10% of newborns. Classically, it is differentiated from a hip "clunk," which is heard and felt as the hip goes in and out of joint. Most hip clicks are completely benign. The cause of the click is unclear but may be due to movement of the ligamentum teres between the femoral head and acetabulum or the hip adductors as they slide over the cartilaginous greater trochanter. Worrisome features that might warrant evaluation (e.g., hip ultrasound, hip x-ray) include late onset of click, associated orthopaedic abnormalities, or other clinical features suggestive of developmental dysplasia (e.g., asymmetric skin folds/creases, unequal leg length).

16. Why are hip x-rays for DDH often difficult to interpret in the newborn period?

The femoral head and acetabulum are cartilaginous at birth, and significant calcification to permit visualization on x-ray does not occur until 3–4 months of age. Because of this difficulty, some radiologists prefer to use ultrasound, although that, too, has its limitations. There is probably no substitute for a good exam under appropriate conditions!

17. Who is at highest risk for DDH?

Dislocated, dislocatable, and subluxable hip problems occur in about 1–5% of infants. However, 70% of dislocated hips occur in girls, and 20% occur in infants born in a breech position. Other risk associations include:

Congenital torticollis	Calcaneovalgus foot deformities in infants < 2500 g
Skull or facial abnormalities	Amniotic fluid abnormalities (especially
First pregnancy	oligohydramnios)
Positive family history of dislocation	Prolonged rupture of membranes
Metatarsus adductus	Large birth weight

MacEwen GD: Congenital dislocation of the hip. Pediatr Rev 11:249–252, 1990.

18. How is DDH treated?

The recommended treatment is to keep the legs abducted and the hips and knees flexed so that the developing head of the femur is kept within the acetabulum. Two commonly used devices are the Pavlik harness and the Frejka pillow splint. The use of multiple diapers to keep the hip adducted does not provide adequate stabilization and is usually not effective. Also, the use of diapers to treat a hip click is not warranted because the click is usually benign and the true DDH patient is not adequately treated by this approach.

19. What are the most common bacterial agents in neonatal osteomyelitis?

Staphylococcus aureus, group B *Streptococcus*, *Escherichia coli*, *Klebsiella*, *Salmonella*, and *Pseudomonas*. As opposed to osteomyelitis (which is not very common), septic arthritis is extremely rare. *Staphylococcus* is the most common organism, but one should always think of gonococcus as well with early septic arthritis.

20. What bone is most frequently fractured in the newborn?

The clavicle. This injury, which stems from excessive traction during delivery, generally results in a greenstick fracture. This fracture usually heals quite nicely without any therapy, although the callus formation may be notable.

21. How long should fractures in neonates be immobilized?

Neonatal fractures generally heal more quickly than their counterparts in children or adults. Because of this, and because of the difficulty in casting neonates, some fractures that would be severely problematic in an adult are barely treated in a neonate. A clavicular fracture will heal within 3 weeks in a newborn infant, as opposed to 6–8 weeks in an adult, and does not need to be immobilized in most cases. Femoral fractures, common in premature infants with rickets, are usually well healed within 3 weeks, compared with the 6–10 weeks in an older child or adult with this fracture. Femoral fractures usually are splinted to help healing, but not always if there is minimal displacement.

22. Discuss the features of constriction ring syndrome (Streeter's dysplasia).

Constriction ring syndrome is a rare syndrome that is characterized by ring-like constriction bands around the upper and lower extremities or the trunk. The etiology is unknown, and it is not hereditary. The extent and depth of the rings vary. The bands may be subcutaneous or may extend down to bone. These bands may interfere with lymphatic and venous return. This causes edema and enlargement of the distal part with decreased capillary refill. If there is great disruption to the local circulation, the part may undergo autoamputation in utero. Often there are other concomitant anomalies of the hand including syndactyly, acrodactyly, hypoplasia, camptodactyly, and symphalangia. Other associated anomalies include cleft palate and lip and talipes equinovarus deformity of the foot.

23. The foot of a newborn appears to be dorsiflexed such that the top of the foot lies directly against the anterior portion of the lower leg. What are the two diagnostic considerations, and how would you differentiate between the two?

Calcaneovalgus foot deformity is the most likely diagnosis. It is believed that there is no intrinsic problem with bone or joint development and that the deformity results from intrauterine positioning. The natural history of the untreated condition is one of spontaneous correction with no long-term sequelae. The second possibility is **posteromedial bowing of the distal tibia**. The foot is folded on the anterior surface of the leg, but the flexibility of the foot and ankle are normal. There is significant shortening of the affected side and decreased soft tissue. Because the physical findings may be difficult to distinguish from calcaneovalgus foot deformity in the newborn, anteroposterior (AP) and lateral radiographs of the leg should be obtained. This condition improves with time, usually during the first 3 years of life. However, long-term orthopaedic care is required because the affected limb always shows significant growth discrepancy and internal tibial torsion at maturity.

24. Discuss the orthopaedic manifestations of the TAR syndrome.

Thrombocytopenia with **absent r**adius (TAR) syndrome presents with several orthopaedic findings. In the upper extremity, there is bilateral absence of the radius usually with all five fingers present. The thumbs may be hypoplastic. Abnormalities of the fingers may include absence of the middle phalanx of the fifth finger, clinodactyly, or partial syndactyly. In almost one half of the patients, shortening or bowing of the ulna with deficiency of the extensor tendons may occur. In addition, the humerus may be short or absent. In almost 40% of patients, there are associated lower extremity anomalies. These mainly involve the knee and include subluxation or dislocation of the patella and hypoplasia of the knee. The most common deformity of the lower extremities is genu varum with a flexion contracture and internal tibial torsion. These patients also may have hip dislocations, varus or valgus deformities of the hips, and shortening of the legs with hypoplastic or absent tibiae or fibulae.

25. A newborn baby exhibits swelling over the midshaft of the right clavicle. What are the two most common diagnostic considerations?

Birth fractures of the clavicle are extremely common, but most often are accompanied by pseudoparalysis of the extremity (secondary to "splinting" from pain) for at least 3–5 days. There is pain with passive movement. Radiographs show the fracture, which usually heals with massive callus. In the absence of pain, one must consider congenital pseudarthrosis of the clavicle. The pseudarthrosis is fully present at birth. There is no history of birth injury or other trauma. The right clavicle is almost always affected. At the pseudarthrosis, the clavicular ends are enlarged, and there is painless motion between the two fragments. The etiology remains unknown, but several theories have been proposed including exaggerated arterial pulsations and pressure on the clavicle by the subclavian artery that is normally more cranial on the right side. In bilateral cases, it is thought that there is an abnormally high subclavian artery on both sides. With growth, the deformity increases, and the overlying skin becomes thin and atrophic. The affected shoulder often droops, and there is asymmetry between the two shoulders. No functional impairment is noted. Treatment involves resection of the nonunion and internal fixation with bone grafting.

26. True or false? Neonates do not perceive pain.

False. Although it has been a common conception that responses to noxious stimuli in neonates represented only decorticate responses, more recent studies demonstrate definite behavioral responses with nociception. Neonates (both term and preterm) exhibit flexion and adduction of the affected limb as well as distinct facial expressions. In older infants, there is also a pain "cry" with distinct spectrographic characteristics that distinguish it from other types of crying.

27. When does the fetus have the ability to perceive tactile stimuli?

Cutaneous sensory receptors first appear in the perioral area during the 8th week of gestation. They are present in all cutaneous and mucous surfaces by the 20th week of gestation. Synapses between the sensory fibers and neurons in the dorsal horn first appear at the 6th week of gestation.

28. What are signs of opiate withdrawal in neonates?

• **Neurologic:** high-pitched crying, irritability, increased wakefulness, hyperactive deep tendon reflexes, increased muscle tone, tremors, exaggerated Moro reflex, generalized seizures, intraventricular hemorrhage

- **GI:** poor feeding, uncoordinated and constant sucking, vomiting, diarrhea, dehydration
- **Autonomic signs:** increased sweating, nasal congestion, fever, mottling
- **Other:** poor weight gain, increased REM sleep, disorganized sleep states, skin excoriation

Many of these signs are components of scoring systems designed to quantify withdrawal in neonates and infants.

29. Is there any hazard in the use of fentanyl in neonates?

Fentanyl has numerous side effects. Many of these are common among all of the opiates, such as respiratory depression, sedation, dysphoria, seizures, nausea, vomiting, urinary retention, ileus, biliary tract spasm, and histamine release. The histamine release associated with fentanyl is thought to be less than that associated with other opiates, which may explain why large doses of fentanyl (25–50 µg/kg) may have little hemodynamic impact. Chest wall rigidity is a unique feature of fentanyl and appears to occur more frequently with rapid administration of large doses. It has also been observed that tolerance occurs more rapidly with fentanyl in neonates. This may be because of the shorter duration of action of fentanyl and its less potent sedating effects.

30. Is there a difference between the use of morphine and fentanyl infusions to sedate neonates on extracorporeal membrane oxygenation (ECMO)?

This is a topic of some controversy. Morphine might be a better choice than fentanyl because there are data to suggest that fentanyl binds extensively to the membrane in the ECMO lung. There are also data to suggest that morphine does not. Consequently, much higher doses of fentanyl may be required to achieve adequate sedation for a neonate on ECMO as opposed to a neonate being sedated for mechanical ventilation alone. However, the pharmacokinetics of morphine may not be straightforward on ECMO. Some data indicate that morphine clearance may increase after a patient is taken off ECMO. The etiology for this change is unclear but may relate to increased hepatic blood flow (and thus hepatic clearance) after a patient is removed from the ECMO circuit.

31. Is it practical to administer epidural analgesia in infants?

Yes, it can be. Most commonly, epidural analgesia is administered by placement of a caudal epidural catheter. With this approach, the epidural space is accessed by the sacrococcygeal hiatus, and the catheter is advanced into the caudal canal. Catheters introduced this way can sometimes be advanced so that the catheter tip is at the lumbar or thoracic level, although this can be quite difficult to do. The caudal approach minimizes risk of damage to the spinal cord. Sometimes anesthetic is administered in a single dose, rather than by using a catheter. The efficacy of the single dose can be variable.

32. Are there any adjunctive agents that can be used to help manage opioid withdrawal in infants?

Several pharmacologic agents are available. The opioid agents that are used tend to have a long half-life. Examples include paregoric, tincture of opium, and methadone. **Paregoric** has fallen out of favor because of the unclear side effects of its nonopiate ingredients (camphor, benzoic acid). **Tincture of opium** is widely used, but standardization with comparable morphine doses (estimated to be 0.04% morphine sulfate) is problematic. **Methadone** is becoming more popular because it can be administered intravenously or enterally and has a long half-life. It is equipotent with morphine. Its enteral bioavailability is virtually 100%.

Benzodiazepines, such as diazepam, are sometimes used, but they are not cross-tolerant with opiates. In addition, diazepam may also be addicting and thus is best used as an adjunct.

Phenobarbital can be useful for sedating and assistance in withdrawal but causes problems with hyperalgesia and alteration of drug metabolism. It also does not control the GI side effects of opiate withdrawal.

Chlorpromazine also has been useful because of its sedating effects. However, with improvements in long half-life opiates, it offers fewer advantages and has many adverse cardiovascular, endocrine, and autonomic side effects.

Clonidine is becoming a useful adjunct because it seems to allow the weaning process to take place more quickly. It is a centrally acting α_2-adrenergic agonist that has sedating effects and acts in tandem with other α-agonists. It is also now available in a transdermal patch form.

33. Is there any evidence that infants can have memory of painful events?

Yes. A recent study looked at how infants who had received topical anesthetic with EMLA prior to circumcision and how those who received no anesthetic prior to circumcision responded to immunization. Those who received EMLA did better with their immunizations in terms of their response to this painful experience!

Taddio A, Katz J, Ilersich AL, Koren G: Effect of neonatal circumcision on pain response during subsequent routine vaccination. Lancet 349(9052):599–603, 1997.

34. Chloral hydrate is a commonly used sedative in children. Can it be used in neonates?

Chloral hydrate (CH) is used in adults and children as a short-acting sedating agent that can be given enterally, has a short half-life, and has minimal effects on respiratory drive. This agent is thought to be a prodrug, which is metabolized to the active form trichloroethanol (TCE). It is cleared principally by glucuronidation and then by metabolism to trichloroacetic acid (TCA). Neonates respond to CH differently: the more active agent seems to be the prodrug and not TCE. TCE competes for hepatic glucuronidation and can displace bilirubin and other protein-bound drugs. Some studies suggest that clearance of CH and its metabolites is much slower in neonates and that these compounds can accumulate to toxic levels with repeated dosing, especially in the setting of hepatic or renal failure. In neonates, clinically detectable concentrations of metabolites can be measured 4–5 days after dosing of CH is stopped. Signs of CH toxicity can include GI irritability, hyperbilirubinemia, cardiac arrhythmias, hypotension, CNS depression, paradoxical agitation, and renal failure. There have also been some reports about potential carcinogenic effects.

Given all these caveats, chloral hydrate is probably safe in single doses but not given in repeated doses over a long period.

Sethna N: Regional anesthesia and analgesia. Semin Perinatol 22:180–389, 1998.

35. Why should EMLA be used with caution in infants/

EMLA is an acronym for eutectic mixture of local anesthetics. The two anesthetic agents in EMLA are lidocaine (2.5%) and prilocaine (2.5%). Prilocaine is metabolized to ortho-toluidine, which can oxidize clinically significant amounts of hemoglobin to methemoglobin in neonates and premature infants. This occurs because the stratum corneum is thinner, causing increased absorption and higher serum levels, and the activity of the NADH-dependent methemoglobin reductase enzyme is 40% lower in neonates than adults. Other factors that can contribute to systemic toxicity with prilocaine include sepsis, metabolic acidosis, anemia, hypoxia, glucose-6-phosphate dehydrogenase (G6PD) deficiency, and coadministration of other agents that produce oxidative stress such as sulfonamides, phenobarbital, phenytoin (Dilantin), and acetaminophen.

BIBLIOGRAPHY

1. Anand K, Arnold JH: Opioid tolerance and dependence in infants and children. Crit Care Med 22:334–342, 1994.
2. Anand K, Hickey P: Pain and its effects in the human neonate and fetus. N Engl J Med 317:1321–1329, 1987.
3. Arnold JH, Truog RD, Orav EJ, et al: Tolerance and dependence in neonates sedated with fentanyl during extracorporeal membrane oxygenation. Anesthesiology 73:1136–1140, 1990.
4. Arnold JH, Truog RD, Scavone JM, Fenton I: Changes in the pharmacodynamic response to fentanyl in neonates during continuous infusion J Pediatr 119:639–643, 1991.
5. Franck LS, Vilardi J, Durand D, Powers R: Opioid withdrawal in neonates after continuous infusions of morphine or fentanyl during extracorporeal membrane oxygenation. Am J Crit Care 7:364–369, 1998.
6. Geiduschek JM, Lynn AM, Bratton SL, et al: Morphine pharmacokinetics during continuous infusion of morphine sulfate for infants receiving extracorporeal membrane oxygenation. Crit Care Med 25:360–364, 1997.

7. Jackson ST, Hoffer MM, Parrish N: Brachial plexus palsy in the newborn. J Bone Joint Surg 70A:1217–1220, 1988.
8. Jacqz-Aigrain E, Burtin P: Clinical pharmacokinetics of sedatives in neonates. Clin Pharmacokinet 31:423–443, 1996.
9. Koren G, Crean P, Klein J, et al: Sequestration of fentanyl by the cardiopulmonary bypass (CPBP). Eur J Clin Pharmacol 27:51–56, 1984.
10. Kornblum M, Stanitski DF: Spinal manifestations of skeletal dysplasias. Orthop Clin North Am 30:501–520, 1999.
11. Leuschen MP, Willett LD, Hoie EB, et al: Plasma fentanyl levels in infants undergoing extracorporeal membrane oxygenation. J Thorac Cardiovasc Surg 105:885–891, 1993.
12. MacEwen GD: Congenital dislocation of the hip. Pediatr Rev 11:249–252, 1990.
13. Sethna N: Regional anesthesia and analgesia. Semin Perinatol 22:180–389, 1998.
14. Suresh S, Anand K: Opioid tolerance in neonates: Mechanisms, diagnosis, assessment, and management. Semin Perinatol 22:425–433, 1998.
15. Taddio A, Katz J, Ilersich AL, Koren G: Effect of neonatal circumcision on pain response during subsequent routine vaccination. Lancet 349(9052):599–603, 1997.

14. PULMONOLOGY

DIFFERENTIAL DIAGNOSIS OF NEONATAL PULMONARY DISORDERS

1. Although apnea in premature infants is often due to the degree of immaturity (so-called apnea of prematurity), what are other causes of apnea in this population?

SYSTEM	PERTURBATION
Central nervous system	Intracranial hemorrhage, hypoxic-ischemic encephalopathy, seizures, congenital anomalies, maternal drugs, drugs used to treat the infant
Respiratory	Pneumonia, obstruction with lesions, anatomic obstruction (pharynx or tongue blocking airway), upper airway collapse (tracheal or laryngomalacia), severe respiratory distress syndrome, atelectasis
Infections	Septicemia or meningitis due to bacterial, fungal, or viral agents
Gastrointestinal	Necrotizing enterocolitis, gastroesophageal reflux, Valsalva during bowel movements
Metabolic	Hypoglycemia, hypocalcemia, hypo- or hypernatremia, inborn errors of metabolism, increased ambient temperature, hypothermia
Cardiovascular	Hypotension, congestive heart failure, hypovolemia, patent ductus arteriosus
Hematologic	Anemia

2. Of all newborn infants who die from culture-proven bacteremia, what proportion has pneumonia?

Ninety percent of infants dying from bacteremia have evidence of pneumonia on postmortem examination. Many of these infants, however, will not have positive blood cultures during life, making the bacteriologic diagnosis of pneumonia a very difficult one in the newborn. If pneumonia is suspected from clinical examination or chest x-ray, it should be treated aggressively until it has clinically resolved or the child has been treated for a minimum of 10 days.

3. What are the most common radiographic features of group B streptococcal (GBS) pneumonia in premature infants? In full-term infants?

In premature infants, GBS often mimics respiratory distress syndrome (RDS) with a diffuse reticulogranular pattern and air bronchograms. It is unclear whether this is an indication of simultaneous disease processes (RDS and GBS) or whether the GBS disease causes a secondary surfactant deficiency that produces a radiographic appearance similar to RDS when the premature infant is infected.

In term-gestation neonates, the most common GBS appearance mimics that of transient tachypnea of the newborn, with increased perihilar interstitial markings, hyperexpanded lung fields, and small pleural effusions.

4. Is apnea of prematurity correlated with an increased incidence of sudden infant death syndrome (SIDS)?

No. Although apnea is often believed to be a provocative factor for SIDS, this relationship has never been causally established. It appears that premature infants with apnea of prematurity are no more likely to die from SIDS than those of comparable gestational age who do not have apnea of prematurity. Premature infants do, however, have a higher SIDS rate than do term infants, suggesting that immaturity of respiratory control may be a component of SIDS. Furthermore, several studies have indicated that unless one records respiratory patterns of premature infants, apnea will not be detected because the respiratory abnormalities in these babies are very difficult to see clinically.

5. What is the differential diagnosis of infants who are unable to expand their lungs at birth, even with positive pressure ventilation?
- Massive meconium aspiration syndrome (MAS)
- Congenital (intrauterine) pneumonia
- Pulmonary hypoplasia
- Congenital diaphragmatic hernia (CDH)
- Massive pleural effusions (e.g., with hydrops fetalis)
- Cystic adenomatoid malformation
- Anatomic malformations: tracheal or laryngeal webs, hypoplasia, or agenesis

NEONATAL RESUSCITATION

6. What is the maximum concentration of oxygen that a self-inflating anesthesia bag not connected to an oxygen reservoir can deliver?

Only about 40% oxygen can be delivered without a reservoir. Each time a self-inflating bag is squeezed, room air is drawn into the bag, diluting any oxygen that is connected. When a reservoir is connected, concentrations up to 90% or more of oxygen may be delivered. One of the limitations of the self-inflating bag is that the desired concentration of oxygen cannot be altered easily.

7. What are the approximate endotracheal (ET) tube sizes that would be appropriate for premature infants of varying birth weights?
- 2.5 mm internal diameter (ID) for infants < 1000 g
- 3.0 mm ID for infants 1000–2000 g
- 3.5 mm ID for infants 2000–3500 g

These sizes are reasonable approximations for most infants, but attention should be paid to the ease of introduction of the ET tube into the airway. A 2.5-mm ET tube may be too small for some babies < 1000 g, and it may be too large for a few infants with birth weights > 1000 g. The ET tube should go easily into the airway, and a small leak should be audible around the ET tube when pressures of 25–30 cm H_2O are exceeded. Too snug of an ET tube may lead to tracheal inflammation and stenosis, whereas too small an ET tube simply may not allow adequate gas delivery to the lungs.

8. Prior to radiographic verification, how far should an ET tube be inserted to be in the appropriate position for infants of varying birth weight?

The "tip-to-lip" rule for placement is the distance from the ET tube tip to the centimeter marking on the tube itself. Good approximations are:
- 7 cm for a child of 1000 g birth weight
- 8 cm for a child of 2000 g birth weight
- 9 cm for a child of 3000 g birth weight
- 10 cm for a child of 4000 g birth weight

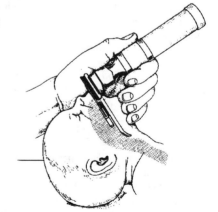

Appropriate position for ET tube insertion. (From Goldsmith JP, Karotkin EH (eds): Assisted Ventilation of the Neonate. Philadelphia, W.B. Saunders, 1996, p 108, with permission.)

9. Which of the following is currently recommended by the Neonatal Resuscitation Program (NRP): (a) calcium chloride for asystole; (b) atropine for bradycardia; (c) epinephrine for heart rate < 60/minute; (d) 5% albumin for hypovolemia; (e) room air ventilation instead of 100% oxygen ventilation?

Only (c) epinephrine for heart rate < 60/minute is currently recommended by the NRP. The other therapies have their advocates, but most studies have not shown them to be effective adjuncts to neonatal resuscitation. Room air resuscitation, in particular, has been suggested recently as an alternative to oxygen resuscitation in order to reduce free oxygen radical exposure, but no large-scale, prospective studies have, as yet, demonstrated its safety and efficacy.

10. Name some important historical figures who needed resuscitation after birth.

Voltaire, Samuel Johnson, Goethe, Thomas Hardy, Pablo Picasso, and Franklin D. Roosevelt. The world would have been a very different place had these individuals not had the benefit of resuscitation, rudimentary as it was. Remember, there were no board-certified neonatologists until the mid-1970s!

11. Who was the first to use a mechanical device for intubation and resuscitation of neonates?

Blundell (1790–1878), a Scottish obstetrician, used a "silver tracheal pipe" that had a blunt distal end with two side holes. He would slide his fingers over the tongue to feel the epiglottis and guide the tube into the trachea. Blundell would blow air into the tube approximately 30 times a minute to ventilate the baby.

12. Name the three initial steps in neonatal resuscitation.

1. Thermal management—the infant should be dried and kept warm to avoid breakdown of brown fat.
2. The airway should be cleared of fluid and birth debris.
3. The baby should receive tactile stimulation. One does not need to spank the baby's bottom. Gentle stroking and rubbing of the skin of the legs and buttocks should suffice. The thorax should not be rubbed because it may interrupt a respiratory effort.

13. What is primary apnea, and how is it distinguished from secondary apnea?

A regular sequence of events occurs when an infant becomes hypoxemic and acidemic. Initially, gasping respiratory efforts increase in depth and frequency for up to 3 minutes, followed by approximately 1 minute of primary apnea. If oxygen (along with stimulation) is provided during the apneic period, respiratory function spontaneously returns. If asphyxia continues, gasping then resumes for a variable period of time, terminating with the "last gasp" and followed by secondary apnea. During secondary apnea, the only way to restore respiratory function is with positive pressure ventilation and high concentrations of oxygen. Thus, a linear relationship exists between the duration of asphyxia and the recovery of respiratory function following resuscitation. The longer the artificial ventilation is delayed after the last gasp, the longer it will take to resuscitate the infant. However, clinically, the two conditions are indistinguishable.

Recently, it has been suggested that resuscitation with room air may be as effective as high oxygen resuscitation. The concept is that the use of high oxygen may provoke free radical injury to the brain during resuscitation. More work needs to be done in this area before oxygen can be abandoned, however, because apneic infants are often quite hypoxemic.

14. How much pressure does it take to inflate the lungs of a normal infant at the moment of birth?

The first breath of an infant has been measured in the delivery room and is reported to be between –30 and –140 cm H_2O. These pressures are needed to overcome the substantial fluid and elastic forces in the airway. As surfactant is deposited, however, subsequent breaths rapidly decrease to –4 to –10 cm H_2O. If surfactant is decreased, as in RDS, the baby must continue to exert the original very high effort to continue to inflate the lung. With limited energy reserves, this effort soon deteriorates, and respiratory failure ensues.

15. Should infants be intubated nasally or orally?

Studies support both routes of intubation for newborn infants. The oral intubation school argues that, because neonates are obligate nose breathers, they will demonstrate increased work of breathing and atelectasis following removal of nasotracheal tubes. On the other hand, the nasal intubation school asserts that orotracheal intubation results in grooving of the palate with subsequent orthodontic problems. Nasal tubes, however, have been associated with injury to the nasal cartilage. Therefore, operator skill and institutional tradition are primary considerations in this clinical decision.

TRANSITIONAL PHYSIOLOGY AND THE ASPHYXIATED FETUS

16. Asphyxia is a condition of impaired gas exchange characterized by what blood gas abnormalities?

A. Hypoxemia
B. Hypercapnia
C. Metabolic acidosis

C. Metabolic acidosis. Asphyxia has become a controversial subject because so much litigation has been initiated over difficult deliveries of babies. *Asphyxia* often is used inappropriately to describe infants who experience transient depression or delayed transition, much to the dismay of obstetricians because of the medicolegal problems associated with birth asphyxia. In general, it is better not to label infants as "asphyxiated," but simply to describe numerically the metabolic derangements that are present following birth.

17. A child is depressed and requires vigorous resuscitation in the delivery room. Subsequently he demonstrates labile oxygenation and right-to-left shunting. A heart murmur is auscultated. What is the most likely anatomic or physiologic basis for the murmur?

Tricuspid regurgitation is the most likely source of the murmur. Tricuspid regurgitation is due to increased pulmonary pressure and the back-flow of blood into the right atrium. Although two fetal channels often remain open in this situation of transitional circulation (the foramen ovale and the ductus arteriosus), the source of heart murmurs is most likely from the associated tricuspid regurgitation.

18. In the American Academy of Pediatrics–American College of Obstetricians and Gynecologists' guidelines regarding intrapartum asphyxia as a cause of brain injury, what criteria must be present?

A neonate who has had severe enough hypoxia proximal to delivery to result in hypoxic ischemic encephalopathy should show evidence of all of the following:

- Profound metabolic or mixed acidemia (pH < 7.00) on an umbilical cord arterial blood sample
- Persistence of an Apgar score of 0–3 for longer than 5 minutes
- Neonatal neurologic sequelae (e.g., seizures, coma, or hypotonia)
- Multiorgan system dysfunction (e.g., renal, cardiovascular, gastrointestinal, pulmonary, or hematologic)

American Academy of Pediatrics, American College of Obstetricians and Gynecologists: Guidelines for Perinatal Care, 4th ed. Elk Grove Village, IL, AAP/ACOG, 1997.

19. What are the established relationships between Apgar scores and subsequently diagnosed cerebral palsy (CP)?

- 73% of children who develop CP have 5-minute Apgar scores of 7–10.
- A child with a 1-minute Apgar Score of 0–3, but a 10-minute Apgar score of ≥ 4 has a 1% chance of subsequently developing CP.

- Of children with a 15-minute Apgar score of 0–3, 53% die and 38% of survivors will subsequently develop CP.
- Of children with a 20-minute Apgar score of 0–3, 59% die and 57% of survivors will subsequently develop CP.

20. True or false: Mental retardation or seizures that are not associated with cerebral palsy are not likely to be due to asphyxia or other intrapartum events?

True. The etiology of mental retardation and seizures is not known in most cases.

21. In 1862, William John Little concluded that "spastic rigidity" (cerebral palsy) was due exclusively to perinatal events. This led to the general belief of the next 100 years that cerebral palsy was a preventable disorder due to obstetric events. What was Dr. Little's medical specialty?

Dr. Little was an orthopaedic surgeon. He saw children with the spasticity and mobility problems associated with CP. Only in the past two decades has it been recognized that only 4–10% of CP can be attributed to intrapartum events. That understanding has not, however, prevented the initiation of litigation in many cases of CP, even when no obstetric or neonatal malpractice exists!

22. What prominent neurologist in 1897 came to the conclusion that most CP was not due to intrapartum events?

Sigmund Freud. Although he is most well-known for his work in psychiatry, Freud was a prominent neurologist who made many astute observations in the field.

23. True of false: Electronic fetal monitoring of the fetal heart rate has resulted in decreased deaths and a decrease in the incidence of cerebral palsy?

False. Electronic fetal monitoring has not been shown to be any better than intermittent auscultation of the fetal heart rate. There are no well-controlled trials that show any decline in deaths or cerebral palsy rates that can be attributed to electronic fetal heart rate monitoring.

24. What are the arterial PO_2 levels in a fetus?

If one were to obtain arterial blood gases in a fetus, the PaO_2 would be in the range of 25–35 mmHg. Although seemingly low, the high affinity of fetal hemoglobin for oxygen results in a highly saturated blood that is sufficient to meet the metabolic needs of the fetus. There is, however, little additional room for the PO_2 to decrease, and the fetus who begins to decrease his oxygen level even a small amount may develop problems quickly.

25. Isn't fetal distress the same thing as "asphyxia" of the fetus?

No. Fetal distress will often manifest as nonreassuring fetal heart rate patterns, meconium staining of the amniotic fluid, or low 1-minute Apgar score. None of these have any predictive value for long-term neurologic outcome. However, the presence of signs of fetal distress is a good predictor of the need for resuscitation after delivery.

26. Is asphyxia reversible?

Shorter and less severe periods of asphyxia often reverse spontaneously and may not lead to any long-term damage unless they occur repeatedly. However, complete failure of gas exchange can cause death in as little as 10 minutes.

The outcome of infants with asphyxia depends on several factors:

Speed of onset of asphyxia

Duration and extent of asphyxia

Presence of ischemia in addition to hypoxia

Resuscitative efforts

The significance of ischemia, in particular, cannot be overstated. Unless circulation is restored, the administration of oxygen will not be effective and acidemia will increase. The ABCs of resuscitation—**a**irway, **b**reathing, **c**irculation—remain the key to successful outcome in resuscitation.

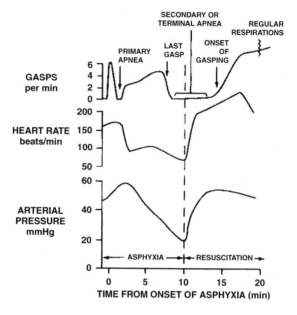

Asphyxial changes and the effects of resuscitation. (From Goldsmith JP, Karotkin EH (eds): Assisted Ventilation of the Neonate. Philadelphia, W.B. Saunders, 1996, p 84, with permission.)

27. Who was Virginia Apgar?

Virginia Apgar, an anesthesiologist at Columbia Presbyterian Medical Center in New York City, introduced the Apgar scoring system in 1953 to assess the newborn infant's response to the stress of labor and delivery.

28. If Apgar scores are not useful in predicting long-term outcome, why do we even bother recording them?

Apgar scores are useful for assessing and describing the condition of neonates after birth and their subsequent transition to extrauterine state.

ASSESSMENT	0	1	2
Breathing	No spontaneous respirations	Weak respiratory effort	Vigorous respiratory effort
Heart rate	No heart rate (HR)	HR < 100 bpm	HR > 100 bpm
Color	Generalized cyanosis	Acrocyanosis	Pink, including extremities
Reflex irritability	None	Weakly responsive	Vigorously responsive
Tone	Flaccid	Weak tone	Good tone

The Apgar scores are generally obtained and totaled at 1 minute and 5 minutes following birth, and scores should be recorded for longer periods (at 10, 15, and even 20 minutes) if they are low (until the score is ≥ 7). Low Apgar scores are useful in identifying neonates who are depressed, and the change in score at 1 minute, 5 minutes, and subsequent time intervals is helpful in assessing the efficacy of resuscitation. Low Apgar scores (< 3) that persist beyond 5 minutes have a better correlation with a poor long-term outcome than Apgar scores at 1 minute.

29. What is the long-term outcome of infants who are severely asphyxiated?

The mortality among severely asphyxiated infants is high and can vary from 50% to 75%. Among survivors, long-term neurodevelopmental sequelae are common and occur in approximately one-third of infants. Currently, there are no dependable predictors of long-term outcome. Presence and extent of neurologic abnormalities in the early postasphyxial phase and the persistence of abnormal neurologic findings at the time of discharge are the simplest and most effective predictors of long-term outcome. One measure of the severity of early neurologic dysfunction is the clinical staging system developed by Sarnat. Infants with Sarnat stage 1 encephalopathy are the ones who have mild asphyxia and recover without any significant neurologic sequelae. However, among infants with Sarnat stages 2 and 3 encephalopathy, the incidence of long-term neurodevelopmental handicaps can range anywhere from 50% to 100%. In one study of infants who had no detectable heart rate at birth and at 1 minute of age, two-thirds died prior to discharge, and 33% of the survivors had severe neurologic handicaps.

Sarnat Classification of Postanoxic Encephalopathy

SARNAT STAGE	SIGNS/SYMPTOMS	EEG RESULTS	OUTCOME
I	Lasts < 24 hours; hyperalert; uninhibited Moro and stretch reflexes; sympathetic effects	Normal	Normal
II	Obtundation; hypotonia; strong distal flexion; multifocal seizures	Periodic EEG pattern, occasionally preceded by continuous delta activity	Normal if < 5 days; abnormal if > 7 days
III	Stuporous; flaccid; suppressed autonomic and brain stem functions	Isopotential EEG or burst-suppression	Likely neurologic impairment or death

From Sarnat HB, Sarnat MS: Neonatal encephalopathy following fetal distress. A clinical and electroencephalographic study. Arch Neurol 33:696–705, 1976, with permission.

Jain L, Ferre C, Vidyasagar D, et al: Cardiopulmonary resuscitation of apparently stillborn infants. J Pediatr 118:778–782, 1991.

30. Are newborn brains more resistant to perinatal hypoxic and ischemic injury?

Younger animals have been shown to have greater resistance to hypoxic-ischemic injury than older animals. However, certain areas of the brain appear to be more vulnerable to injury in neonates than in adults and in preterm as compared with term infants. The neonatal brain is often described as having some degree of "plasticity," in which some areas may assume function of other areas of the brain following injury. To what degree this phenomenon actually takes place is not known, but it may explain why prediction of outcome following neurologic injury in the neonate is so fraught with error.

31. What are the differences in the pattern of neurologic injury after hypoxic-ischemic insult in preterm and term infants?

In preterm infants who survive with hypoxic-ischemic injury, periventricular leukomalacia (PVL) is the most common (and most devastating) neuropathologic lesion. A large percentage of infants with PVL develop spastic diplegia later on in their lives. In term infants, patterns of neuropathologic injury commonly seen are "watershed infarcts" and diffuse cortical necrosis. These infants are at high risk for developing spastic monoplegia, hemiplegia, or quadriplegia.

32. Asphyxiated infants who are successfully resuscitated often show signs of injury to multiple organ systems. What other organs are involved? Is the injury permanent?

In asphyxiated infants who have been successfully resuscitated, the central nervous system (CNS) is the most frequently involved site (72%), followed by the kidneys (62%), heart (29%), intestines (29%), and lungs (26%). Multiple organ involvement occurs even as the asphyxiated fetus or neonate tries to redistribute blood to vital organs as a part of the diving reflex. Fortunately, injury to these organs (except CNS) is not permanent, and complete recovery of function can be expected in most infants who survive. However, the presence of multiorgan failure can seriously jeopardize chances of survival in the immediate postnatal period.

Martin-Ancel A, Garcia-Mix A, Gaya F, et al: Multiple organ involvement in perinatal asphyxia. J Pediatr 127:786–793, 1995.

33. What is the cause of oliguria in infants with hypoxic-ischemic perinatal injury?

Oliguria is commonly seen in asphyxiated infants and can result from one or more of the following causes:

• Acute renal failure (either acute tubular necrosis or acute cortical necrosis)
• Asphyxiated bladder syndrome
• Syndrome of inappropriate antidiuretic hormone secretion (SIADH)

Although recovery from acute tubular necrosis is common, acute cortical necrosis is usually fatal. Infants with asphyxiated bladder syndrome, with marked distention, usually recover within a few days, as do most infants with SIADH, unless there has been a pituitary infarct.

34. Prolonged resuscitation in the delivery rooms often makes resuscitated infants very cold. Is hypothermia harmful to these infants?

Until recently, the presence of hypothermia in resuscitated infants was thought to correlate with poor survival and higher occurrence of complications. However, recent studies have shown that selective cooling of the brain in infants suspected of having severe hypoxic-ischemic brain damage can improve long-term outcome. Initial pilot studies from several nurseries around the world have been very promising in this regard. Hypothermia trials are currently being conducted, and we hope to have the answer to this question before the next edition of this book is published.

35. What is the outcome of infants receiving various forms of resuscitation?

Outcome of depressed infants is usually determined by the degree of resuscitative efforts that are necessary. In one study, infants who required chest compressions and epinephrine had the worst outcome, with up to 56% dying in the neonatal period and 21% with intracranial hemorrhage. Other complications noted in recipients of chest compressions included seizures (18%), respiratory distress (68%), and pneumothorax (24%).

Jain L, Vidyasagar D: Cardiopulmonary resuscitation of newborns: Its application to transport medicine. Pediatr Clin North Am 40:287–301, 1993.

36. How is the outcome of resuscitation affected by prematurity and birth weight?

Very low birth weight (VLBW) infants have the greatest need for resuscitation at birth, with up to two-thirds of infants less than 1500 g requiring some form of resuscitation. The morbidity and mortality in VLBW infants requiring cardiopulmonary resuscitation (CPR) are inversely related to their birth weight. Recent data indicate that VLBW infants do better if they are delivered and cared for at tertiary care centers. The speed of an in-house response team to the delivery room for resuscitation unquestionably is a great advantage of the tertiary care center compared to a community hospital.

37. What are the absolute indications for initiating positive pressure ventilation through a bag and mask apparatus in a newborn?

• Apnea
• Ineffective or gasping respirations
• Bradycardia (heart rate < 100 bpm)
• Intractable cyanosis

38. What are two contraindications to immediate bag-mask ventilation?

Immediate bag and mask ventilation is contraindicated when there is thick meconium in the hypopharynx and trachea or if a congenital diaphragmatic hernia is known or suspected. In all instances, however, the resuscitator must weigh the advantages of bag and mask therapy with the risks. At times, immediate intubation for either suctioning or avoidance of abdominal distention may be required.

39. What are some indications for endotracheal intubation during the resuscitation of a newborn?

- Need for prolonged bag and mask ventilation
- Prolonged chest compressions (> 1 minute)
- Ineffective bag-mask ventilation
- Delivery through thick or particulate meconium-stained amniotic fluid
- Congenital diaphragmatic hernia (avoid insufflating the bowel with bag-mask ventilation, if possible)

40. What causes persistent bradycardia or cyanosis in an infant who is receiving bag-mask ventilation?

- Improper mask size or fit (mask should fit snugly from the bridge of the baby's nose to the base of the chin)
- Poor seal of mask over the baby's face
- Improper positioning of the infant (remember to place the baby in the "sniffing" position, with the neck slightly extended and the chin up)
- Airway obstruction or need for suctioning
- Ineffective manual ventilation (remember to watch for that chest rise and to use just enough positive pressure ventilation—about 15–20 cm H_2O pressure for the average term infant— to see good chest rise)
- Make sure the oxygen source is turned on to the bag apparatus: "the heart and lungs can't run if there's no gas"

41. What are the appropriate steps for intubation of a neonate?

1. Always check the equipment to assure proper functioning (e.g., laryngoscope blade bulb works, suction is on, 100% free flow oxygen is turned on, tape for ET tube is available).

2. Be sure that the warmer bed is flattened and not at an angle, which will distort landmarks.

3. Choose the appropriately sized ET tube.

4. Position the baby with his neck slightly extended and his chin up (use a roll under the shoulders to achieve proper extension if necessary). Do not hyperextend the neck!

5. Make sure the hypopharynx has been suctioned to clear debris.

6. Using the laryngoscope blade to visualize the vocal cords, insert the ET tube to the appropriate depth. (Limit intubation attempts to approximately 20 seconds to avoid reflex bradycardia.)

7. Institute manual ventilation while holding the tube in a secure position.

8. Listen for equal breath sounds on both sides of the chest.

9. Auscultate over the stomach to make sure there is not an esophageal intubation.

10. Watch for symmetric chest rise. Give just enough positive pressure to initiate chest rise.

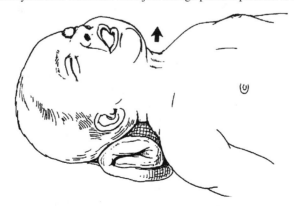

The infant in the sniffing position. Note that the neck is not hyperextended. (From Goldsmith JP, Karotkin EH (eds): Assisted Ventilation of the Neonate. Philadelphia, W.B. Saunders, 1996, p 142, with permission.)

42. When should epinephrine be given during a resuscitation in the delivery room?

In a depressed infant with gasping or absent respirations, 100% oxygen should be given via positive pressure ventilation (PPV). Depending on the extent of asphyxia (and depression of heart rate), cardiac compressions are usually initiated within 30 seconds. If there is no response (i.e., increased heart rate) after at least 30 seconds of PPV with 100% oxygen and chest compressions, epinephrine is indicated. Epinephrine 1:10,000 can be given through an IV, umbilical vein, or ET tube at a dose of 0.1–0.3 ml/kg.

43. When is sodium bicarbonate administered in a resuscitation?

If there is no response to epinephrine in a severely asphyxiated infant (with continued apnea and a heart rate < 100 bpm), sodium bicarbonate (and/or a volume expander) should be considered. If an infant is being adequately ventilated, the partial correction of metabolic acidosis may improve pulmonary blood flow and improve oxygenation. Half-strength (4.2% solution or 0.5 mEq/ml) bicarbonate is preferable, given in a dose of 2 mEq/kg slowly over 2–5 minutes.

44. Are there complications of sodium bicarbonate therapy in infants?

The relative risks of sodium bicarbonate therapy in infants are related to dosage (higher > lower), rapidity of administration (faster > slower), and osmolality (higher > lower). Physiologic complications include a transient increase in $PaCO_2$ and fall in PaO_2. The sudden expansion of blood volume and increase in cerebral blood flow may increase the risk of periventricular and intraventricular hemorrhage in preterm infants. Other potential complications include the development of hypernatremia and metabolic alkalosis.

45. If the newborn is stabilized and the extent of acidosis is determined by an arterial blood gas, how is the therapeutic correction calculated?

$$\text{Dose of NaHCO}_3 \text{ (mEq)} = \text{Base deficit (mEq/L)} \times \text{body weight (kg)} \times$$
$$0.3 \text{ (bicarbonate space)} \times 0.5 \text{ (half correction)}$$

Generally, it is safest to correct half the base deficit initially and then reassess acid-base status to determine if further correction is necessary. Under optimal circumstances, sodium bicarbonate should be infused in small doses over 10–20 minutes as a dilute solution (0.5 mEq/ml). It is sometimes not possible to take that long to give bicarbonate. These authors have not found that more rapid infusion (over 5 minutes) in a hypoxemic, acidemic baby is especially deleterious.

46. What are the side effects of naloxone?

Naloxone has a history of being remarkably free of side effects, except for the possible precipitation of sudden drug withdrawal in infants born to drug-addicted mothers. Other reported side effects relate to the sudden release of catecholamines, which can cause hypertension, sudden cardiac arrest, and cardiac dysrhythmias. It is important to remember that the half-life of naloxone is significantly shorter than that of opioids.

47. Should umbilical arterial catheters be kept in a "low" or "high" position?

Umbilical catheters kept in a low position (L3–5) have a somewhat higher incidence of lower limb blanching and cyanosis compared with high lines (T6–10). However, it may be preferable to see a lower limb blanch and be able to remove a catheter than to have a renal or mesenteric vessel blanch about which no one is aware! Also, high lines may be associated with a slightly increased risk of periventricular or intraventricular hemorrhage and embolization of clots to arterial vessels distal to the catheter site. No differences in the development of sepsis or necrotizing enterocolitis have been noted between infants with low or high umbilical catheters.

48. What is the primary way by which an infant regulates cardiac output?

Heart rate is the main variable through which an infant can increase cardiac output. A baby cannot significantly change stroke volume. Bradycardia will significantly reduce a newborn's cardiac output.

49. What are the indications for chest compressions in an infant, and how should they be done?

If the infant's heart rate is < 60, or 60–80 and not rising after 30 seconds of positive pressure ventilation, external cardiac massage should be initiated. Compressions are stopped when the heart rate rises above 80 bpm. To do compressions on an infant correctly, place the hands around the chest, compress the mid to lower sternum with the thumbs, and press down firmly by $\frac{1}{4}$ to $\frac{3}{4}$ of an inch. Compression should continue at $\frac{1}{4}$-second intervals with ventilation interposed after every third compression in a 3:1 ratio (i.e., 90 compressions and 30 ventilations per minute).

50. What is a good source of emergent venous access in the newborn?

An umbilical venous catheter (UVC). A UVC can be placed quickly by trimming the umbilicus to approximately 1 cm in length and inserting the catheter just far enough to obtain blood flow (usually about 4–5 cm in term infants). All medications (including vasopressor agents) and fluids can be given through this line. This source of access is often available for many days after birth with appropriate preparation of the cord.

51. What are the common medications used for newborn resuscitation? How are they given and in what doses?

Neonatal Resuscitative Drugs

DRUG	CONCENTRATION	DOSE	ROUTE(S)
Epinephrine	1:10,000	0.1–0.3 ml	Intratracheally Intravenously Intracardiac
NaHCO$_3$	0.5 mEq/ml	1–2 mEq/kg	Intravenously, slowly
Naloxone	0.4 mg/ml	0.25–0.5 ml/kg	Intravenously Intramuscularly Subcutaneously Endotracheally (dilute)

52. What fluids are appropriate to use in newborn resuscitation?
- **Colloids:** 5% albumin, plasma derivatives, and blood
- **Crystalloids:** normal saline and lactated Ringer's solution. Avoid the use of glucose solutions for acute volume expansion if possible.

53. Why is it important to check blood glucose concentration during resuscitation?

Hypoglycemia can be very damaging to the developing nervous system. It can result when hepatic glycogen stores are depleted from stress. A blood glucose level < 45 mg/dl should be treated immediately. Ten percent dextrose in water should be infused at a dose of 2–4 ml/kg over 10–15 minutes in an attempt to correct hypoglycemia. It is not necessary to use higher concentrations of glucose in such circumstances, such as D$_{25}$W. After correction of hypoglycemia has been achieved, normoglycemia can be maintained by an infusion rate of 4–8 mg/kg/min.

54. Following resuscitation, a decision is made to insert an umbilical artery catheter. Describe procedural complications that could result in hypothermia.
- Room temperature has been chosen for the comfort of health care providers, not the baby.
- Care providers block overhead radiant warmth from reaching the infant.
- The infant is inadequately dried.
- The infant is restrained in a "spread eagle" position, increasing surface area exposed to radiant and convective heat loss.
- The baby may receive sedative or analgesic drugs, which interfere with thermoregulation (e.g., diazepam).
- The abdomen is "prepped" with cold iodophor solution.

• Excess iodophor solution remains in contact with the infant's skin.
• The infant is draped with a surgical towel, blocking overhead radiant warmth.
• The catheter is flushed with cold solution.
• Inspired gas is insufficiently humidified and heated.

55. Why is sodium bicarbonate not administered to treat respiratory acidosis?

Unless ventilation is adequate, the carbon dioxide produced by the buffering reaction will not be consumed and will act as a weak acid, further reducing the pH ("closed flask" phenomenon). It is therefore inappropriate and even dangerous to give bicarbonate until ventilation has been established and is found to be adequate.

56. Why is measurement of hematocrit following acute blood loss not a good indicator of blood volume?

The immediate response to acute blood loss is vasoconstriction to maintain blood pressure. The blood that has been lost contains the same percentage of red blood cells as the blood that is retained. The hematocrit will not drop until fluid repletion of the intravascular volume occurs.

57. List the important clinical signs used to assess tissue perfusion.

Pulse rate and quality, capillary refill time, and urine output.

58. After a traumatic delivery, what are the most commonly injured systems?

• Cranial injuries: caput succedaneum, subconjunctival hemorrhage, cephalohematoma, skull fractures, intracranial hemorrhage, cerebral edema
• Spinal injuries: spinal cord transection
• Peripheral nerve injuries: brachial palsy (Erb-Duchenne paralysis, Klumpke paralysis), phrenic nerve, and facial nerve paralysis
• Visceral injuries: liver rupture or hematoma, splenic rupture, adrenal hemorrhage
• Skeletal injuries: fractures of the clavicle, femur, and humerus

59. When should neonatal resuscitation be stopped?

No precise answer is possible because clinical circumstances and responses are variable. However, in one study of 58 newborns with an Apgar score of 0 at 10 minutes despite appropriate resuscitative efforts, only 1 of 58 survived, and that infant had profound CP. Currently, a study is underway that is examining the effects of hypothermia and brain cooling on posthypoxic cerebral injury. It is hoped that this technique may alter outcome in such cases.

Prolonged resuscitation has a very high risk of ischemic injury to the brain resulting in cystic encephalomalacia, CP, severe microcephaly, and developmental delay. Failure of response after > 10–15 minutes should prompt consideration of cessation.

Jain L: Cardiopulmonary resuscitation of apparently stillborn infants: Survival and long-term outcome. J Pediatr 118:778–782, 1991.

60. An infant who requires an extensive resuscitation should be observed closely for the development of hypoxic-ischemic encephalopathy. What are the acute neurologic components of this syndrome?

Persistent and prolonged hypotonia   Depressed reflexes
Altered level of consciousness   Convulsions

RADIOLOGY OF PULMONARY DISORDERS OF THE NEONATE

61. Where should the tip of an umbilical arterial (UA) catheter in satisfactory position project on an AP radiograph of the chest and abdomen?

There are two major schools of thought on this subject. For many years, the preferred position was between the third and fourth lumbar vertebrae, as projected on an AP radiograph. The tip lies below the take-off points for the renal and mesenteric arteries, theoretically reducing the risk of injecting fluids or drugs directly into those vessels. With this catheter placement, however, it has been shown that, even with relatively low pressure, injectable material can ascend retrograde into the aorta for quite some distance. Other neonatologists prefer a higher placement, in the thoracic aorta at approximately T10–T12, again avoiding placement of the catheter near the major tributaries off the descending aorta. Positioning the tip there, however, means that anything injected will flow past major vessels. Several papers have argued for one placement versus the other, but both are probably safe as long as one takes the following precautions:

- Careful placement until sterile conditions
- Daily evaluation of ease of injection and withdrawal of blood
- Assessment of the pressure waveform on the monitor screen
- Inspection of the site for erythema and induration
- Daily evaluation of urine output and blood pressure
- Prompt removal of the line as soon as it is no longer needed

Umbilical catheters may be left in place for many days as long as the above conditions are satisfactorily met. In extremes, a catheter can be kept in place for 3 weeks without complication.

62. Where should the tip of an umbilical venous (UV) catheter be placed for satisfactory projection on an anteroposterior (AP) radiograph of the chest and abdomen?

The UV catheter should be kept at the lower margin of the cardiac silhouette, approximately at the level of the right diaphragm, which would correspond to the junction of the inferior vena cava and right atrium of the heart. UV catheters should not be allowed to remain below this level or within any of the branches of the portal system of the liver. Infusion of calcium or hyperalimentation into catheters in these incorrect positions may lead to liver toxicity, portal necrosis, cirrhosis, and cavernous transformation of the portal vein. Umbilical venous lines may also inadvertently cross the foramen ovale and enter the left heart. Catheters in this location occasionally will cause rhythm disturbances of the heart. This incorrect placement can be detected by the high levels of pO_2 obtained on a venous sample of blood.

63. What is the best position, as seen on an AP radiograph of the chest, for the tip of an ET tube in an intubated neonate?

The optimal position for an ET tube is approximately halfway between the thoracic inlet (look for the medial ends of the baby's clavicles to get a good approximation) and the carina or level of tracheal bifurcation. In small neonates, ET tubes often enter the right mainstem bronchus and produce left-sided atelectasis. They may also exert vagal effects and cause bradycardia or irritation if they strike the carina frequently. Tubes that are excessively high also may produce vagal effects and loss of effective ventilation.

64. What is the most common radiographic appearance of the lungs in a premature neonate with respiratory distress syndrome?

The classic RDS picture in a premature neonate has a diffuse increase in lung density (opacity) with a fine, reticulogranular (grainy) or ground-glass appearance, air-bronchograms (a darker appearance to the branching central airway as contrasted with the opacity of the lungs), and low lung volumes.

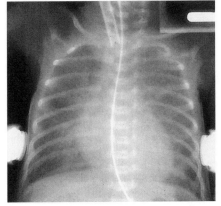

An infant with RDS showing air bronchograms and reticulogranular appearance. An endotracheal tube and nasogastric tube are present.

65. What disease process can produce a radiographic appearance to the lungs that is identical to respiratory distress syndrome?

GBS pneumonia in the premature infant is reported to have an appearance similar to RDS. It may be, however, that premature babies with GBS disease can also have surfactant inactivation or deficiency with true RDS as well as GBS septicemia. Although Sir William Osler might not like the concept of two diagnoses in one little patient, it probably happens more often than not!

66. What would be a typical appearance to the lungs in a newborn with significant meconium aspiration?

These babies often have a coarse, irregular increase in lung markings accompanied by hyperinflation of the lungs. The pneumonic process here is one of patchy atelectasis and overdistention. Pneumothorax is a frequent accompanying abnormality as well.

67. In a newborn with suspected transient tachypnea of the newborn ("wet lung syndrome," "transient respiratory distress of the newborn," "delayed reabsorption of fetal lung fluid"), about how long should it take for the chest radiograph to return to a normal appearance in order to be consistent with this diagnosis?

The typical textbook description of this clinical condition is a hazy-appearing lung, often with fluid in the right horizontal fissure, and increased perihilar markings. The babies have rapid shallow breathing, in contrast to the retractions of RDS or meconium aspiration syndrome. It usually is reported to last approximately 24 hours, with 48–72 hours considered the maximum. Some infants, however, seem to have this clinical problem for many more days, with subsequent uneventful recovery. What immediately turns off fetal lung fluid production at birth has not been established. One theory is that some babies may continue to produce a low level of lung fluid for a period of time after they are born.

68. What should I look for on the chest radiograph of a newborn in whom congenital diaphragmatic hernia (CDH) is suspected (usually by antenatal sonography of the fetus)?

The CDH patient rarely presents at birth as the diagnostic dilemma in the delivery room that it once was. With fetal ultrasound, most of these infants are diagnosed before birth, and some even have surgery before they are born at specialized fetal treatment centers. Radiographically, they have a complex pattern of lucency in one hemithorax (usually the left side, and reflecting air-containing loops of intestine), contralateral shift of the heart and other mediastinal structures, and a lack of expected air-containing intestine in the abdomen.

69. If a unilateral pneumothorax is suspected in a newborn, what is the best projection of the chest to confirm or exclude this diagnosis?

Early air leaks are often difficult to diagnose. The most obvious finding, however, is a separation of the edge or margin of the lung from the inner margin of the chest wall, with no lung markings definable in that space. An AP decubitus view of the chest with the side of suspected pneumothorax to the top (nondependent) is also helpful. For example, if you suspect a left-sided pneumothorax, you should order a "right decubitus AP chest radiograph," which means the right side of the patient will be dependent and the left side nondependent. If a pneumothorax is present, look for a zone of lucency representing pleural air collecting between the lateral chest margin and the adjacent lung.

RESPIRATORY DISTRESS SYNDROME

70. Which collapses faster, a small bubble or a larger one?

The small one, because of surface tension. The LaPlace relationship states $P = 2T/R$, where P is the pressure across the wall of the sphere, T is surface tension of the substance forming the bubble (i.e., its tendency to collapse), and R is the radius of the sphere. The smaller the radius, the greater the collapsing pressure.

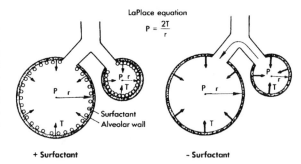

The LaPlace relationship. In the absence of surfactant, the smaller alveolus has a greater surface tension than the larger and tends to empty into the larger alveolus. In the presence of surfactant, the compacting of surface-tension reducing surfactant acts to "splint" the lung against further collapse. (Courtesy of F. Netter, CIBA-Geigy Corp., Ardsley, New York.)

When the bubbles are alveoli without surfactant, pressure on the alveolar surface is quite high because the surface tension is high. As the surfactantless alveolus collapses during exhalation, pressure increases as the radius of the alveolus decreases.

Avery and Mead described the absence of a surface tension–reducing substance in the alveolar fluid of infants who died of hyaline membrane disease. The substance turned out to be surfactant, which greatly lowers the alveolar surface tension and, therefore, the alveolus's tendency to collapse. Surfactant also lowers surface tension as the diameter of the alveolus decreases, allowing for stable alveoli at end expiratory volumes.

71. What are the physiologic, physical, and biochemical factors that result in pulmonary vasodilatation at the time of birth?

Within minutes after delivery, pulmonary artery pressure falls, and blood flow increases in response to birth-related stimuli, such as ventilation, increased pO_2, and shear stress. Physical stimuli, including increased shear stress, ventilation, and increased oxygen, cause pulmonary vasodilation in part by increasing production of vasodilators, nitric oxide, and prostacyclin. Pretreatment with the nitric oxide synthase inhibitor, nitro-L-arginine, attenuates pulmonary vasodilation after delivery by 50% in near-term fetal lambs. These findings suggest that a significant part of the rise in pulmonary blood flow at birth may be related directly to the acute release of nitric oxide. Each of the birth-related stimuli can stimulate nitric oxide release independently, followed by vasodilation through cyclic guanosine monophosphate (cGMP) kinase–mediated stimulation of K+ channels. Although the endothelial isoform of nitric oxide synthase III has been presumed to be the major contributor of nitric oxide at birth, recent studies suggest that other isoforms (neuronal type I and inducible type II) may be important sources of nitric oxide release in utero and at birth. Other vasodilators, especially prostacyclin, also modulate changes in pulmonary vascular tone. Rhythmic lung distention and shear stress stimulate both prostacyclin and nitric oxide production in late gestation. Increasing oxygen tension also triggers nitric oxide activity and overcomes the effects of prostacyclin inhibition at birth. Thus, although nitric oxide does not account for the entire fall in pulmonary vascular resistance at birth, nitric oxide synthase activity appears important in achieving postnatal adaptation of lung circulation.

Abman SH, Stevens T: Perinatal pulmonary vasoregulation: Implications for the pathophysiology and treatment of neonatal pulmonary hypertension. In Haddad G, Lister G (eds): Tissue Oxygen Deprivation: Developmental, Molecular, and Integrative Functions. New York, Marcel Dekker, 1996, pp 367–432.

72. What is the composition of surfactant?

Surfactant, from "surface active material," is 80% phospholipids and 8% neutral lipids. The phospholipid most responsible for surface tension reduction is dipalmitoyl phosphatidylcholine (DPPC). Twelve percent of surfactant is protein, half of which are most likely serum contaminants. Surfactant proteins A, B, C, and D (SP-A, SP-B, SP-C, SP-D) are active in surfactant's surface tension reduction, secretion, absorption, and immune function. SP-A works with other proteins and lipids to improve surface actions and regulate secretion and reuptake. It also works with host defense in the alveolus. Lipophilic SP-B and SP-C facilitate adsorption and spread of lipid across the alveolar surface. SP-D is known to be a ligand for pathogens.

73. How is surfactant manufactured?

Surfactant is made in alveolar type II cells. The endoplasmic reticulum and Golgi apparatus package the lipid and protein precursors. Lamellar bodies are formed, including more protein with increasing gestational age. Catecholamines, corticosteroids, and other hormones stimulate the type II cell's secretion of lamellar bodies. These unravel to form tubular myelin. Tubular myelin then adsorbs as a lipid-protein monolayer on the alveolar surface, giving maximum surface support to the alveolus. The interaction between intact protein and phospholipid allows optimal surfactant functioning.

Surfactant is inactivated in the alveolar space without large changes in amounts of its components. The monolayer does break down as protein and lipid dissociate. Surfactant changes to a small aggregate form that minimally reduces surface tension. These aggregates are then absorbed by macrophages and type II cells, which recycle lipid and protein components.

74. If you could only receive one treatment, antenatal steroids or surfactant replacement, which would you pick?

The therapies seem to be additive. If one had to pick, however, one might side with Mary Ellen Avery, the person who first described the deficiency of surfactant in the lungs of babies with RDS, who would choose the steroids because of their multisystem maturational effects.

75. When should surfactant be given?

Most agree, earlier is better. "Prophylactic" versus "treatment" produces lower mortality, fewer pneumothoraces, less pulmonary interstitial emphysema, and perhaps less bronchopulmonary dysplasia (BPD; O_2 at 28 days), especially for infants < 29 weeks. By prophylaxis, most agree that for babies < 27–29 weeks, treatment should be given soon after birth, following initial stabilization. It is better not to wait for x-rays to show the ground-glass appearance or other markers for definite RDS. With increased use of antenatal steroids, the need to intubate babies, much less give additional surfactant, is decreased in infants > 27 weeks.

76. What are the advantages of prophylactic surfactant?

Four major randomized trials have addressed the issue of preventive versus rescue treatment strategies for exogenous surfactant administration in VLBW infants. In studies using synthetic surfactant, there were significant reductions in pneumothorax and pulmonary interstitial emphysema when surfactant was administered at or soon after birth compared with selective administration in infants with established RDS. Infants randomized to early selective surfactant administration demonstrated a decreased risk of neonatal mortality, chronic lung disease, and death at 36 weeks. No differences in other complications of RDS or prematurity were noted. In the meta-analysis of Soll, prophylactic rather than delayed administration of surfactant to all infants deemed at high risk for RDS reduced the risk of pneumothorax, pulmonary interstitial emphysema, bronchopulmonary dysplasia, and death. Similar benefits are associated with early selective rather than delayed surfactant administration in premature infants intubated for respiratory distress within the first 2 hours of life. Although no randomized trials compare prophylactic surfactant treatment with early selective surfactant treatment, studies suggest that the greatest benefit may come from the earliest care. Kendig et al. demonstrated that the benefits of prophylactic treatment remain even if initial surfactant therapy is delayed until 10–15 minutes after birth. This distinction is important in that attention to neonatal resuscitation, ET tube positioning, and adequate oxygen saturation can be assessed prior to intratracheal bolus surfactant administration.

OSIRIS Collaborative Group: Early versus delayed neonatal administration of a synthetic surfactant: The judgment of OSIRIS. Lancet 340:1363–1369, 1992.

Soll SR, Morley CJ: Prophylactic versus selective use of surfactant for preventing morbidity and mortality in preterm infants. In Cochrane Library, Issue 1. Oxford, Update Software, 1999.

77. What can be done besides surfactant therapy in RDS?

The goal of therapy is to maintain minute volume by maintaining functional, open alveoli for gas exchange. When atelectasis occurs in infants with RDS, CO_2 cannot get out, and O_2 cannot get in. To maintain alveolar volume and, therefore, gas exchange, positive end expiratory pressure (PEEP) can be very helpful. Continuous positive airway pressure (CPAP) can be used to maintain alveolar volume during exhalation despite inadequate surfactant. It works if the pressure delivered to the alveoli prevents closing pressure (remember P = 2T/R) from completely collapsing alveoli, but it should not be so great that it hinders adequate exhalation.

When alveolar collapse is too rapid or widespread, positive pressure ventilation is the best tool. Positive pressure opens the alveoli for inhalation. End expiratory pressure maintains alveolar volume during exhalation. Positive pressure ventilation will be necessary until adequate surfactant reduces surface tension and enough alveoli are inflated for adequate minute ventilation.

A word about high-frequency ventilation: the primary pathology of RDS comes from an inability to maintain lung inflation and fluid leak into the alveolar space. Secondary pathology originates from positive pressure re-expansion of collapsed alveoli. A ventilation strategy that maintains lung volume and avoids large distending pressure seems ideal. That is the idea behind high-frequency ventilation for RDS. The lung is inflated, and lung volumes are maintained while gas exchange occurs using tidal volumes less than dead space. High-frequency ventilator technology is improving, and its applicability as the first-line treatment for RDS is under investigation. Several prior trials, however, have suggested that high-frequency ventilation may be better as a rescue therapy than as an initial treatment. The jury is still out, however.

78. Are there complications and problems with surfactant therapy?

U.S. mortality from RDS and prematurity declined significantly with the introduction of exogenous surfactant. By 1994, the combination of congenital and chromosomal defects had become the leading cause of infant mortality, and RDS with prematurity fell, for the first time, to number two on the list. Although bronchopulmonary dysplasia (BPD) has not significantly decreased in numbers, the severity of chronic lung disease has declined for most surviving premature infants with RDS.

The only pulmonary complication that has increased with therapy is a small but noticeable increase in pulmonary hemorrhage. Other nonpulmonary complications have not been significantly affected. Clinicians have noticed an earlier unmasking of significant left-to-right flow through the patent ductus arteriosus after surfactant therapy.

79. What is CPAP?

Continuous positive airway pressure can be applied to an infant's airway using a variety of devices to maintain positive pressure in the airway during spontaneous breathing. These devices include headhood, face chamber, face mask, several types of nasal prongs, nasopharyngeal tube, and endotracheal tube. Nasal prongs are used most often. Not all CPAP devices are equal, and they have varying degrees of success. They have been associated with a number of problems such as difficulty with access to the baby, maintaining connection to the airway, increase in dead space, and increase in airway resistance.

80. What is the effect of CPAP?

Like many things in life, the right amount is beneficial and too much is detrimental. When the proper amount of positive pressure is used, CPAP will:
- Increase transpulmonary pressure and functional residual capacity (FRC)
- Prevent alveolar collapse and decrease intrapulmonary shunting
- Increase compliance
- Conserve surfactant
- Increase airway diameter and splint the airway
- Splint the diaphragm

However, if too much CPAP pressure is applied, it can cause overdistention of the alveoli, worsen ventilation-perfusion match, increase pulmonary vascular resistance, decrease compliance, and impede venous return to the right side of the heart, thereby decreasing cardiac output.

81. What are the indications for using CPAP in the neonate?

The indications for CPAP include but are not limited to:
- Diseases with a low FRC (e.g., respiratory distress syndrome)
- Apnea and bradycardia of prematurity
- MAS
- Airway closure disease (e.g., bronchiolitis, BPD)
- Tracheomalacia
- Partial paralysis of the diaphragm
- Respiratory support after extubation

82. What are the complications of nasal prong CPAP?

Pneumothorax ($< 2\%$) usually occurs in the acute phase and is usually more benign than when it occurs during mechanical ventilation. Pneumothorax is *not* a contraindication for CPAP therapy.

Nasal obstruction from secretions or improper positioning of CPAP prongs. Secretions in nasal cavities should be suctioned every 4 hours or as needed.

Abdominal distention from swallowed air is usually benign and occurs more commonly in the chronic than acute phase, especially in infants treated with aminophylline. Abdominal distention can be treated by intermittent aspiration of the stomach. For severe distention, an indwelling orogastric tube may be required.

Nasal or septal erosion or necrosis is a concern in a VLBW premature infant with sensitive skin, who may need CPAP therapy for weeks. However, this can be prevented by choosing the proper size CPAP cannula and avoiding compression of the septum. A snug cap is used to hold the tubings securely in place, and self-adhesive Velcro is used to keep the cannulae away from the septum.

83. What is OI?

OI stands for the oxygen index. It is used to express the severity of the respiratory disease.

$$OI = MAP \times FiO_2 / PaO_2 \text{ and MAP} = (PIP - PEEP) \times T_I / (T_I + T_E) + PEEP$$

where MAP = mean arterial pressure; FiO_2 = fractional concentration of oxygen in inspired gas; PaO_2 = partial pressure of oxygen in arterial blood; PIP = peak inspiratory pressure; PEEP = positive end expiratory pressure; T_I = inspiration time; T_E = expiration time.

Note that the MAP is influenced by all respirator controls except the FiO_2. However, without a uniform ventilation strategy, the OI cannot be universally applied as an expression of severity of respiratory disease. This is especially true in the unit, where patients may be hyperventilated; in these patients, the MAP, and thus the OI, is elevated regardless of the severity of disease.

MECONIUM-STAINED AMNIOTIC FLUID AND MECONIUM ASPIRATION SYNDROME

84. Do vigorous meconium-stained infants need to be intubated and suctioned in the delivery room?

No. Those who have an initial heart rate > 100 bpm, good respiratory effort, and reasonable tone will not benefit from intubation and suctioning. In fact, some vigorous infants may be injured in the process of suctioning because they are so difficult to restrain. Only when it is essential to remove significant meconium from the airway should big babies be suctioned; otherwise the risks appear to outweigh the benefits, particularly if less experienced individuals are attempting the intubation.

85. How long has meconium been present in the amniotic fluid if an infant has evidence of meconium staining?

Gross staining of the infant is a surface phenomenon proportional to the length of exposure and meconium concentration. With heavy meconium, staining of the umbilical cord begins in as little as 15 minutes, and with light meconium, after 1 hour. Yellow staining of the newborn's nails requires 4–6 hours. Yellow staining of the vernix caseosa takes about 12–14 hours.

86. Is meconium staining a good marker for neonatal asphyxia?

Because 10–20% of all deliveries have in utero passage of meconium, meconium staining alone is not a good marker for neonatal asphyxia. For an infant to pass meconium, however, there does need to be a period of hypoxemia that initiates increased bowel contractility prior to birth. Simply having hypoxemia, however, is not the same thing as having perinatal asphyxia.

87. If meconium is noted prior to or at the time of delivery, what is the recommended course of action?

Regardless of the nature of the fluid, the obstetrician should attempt to suction the infant's oro- and nasopharynx prior to delivery of the shoulders. An 8- or 10-French flexible catheter is much more effective than bulb syringing. The next course of action depends on the thickness of the meconium and the clinical appearance of the baby. With thin meconium, it the infant is crying and vigorous, visualization of the larynx and intubation are probably not necessary and may, in fact, be harmful to the child if the airway is injured. With thick meconium in a depressed infant, the infant's pharynx should be suctioned followed by endotracheal intubation with suctioning below the vocal cords. If the infant is vigorous, visualization of the cords may suffice, and if no meconium is noted at that level, intubation may be deferred. However, many clinicians recommend that the trachea be suctioned whenever there is thick meconium.

88. What underlying disorder is associated with 50–67% of all cases of infants diagnosed with persistent pulmonary hypertension of the newborn (PPHN)?

MAS is associated with the majority of cases of PPHN. Other associated disorders include RDS, sepsis or pneumonia, idiopathic PPHN, and lung hypoplasia (including CDH). In all instances, the pulmonary vascular resistance remains near systemic levels and results in right-to-left shunting of blood.

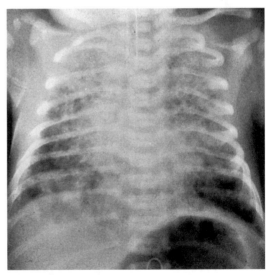

An infant with severe MAS. There are diffuse patchy infiltrates throughout the lung fields.

89. What factors are involved in the pathophysiology of MAS?

Once meconium is aspirated into the lungs, the following processes occur:
- Airway obstruction
- Alveolar and parenchymal inflammation
- Alveolar and parenchymal edema

- Altered pulmonary vasoreactivity leading to pulmonary vasoconstriction, increased pulmonary resistance, and right-to-left shunting
- Direct toxicity of meconium constituents on pulmonary parenchyma leading to ischemia and necrosis
- Surfactant dysfunction (inactivation and decreased production of surfactant proteins A and B [SP-A and SP-B])
- Pulmonary vascular remodeling
- Altered lung elastic forces (increased resistance, decreased compliance)

90. What background disorder makes up the largest proportion of neonates who are treated with extracorporeal membrane oxygenation (ECMO)?

Infants with MAS make up 35–40% of infants who are treated with ECMO. Many of the infants who subsequently need ECMO for MAS might have avoided this therapy with more aggressive early management of their aspiration. Unfortunately, the circumstances that lead to MAS in many cases are precipitous and unavoidable. As a result, by the time therapy can be started, the pathophysiology is sufficiently far advanced and can be halted only by the use of ECMO. Other disorders that are managed with ECMO include sepsis, pneumonia, pulmonary hypoplasia, and RDS. MAS patients tend to have the shortest ECMO courses and the highest survival rates, approaching 100% in the most experienced ECMO centers.

91. Meconium happens! Meconium-stained amniotic fluid (MSAF) is found across all races and socioeconomic strata in humans. Additionally, MSAF and MAS are noted frequently in domestic animals. How do farmers and veterinarians manage MSAF in an effort to prevent MAS?

Farmers and veterinarians grab newborn animals by their hindquarters and swing them in a circular motion. Centrifugal forces move meconium-stained fluid outward into the upper airway and oropharynx. Caretakers then manually remove the material.

92. Is thin-consistency MSAF more likely to enter the airways and cause MAS or other respiratory distress compared with thick-consistency MSAF?

No. The thicker the consistency of MSAF, the greater the likelihood of MAS or other respiratory distress. There is at least a seven-fold increase in the incidence of respiratory disorders among infants born through "pea-soup" MSAF compared with those born through watery-consistency MSAF.

93. Which of the following therapies have been approved by the Food and Drug Administration (FDA) specifically for the management of MAS: (a) systemic corticosteroids, (b) exogenous surfactant, (c) inhaled nitric oxide, (d) high-frequency ventilation, (e) ECMO?

None! Although all of these therapies are commonly used to treat the child with respiratory disease, only exogenous surfactant, inhaled nitric oxide, and high-frequency ventilation have received FDA approval. These therapies have been approved for use in RDS or persistent pulmonary hypertension, but not specifically for the treatment of MAS.

94. Oropharyngeal suctioning by an obstetrician prior to delivery of an infant's trunk and shoulders plays an important role in preventing MAS. Which method of suction is better: bulb syringe or suction catheter?

Neither. Both in vitro and in vivo studies have assessed these methods. There are no clearcut advantages to either approach. The key to success is the effective removal of meconium.

95. What mechanisms of meconium aspiration into the lungs contribute to ventilatory failure, and what is the role of surfactant therapy in treatment of this condition?

Meconium-induced lung injury is associated with many pulmonary changes that contribute to respiratory failure. These include airway obstruction, inflammation with release of vasoactive substances, and surfactant dysfunction. Meconium has the ability to inactivate surfactant both in vivo and in vitro and has direct effects on type II pneumocyte function. In both animal models and human infants who have aspirated meconium and who are undergoing pulmonary fluid analysis, inflammatory cell numbers and total protein are significantly elevated compared with control infants. Various inflammatory mediators including myeloperoxidase and interleukin-8 are increased. Maximal influx of inflammatory cells occurs by 16 hours of age with some recovery by 72 hours. These findings support the role of surfactant replacement in infants with meconium aspiration syndrome that requires ventilatory support. The optimal method of surfactant treatment is currently under refinement, however, with some evidence supporting a surfactant lavage of the airways that is distinct from bolus administration of surfactant as used in preterm infants with RDS.

PULMONARY HYPERTENSION

96. What is persistent pulmonary hypertension of the newborn?

Successful transition from intrauterine to extrauterine life requires that the pulmonary vascular resistance decreases precipitously at birth. In infants with PPHN, this decrease does not occur. Pulmonary arterial pressure remains elevated, and blood continues to shunt right to left across the ductus arteriosus and foramen ovale, resulting in significant hypoxemia.

97. When was PPHN first described? Why is persistent fetal circulation not an accurate term to describe PPHN?

Gersony and coworkers (1969) described a group of term infants without structural heart disease who became cyanotic shortly after birth and had only mild respiratory distress. These infants all had suprasystemic pulmonary arterial pressures with right-to-left shunting across persistent fetal pathways (ductus arteriosus and foramen ovale). Hence, this condition was called *persistent fetal circulation.*

The shunting across the foramen ovale and ductus arteriosus as a result of suprasystemic pulmonary arterial pressure seen in PPHN is very similar to fetal circulation. However, the exclusion of placental circulation and the fact that ductus venosus may or may not be patent preclude the use of the term *persistent fetal circulation* to describe this condition. The term *persistent pulmonary hypertension of the newborn* describes the pathophysiology of the disease more accurately, indicating that the critical problem in this situation is the failure of the pulmonary circulation to decrease to normal pressures.

98. What are the clinical features of PPHN?

Infants with PPHN are usually delivered at term or post-term. Often they are born through MSAF. The typical clinical manifestations of a neonate with PPHN are as follows:

- Labile hypoxemia or cyanosis disproportionate to the level of respiratory distress. These infants are extremely sensitive to environmental stimuli.
- Infants with significant ductal shunting have higher oxygen saturation in the right hand (preductal) than in the legs (postductal). Similarly, PaO_2 in the right radial artery is significantly greater than that obtained from the umbilical artery. Infants with predominant shunting at the level of foramen ovale have similar pre- and postductal oxygen levels.
- Cardiac murmur compatible with tricuspid insufficiency.
- Chest radiograph may reveal cardiomegaly. The underlying disease (such as CDH or RDS) alters the radiologic picture. Infants with idiopathic PPHN have clear and undervascularized lung fields ("black-lung" PPHN).
- Echocardiography is important to rule out cyanotic congenital heart disease and to establish the diagnosis. In infants with PPHN, shunting at atrial and ductal level can be demonstrated. Tricuspid insufficiency, right ventricular hypertrophy, septal deviation to the left, and prolonged right ventricular systolic intervals support the diagnosis of PPHN.

99. What are the common causes of PPHN?

The common causes of PPHN are summarized in the mnemonic **DIAPHRAGMATIC:**

Diaphragmatic hernia (hypoplastic lungs)
Infection (including pneumonia)—especially group B streptococci
Aspiration syndromes (e.g., meconium, amniotic fluid)
Postmaturity
Hyperviscosity (polycythemia, hyperfibrinogenemia)
Respiratory distress syndrome (hyaline membrane disease)
Asphyxia
Growth retardation (placental insufficiency)
Maternal nonsteroidal anti-inflammatory drug (NSAID) ingestion
Air leak, **a**lveolar-capillary dysplasia
Transient tachypnea of newborn
Idiopathic ("black lung" PPHN)
Congenital anomalies of the lung

The causes of PPHN can also be classified depending on the predominant abnormality involved (see figure).

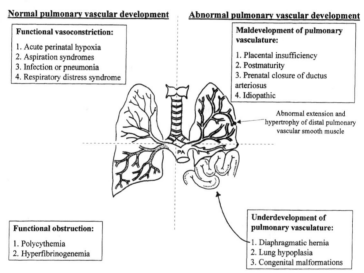

Classification of persistent pulmonary hypertension of the newborn (PPHN) based on predominant abnormality involved. PPHN associated with normal pulmonary vascular development is depicted on the left half of the figure. This includes conditions associated with functional vasoconstriction (left upper quadrant) and functional obstruction secondary to hyperviscosity (left lower quadrant). PPHN secondary to abnormal pulmonary vascular development is shown in the right half of the figure and includes maldevelopment with increased muscularization (right upper quadrant) and underdevelopment with decreased number of vessels (right lower quadrant) of pulmonary vasculature. (PA = pulmonary artery.)

100. Why is the right hand a preferred site to obtain preductal pulse oximetry readings?

In some infants, the left subclavian artery arises from the arch of aorta just distal to the level of the insertion of ductus arteriosus (see figure in question 101). In these infants, a pulse oximetry probe applied to the left hand indicates postductal saturations. Hence, it is always better to obtain preductal oxygen saturation from the right upper limb, a site that indicates preductal saturation.

101. What is the pathophysiology of PPHN?

Persistent elevation of pulmonary arterial pressure in PPHN is secondary to active constriction of pulmonary vessels (as in pneumonia), underdevelopment of the pulmonary vessels (as in congenital diaphragmatic hernia), or maldevelopment of the pulmonary vasculature (as in prenatal ductal closure from maternal ingestion of NSAID and idiopathic PPHN).

Vascular remodeling. In infants dying from PPHN secondary to maldevelopment of the pulmonary vessels, pulmonary arterial smooth muscle hypertrophies and extends from pre-acinar arteries into normally nonmuscular intra-acinar arteries, even to the level of the alveolus. This thickened muscle encroaches on the vessel lumen and results in mechanical obstruction to blood flow.

Functional abnormalities in the pulmonary vessels (reduced nitric oxide synthase, reduced soluble guanylyl cyclase, and increased levels of vasoconstrictors such as endothelin) have been described.

Persistently elevated pulmonary vascular resistance increases right ventricular afterload and oxygen demand and impairs oxygen delivery to cardiac muscle. Ischemic damage to the myocardium, papillary muscle necrosis, and tricuspid regurgitation can occur. Increased right ventricular pressure displaces the septum into the left ventricle, impairs left ventricular filling, and decreases cardiac output. Myocardial dysfunction is an important cause for mortality in PPHN.

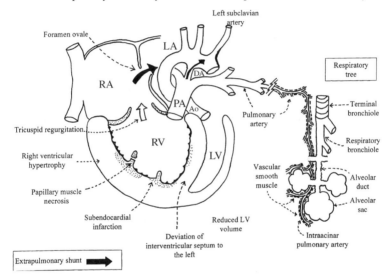

Pathology of persistent pulmonary hypertension of the newborn (PPHN): Suprasystemic pulmonary arterial pressure results in right ventricular (RV) hypertrophy and deviation of interventricular septum to the left. This reduces the left ventricular (LV) volume and decreases systemic output. Extrapulmonary right-to-left shunt occurs at the foramen ovale from the right atrium (RA) to the left atrium (LA) and at the level of ductus arteriosus (DA) from the pulmonary artery (PA) to the aorta (Ao). Normally, pulmonary arteries distal to the level of terminal bronchioles are not muscular. Abnormal extension and hypertrophy of distal pulmonary vascular smooth muscle (shown as interrupted lines), sometimes to the level of intra-acinar arteries, is seen in severe PPHN.

102. How do you differentiate cyanotic congenital heart disease from PPHN?

It is often very difficult clinically to differentiate between these two conditions. Patients with PPHN are more labile with wide swings in oxygen saturations. A significant difference between the pre- and postductal oxygen saturations is also a clinical finding in favor of PPHN. The response to respiratory and metabolic alkalosis also has been used to confirm the diagnosis. If systemic arterial oxygenation improves when the newborn is hyperventilated to an alkalotic pH, it is presumed that the hypoxia is due to pulmonary vasospasm and PPHN. However, these results must be interpreted with caution. The best way to differentiate between these two entities is by echocardiography.

An additional test that is sometimes used in this clinical situation is the **hyperoxia test**. The child to be tested is placed on an inspired oxygen level of 100%. On an arterial blood gas determination, if the PaO_2 rises above 100 mmHg, it is unlikely that the infant has significant cyanotic heart disease and more likely has pulmonary hypertension or pulmonary parenchymal disease.

This test, however, is not infallible, and some children with PPHN may not be able to increase their PaO_2 above 100 mmHg. In addition, it may be necessary to give positive pressure ventilation to a baby to be sure that one is ventilating the lungs of a child with pulmonary disease adequately to maximize the arterial oxygen levels.

103. What are the principles of management of PPHN?

In patients in whom PPHN is secondary to an underlying cause such as pneumonia, aggressive therapy directed at the predisposing condition is very important. The basic principles used to manage PPHN to date are summarized in the mnemonic **SOAPSTONE:**

Sedation and minimal stimulation

Oxygen

Acidosis correction

Pressors and volume to maintain blood pressure

Surfactant

Tolazoline (currently not recommended)

Oscillatory or jet ventilation

Nitric oxide

Extracorporeal membrane oxygenation (ECMO)

104. What is the long-term outcome of infants treated for PPHN?

In the past, the mortality for infants with PPHN ranged from 20% to 40%, and the incidence of neurologic handicap ranged from 12% to 25%. With recent advances in conservative management, survival and neurodevelopmental outcome have improved considerably. In most centers, ECMO has further reduced mortality from severe PPHN. Survival rates between 76% and 93% have been reported for infants with pneumonia, meconium aspiration, and idiopathic PPHN who require ECMO. The outlook for infants with diaphragmatic hernia requiring ECMO has not been as dramatic, and survival is still only 58%.

Currently, most infants treated for PPHN have few respiratory symptoms or neurologic or developmental sequelae by 1 year of age. However:
- Infants presenting with more severe parenchymal disease may have persistent tachypnea and bronchospasm
- Neurologic development may be impaired in children with PPHN, especially if severely asphyxiated.
- An increased incidence of sensorineural hearing loss among infants with PPHN treated with hyperventilation and alkalization has been reported.

105. What are the future prospects for treating infants with PPHN?

Although ECMO has considerably reduced the mortality from PPHN, it is an invasive procedure limited to a few tertiary care centers. Inhaled nitric oxide has reduced the need for ECMO from 64–71% to 40–46% in two randomized, controlled trials without significant improvement in survival. Two possibilities for enhancing the effect of inhaled nitric oxide are being currently investigated.

1. Nitric oxide acts by stimulating soluble guanylyl cyclase and producing cyclic guanosine monophosphate (GMP) in vascular smooth muscle. Cyclic GMP induces smooth muscle relaxation but is rapidly broken down by phosphodiesterase-5 (PDE-5) enzyme. PDE-5 inhibition should increase the level of cyclic GMP in vascular smooth muscle and enhance nitric oxide–induced relaxation. An inhibitor of this enzyme, sildenafil (Viagra), is currently used in the treatment of impotence. Several other PDE-5 inhibitors (Zaprinast, dipyridamole, and E4021) have been used successfully in animal models of PPHN.

2. High levels of oxygen free radicals are present in many disease states that cause PPHN. Superoxide anion combines nitric oxide to produce the toxic free radical peroxynitrite. Antioxidants such as superoxide dismutase (SOD) remove these toxic free radicals and enhance nitric oxide–mediated vasorelaxation in isolated pulmonary vessels. Similar results might be obtainable in vivo.

106. The use of inhaled nitric oxide acts substantially like endothelium relaxing factor and acts as the major regulator of vascular smooth muscle tone. Why doesn't it also dilate the systemic vascular system?

Nitric oxide has a high affinity for the iron of all heme proteins, including reduced hemoglobin, with which it forms nitrosyl-hemoglobin (NOHb). The NOHb is then oxidized to methemoglobin with the production of nitrate. As a result, when given by inhalation, NO is inactivated before acting on any systemic vascular bed, while relaxing the pulmonary vascular smooth muscle through the cyclic GMP production. In normal development and in near deliveries, endogenous NO produced in endothelial cells from oxygen and L-arginine diffuses into smooth cells in the vascular wall and causes vasodilatation. NO that diffuses into the blood vessel lumen is avidly bound by hemoglobin and does not cause systemic vasodilatation.

107. Use of inhaled nitric oxide has been shown in randomized, controlled clinical trials to improve neonatal outcomes in patients with hypoxic respiratory failure (meconium aspiration, pneumonia with or without sepsis, and RDS) in term infants. What have been the outcomes of infants with congenital diaphragmatic hernia?

Eleven randomized, controlled clinical trials have been completed in term and near-term infants with pulmonary hypertension. One trial was a randomized comparison of NO versus prostacyclin for postoperative pulmonary hypertension after cardiac surgery, and one was a randomized trial using various doses. Not including the latter studies, meta-analysis performed by Barrington and Finer showed that 54% of hypoxic near-term infants responded to inhaled NO within 30–60 minutes with a significant increase in PaO_2, compared with 29% of controls (relative risk 2.02). After 30–60 minutes of treatment, PaO_2 in the NO-treated infants was 46.4 mmHg higher than in the controls, and the oxygenation index was 10.7 units less than in control infants. The incidence of death or need for ECMO was significantly reduced by treatment with inhaled NO (relative risk 0.72). This reduction was primarily in the numbers of infants who go on to require ECMO, as there did not appear to be a reduction in mortality.

Infants with congenital diaphragmatic hernia are unique in their presentation in that symptoms include pulmonary hypertension. In the NINOS trial, 53 infants with congenital diaphragmatic hernia were enrolled (28 control, 25 inhaled NO–treated). No significant difference in the occurrence of death occurred with NO therapy. More inhaled NO–treated infants required ECMO (80% versus 54% in controls). There were no significant improvement in PaO_2, no reduction in oxygenation index associated with inhaled NO, and no other important differences between groups. Current data from randomized, controlled clinical trials indicate that treatment with inhaled nitric oxide (in an initial dose of 20 ppm) appears to be a safe and effective therapy that decreases the need for ECMO in the non-CDH near-term infant with hypoxic respiratory failure with or without echocardiographic evidence of persistent pulmonary hypertension of the newborn.

108. Inhaled nitric oxide has been studied extensively and shown to improve oxygenation and reduce the need for ECMO. However, weaning strategies for both nitric oxide and oxygen supplementation have not been as well defined. What are the major concerns regarding the weaning of both ppm NO and oxygen in infants with persistent pulmonary hypertension of the newborn?

When NO and O_2 come into contact, ONO (peroxynitrite), a potent oxidant, is formed. The relative amount of NO, O_{2-} and ONO^-, and antioxidants in the airway will determine whether NO will be beneficial or potentially toxic. These oxidants can contribute to lung injury by enhancing lung inflammation, producing pulmonary edema, and reducing surfactant function. Furthermore, recent findings have shown that abrupt withdrawal of inhaled NO, even in infants with minimal or no response, can induce worsening pulmonary hypertension. Thus, many infants with pulmonary hypertension continue to require inhaled NO at less than 5 ppm for a considerable time. The potential for pulmonary inflammatory injury can be decreased as the concentration of either inhaled NO or O_2 are lowered, although many infants will continue to require several days of inhaled NO in order to prevent recurrence of pulmonary hypertension.

109. Infants with fetal akinesia syndrome (Pena-Shokeir phenotype) frequently have pulmonary anomalies. Describe the pulmonary anomalies in this disorder.

Infants with Pena-Shokeir phenotype (also termed arthrogryposis multiplex congenita with pulmonary hypoplasia) have gracile ribs and reduced thoracic volume. Lack of fetal breathing activity, polyhydramnios secondary to lack of fetal swallowing, and intrauterine constraint result in muscular hypoplasia involving both intercostal and diaphragmatic musculature. Thoracic wall weakness, hypotonia of the muscles of respiration, and anterior horn cell atrophy or deficiency lead to reduced ventilatory drive, which may improve over time in selected infants.

110. Fetal airway obstruction can be the direct result of intrinsic defects in the larynx or trachea resulting in congenital high airway obstruction syndrome. What is the differential diagnosis of extrinsic fetal obstruction?

Conditions that have been reported to compromise the fetal airway by extrinsic compression or mass effect are listed. The two major causes of extrinsic fetal airway obstruction are cervical lymphangioma and teratoma.

Cervical teratoma	Thyroglossal duct cyst
Lymphangioma	Thyroid cyst or tumor
Congenital goiter	Occipital encephalocele
Branchial cleft cysts	Cervical myelomeningocele

111. What precautions should be taken for the child with suspected fetal airway obstructive syndromes during pregnancy and at the time of delivery?

As fetuses with fetal airway obstruction reach viability, they should be monitored closely for development or progression of hydrops (for intrinsic obstruction cases) or polyhydramnios (when extrinsic obstruction is present). The fetus should be delivered by using the ex utero intrapartum treatment (EXIT) procedure, with maintenance of uteroplacental circulation and gas exchange. This approach provides time to perform procedures such as direct laryngoscopy, bronchoscopy, or tracheostomy to secure the fetal airway, thereby converting an emergent airway crisis into a controlled situation.

112. What are the indications and the risks associated with the use of inhaled nitric oxide for the treatment of ventilatory failure in preterm infants?

Based primarily on studies in the preterm lamb (78% gestation) representative of human gestation of approximately 31 weeks, inhibition of endogenous NO production increases fetal pulmonary vascular resistance. When endogenous NO production is blocked during delivery of the preterm lamb, the normal increase in pulmonary blood flow associated with mechanical ventilation and lung inflation is attenuated markedly. Animal studies also have found that inhaled nitric oxide at 5 ppm reduces neutrophil recruitment into the airways and decreases pulmonary edema. In studies of human infants, low-dose (5 ppm) inhaled nitric oxide has been employed in infants with GBS sepsis, pulmonary hypertension, severe hypoxemia associated with prolonged oligohydramnios, and pulmonary hypoplasia. Five infants survived in the study by Kinsella, although intracranial hemorrhage occurred in 60%. Data in the preterm infant, however, are currently very limited, and the risk of intracranial hemorrhage seems high. At present, the FDA does not believe that NO use in premature babies is indicated.

Kinsella JP, Ivy DD, Abman SH: Inhaled nitric oxide lowers pulmonary vascular resistance and improves gas exchange in severe experimental hyaline membrane disease. Ped Res 36:402–408, 1994.

MECHANICAL VENTILATION OF THE NEONATE

113. What are the two basic ways of cycling conventional mechanical ventilators?

1. **Time-cycled, pressure-limited** ventilators have become the standard in neonatal mechanical ventilation because of the problems associated with volume-cycled ventilators. Time-cycled,

pressure-limited ventilators have the advantage of providing continuous flow through the circuit, which allows the infant to take spontaneous breaths of fresh gas between mechanical breaths (the mechanical breaths are referred to as intermittent mandatory ventilation [IMV]). The system gives the operator direct control over the delivered peak inspiratory pressure (PIP) and allows easy compensation for leak around endotracheal tubes, and the decelerating flow pattern allows better gas distribution within the lungs.

2. **Volume-cycled** ventilators deliver a preset tidal volume, usually in a constant flow fashion, generating whatever pressure is necessary to deliver the gas into the lungs. This results in a triangular pressure and volume waveforms with maximum volume and pressure being reached just before the onset of exhalation.

114. What are the disadvantages of time-cycled, pressure-limited ventilators?

The chief disadvantage is the fact that tidal volume is not directly controlled. The delivered tidal volume is determined by the interaction between PIP and lung compliance. Consequently, as compliance changes, so will the delivered tidal volume. Improving lung compliance can lead to excessive tidal volume and cause lung injury. Conversely, worsening compliance can lead to hypoventilation and loss of lung volume. In addition, if an infant is breathing asynchronously with the ventilator, peak pressures are reached quickly and volume is reduced. This situation may result in a serious deterioration of blood gases.

115. What unique problems make volume-cycled ventilation difficult in newborn infants?

Uncuffed endotracheal tubes that are used in newborn infants result in a variable degree of air leak around the tube, causing variable loss of tidal volume. Additional tidal volume is lost through gas compression within the relatively large volume of gas in the ventilator circuit and humidifier, and to stretching of the relatively compliant circuit during inspiration. As a result, the tiny premature infant with poorly compliant lungs receives only a small and variable fraction of the tidal volume generated by the ventilator. In essence, one ends up ventilating the circuit rather than the baby!

116. What are the ways to increase ventilation (improve CO_2 removal) in an infant on time-cycled, pressure-limited ventilation?

- Increase IMV
- Increase PIP
- Decrease PEEP
- Decrease dead space (e.g., by shortening the endotracheal tube)

Keep in mind that there is an upper limit to the effective respiratory rate. An excessively rapid IMV rate may lead to inadequate expiratory time with incomplete exhalation and air trapping. Thus, paradoxically, when the IMV is > 90–120 breaths/minute, further increases in rate may lead to CO_2 retention. This situation is most likely to occur in infants with increased airway resistance and prolonged time constants. In such infants, the best way to improve ventilation is to *decrease* the IMV rate.

Remember that the tidal volume is proportional to the difference between PIP and PEEP. This is referred to as ΔP. Thus, lowering PEEP will increase ΔP and improve ventilation (although it can lead to loss of lung volume with deterioration of oxygenation). Occasionally, excessively high PEEP in a patient with relatively compliant lungs can lead to incomplete exhalation and CO_2 retention. This is not a common problem but should be considered in a patient with improving oxygenation and a worsening respiratory acidosis.

117. Name the two major factors that affect oxygenation in neonatal mechanical ventilation?

Mean airway pressure (Paw)

FiO_2

Mean airway pressure has been shown to be a major determinant of oxygenation. Adequate distending pressure is needed to maintain lung volume and avoid the diffuse microatelectasis that would lead to ventilation-perfusion imbalance with consequent hypoxemia.

118. List the key ventilator variables that affect mean airway pressure in conventional time-cycled, pressure-limited ventilation.

- PIP
- PEEP
- Inspiratory to expiratory ratio (I:E ratio)
- Inspiratory flow

Mean airway pressure is the area under the pressure curve (see figure). Increasing the PEEP is usually the most effective means of increasing the Paw. The least well recognized factor affecting the area under the curve is the slope of the upstroke of pressure, which determines the shape of the pressure waveform. Higher flow leads to more rapid upstroke and a more square-shaped curve, which has a larger area than one with a gradual upstroke and a more triangular shape.

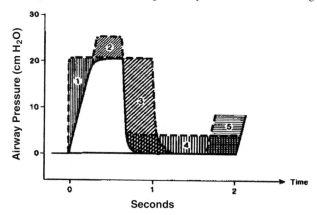

The effects of changes in mean airway pressure (MAP) on the respiratory waveform. The figure shows the many ways that MAP can be changed, all of which will have a different effect on arterial blood gases. (From Reynolds EOM: pressure waveform and ventilator settings for mechanical ventilation in severe hyaline membrane disease. Int Anesthesiol Clin 12:259, 1974, with permission.)

119. When placing an infant on conventional time-cycled, pressure-limited ventilation, how do you choose the initial PIP?

For any given PIP, the delivered tidal volume will be determined by the compliance of the baby's lungs. Select a pressure based on your best estimate of what the infant will need and observe the result. If there is adequate chest rise, good breath sounds, and oxygenation, the pressure is appropriate. If the chest rise is excessive, reduce the PIP, and if the chest movement is inadequate, higher PIP is needed (assuming the endotracheal tube is correctly placed).

Most modern infant ventilators now have the means to directly measure tidal volume (V_T), eliminating the dependence on subjective assessment of adequacy of chest wall movement and allowing more accurate determination of optimal PIP. The target V_T measured at the airway opening should be 4–6 ml/kg in the acute phase of the disease. *Note:* Some devices measure V_T at the point where the circuit attaches to the ventilator. This position is undesirable because it will give an artificially large V_T measurement, ignoring the loss of V_T to compression of gas in the circuit and circuit stretching. Furthermore, gadgets do malfunction, so continue to use your eyes and ears to verify that the "numbers" are believable!

120. List as many possible causes of acute CO_2 retention in an infant on mechanical ventilation as you can (there are many more than you may think!).

- The endotracheal tube is dislodged
- The endotracheal tube is occluded with secretions
- The endotracheal tube is up against the carina
- Accumulation of secretions in the airways (patient needs suctioning)
- The patient has a pneumothorax and some other condition that acutely decreased lung compliance

• Acute bronchospasm
• Oversedation with suppression of spontaneous respiratory effort
• Ventilator malfunction (e.g., leak in circuit, partial disconnection)
• Acute onset of sepsis with loss of spontaneous respiratory effort
• Acute abdominal distention leading to decreased diaphragmatic excursion

Most of these should be readily recognizable clinically. If the chest is not moving, the first priority is to make sure that the airway is patent, the ET tube is in place, and the ventilator is cycling. Many modern infant ventilators have the ability to display flow and pressure waveforms, which should help diagnose or confirm the problem. When in doubt, **reintubate**. Manual ventilation may be appropriate if a circuit or ventilator problem is suspected, but be careful to avoid using excessive pressure that may cause lung injury.

121. What are some adverse effects associated with mechanical ventilation?
• Acute lung injury (baro- or volutrauma, such as pneumothorax, pneumomediastinum, pneumopericardium, pulmonary interstitial emphysema)
• Chronic lung injury (chronic lung disease, bronchopulmonary dysplasia)
• Hemodynamic impairment due to increased intrathoracic pressure
• Intraventricular hemorrhage and periventricular leukomalacia
• Tracheitis or pneumonia
• Tracheal damage with subglottic stenosis
• Palatal groove and damage to tooth buds of the upper incisors

Some degree of impairment of venous return to the heart is inevitable because, unlike spontaneous breathing, intrathoracic pressure is above ambient pressure during positive pressure ventilation. The problem becomes more severe when high or excessive pressures are used. Intraventricular hemorrhage can be triggered by hemodynamic instability, elevated venous pressure, and sudden increases in cerebral blood flow (as might occur with retention of CO_2). Periventricular leukomalacia is associated with hypotension and with marked respiratory alkalosis.

122. Which of the following scenarios is more likely to lead to acute air leak, such as a pneumothorax?
A. PIP of 25 cm in H_2O in a 3.5-kg infant with normal lungs who is ventilated because of neurologic dysfunction
B. PIP of 32 in a 1.2-kg, 28-week premature infant with "whiteout" lungs on chest x-ray secondary to severe RDS

The correct answer is A. Normal lungs are quite compliant, and a PIP of 12–14 cm H_2O is usually sufficient to produce normal tidal volume. A pressure of 25 cm H_2O would produce an excessively large tidal volume in this infant, leading to overstretching of the tissues and air leak. Excessive tidal volume has been shown to be more important than pressure in the genesis of lung injury. The term *volutrauma* is increasingly used in place of *barotrauma* for this reason. On the other hand, the high PIP in scenario B is most commonly necessary to achieve an adequate tidal volume, given the disease severity, and is less likely to cause pneumothorax.

123. Which of the following infants, each ventilated with PIP of 25 cm H_2O, PEEP of 5 cm H_2O, IMV of 90 breaths/minute, and an inspiratory time of 0.3 seconds, is *least* likely to experience hypercarbia, hemodynamic impairment, and air leak secondary to incomplete exhalation (air-trapping)?
A. A 12-hour-old, 760-g, 26-weeks' gestation premature infant with RDS
B. A 2-hour-old, 3.8-kg, 41-weeks' gestation infant with meconium aspiration syndrome
C. A 6-week-old, 1420-g, former 25-weeks' gestation premature infant with severe chronic lung disease

The correct answer is A. Hypercarbia, hemodynamic impairment, and air leak secondary to incomplete exhalation (air-trapping) occur when the expiratory time is too short to allow complete exhalation before the next mechanical breath occurs. This situation is most likely to occur in infants who have increased airway resistance, such as is seen in meconium aspiration with acute airway obstruction or in chronic lung disease in which airway edema, copious secretions, and bronchospasm are typically seen. Both infants will have prolonged time constants. **Time constant** is the product of lung compliance and airway resistance. Conceptually, time constants reflect the time it takes for gas flow to cease and pressure to be fully equilibrated between the large airways and the alveoli when a sudden pressure change is applied to the airway opening (three time constants are needed for 95% equilibration).

In acute RDS, compliance is low and airway resistance is also low (normal). Therefore, short inspiratory times can be used. In addition, time constants are also a function of size (total compliance, not compliance/kg are used). Consequently, large subjects such as adults or horses have long time constants, and small premature infants and hummingbirds have short time constants. Time constants are a major determinant of resting respiratory rate, which turns out to fall exactly where work of breathing is lowest. This is why, at rest, adults breathe at a rate of 14 breaths/min, term infants breathe at 40 breaths/min, and small premature infants at about 60 breaths/min. Mice and hummingbirds breathe a lot faster than that! In infants with acute respiratory distress, tachypnea is a reflection of shorter time constants as lung compliance decreases because of various causes. Asthmatics, on the other hand, prefer to breathe rather slowly because of their prolonged expiratory phase. *The bottom line:* consider the underlying disease process and its pathophysiology before making decisions about ventilator settings.

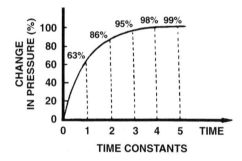

Time constants of the lung. A percentage change in pressure in relation to the time (in time constants) allowed for equilibration. As a longer time is allowed for equilibration, a higher percentage change in pressure occurs. (From Carlo WA, Martin RJ: Principles of assisted ventilation. Pediatr Clin North Am 33:221, 1986, with permission.)

124. What are some of the advantages of synchronized mechanical ventilation?
• Avoidance of asynchrony (baby "bucking" or "fighting" the ventilator)
• Less need for paralysis and sedation
• Lower airway pressures, because the baby and the ventilator work in tandem
• Decreased risk of baro/volutrauma and intraventricular hemorrhage
• Preservation of respiratory muscle training (compared to muscle paralysis)
• Greater ease of weaning from mechanical ventilation

125. What is assist-controlled (A/C) ventilation? How does it differ from synchronized intermittent mechanical ventilation (SIMV)? When should it be used?
A/C ventilation is a form of mechanical ventilation in which the infant triggers the ventilator to cycle with each breath. With a small triggering effort, therefore, the baby can achieve a much higher level of ventilatory support than with spontaneous breathing. In general, A/C ventilation can be used very successfully to treat VLBW babies with RDS or pulmonary insufficiency of prematurity. It has become the most common way to initiate mechanical ventilation therapy in these clinical situations. It often enables patients to be ventilated at lower PIP levels than with conventional mechanical ventilation or SIMV. It differs from SIMV in that with A/C the baby will trigger a ventilator breath with each respiratory effort. In SIMV, the ventilator is synchronized to the baby's respiratory cycle so as to avoid stacking of ventilator and infant breaths, but the baby does not actually trigger ventilator breaths during SIMV ventilation. With modern ventilators, if the baby becomes apneic during either A/C ventilation or SIMV, the machine will deliver a preset number of breaths per minute.

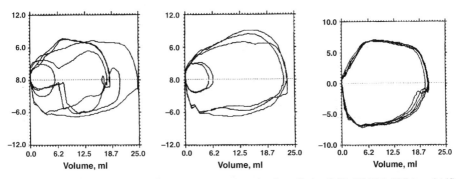

Flow-volume loops indicating the differences among conventional ventilation (left), SIMV (middle), and A/C ventilation (right). The loops at the top are erratic with CMV. With SIMV, the loops are either ventilator generated or infant generated. In A/C mode, all loops are ventilator generated with the infant triggering breaths above the set rate or the ventilator delivering a breath below the set rate. (From Goldsmith JP, Karotkin EH (eds): Assisted Ventilation of the Neonate. Philadelphia, W.B. Saunders, 1996, p 221, with permission.)

126. An infant is now on PIP of 18 cm H_2O, IMV rate of 30 breaths/min, and FiO_2 of 0.3. Which is the correct say of weaning an infant from mechanical ventilation in A/C mode?
   A. Progressively decrease the PIP and IMV
   B. Progressively lower the IMV leaving the PIP unchanged
   C. Progressively lower the PIP leaving the IMV unchanged

The correct answer is C. In A/C mode, every breath that the infant takes triggers a ventilator breath—every breath is supported. As a result, the baby is in control of the ventilatory rate. The IMV rate is only a backup rate in case the infant is apneic or the triggering mechanism is not functioning. Decreasing the IMV rate does not actually decrease the level of support the infant is receiving. Weaning occurs by lowering the degree of support for each breath, i.e., the PIP. Ultimately, when the PIP is down to where the ventilator is generating only enough pressure to overcome the resistance of the endotracheal tube and circuit, the baby is ready for extubation (usually about 10 cm H_2O).

127. Why does hand-ventilation with a bag usually work when mechanical ventilation is failing?

Because with manual ventilation we usually use much higher PIP levels than that we would dare to set on the ventilator! It is easy to inadvertently generate pressures > 40 cm H_2O with all the adrenaline flowing in a crisis. Beware of the risk of pneumothorax! Using a manometer may be helpful, but most of the mechanical gauges grossly underestimate the actual PIP and the actual duration of inspiration, especially when the ventilatory rate is rapid. This explains, in part, why when you place the baby back on the ventilator, ostensibly on the same settings as the pressures that were used with hand ventilation, the saturation usually drifts down again (because the ventilator PIP is actually lower than that with which you were bagging). It is sometimes preferable to maintain the infant on the ventilator and simply increase the level of support (PIP and IMV) as needed to achieve the desired result. This approach allows you to continue to use the monitoring function of the ventilator to provide feedback regarding the tidal volume and other parameters, and it provides controlled and accurate pressure delivery. However, if the baby is still doing poorly, hand ventilation is an acceptable alternative.

128. What do you do when an infant seems to deteriorate on a ventilator?

When a baby is doing poorly on a ventilator, one should remove the baby from the machine and hand ventilate with an anesthesia (preferably) or self-inflating bag. The chest excursion should be carefully examined and breath sounds auscultated to be sure that the ET tube is still well positioned and not plugged. If there is any question about the tube, it should be replaced promptly. A chest radiograph is often helpful to be certain about position of the tube and that there is not an air leak. If the tube seems fine and there are no radiologic changes, the ventilator itself must be carefully checked for malfunction. Respiratory therapists should be available around the clock in any intensive care nursery in which infants are ventilated.

129. How does one prepare to extubate a baby?

Although there is a great deal of literature on neonatal intubation, few articles describe the risks of extubation. Nothing is more frustrating than successfully completing a course of neonatal mechanical ventilation on a sick baby, only to have a serious setback from a poor effort at extubation. When a child has reached the predetermined levels for extubation, the following should be done:

- A chest x-ray should be obtained as a baseline so that postextubation changes can be compared.
- The child should be NPO for at least 4 hours prior to extubation and placed on IV fluids during that time.
- A CPAP set-up or oxygen should be available to transition the child to spontaneous breathing.
- A laryngoscope and a new ET tube should be at hand in case the child does poorly.
- It is not necessary to initiate steroids prior to routine extubation. Nor is the routine use of methylxanthines prior to extubation for respiratory stimulation needed in all children. These adjuncts, however, may be useful if a child has failed one or two prior attempts at extubation.

130. How does one proceed to extubate the infant following these preparations?

When the child is ready to be extubated, the tube should be untaped from the face carefully to avoid causing any abrasions. An anesthesia bag should be attached to the ET tube, and a long, slow low-level (15 cm H2O) positive pressure breath should be administered as the ET tube is withdrawn from the airway. This breath overcomes the natural negative pressure created as the tube is withdrawn from the airway. The child should be placed on CPAP or in oxygen and observed closely. Stridor or hoarseness is common and typically indicates upper airway edema. Marked retractions also may be seen and are worrisome, indicating either volume loss in the lung or upper airway obstruction. If the child has difficulty, the tube should be replaced immediately and another extubation attempt made in 2–3 days. Adequate humidification of inspired gas is essential after extubation. Because of the initial inability to oppose the vocal cords, feeding should not be resumed for at least 6–12 hours postextubation. Clinical deterioration that occurs 24–48 hours after extubation may be due to a number of factors: increased atelectasis, upper airway edema and obstruction, or muscular fatigue. If reintubation is deemed necessary, it should be carried out promptly. "Cheerleading" the child to recovery rarely works, and occasionally significant pulmonary hypertension appears when the work of breathing leads to increased acidosis following a trial of extubation. This setback can be frightening and extremely difficult to manage.

NEONATAL HIGH-FREQUENCY VENTILATION

131. What is neonatal high-frequency ventilation?

Neonatal high-frequency ventilation uses devices that provide respiratory support for critically ill neonates with the use of small tidal volume, rapid rate assisted ventilation. Generally this means rates > 150 breaths per minute and tidal volumes < 2–3 ml/kg.

132. Name the three different types of high-frequency ventilation and what makes each distinct.

(1) High-frequency oscillation (Sensormedics); (2) high-frequency jet ventilation (Bunnel, Inc.); and (3) high-frequency flow interruption (Infant Star). Oscillation exchanges gas by producing positive and negative flow in the ventilator circuit through the use of a vibrating diaphragm. Jet ventilation delivers high-frequency breaths through the interruption of a continuous gas flow directly into the airway through a unique ET tube located in the airway. The interruption takes place in a patient box located close to the baby, by a pincher valve that opens and closes on a piece of plastic tubing. With jet ventilation, inspiration is active; exhalation is passive. High-frequency flow interruption generates the signal by interrupting the flow of gas. It is similar to the jet ventilator except that the interruption of the gas flow occurs at a site much farther from the infant.

133. Have the three types of high-frequency ventilation been compared in clinical trials?

No. Because there have been no comparison trials, each type has its advocates and critics.

134. What happens to tidal volume delivery to the alveolus when frequency is increased during high-frequency oscillation?

It decreases. Impedence of the airway and ET tube are frequency dependent. As rate is increased, impedence to transmission of pressure swings increases. Thus, tidal volume decreases as frequency is increased.

135. How is minute ventilation estimated on high-frequency ventilation?

Normally, with standard mechanical ventilation or spontaneous breathing, minute ventilation = frequency × tidal volume. In high-frequency ventilation, minute ventilation = (frequency) × (tidal volume)^2.

These questions emphasize the importance of understanding the differences between high-frequency oscillation and conventional ventilation. In conventional ventilation, increasing the rate will increase carbon dioxide elimination in most cases. With high-frequency ventilation, turning up the rate generally causes a decrease in minute ventilation due to the loss of tidal volume delivery. When ventilation is inadequate during high-frequency ventilation, turning the rate down can increase carbon dioxide elimination.

136. How does high-frequency ventilation work?

No one really knows. Modeling of the wave flow in high-frequency ventilation is exceedingly complex. Several theories have been proposed, however, to explain high-frequency ventilation.

1. The **spike theory.** This theory postulates that the resistance along the periphery of the airway is higher than in the center so that a spike is produced that extends far down the center of the airway, bypassing much of the lung's dead space.

2. **Pendeluft.** The rapid to-and-fro movement of air between lungs or between lung segments may be enhanced at higher frequencies.

3. **Brownian diffusion** may increase at higher frequencies.

4. **Coaxial flow.** This theory speculates that gas flow in the airway is not simply a to-and-fro movement. Rather, inhaled gas spikes down the center of the airway, while the exhaled carbon dioxide moves along the periphery in a circuitous fashion. As frequencies increase, a whirlpool may actually arise within the airway that literally pulls the small volume puffs of gas to a very deep region of the lung (see figure).

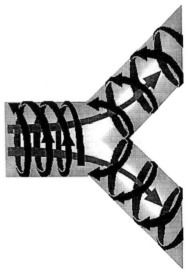

Coaxial flow during high-frequency ventilation. Fresh gas is pulled sharply down the center of the airway, while exhaled CO_2 is removed along the periphery. (From Spitzer AR: High-frequency jet ventilation. In Spitzer AR (ed): Intensive Care of the Fetus and Neonate. St. Louis, Mosby, 1996, p 573, with permission.)

137. What factors affect ventilation during high-frequency ventilation?

Just as in conventional ventilation, changes in respiratory system impedance affect carbon dioxide elimination during high-frequency ventilation. The important distinction is that high-frequency ventilation is more sensitive to changes in impedance than conventional modes of ventilation. Changes in ET tube size, respiratory system compliance, airway patency, and mucus plugging can all have a profound effect on tidal volume delivery and therefore ventilation. Because of the frequencies used and the small tidal volumes, these changes seem to be significantly magnified with high-frequency ventilation compared with conventional ventilation.

138. In neonates with poor lung inflation, should high-frequency oscillation be used at lower, the same, or higher mean airway pressure than that being used on conventional ventilation?

The strategy with which high-frequency oscillation is used is important. Patients with diffuse loss of lung volume (atelectasis) should be treated with lung recruitment strategy. High-frequency oscillation allows the use of higher mean airway pressures than conventional ventilation because the small tidal volumes promote ventilation without causing lung overinflation. This approach has been studied in animal models of hyaline membrane disease and had been shown to improve lung inflation, decrease acute lung injury, decrease pulmonary air leaks, and promote survival. Often referred to as a "high mean airway pressure strategy," the real goal is not a high mean airway pressure, but rather optimal lung inflation. Unfortunately measures of optimal lung inflation are not available. Clinically, the goal is to promote lung recruitment while avoiding lung overinflation, cardiac compromise, and lung atelectasis.

The chest radiograph and the PaO_2/FiO_2 ratio can be used to help guide therapy. If the chest x-ray shows more than nine posterior ribs of inflation, flattened diaphragms, a small heart, or very clear lung fields, the lung may be overinflated. Similarly, if the mean airway pressure is high and the FiO_2 is low, then mean airway pressure should be decreased before FiO_2. If the chest x-ray shows less than seven posterior ribs of inflation, domed diaphragms, a normal heart size, or diffuse radioopacification, the lung may be underinflated. Therefore, if the mean airway pressure is low and the FiO_2 is high, mean airway pressure should be increased. The assessment of cardiac function is also important for the safe use of high-frequency ventilation. Monitoring heart rate, blood pressure, urine output, and capillary refill can help to alert the care provider to changes in cardiac output.

139. What adverse events have been reported with the use of high-frequency ventilation?

Several studies have shown evidence of increased brain injury (periventricular leukomalacia and intraventricular hemorrhage) associated with high-frequency ventilation, particularly when initiated as an initial treatment modality in the VLBW baby. Although meta-analysis does not confirm this finding, the concern remains and further studies are needed in this regard. Necrotizing tracheobronchitis was a complication reported with early models of high-frequency ventilation. This complication has disappeared with the development of improved humidification systems.

140. What are the variables used to alter oxygenation during high-frequency ventilation?

Altering mean airway pressure to optimal levels will change lung volume, improve ventilation-perfusion matching, and decrease intrapulmonary shunt. FiO_2 is used to change the alveolar oxygen concentration.

In oscillatory ventilation, mean airway pressure can be altered directly by changing that setting on the ventilator. With jet ventilation, mean airway pressure is a measured value that is a combination of several factors: PIP, PEEP, duration of inspiratory phase (jet valve on time), and background sigh rate.

141. Has high-frequency ventilation been conclusively shown to reduce the use of ECMO in neonates with MAS?

No. Only anecdotal evidence exists to support the efficacy of high-frequency ventilation in neonates with MAS. In fact, in neonates with MAS and signs of air trapping, high-frequency ventilation may be dangerous. Reported success in MAS with high-frequency ventilation appears to be about 30–40%.

142. Theoretically, how does high-frequency ventilation prevent acute lung injury in hyaline membrane disease?

Volutrauma occurs most rapidly when the lung is repeatedly cycled from a low volume to a high volume. Use of zero end-expiratory pressure and excessive tidal volumes can create acute lung injury within minutes. Application of end-expiratory pressure reduces "atelectotrauma" by preserving functional residual capacity at the end of each assisted breath. Lung overinflation is avoided by using small tidal volumes. Thus, the extremes of low and high lung volumes are avoided with high-frequency ventilation.

143. What other tools do we use in neonatology to promote better lung inflation and reduce the injury associated with ventilating a collapsed lung?

The use of end-expiratory pressure, surfactant, prone positioning, and liquid ventilation all promote lung recruitment over time. They work by stabilizing recruited alveoli at the end of exhalation.

144. To use high-frequency ventilation safely, what factors must be carefully monitored?

Hyperventilation must be avoided. Data on brain injury in neonates suggest that hyperventilation may cause brain injury through ischemia as CO_2 is lowered. This finding has been observed in a number of published studies, both with conventional and high-frequency ventilation.

Lung over- or underinflation also may have adverse affects on the baby. Currently, no good methods are available for defining optimal lung volume during high-frequency ventilation. Evaluating cardiac performance, chest radiographs, and PaO_2/FiO_2 ratio can help the clinician avoid extremes, but the Holy Grail of high-frequency ventilation is defining when the lung is optimally inflated.

145. In what pulmonary disease states has high-frequency ventilation been shown to promote improved oxygenation compared with conventional modes of ventilation?

The most dramatic improvements in oxygenation have been reported in patients with poor lung inflation. In general this means neonates with RDS or pneumonia. Lung disease in which there is a significant amount of airway debris or resistance does not seem to respond as well to high-frequency ventilation.

146. What is ECMO?

Extracorporeal membrane oxygenation (ECMO) is a modification of standard cardiopulmonary bypass techniques used in the operating room during open heart surgery. It was adapted in a simplified circuit to provide artificial life support to pulmonary patients in an ICU setting. Neonatal ECMO was the first clinically successful application of this technology to treat severe and progressive cardiorespiratory failure caused by meconium aspiration syndrome complicated by persistent pulmonary artery hypertension occurring in the first week of life. Babies qualifying for early ECMO support had failed to respond to more conventional life support techniques such as mechanical hyperventilation–induced alkalosis, cardiotonic pressor infusions, and priscoline. Subsequently, other life-threatening neonatal conditions were treated with ECMO, including RDS in near-term babies, sepsis or pneumonia, and congenital diaphragmatic hernia. ECMO was also applied to older infants and to pediatric and adult patients. At the core of ECMO technology are the heart-lung pump (a semiocclusive roller device) and the innovative Kolobow polycarbonate-spooled, silicone membrane oxygenator (see figure, top of next page). Both devices are powerful enough to completely support cardiac output and lung function in neonates.

147. What is ECLS?

Extracorporeal life support includes ECMO, hemofiltration, hemodialysis, and indwelling oxygenator filaments (IVOX or intravenous oxygenator). Many of these other techniques can be incorporated with an ECMO circuit or can be applied separately.

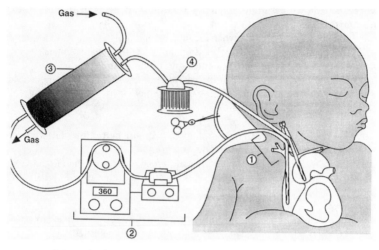

Schematic of ECMO apparatus. (Courtesy of S. Baumgart, M.D.)

148. What evidence suggests that ECMO actually works?

The definitive randomized trial establishing the effectiveness of neonatal ECMO was conducted by the National Health Service in the United Kingdom. Thirty of 93 infants (32%) referred to ECMO centers died compared to 54 of 92 (59%) receiving conventional care. The relative risk for reduced mortality with ECMO was 0.55 (0.39–0.77, 95% confidence limits, P < 0.0005). Of survivors, 1 child in each group was severely disabled at 1 year, and 10 ECMO patients, compared to 6 conventionally treated infants, were disabled to a lesser degree. The UK Collaborative ECMO Trial Group concluded ECMO support should be actively considered for mature neonates with severe but potentially reversible respiratory failure.

UK Collaborative ECMO Trial Group: UK collaborative randomised trial of neonatal extracorporeal membrane oxygenation. Lancet 348(9020):75–82, 1996.

149. Who is a neonatal ECMO candidate?

ECMO's success relies on the physician's ability to recognize within the first week of illness those near-term or term newborn infants with reversible pulmonary disease and to exclude infants with irreversible pulmonary disease. The ECLS Organization's Registry data estimate that only 1 in about 1700 infants can benefit from ECMO. Criteria for ECMO patient selection have been widely debated during the past decade, and two controversial questions have arisen: (1) Is less invasive therapy likely to succeed? (2) With constantly improving neonatal ventilatory and pharmacologic techniques, must physicians continually reassess ECMO criteria? In general, the earlier the ECMO physician can identify the infant with a high probability of dying from his or her disease prior to iatrogenic consequences of conventional therapy, the better the patient selection and outcome. The following inclusion and exclusion criteria provide general neonatal ECMO guidelines that are currently widely accepted:

- \> 34 weeks' gestational age
- \> 2.0 kg birth weight
- < 2 weeks' postnatal age (or ≤ 10 days high-pressure mechanical ventilation, relative age)
- Reversible cardiopulmonary condition
- No major cardiac malformation
- No syndromes with unsurvivable prognosis
- No uncontrollable bleeding diathesis (e.g., disseminated intravascular coagulation with bleeding uncontrolled despite multiple component transfusions or progressive parenchymal brain hemorrhage
- No irrecoverable brain injury

Once the above inclusion and exclusion criteria have been considered, one of several pulmonary indices is used to assess the severity of respiratory illness and the likelihood of death if the infant is treated conventionally. The simplest and most popular index is the **oxygen index** (OI) shown in the figure. Briefly, the OI is equivalent to the mean airway pressure generated during mechanical ventilation multiplied by the FiO_2 (both of these values indicate level of conventional ventilatory support) and then divided by the postductal arterial oxygen tension in the blood (a sensitive indicator of both ventilation and perfusion of the baby's lung). The resulting value is multiplied by 100. The relative importance of the ratio between mean airway pressure and arterial oxygen tension in the calculation of OI performed at 1.00 (FiO_2) is further demonstrated graphically in this figure. Once the PaO_2 is below 40 mmHg in the denominator of the OI equation, a geometric rise in OI occurs. This rise parallels increased pulmonary vascular resistance with increased right-to-left shunting in the patient with severe pulmonary arterial hypertension.

Oxygen index (OI) versus PaO_2 and mean airway pressure (MAP).

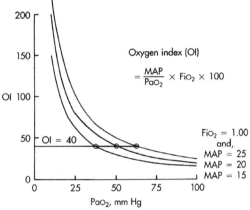

150. How may vascular access for ECMO be achieved, and what are the benefits and liabilities of venoarterial versus venovenous bypass?

1. **Venoarterial bypass.** The gold standard for ECMO therapy is venoarterial (VA) bypass. An internal jugular drainage cannula and a second common carotid arterial infusion cannula are placed surgically through a right neck incision performed at the bedside. VA-ECMO provides complete cardiopulmonary support to an infant's native heart and lungs when either or both are failing.

Advantages:	*Disadvantages:*
Complete cardiopulmonary support	Carotid artery ligation
Used for heart and lung failure	Embolism (clot, air) infused into arterial
Cardiac function not essential	circulation
	Potential hyperoxic reperfusion injury

2. **Venovenous bypass.** A less-invasive technique for augmenting systemic oxygenation using ECMO is venovenous (VV) bypass. In neonates, a novel double-lumen cannula (12 or 14 French) is surgically inserted into the internal jugular vein and positioned within the right atrium. Blood is withdrawn from the lateral lumen, reoxygenated, and infused back into the medial lumen. The right atrial admixture of oxygenated and deoxygenated blood then crosses through fetal channels (the foramen ovale and the ductus arteriosus) in the infant with severe pulmonary arterial hypertension to supply systemic oxygenation via shunt flow. Because systemic blood supply is delivered entirely by the infant's native left ventricle, sufficient ventricular force must be available to circulate this oxygenated admixture against systemic vascular resistance, which is usually increased in the critically ill patient. Frequently, both cardiotonic pressors and generous volume infusions of saline, albumin, or plasma along with blood transfusions are required to

maintain an infant's circulation on VV-ECMO. Venovenous access avoids invasion of the carotid artery; therefore, systemic embolism is less risky and the right common carotid artery is left intact following decannulation from bypass.

Advantages:	*Disadvantages:*
Spares carotid artery	Less effective cardiac support
Embolism less risky	Lower PaO_2 with mixing in right atrium
One double-lumen cannula	Recirculation into double-lumen cannula
sufficient	SvO_2 and SaO_2 monitors unreliable; must follow PaO_2,
	pH to judge oxygen sufficiency

151. What is the single most important parameter for monitoring the effectiveness of ECMO?

The mixed venous saturation (SVO_2) from the jugular venous cannula drain is monitored continuously during bypass using a fiber-optic device inserted directly into the blood path coming out of the patient. Mixed venous saturation does not so much reflect pulmonary function (as does the systemic arterial saturation) as represents the adequacy of tissue oxygen delivery from the native heart and the ECMO circuit combined. If the oxygen delivered by ECMO is enough to meet tissue oxygen demand, then the SVO_2 is generally > 70–75%. Failure to meet tissue oxygen demand results in the progressive desaturation of venous blood returning from the capillary beds into the right atrium. An SVO_2 < 65–70% indicates marginal oxygen delivery, and an SVO_2 < 60% is associated with lactic acid production through anaerobic metabolism. Therefore, the single most important parameter monitored during ECMO and used to assess the adequacy of bypass is the SVO_2. Notably, during venovenous ECMO the SVO_2 may be artificially elevated because of recirculation of arterialized blood back into the drainage side of the double lumen cannula; however, trends in SVO_2 may still be useful, and the patient may be taken off bypass briefly to assess a true SVO_2.

152. How long do babies stay on bypass? How do you know when to wean ECMO flow?

The average ECMO course proceeds over 3–7 days, awaiting spontaneous lung recovery. Cardiac recovery and mobilization of capillary leak edema usually precede lung recovery and weaning the ECMO pump flow rate. As the tissue edema is mobilized, fluid is transferred back into the intravascular space, increasing the baby's native cardiac output. Therefore, the infant's systemic arterial saturation and PaO_2 may actually decrease during recovery (as ECMO support is weaned and the infant's native cardiac output drives right-to-left shunting of deoxygenated blood through fetal channels in an accelerated fashion). During this early improvement phase on ECMO, diuretic therapy (furosemide, mannitol) or hemofiltration may assist in reducing this native circulation of desaturated blood. Thereafter, as the mixed venous saturation improves in the jugular venous cannula (above 80%), the ECMO pump flow is reduced in 10 ml/min decrements until a pump idle rate is reached of approximately 100 ml/min minimum flow (to prevent stasis and clotting within the circuit). Frequent arterial *and* venous blood gas assessments are important during the weaning process. Recent reports have suggested that pulmonary function testing demonstrating increased functional residual capacity (> 15 ml/kg) and improved dynamic lung compliance may be useful in determining more exactly when lung recovery is sufficient to warrant coming off bypass.

153. What is liquid ventilation?

Liquid ventilation refers to the process of filling the lung with a "breathable" liquid through which gas exchange can take place. Perfluorochemicals are nontoxic, poorly absorbed, and capable of carrying respiratory gases. It is possible to breathe a perfluorochemical liquid, but because of the density and viscosity of the fluid, support from a ventilator is required. The two forms of liquid ventilation generally discussed are partial liquid ventilation, in which a conventional ventilator is used on the liquid-filled lung, and total liquid ventilation, which uses a special liquid ventilator to push and pull tidal volumes of liquid.

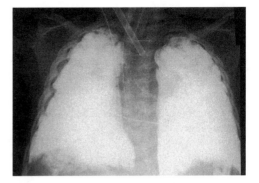

Liquid ventilation. The lung is filled with per-fluorocarbon, which is highly radiopaque.

154. What is the effect of filling the lung with a liquid on lung compliance?
Compliance markedly increases as surface tension is reduced to near zero. Compliance refers to the change in volume divided by the change in pressure ($C_L = \Delta V / \Delta P$). When the air-liquid interface is eliminated and replaced with a liquid-liquid interface, virtually all surface tension is eliminated, and the lung becomes significantly more compliant.

155. Name some diseases that might benefit from liquid ventilation.
• RDS (improves compliance and recruits lung volume)
• MAS (removes debris and recruits lung volume)
• Pneumonia (removes debris, may be a vehicle to deliver drugs such as antibiotics)
• Congenital malformations (may act as a good contrast media for radiographs and magnetic nuclear imaging)

156. How long has the technique of liquid ventilation been studied?
Breathing liquids was introduced into the medical literature in the 1920s as a way to cleanse the lung after poisonous gas inhalation. Later, liquid ventilation was evaluated in animals to reduce surface tension in the surfactant-deficient lung and as a means to improve underwater diving for adults. In the last three decades, animal studies have been specifically directed at the clinical applications in the pathologic lung. Clinical trials began in 1989 and continue today.

157. Liquid ventilation worked in the movie *The Abyss*. Does it work in humans?
The human trials to date have been encouraging, but enrollment has been slow. The publications on phase 1 and 2 trials have suggested that this may be safe and very effective. The pivotal phase 3 trials are underway in adults only. There has been a reluctance to move forward in infants because of the unknown potential for long-term problems. To date, in neonates who have been treated, the problems have been minor, and the potential advantages appear significant.

158. When will liquid ventilation be clinically available?
A lot of work still needs to be done before this technique can be used widely to treat neonatal lung diseases.

AIR LEAK SYNDROMES

159. The incidence of air leak is highest in the newborn in association with which respiratory conditions?
Air leak occurs in 41% of babies with MAS, 27% with RDS, 10% with transient tachypnea, and 1–2% of all newborns. The reason for the increase with MAS is the viscosity of meconium, which results in a ball-valve mechanism that leads to air trapping. Newborns in general have a

higher incidence of air leaks than the general population because of the high transpulmonary pressure (-30 to -150 cm H_2O) associated with the onset of breathing.

160. What is the least common form of neonatal air leak syndrome?

Fortunately, pneumopericardium is the least common, occurring in 2% of babies with air leak. Pneumopericardium must be recognized promptly because of its high morbidity and mortality. Interstitial emphysema is quite common (35%) and in many cases precedes the other forms of air leak. Pneumothorax accounts for 20% of neonatal air leaks, and 3% of babies have a pneumomediastinum.

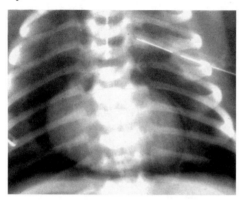

An infant with a pneumopericardium. The pericardium is separated from the epicardium of the heart, and air can be seen within the pericardial space surrounding the heart. Overall contrast has been increased to better visualize the pericardial air.

161. Reports over the past decade have suggested a decline in the incidence of neonatal air leak syndromes. Give two reasons why this is occurring.

One of the major factors has to be the "kinder, gentler" approach to neonatal ventilation. Permissive hypercapnia was all the rage of the 1990s and has lead to more conservative ventilatory management strategies. Examples include early and aggressive use of CPAP, shorter inspiratory times, and lower PIP.

A second important change was the introduction of surfactant replacement therapy in the later 1980s. Most of the early surfactant trials documented about a 30–50% reduction in the rate of neonatal air leaks.

162. You are called to the bedside of a baby who has suddenly become cyanotic while on a ventilator. You listen to the chest and you hear better breath sounds on the right side. You call for a chest radiograph, but the x-ray technician is on a break. Neither the senior resident nor the neonatologist is available, and you are on your own. What do you suspect, and how do you tell if you are correct?

Your suspicion should be high for a tension pneumothorax in this clinical situation. Before you place a needle into the chest, however, consider the following:
- You could transilluminate the chest with a high-intensity fiber-optic light. If a pneumothorax is present, the left side should "light up" whereas the right will transilluminate less.
- Gently retract the ET tube while auscultating. If breath sounds improve, it means the ET tube had advanced into the right mainstem bronchus. After repositioning the tube, the patient should improve immediately.

163. A baby is breathing asynchronously on a conventional ventilator, and you are concerned that she is at risk for a pneumothorax. Name some things you can do to decrease the risk of air leak in this patient.

- Increasing the gas temperature may slightly decrease the incidence of air leak.
- Decreasing the inspiratory time will decrease mean airway pressure and could decrease the risk of pneumothorax, but may reduce oxygenation.

- Increasing the ventilatory rate may allow you to take over ventilation and decrease the baby's effort, but you need to watch for air trapping.
- Utilization of a synchronized mode of ventilation (SIMV or A/C) will help the baby to breathe with the ventilator breaths.
- Sedation and pain relief may help significantly.
- Paralytic agents such as pancuronium prevent pneumothoraces in premature babies who are actively expiring against positive pressure ventilation, but should be used as a last resort.

164. Name several possible ways to treat unilateral pulmonary interstitial emphysema (PIE).

The primary goal of treatment of unilateral PIE is to allow the affected lung to deflate. Selective bronchial intubation will allow the contralateral lung to deflate (of course, selective left mainstem intubation may be technically difficult), but may pose problems because the perfusion to the ventilated lung may not be sufficient for gas exchange in all cases. A randomized trial of high-frequency jet ventilation did show effectiveness in treating PIE by lowering the mean airway pressure, which may allow PIE to resolve. In infants, the lung in the superior position will receive more of the ventilation. Placing the affected lung in the downward position may be helpful in deflating that lung.

165. What important sign distinguishes a tension pneumothorax from one without tension?

There is no specific sign. In a tension pneumothorax, an ongoing air leak contributes to a progressive increase in intrathoracic pressure. Shift of the trachea or the point of maximal impulse, decreased breath sounds, pallor, or cyanosis and retractions may occur in either tension or non-tension pneumothoraces. In a tension pneumothorax, the critical factor is the ongoing increase in cardiopulmonary embarrassment to the patient. In most instances, when a pneumothorax is first detected, it is very difficult to tell whether a pneumothorax is under tension. If the child appears clinically stable for the moment, one can wait for a period of time (30–60 minutes) and repeat a chest radiograph prior to the insertion of a chest tube. In some cases, however, one cannot wait and a thoracentesis must be done immediately.

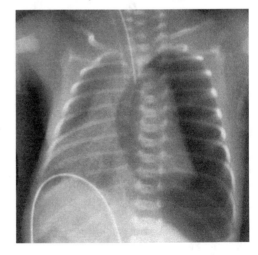

Severe tension pneumothorax on the left side.

166. Why do neonates have an increased susceptibility to alveolar rupture?

Neonates are subject to air leaks because of uneven alveolar ventilation in RDS or MAS. Air trapping also frequently occurs because of small airway plugs. The areas that are more distensible receive more ventilation, which leads to high transpulmonary pressure that, in turn, increases the likelihood of alveolar rupture. Another factor is that the neonate has fewer alveolar connecting channels (pores of Kohn), which allow air to redistribute between ventilated and nonventilated alveolar spaces. Lastly, resuscitation by an overzealous, inexperienced practitioner also increases the newborn's susceptibility to air leaks.

167. Where do you place a chest tube for best drainage of an air leak?

Ideally, one wants to place a chest tube in the thoracic cavity where it will do the most good with the least risk to the infant. Positioning of the infant is the key to the entire procedure. All too commonly, the baby is allowed to remain supine. When one enters the chest in that position, the catheter hits the lung and moves posteriorly (see figure). If the child, however, is placed nearly vertical to start the procedure, it is easy to angle the catheter anteriorly for optimal placement. The thoracostomy tube is inserted through an incision made in the fifth interspace in the midaxillary line. After the incision is made, one tunnels up an interspace with a hemostat, which is used to pop through the strong muscular wall of the chest (yes, it is tough even in a tiny premature infant!). If a pneumothorax is present, a gush of air should be seen when the chest is opened. The catheter should be advanced so that no end holes lie outside the chest wall. If the catheter is inserted too far, it must be pulled back. The chest tube is then connected to a suction apparatus. The suction rarely needs to be greater than –10 to –15 cm H_2O. Noisy bubbling from the drainage apparatus at the bedside from high wall suction is also unnecessary and only gives the nurse and the baby's parents a headache!

The use of anterior catheter insertions in the second interspace is not advocated, except in rare circumstances. It is too easy to hit the breast bud, which may damage future breast development or leave unsightly scars in any patient.

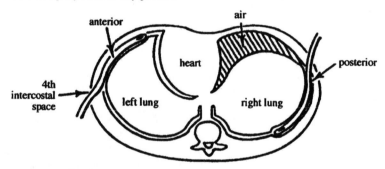

Appropriate chest tube placement is shown on the left side of the figure, with the chest tube in the proper position to reach air in the superior part of the thorax. On the right side of the figure, the chest tube has hit the lung and migrated posteriorly, preventing it from evacuating the air lying superiorly.

168. How can renal malformations increase the likelihood of pneumothorax in newborns?

Obstructive uropathies lead to oligohydramnios. Insufficient amniotic fluid volume leads to pulmonary hypoplasia. The mechanism is not completely understood but in part is due to external compression of the neonate's thorax that impedes fetal lung growth. It is also believed that fetal breathing movements against an intrauterine fluid volume may be critical for normal lung development.

169. A term infant with a nontension air leak may be treated by placing the baby in 100% oxygen. Explain how this works.

The air in a spontaneous or nontension pneumothorax will have the same nitrogen concentration as room air. By allowing the baby to breathe pure oxygen, a gradient for nitrogen is created from the extrapulmonry to the intrapulmonary spaces. Nitrogen will naturally diffuse across this gradient, allowing the pneumothorax to reabsorb more rapidly. Caution should be used when considering this approach in the preterm infant who is more subject to oxidant injury.

BRONCHOPULMONARY DYSPLASIA

170. What is bronchopulmonary dysplasia (BPD)?

BPD is the chronic lung disease that often follows RDS in the VLBW baby. First described by Northway in 1967, it has become the greatest foe of all neonatologists and the focal point of perhaps more studies than any other clinical syndrome in neonatology. BPD was not a disease until the neonate became a patient. Once people attempted to save critically ill neonates with lung disease, a certain percentage developed BPD. In most nurseries, the BPD rate is about 30%. The more immature the infant, the more likely it is that BPD will develop. BPD is defined as a need for oxygen at either 28 days of life or, more recently, at 36 weeks postconception, with radiographic changes consistent with chronic lung disease. This latter definition emerged when incredibly tiny premature infants began to survive, virtually all of whom needed oxygen at 28 days.

171. Describe the histopathologic features of infants with BPD.

In a series of open lung biopsies from VLBW infants, aged 14 days to 7 weeks, on ventilatory support with radiographic changes consistent with chronic lung disease, Coalson et al. described a consistent lack of alveolarization with variably widened alveolar septae and minimal changes in the airways. Mild to moderate septal fibrosis was also apparent. These widened alveolar septae were hypercellular with disordered capillary growth. Typically, the alveolar spaces were laden with numerous alveolar macrophages and neutrophils.

Transmission electron microscopy demonstrated poor differentiation of type I and type II lung epithelial cells. These epithelial cells had relatively abundant cytoplasm and extensive glycogen stores; however, lamellar bodies were extremely rare to totally absent. There was no progression of alveolarization with enlarged simplified terminal airspaces, minimal and focal saccular fibroplasia. The interstitium of the lung contained myofibroblasts, and there was focal deposition of elastin and collagen fibers. Most saccular walls showed blunted "outpouchings" or secondary crest formation.

Coalson I, Kuehl T, Prihoda T, et al: Diffuse alveolar damage in the evolution of bronchopulmonary dysplasia in the baboon. Pediatr Res 24:357–366, 1988.

172. How does BPD develop?

The etiology of BPD is not clear, but several factors likely contribute to its development (the 6 Ps of BPD):

1. Prematurity
2. Positive pressure ventilation
3. Prolonged oxygen exposure
4. Protracted use of endotracheal tubes
5. Pulmonary edema (from a patent ductus arteriosus [PDA], overhydration, or delayed diuresis)
6. Pulmonary air leak (e.g., interstitial emphysema, pneumothorax)

Other factors, such as free oxygen radical exposure and sepsis, also seem to be contributory in many instances. Sepsis, in particular, has recently become an increasingly important piece of the puzzle of BPD. The key to this disease, however, appears to be the chronic exposure that babies have to the 6 Ps.

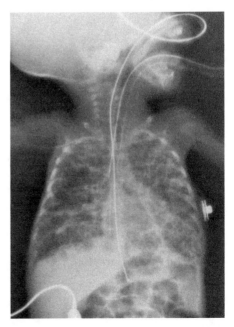

Severe stage IV bronchopulmonary dysplasia (BPD).

173. One of your patients is now being treated with dexamethasone for BPD. The child is on a 6-week course of therapy. Should you be concerned about adrenal suppression when treatment is discontinued?

Adrenal suppression in the newborn usually does not seem to pose as many problems as it does in older children or adults. After 30 days, however, there is a high likelihood of some adrenal insufficiency. It may therefore be better to try to limit steroid use to less than 14 days, which seems to have a lesser effect on adrenal suppression. If longer courses are used, however, some of the effects can be minimized by giving every-other-day treatment for the last week or 2 of a course of steroids in BPD.

Perhaps more important is the effect of steroids on subsequent neural development. Both animal and human studies indicate that chronic steroid use may result in reduced amounts of neural tissue mass. Neurologic handicaps may be higher in infants treated with dexamethasone.

174. When should steroids be started for BPD?

There is good evidence that the optimal use of steroids for BPD occurs between 10 days and 4 weeks of life. Children who appear to respond optimally are those with a pattern of alveolar haziness on chest radiograph. This radiographic appearance probably represents interstitial and alveolar edema from the inflammatory reaction to oxygen and positive pressure, which seems to respond well to the use of early dexamethasone treatment. Because of the increasing concern about the effects of steroids on neurologic development, however, steroid use should be restricted to those infants with more severe disease courses, who are likely to remain chronically ventilator dependent.

175. What drug and what doses should be administered to treat BPD?

About the only agreement among neonatologists about treatment of BPD is the choice of drug—dexamethasone. The optimal dosing schedule has yet to be firmly established. Many textbooks cite 0.5 mg/kg/day as the optimal starting dose, but some researchers have found that an initial dose of 1.0 mg/kg/day is far more effective. The drug taper can occur rapidly, and the course of treatment can be reduced to less than 2 weeks. A subsequent week of every-other-day therapy can be used if needed. Our usual approach is as follows:

Dosing Schedule for Treatment of Bronchopulmonary Dysplasia

Days 1–3	1.0 mg/kg/day
Days 4–6	0.5 mg/kg/day
Days 7–8	0.25 mg/kg/day
Days 9–10	0.1 mg/kg/day
Days 11–17	0.1 mg/kg/every other day (if needed)

Again, this is only one suggested approach that has appeared to work well. Many other treatment courses are equally effective in many instances.

Treatment after 4 weeks of life is less effective, and discontinuation of steroids is often met with a significant rebound effect; at times, the infant may become even more oxygen dependent than prior to steroid therapy. When an infant is started on steroids after 4 weeks of life, a more prolonged course of every-other-day treatment may be needed.

176. Why can a child recover from BPD when an adult cannot repair the lung injury seen in emphysema?

Children continue to add new alveoli until approximately 8 years of age. After that time, surface area and volume within the lung continue to increase with growth, but new alveoli are no longer added. Although scarring does occur in the lungs of BPD patients, there appears to be sufficient healthy tissue to regenerate an adequate new alveolar volume.

177. What other treatments besides steroids help in BPD?

The key to recovery from BPD is growth of alveoli and overall growth. As a result, optimal nutritional support is critical in BPD, perhaps more than anything else. Other therapeutic adjuncts that help are:

- Optimal ventilator management
- Provision of optimal PEEP for tracheobronchomalacia
- Bronchodilators
- Fluid restriction (it is difficult in neonates to give many calories and restrict fluids at the same time!)
- Diuretic therapy
- Chloride supplementation to prevent metabolic alkalosis from diuretics
- Prompt closure of a PDA, if present
- Methylxanthines (both caffeine and theophylline decrease work of breathing and apnea)
- Sedation and pain relief

178. What are BPD spells and how should they be treated?

BPD spells are acute episodes of deterioration encountered during the course of treatment of a child with BPD. The baby typically becomes increasingly cyanotic, agitated, and inconsolable, with a marked deterioration in overall pulmonary status. Oxygen and ventilatory assistance often need to be increased during these episodes. They may, at times, be very acute and severe and occasionally result in sudden death.

BPD spells frustrate even the best of neonatologists with respect to their management. Bronchospasm is often cited as the cause of this deterioration, but the authors' personal experience suggests that many such episodes, especially the more acute, severe forms, are more commonly the result of airway collapse from tracheobronchomalacia. Increasing the PEEP to stabilize an airway (assuming the child is intubated) can be beneficial in such cases. Computerized pulmonary function testing readily allows determination of optimal PEEP in this clinical situation. If one does suspect bronchospasm, pre- and postbronchodilator therapy can be evaluated with pulmonary function testing. Flexible fiber-optic bronchoscopy is also valuable, and one can see the airway open to a more normal size and configuration when one reaches an optimal PEEP.

179. Why are chlorothiazide and spironolactone preferred as diuretics in BPD as opposed to furosemide? Isn't furosemide a better diuretic?

There is no question that furosemide is a more potent diuretic than either chlorothiazide or spironolactone. In chronic situations such as BPD in the neonate, however, calcium sparing is important to prevent rickets, and thiazide diuretics are thought to be more effective in this regard. Spironolactone helps prevent potassium loss and reduces the severity of metabolic alkalosis from diuretics. It is always a good idea, however, to initiate KCl supplementation whenever diuretics are initiated for BPD, because so many of these children develop a significant metabolic alkalosis. Furosemide also has a greater tendency to produce nephrocalcinosis when used on a chronic basis, which is less likely with thiazides, because they reduce calcium excretion in the kidney.

APNEA OF PREMATURITY

180. What is apnea of prematurity?

Apnea is the cessation of breathing. Although this problem affects people of all ages in many different forms, it is most prevalent in premature infants prior to 36 weeks' gestation. Pathologic apnea refers to cessation of breathing for > 20 seconds; < 20 seconds and accompanied by bradycardia 20% below the baseline heart rate; or < 20 seconds with oxygen desaturation below 80%. Most apnea of prematurity is classified as **central** apnea (see figure, top), characterized by complete absence of respiratory effort. Other types of apnea commonly seen are **obstructive** apnea and **mixed** apnea. Obstructive apnea occurs when the infant makes a respiratory effort, but no airflow is present secondary to obstruction (see figure, bottom). Obstructive apnea is often associated with gastroesophageal reflux. Mixed apnea is a combination of central and obstructive apnea.

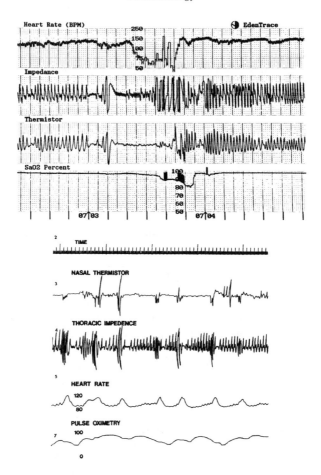

181. What is periodic breathing?

Periodic breathing is a type of central apnea characterized by brief pauses in breathing of < 10 seconds, followed by periods of regular respiration of < 20 seconds' duration. This pattern repeats itself for at least three cycles and often many more (see figure). The significance of this form of breathing is unknown at present. Many prematurely born infants demonstrate periodic breathing,

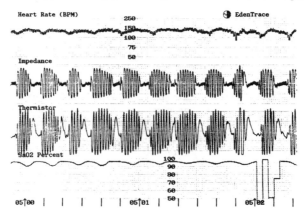

often as much as 20–30% of total sleep time. Because of the frequency of this finding, some neo-natologists consider periodic breathing to be a normal maturational process. On the other hand, it also may be a reflection of significant immaturity of respiratory control and a variant of apnea.

182. What is the incidence of apnea of prematurity?

Virtually all premature infants have some degree of apnea. At 34–35 weeks' postconceptional age, about 65% of infants have demonstrable apnea. About two-thirds of these children have central apnea or periodic breathing, and one-third have obstructive or mixed apnea.

183. What is the significance of apnea of prematurity?

In the short term, particularly in the intensive care nursery, extremely premature infants can have prolonged apneic episodes that may be fatal. As they mature, most infants will have more self-limited episodes. Less clear are the long-term effects on infants who have had a history of severe apnea of prematurity. Investigators are beginning to explore whether apnea of prematurity, particularly with oxygen desaturation, may affect learning and other aspects of childhood development.

184. When does apnea of prematurity resolve?

Although the majority of apnea of prematurity is gone by 37 weeks' postconceptional age, in many cases it can persist even beyond 45 weeks' postconceptional age, occasionally longer. Recent evidence has demonstrated that the earlier the gestational age at birth, the longer the apnea persists postnatally.

185. Does apnea of prematurity need treatment?

In the most severe cases, infants with severe apnea of prematurity may need endotracheal intubation and mechanical ventilation, CPAP, or oxygen therapy. Some infants may have their apnea controlled by the methylxanthines, caffeine, or theophylline. Caffeine is the preferred treatment because of its once-a-day dosing and fewer side effects. Patients are typically loaded with 20 mg/kg of caffeine citrate and maintained on 7–8 mg/kg/day. The therapeutic range is between 12 and 20 μg/ml. Some patients may be controlled at very low levels, under 5 μg/ml, whereas others need to be near or above 20 μg/ml. At these authors' institution, caffeine is maintained until the infant is > 1500 g and apnea-free for 5 days. At that point, the medication is discontinued. The half-life of caffeine is over 100 hours, and the level drops slowly. In rare instances, infants develop apnea after caffeine discontinuation, and they may need to be restarted, and sometimes discharged, on the medication. This occurs in approximately 2% of NICU patients.

186. Do premature infants with apnea need to be discharged on home monitors?

Home cardiorespiratory monitoring is a technology developed in the 1970s after several studies suggested a possible relationship between apnea and sudden infant death syndrome (SIDS). Since that time, hundreds of thousands of premature infants have been discharged on these monitors. Although anecdotal evidence has shown that these devices are effective in decreasing SIDS, no large, controlled study has demonstrated this conclusively. Many physicians feel that monitoring at home is an important aspect of infants' care. Others feel that it is useless. There is tremendous variation around the United States and the world in home monitor utilization, and no established standard of care for prescribing, maintaining, or discontinuing monitors exists.

SUDDEN INFANT DEATH SYNDROME

187. What is SIDS?

SIDS is unexpected death of an infant under 1 year of age that remains unexplained after a thorough autopsy, history, and investigation of the scene of the death. It was given the name SIDS in 1969. Although people of all ages die suddenly, the rate of sudden death is highest under 1 year of age. The 1-year cutoff has been arbitrarily assigned; in actuality, the overwhelming majority of SIDS deaths occur prior to 6 months of life.

188. How many infants die of SIDS each year?

In the United States, there were about 3000 deaths from SIDS in 1998. This represents a rate of approximately 0.75 deaths from SIDS per 1000 live births. The peak age of SIDS is 2–5 months. The rate is substantially higher in urban areas, particularly among African-American infants. Interestingly, the SIDS rates in the Hispanic and Asian populations are equal, or lower than, the caucasian population. In the developed nations of Europe and Asia, SIDS rates are slightly lower than in the U.S. SIDS rates are also lower for Australia and New Zealand.

189. Has the rate of SIDS changed over the past 30 years since it was first recognized as an entity?

The SIDS rate slowly declined from 1985 to 1994, then began to drop precipitously from about 2 deaths per 1000 births in 1992 to the present 0.75 per 1000 births. This rapid decline paralleled the institution of the "Back to Sleep" campaign, sponsored by the National Institutes of Health, the SIDS Alliance, and the American Academy of Pediatrics. This initiative followed the discovery that the simple act of changing infants' sleeping positions from the stomach to the back in England and Australia was responsible for a dramatic reduction in the SIDS rate. The rate of infants sleeping on their backs has risen from 15% to over 70% in the past 5 years in the U.S. It is likely that the SIDS rate will decrease even lower as more and more infants sleep on their back.

190. How did such a simple change have such a great effect?

Good question! In medicine, as in all aspects of life, uncomplicated and elegant observations can make great differences. Although the exact physiology is unclear, it is likely that sleeping on the back reduces the re-breathing of carbon dioxide, adjusts the position of the airway, thus reducing obstruction, or reduces the possibility of poor oxygenation-ventilation through the mattress. The effects on the baby's thermal environment and the ability to eliminate heat may also be important. It may be a combination of all of these changes or a completely different factor as yet undiscovered.

191. Is SIDS a form of child abuse?

There has been a great deal of publicity about infants originally diagnosed with SIDS who were ultimately found to be the victims of a homicidal parent. These children included the case that established the supposed link between SIDS and apnea. Again, like many things in the news, this represents an extremely small number of cases and is the exception rather than the rule. Although it is impossible to quantify, it is thought that less than 2% of SIDS cases are probable homicides.

192. What are the risk factors for SIDS?

The greatest known risks for SIDS appear to be prone sleeping and maternal smoking, both prenatally and postnatally. It has been estimated that if all infants slept on their back, and no mothers smoked, the SIDS rate would be about 60% lower than it is now! Other apparent risk factors include African-American race, low socioeconomic status, young maternal age, winter season, and prematurity. The SIDS rate for premature infants is about 2.25 times that for full-term infants. Infants with apnea of prematurity are at no greater risk for SIDS than premature infants without apnea of prematurity.

LUNG ABNORMALITIES

193. What are the different types of congenital cystic lesions of the lung?

Congenital cystic lesions of the lung generally include those diseases that result from a problem in the formation of mesodermal and ectodermal tissue during lung development. These lesions include pulmonary sequestrations, congenital cystic adenomatoid malformations, congenital lobar emphysema, and bronchogenic pulmonary cysts.

194. What is the most common congenital lung malformation?

Pulmonary sequestration is thought to be the most common congenital lung malformation. A pulmonary sequestration is an area of nonfunctioning lung tissue with no connection to the tracheobronchial tree but with a systemic arterial supply. Pulmonary sequestrations can be diagnosed antenatally. They can be asymptomatic in the newborn or can cause respiratory distress secondary to lung compression or congestive heart failure. Resection is generally recommended, even if asymptomatic, to reduce secondary risk of recurrent infection.

195. How are pulmonary sequestrations classified?

Pulmonary sequestrations are either **extralobar** or **intrapulmonary**. Extralobar pulmonary sequestrations include lesions with lung tissue surrounded by its own pleura. Intrapulmonary sequestrations, also known as intralobar sequestrations, have no discernible pleural tissue.

196. What is a congenital cystic adenomatoid malformation of the lung, and how does it generally present?

Congenital cystic adenomatoid malformation originates as an adenomatous growth in the terminal bronchioles early in gestation. In most cases, there is a connection with the tracheobronchial tree that causes these lesions to increase in size. Only one lobe of the lung is usually involved. Congenital cystic adenomatoid malformations are now frequently diagnosed in the antenatal period by sonography. The most common presentation in the postnatal period is respiratory distress. Respiratory distress is caused by a ball-valve effect, which in turn causes an increase in the size of the lesion. Surgical removal of the affected lobe is the treatment of choice.

197. What is the most common cause of mortality from congenital lung malformations?

Persistent pulmonary hypertension of the newborn. Lung malformations such as congenital diaphragmatic hernia and congenital cystic adenomatoid malformation can lead to lung hypoplasia and concomitant PPHN. Recent efforts have been made to identify infants at greatest risk of mortality who might be candidates for fetal surgical intervention.

198. When congenital lung malformations are diagnosed in the antenatal period, what are some poor prognostic signs?

The presence of nonimmune hydrops fetalis, shift of the mediastinum, bilateral lesions, and the presence of other associated congenital abnormalities all portend a poor prognosis for infants with congenital lung lesions.

199. Are there any congenital lung malformations that have been successfully treated antenatally?

Congenital cystic adenomatoid malformation has been treated with some success in the antenatal period. Antenatal surgical repair of congenital cystic adenomatoid malformations is generally limited to infants with fetal hydrops. One series of 13 infants had 8 survivors; 5 infants died in the intraoperative or perioperative period. In all survivors, resection of the malformation led to resolution of fetal hydrops and increased lung growth. The principal operative concern is the initiation of maternal labor. Congenital diaphragmatic hernia repair also has been attempted antenatally by a technique of tracheal plugging, which allows expansion of existing pulmonary tissue.

200. What is the cause of congenital lobar emphysema?

Congenital lobar emphysema is caused by antenatal bronchial obstruction. This obstruction can be either intrinsic or extrinsic to the bronchiole and causes an overinflation of the pulmonary lobe. Intraluminal obstruction can result from a cartilaginous deficiency or inflammatory changes. Extrinsic causes include compression from an adjacent vascular structure or mass. Infants can present with respiratory distress or be asymptomatic in the newborn period. This lesion is more common in males, is usually seen in the left upper lobe, and is frequently associated with other congenital abnormalities of the heart and kidney. The treatment of congenital lobar emphysema is usually lobectomy.

201. What is a bronchogenic cyst?

A bronchogenic cyst results from abnormal budding of bronchial tissue during development. Bronchogenic cysts are single unilocular lesions of 2–10 cm in diameter. The cysts may or may not communicate with the remainder of the tracheobronchial tree. Bronchogenic cysts can be found in the mediastinum or in the peripheral lung tissue. Mediastinal cysts are thought to arise earlier in the development than those found in the periphery. Bronchogenic cysts can be asymptomatic at birth and may not present until adulthood. Other lesions are symptomatic from compression or infection. Surgical resection is generally recommended.

BIBLIOGRAPHY

Neonatal Resuscitation
1. American Heart Association/American Academy of Pediatrics Neonatal Resuscitation Program Steering Committee: Textbook of Neonatal Resuscitation. Elk Grove Village, IL, AAP, 2000.
2. Jain L, Keenan W (eds): Resuscitation of the Fetus and Newborn. Clin Perinatol 26(3), 1999.

Transitional Physiology and the Asphyxiated Fetus
3. Donn SM, Faix RG: Delivery room resuscitation. In Spitzer AR (ed): Intensive Care of the Fetus and Neonate. St. Louis, Mosby, 1996, pp 326–336.
4. Donn SM, Faix RG: Special procedures used in resuscitation. In Donn SM (ed): The Michigan Manual: A Guide to Neonatal Intensive Care, 2nd ed. Armonk, NY, Futura Publishing, 1997, pp 10–17.
5. Faix RG, Donn SM: General principles. In Donn SM (ed): The Michigan Manual: A Guide to Neonatal Intensive Care, 2nd ed. Armonk, NY, Futura Publishing, 1997, pp 5–9.
6. Rennie JM: Neonatal resuscitation. In Sinha SK, Donn SM (eds): Manual of Neonatal Respiratory Care. Armonk, NY, Futura Publishing, 2000, pp 101–105.

Respiratory Distress Syndrome
7. American Academy of Pediatrics Committee on the Fetus and Newborn: Surfactant replacement therapy for respiratory distress syndrome. Pediatrics 103:684–685, 1999.
8. Kendig JW, Ryan RM, Sinkin RA, et al: Comparison of two strategies for surfactant prophylaxis in very premature infants: A multicenter, randomized trial. Pediatrics 101:1006–1012, 1998.

Meconium-Stained Amniotic Fluid and Meconium Aspiration Syndrome
9. Cleary GM, Wiswell TE: Meconium-stained fluid and the meconium aspiration syndrome: An update. Pediatr Clin North Am 45:511–529, 1998.
10. Cochrane CG, Revak S, Merritt TA, et al: Bronchoalveolar lavage with KL4-surfactant in models of meconium aspiration syndrome. Pediatr Res 44:705–715, 1998.
11. Findaly RD, Taeusch HW, Walther FJ: Surfactant replacement therapy for meconium aspiration syndrome. Pediatrics 97:48–52, 1996.
12. Lam BCC, Yeung CY: Surfactant lavage for meconium aspiration syndrome: A pilot study. Pediatrics 103:1014–1018, 1999.
13. Miller PW, Coen RW, Benirschke K: Dating the time interval from meconium passage to birth. Obstet Gynecol 66:459–462, 1985.
14. Moses D, Holm B, Spitale P, et al: Inhibition of pulmonary surfactant function by meconium. Am J Obstet Gynecol 164:477–481, 1991.
15. Wiswell TE: Bronchoalveolar lavage with dilute Surfaxin (KL4-surfactant) for the management of the meconium aspiration syndrome (MAS). Pediatr Res 45:326A, 1999.
16. Wiswell TE, Fuloria M: Resuscitation of the meconium-stained infant. Clin Perinatol 26:659–668, 1999.

Pulmonary Hypertension
17. Fineman J, Heymann MM, Morin FC 3d: Persistent pulmonary hypertension in the newborn. In Allen HD, Gutgesell HP, Clark EB, Driscoll DJ (eds):Moss and Adams' Heart Disease in Infants, Children, and Adolescents. Baltimore, Lippincott Williams & Wilkins [in press].
18. Finer NN, Barrington KB: Nitric oxide for respiratory failure in infants born at or near term. Cochrane Library, Issue 2. Oxford, Update Software, 1999.
19. Hallman M, Waffarin F, Bry K, et al: Surfactant dysfunction after inhalation of nitric oxide. J Appl Physiol 30:2026–2034, 1996.
20. Hansen T, Corbet A: Disorders of transition. In Taeusch HW, Ballard RA (eds): Avery's Diseases of the Newborn, 7th ed. Philadelphia, W.B. Saunders, 1998.
21. Hedrick MH, Ferro MM, Filly RA, et al: Congenital high airway obstruction syndrome (CHAOS): A potential for perinatal intervention. J Pediatr Surg 29:271–274, 1994.
22. Kinsella JP, Neish SR, Ivy E, et al: Clinical response to prolonged treatment of persistent pulmonary hypertension of the newborn with low doses of inhaled nitric oxide. J Pediatr 123:102–108, 1993.

23. Kinsella JP, Shaffer F, Neish SR, et al: Low-dose inhalational nitric oxide in persistent pulmonary hypertension of the newborn. Lancet 340:8819–8820, 1992.
24. Liechty KW, Crumbleholme TM: Management of fetal airway obstruction. Semin Perinatol 23:496–506, 1999.
25. Matalon S, Demarco I, Haddad C, et al: Inhaled nitric oxide injures the surfactant system of lambs in vivo. Am J Physiol 270:L273–L280, 1996.
26. Moerman P, Fryns JP, Goddeeris P, Lauweryns JM: Multiple ankyloses, facial anomalies, and pulmonary hypoplasia associated with severe antenatal spinal muscular atrophy. J Pediatr 103:238–241, 1983.
27. Morin FC 3d, Stenmark R: Persistent pulmonary hypertension of the newborn. Am Rev Respir Crit Care Med 151:2010–2032, 1995.
28. Neonatal Inhaled Nitric Oxide Study Group: Inhaled nitric oxide and hypoxic respiratory failure in infants with congenital diaphragmatic hernia. Pediatrics 99:838–845, 1997.
29. NINOS Study Group: Inhaled nitric oxide for near-term infants with respiratory failure. N Engl J Med 336:602–605, 1997.
30. Robbins CG, Davis JM, Merritt TA, et al: Combined effects of nitric oxide and hyperoxia on surfactant function and pulmonary inflammation. Am J Physiol 269:L545–L550, 1995.
31. Roberts JD Jr, Fineman JR, Morin FC 3d, et al: Inhaled nitric oxide and persistent pulmonary hypertension of the newborn. The Inhaled Nitric Oxide Study Group. N Engl J Med 336:605–610, 1997.
32. Roberts JD, Zapol WM: Inhaled nitric oxide. Semin Perinatol 24:55–58, 2000.
33. Shokeir MHK: Multiple ankyloses, camptodactyly, facial anomalies, and pulmonary hypoplasia (Pena-Shokeir I syndrome). In Vinken PJ, Bruyn GW (eds): Handbook of Clinical Neurology. Amsterdam, North Holland Publishers, 1982, pp 437–439.
34. Steinhorn RH, Morin FC 3d, Fineman JR: Models of persistent pulmonary hypertension of the newborn (PPHN) and the role of cyclic guanosine monophosphate (GMP) in pulmonary vasorelaxation. Semin Perinatol 21:393–408, 1997.
35. Van Meurs KP, Rhine WD, Asselin JM, Durand DJ: Response of premature infants with severe respiratory distress to inhaled nitric oxide. Pediatr Pulmonol 24:319–332, 1997.
36. Whitsett JA, Pryhuber OS, Rice WR, et al: Acute respiratory disorders. In Avery GB, Fletcher MA, MacDonald MG (eds): Neonatology: Pathophysiology and Management of the Newborn, 4th ed. Philadelphia, Lippincott Williams & Wilkins, 1994.

Conventional Mechanical Ventilation of the Neonate
37. Carlo WA, Martin RJ: Principles of assisted ventilation. Pediatr Clin North Am 33:221, 1986.
38. Goldsmith JP, Karotkin EH (eds): Assisted Ventilation of the Neonate. Philadelphia, W.B. Saunders, 1996.

Neonatal High-Frequency Ventilation
39. Clark RH: High-frequency ventilation. J Pediatr 124:661–670, 1994.
40. Clark RH, Dykes FD, Bachman TE, Ashurst JT: Intraventricular hemorrhage and high-frequency ventilation: A meta-analysis of prospective clinical trials. Pediatrics 98:1058–1061, 1996.
41. Dreyfuss O, Saumon G: Role of tidal volume, FRC, and end-inspiratory volume in the development of pulmonary edema following mechanical ventilation. Am Rev Respir Dis 148:1194–1203, 1993.
42. Froese AB, Bryan AC: High-frequency ventilation. Am Rev Respir Dis 135:1363–1374, 1987.
43. Froese AB, McCulloch PR, Sugiura M, et al: Optimizing alveolar expansion prolongs the effectiveness of exogenous surfactant therapy in the adult rabbit. Am Rev Respir Dis 148:596–577, 1993.
44. Gerstmann DR, Fouke JM, Winter DC, et al: Proximal, tracheal, and alveolar pressures during high-frequency oscillatory ventilation in a normal rabbit model. Pediatr Res 28:367–373, 1990.
45. Meredith KS, deLemos IRA, Coalson JJ, et al: Role of lung injury in the pathogenesis of hyaline membrane disease in premature baboons. J Appl Physiol 66:2150–2158, 1989.
46. Michna J, Jobe AH, Ikegami M: Positive end-expiratory pressure preserves surfactant function in preterm lambs. Am J Respir Crit Care Med 160:634–639, 1999.
47. Spitzer AR: High-frequency jet ventilation. In Spitzer AR (ed): Intensive Care of the Fetus and Neonate. St. Louis, Mosby, 1996.
48. Vannucci RC, Brucklacher RM, Vannucci SJ: Effect of carbon dioxide on cerebral metabolism during hypoxia-ischemia in the immature rat. Pediatr Res 42:24–28, 1997.
49. Wiswell TE, Graziani LI, Kornhauser MS, et al: High-frequency jet ventilation in the early management of respiratory distress syndrome is associated with a greater risk for adverse outcomes. Pediatrics 98:1035–1043, 1996.

Air Leak Syndromes
50. Goldberg RN, Abdenour GE: Air leak syndrome. In Spitzer AR (ed): Intensive Care of the Fetus and Neonate. St. Louis, Mosby, 1996.
51. Miller MJ, Fanaroff AA, Martin RJ: The respiratory system: Other problems. In Fanaroff AA, Martin RJ (eds): Neonatal-Perinatal Medicine: Diseases of the Fetus and Infant, 5th ed. St. Louis, Mosby, 1992, p 834.

52. Soil RE, McQueen ME: Respiratory distress syndrome. In Sinclair JC, Bracken MB (eds): Effective Care of the Newborn Infant. Oxford, Oxford University Press, 1992.

53. Tarnow-Mordi WO, Reid E, Griffiths P, Wilkinson AR: Low inspired gas temperature and respiratory complications in very low birth weight infants. J Pediatr 114:438, 1989.

54. Yu VYH, Wong PY, Bayuk B, Szymonowicz W: Pulmonary air leak in extremely low birth weight infants. Arch Dis Child 61:239, 1986.

Bronchopulmonary Dysplasia

55. Husain A, Siddiqui N, Stocker J: Pathology of arrested acinar development in postsurfactant bronchopulmonary dysplasia. Hum Pathol 29:710–717, 1998.

56. Rojas M, Gonzalez A, Bancalari E: Changing trends in the epidemiology and pathogenesis of neonatal chronic lung disease. J Pediatr 126:605–610, 1995.

57. Van Lierde S, Cornelis A, Devlieger H, et al: Different patterns of pulmonary sequelae after hyaline membrane disease: Heterogeneity of bronchopulmonary dysplasia. Biol Neonate 60:152–162, 1991.

Lung Abnormalities

58. Adzick NS, Harrison MR, Crombleholme TM, et al: Fetal lung lesions: Management and outcome. Am J Obstet Gynecol 179:884–889, 1998.

59. Kravitz RM: Congenital malformations of the lung. Pediatr Clin North Am 41:453–472, 1994.

60. Miller MJ, Fanaroff AA, Martin RJ: Respiratory disorders in preterm and term infants. In Fanaroff AA, Martin RJ (eds): Neonatal-Perinatal Medicine: Diseases of the Fetus and Infant, 5th ed. St. Louis, Mosby, 1992, pp 1040–1065.

61. Pilling D: Fetal lung abnormalities: What do they mean? Clin Radiol 53:789–795, 1998.

62. Ribet ME, Copin M, Gosselin BH: Bronchogenic cysts of the lung. Ann Thorac Surg 61:1636–1640, 1996.

63. Schwartz MZ, Ramachandran P: Congenital malformations of the lung and mediastinum: A quarter century of experience from a single institution. J Pediatr Surg 32:44–47, 1997.

64. Takeda S, Miyoshi S, Inoue M, et al: Clinical spectrum of congenital cystic disease of the lung in children. Eur J Cardio Thorac Surg 15:11–17, 1999.

INDEX

Page numbers in **boldface type** indicate complete chapters.

Abdominal masses, 199–201
ABO set-up
  clinical and laboratory features, 240
  incidence, 239
  neonatal management, 239, 240
Accessory nipples, 81–82
Acetazolamide, 122
Achondroplasia, 213
Acid-base balance
  base excess, 119–120
  bicarbonate therapy, 120
  compensation of imbalance, 120, 121
  contraction alkalosis, 121
  dilution acidosis, 121
  measurements, 119, 120
  volume of distribution in derangement correction,
    120
ACTH. *See* Adrenocorticotropic hormone
Acyclovir
  herpes simplex virus management, 300
  safety, 272
  varicella-zoster virus management, 302
Addiction, neonates
  breast-feeding, 332
  cocaine effects, 332, 333
  meconium testing, 333
  narcotic withdrawal, 332
  opiate withdrawal
    management, 346–347
    signs, 345–346
  withdrawal manifestations, 333
ADH. *See* Antidiuretic hormone
Adjusted age, preterm infants, 23
Adrenal hemorrhage, neonates, 105
Adrenocorticotropic hormone (ACTH),
    insufficiency in neonates, 106
Adrenoreceptors
  cardiac, 39
  renal, 39
  vasopressor actions, 40
Air leak syndromes. *See also specific syndromes*
  associated conditions, 387–388
  chest tube placement, 390
  epidemiology, 388
  incidence trends, 388
  saturated oxygen therapy, 390
Alagille syndrome, diagnosis, 187–188
Albumin
  administration in jaundice, 197
  drug displacement of bilirubin from albumin
    binding sites, 194
  levels in hyperbilirubinemia, 193, 194
Alloimmune thrombocytopenia
  definition, 249
  diagnosis, 250
  management, 250

Alloimmune thrombocytopenia *(cont.)*
  presentation, 250
Alpha-fetoprotein, screening, 205, 329
5-Alpha reductase deficiency, 110
Alveolar rupture, neonate susceptibility, 389–390
AMC. *See* Arthrogryposis multiplex congenita
Amniocentesis
  classification, 7
  complications, 7
  definition, 7
  Down syndrome, 210
  early risks, 8
  indications, 7
  intersex disorders, 109, 110
  sampling errors, 108
  test time requirements, 7
  timing, 7
Amphotericin B, 272, 278
Ampicillin, 271, 272
Androgen insensitivity syndrome
  clinical presentation through life, 110–111
  diagnosis, 110
Anemia. *See also* Diamond-Blackfan anemia;
    Fanconi anemia
  causes in neonates, 228
  diagnosis in utero, 229
  laboratory evaluation, 229
  parvovirus B19 effects, 310
  physiologic
    versus pathologic, 234
    preterm versus full-term infants, 234
Anencephaly
  prevalence, 205
  seizure absence, 329
Ankle clonus, 315
Anophthalmia
  features, 208
  neonatal evaluation, 209
Anterior horn cell damage, 337
Anticipation, 335
Antidiuretic hormone (ADH), elevation in neonates,
    106
Antithrombin III, plasma levels, 256
Aortic stenosis, critical
  balloon valvuloplasty, 60
  definition, 59
  diagnosis, 59–60
Apgar score
  assessment, 354
  cerebral palsy risk evaluation, 325, 352–353
  historical perspective, 354
Aplasia cutis congenita, 81
Apnea
  of prematurity, 349
    classification, 393–394
    definition, 393

Apnea *(cont.)*
  of prematurity *(cont.)*
    incidence, 395
    management, 395
    periodic breathing, 394–395
    resolution, 395
    significance, 395
  primary versus secondary, 351
Arnold-Chiari malformations, 329, 330
Arrhythmia. *See also specific arrhythmias*
  cardiac transplantation, 69
  conduction system maturation, 66
  fetal distress etiologies, 66
  maternal risks for congenital complete heart
      block, 66
  neonatal therapy, 66
Arterial blood gas, fetus, 353
Artery cannulation, neonates, 27
Arthrogryposis multiplex congenita, 342
Ascites, neonatal
  diagnosis, 185
  differential diagnosis, 184
  etiology, 184, 185
  exudates, 185
  lipid nutrition, 185
  transudates, 185
Asphyxia. *See also* Hypoxic-ischemic
      encephalopathy
  long-term outcome, 354–355
  metabolic acidosis, 352
  multiple organ injury, 355–356
  reversibility, 353
Asymptomatic bacteriuria, incidence, 289
Atopic dermatitis, 81
Atrial septal defect, surgery, 73
Autosomal dominant polycystic kidney disease, 138
Autosomal recessive polycystic kidney disease, 138

Bag-mask ventilation
  contraindications, 356
  indications, 356
  troubleshooting, 357
Ballard scoring system, 315, 316
Balloon atrial septostomy, transposition of the great
      arteries, 59
Bartter syndrome, 124
Beckwith-Wiedemann syndrome, presentation, 206
Benzyl alcohol, danger to infants, 21–22
Beta-adrenergic agonists, tocolysis, 11
Bicarbonate
  renal metabolism, 126
  resuscitation administration, 358, 359
  therapy, 120
Biliary atresia
  course, 189
  extrahepatic biliary atresia
    histopathology, 188
    imaging, 188
    incidence, 188
    presentation, 188
  hepatitis, differential diagnosis, 189

Biliary atresia *(cont.)*
  importance of early diagnosis, 187
  management, 189
Bilirubin encephalopathy
  brain deposition, 191, 192
  kernicterus, 192
  neurotoxicity mechanisms, 191
  presentation of acute disease, 192
  preterm toxicity, 193
  risks, 192
Biophysical profile
  components, 1
  neonatal outcome relationship, 2
  umbilical venous pH relationship, 2
Bladder extrophy
  development, 139
  incidence, 139
  repair, 139
Blue diaper syndrome, 94
Blueberry muffin baby, 80
Bohn nodules, presentation, 77
Botulism
  differential diagnosis, 336
  infant versus food-borne botulism, 335
  intubation of infants, 336
  supportive care, 336
Bourgeois, Luoyse, 238
BPD. *See* Bronchopulmonary dysplasia
Brachial plexus palsy
  diagnosis, 341, 342
  differential diagnosis, 341–342
  prognosis, 341
  risk factors, 341
  treatment, 341
Bradycardia, differential diagnosis in newborns, 62–64
Brain death
  criteria, 22–23
  duration of observation, 23
  electroencephalography, 22–23
  ethics, 23
Breast-feeding
  Candida infection of nipple, 156
  contraindications, 155
  drug safety, 17
  duration, 155
  fat variation, 157
  Graves' disease, 104
  initiation, 156–157
  jaundice, 198–199
  maternal benefits, 157
  maternal substance abuse, 332
  milk production determination, 155
  necrotizing enterocolitis protection, 179
  preterm infant
    advantages of human milk, 154
    initiation, 157
  public policy issues, 155–156
  sufficiency evaluation, 156
  supplementation, 155
  tandrieres, 157–158
  vitamin content of milk, 159

Breast-feeding *(cont.)*
  whey-to-casein ratio of milk, 150
Breast milk. *See* Breast-feeding
Breast tissue, size in newborns, 315
Bronchogenic cyst, 398
Bronchopulmonary dysplasia (BPD)
  definition, 391
  dexamethasone therapy
    dosing, 392
    initiation, 392
    side effects, 392
  diuretic therapy, 393
  etiology, 391
  histopathology, 391
  management, 393
  recovery, 392
  spells, 393
  vitamin A supplementation, 159

Café-au-lait spots, 334
Calcium antagonists, tocolysis, 11
Calcium metabolism. *See* Hypercalcemia;
    Hypocalcemia
Camptodactyly, 216
Candidiasis
  late-onset disease, 277
  osteomyelitis, 288
  prevention, 278
  retinopathy of prematurity association, 278
  risk factors for neonates, 276
  treatment, 278
  types and clinical features, 277
Carbohydrate
  formula content, 149
  glucose endogenous production, 149
  lactose malabsorption, 149, 164–165
  milk composition, 154
  neonatal requirement estimation, 148–149
  toxicity to neonates, 149
Cardiac catheterization
  access, 58
  congenital heart disease indications, 55, 58
Cardiac dextroversion, 45
Cardiac output
  cardiac transplantation changes, 70
  determinants in neonate, 31
  infant regulation, 358
  low output following cardiac surgery, 54
Cardiac surgery. *See* Cardiac transplantation;
    Congenital heart disease
Cardiac transplantation
  arrhythmias, 69
  cardiac output changes, 70
  complications, 70
  immunosuppressive therapy, 70
  rejection presentation, 70
Cardiac tumor
  mortality, 71
  surgery, 71
  with tuberous sclerosis, 71
  types, 70–71

Cardiology, **31–73**
Cardiomyopathy
  causes, 69
  with Noonan syndrome, 69
  with Pompe disease, 69
  treatment, 69
  types, 69
Catch-up growth, in low-birth-weight infants, 22
CDH. *See* Congenital diaphragmatic hernia
Cefotaxime, 272
Ceftriaxone, 273
Central venous line thrombosis
  diagnosis, 256
  treatment, 257
Cephalohematoma, 319, 320
Cephalosporins, third-generation, 271
Cerebral palsy (CP)
  Apgar score risk evaluation, 325, 352–353
  asphyxia role, 326
  associated problems, 325
  classification, 324
  cytokine levels, 326
  definition, 324
  diagnosis, 324
  differential diagnosis, 326
  electronic fetal monitoring impact, 325, 353
  infection risks, 325
  preterm infants, 24–25
  prevalence trends, 325–326
  risk factors, 25, 324
  types, 24–25
  ultrasound, 325
Cerebrospinal fluid (CSF)
  antibiotic concentrations, 281
  lumbar puncture, 280
  normal neonatal values in examination, 318
Chest tube, placement in newborns, 29, 390
Chickenpox. *See* Varicella-zoster virus
Chimerism, 218
Chlamydia trachomatis
  conjunctivitis
    blindness association, 284–285
    prophylaxis, 285
  diagnosis, 285
  maternal transmission, 285, 286
  neonatal diseases, 286
  pneumonia, 286
  treatment, 285–286
Chloral hydrate, neonatal use, 347
Chloride diarrhea, 166
Choleductal cyst
  epidemiology, 190
  presentation, 190
  types, 190
Cholelithiasis, associated conditions, 188
Cholestatic jaundice
  definition, 186
  evaluation, 186
  hepatologist referral, 187
Chorionic villus sampling (CVS)
  advantages over amniocentesis, 209

Chorionic villus sampling (CVS) *(cont.)*
  amniocentesis comparison, 8
Chromosomal translocations
  Down syndrome, 210–211
  reciprocal versus robertsonian, 219
  representation, 219
Chromosome 22 deletion, congenital heart disease, 43
Chromosome banding, 217–218
Circumcision
  amputation and gender reassignment, 111, 112
  analgesia, 26–27
  benefits and risks, 26
  religion, 26
Cisapride, preterm infant risks, 163
Clavicle
  fracture, 344, 345
  ossification, 3
Cleft lip, heredity, 217
Cleft palate, heredity, 217
Clinodactyly, 216
Clonic seizure, 327–328
CMV. *See* Cytomegalovirus
Coarctation of the aorta
  associated heart defects, 44–45
  hypertension with, 134
Collodion membrane
  ichthyosis association, 79
  management, 79
Complement, neonatal levels, 262
Confined placental mosaicism, 207–208
Congenital adrenal hyperplasia
  androgen exposure effects on female fetus, 105
  diagnosis, 108, 109
  enzyme deficiencies and manifestations, 104
  genitogram, 108
  physical examination, 108
  renal tubular acidosis, 127
  screening, 96, 97
  sequelae, 108–109
Congenital adrenal hypoplasia, 105
Congenital cystic adenomatoid malformation, 397
Congenital diaphragmatic hernia (CDH)
  causes, 207
  management, 4–5
  nitric oxide treatment, 373
  radiography, 362
  surgery assessment, 5–6
Congenital heart disease
  acyanotic, 44–45
  cardiac catheterization, 54, 58
  congenital complete heart block, 66
  cyanotic, 42–44
  initial evaluation, 49
  postoperative management, 52–54
  preoperative stabilization, 48–52
  presentation in neonates, 48–49
  surgery
    atrial septal defect, 73
    Fontan procedure outcome factors, 72
    hypoplastic left heart syndrome, 73
    operations and sequelae, 55–57

Congenital heart disease *(cont.)*
  surgery *(cont.)*
    shunt operations, 71
    switch operation, 72
    ventricular septal defect, 72–73
Congenital hepatic fibrosis, kidney abnormalities
    with, 138
Congenital hip dislocation. *See* Developmental
    dysplasia of the hips
Congenital hypothyroidism. *See* Hypothyroidism,
    congenital
Congenital lobar emphysema, 397
Congenital mesoblastic nephroma, 258
Congenital nephrotic syndrome
  definition, 130
  evaluation of neonates, 131
  genetic diseases with, 131
  infections as cause, 131
  prognosis, 132
  risk factors, 131
Congestive heart failure
  causes, 38
  definition, 37
  differential diagnosis in neonate, 45
  hemodynamics with truncus arteriosus, 60
  high output failure, 38
  susceptibility of newborns, 38
  symptoms, 38
Conjoined twins
  treatment, 13
  types, 13
Conjunctivitis
  blindness, 284–285
  etiology, 283–284
  Gram staining, 284
  prophylaxis, 285
  time of onset, 283–284
  treatment, 284
Consanguineous parents, recessive disorder risks, 218
Constant Spring hemoglobin, 241
Constriction ring syndrome, 344
Contact isolation, 282
Continuous positive airway pressure (CPAP)
  complications, 366
  efficacy, 365
  indications, 366
  respiratory distress syndrome, 365
Contraction stress test, principles, 15
Cor pulmonale
  causes, 67
  definition, 67
  laboratory findings, 67
  prognosis, 68
  signs and symptoms, 67
  treatment, 68
Corticosteroid
  bronchopulmonary dysplasia, dexamethasone
    therapy
    dosing, 392
    initiation, 392
    side effects, 392

Corticosteroid (cont.)
  fetal lung maturation, 11–12, 364
  hypotension management in neonates, 42
  neutrophil effects, 279
Cortisol
  measurement in preterm infants, 106
  secretory pattern in neonates, 107
CP. See Cerebral palsy
CPAP. See Continuous positive airway pressure
Craniosynostosis, types, 318
C-reactive protein (CRP), sepsis levels, 269–270
Creatinine
  birth versus postnatal levels, 123
  neonatal values, 116
  sodium concentration in urine, 123
Cri du chat syndrome, 213
Crown, location in newborns, 217
CRP. See C-reactive protein
CSF. See Cerebrospinal fluid
CVS. See Chorionic villus sampling
Cyanosis, neonates. See also Congenital heart disease
  abnormal oxygen saturation, 35, 43
  chest film, 37
  differential cyanosis, 35–36, 49
  d-TGA, 36
  electrocardiography, 36–37
  hyperoxia test, 36
  maternal history and likely heart abnormalities, 35
  reverse differential cyanosis, 49
Cystic fibrosis
  gastrointestinal manifestations, 176
  incidence, 212
  meconium ileus association, 171, 173, 175
  presentation, 212
  screening, 96
Cystic kidney disease, 137–138
Cytomegalovirus (CMV)
  diagnosis, 297–298
  hearing loss, 298
  incidence, 297
  neurologic sequelae, 298
  presentation in neonates, 297
  transmission by transfusion, 231, 298

Dandy-Walker malformation, 332
D antigen, 238
DBA. See Diamond-Blackfan anemia
Deafness. See Hearing loss
Deep hypothermic circulatory arrest
  advantages in cardiac surgery, 53
  neurologic sequelae, 53
Deformation
  definition, 214
  sequences, 215
Delivery, 7–17
  injured systems after traumatic delivery, 360
Dermatology, 77–84
Developmental delay, versus mental retardation, 25
Developmental dysplasia of the hips
  nomenclature, 343

Developmental dysplasia of the hips (cont.)
  risk factors, 343–344
  signs, 343
  treatment, 344
  x-ray, 343
Dexamethasone therapy, adrenal insufficiency, 105
Dextrose
  diarrhea induction with glucose/galactose
    malabsorption, 165–166
  neonatal administration, 118
Diamond-Blackfan anemia (DBA)
  definition, 242
  presentation, 242
  prognosis, 242
  transient erythroblastopenia of childhood
    comparison, 242
  treatment, 242
Diarrhea
  carbohydrate malabsorption, 165
  chloride diarrhea, 166
  dextrose induction in glucose/galactose
    malabsorption, 165–166
  osmotic versus secretory, 164
  short gut syndrome, 166
DIC. See Disseminated intravascular coagulation
Disruption
  definition, 214
  sequences, 215
Disseminated intravascular coagulation (DIC)
  factor VIII level, 255
  laboratory testing, 255, 256
  treatment, 255
Diuretics, 121–122, 393
Dobutamine, hypotension management, 41
Dopamine
  hypotension management, 41
  neonates
    dosing, 41
    effects, 40
Down syndrome
  amniocentesis, 210
  chromosomal translocations, 210–211
  congenital heart disease, 45
  duodenal atresia association, 171
  features, 209–210
  gastrointestinal anomalies, 171
  incidence trends, 211
  intelligence, 210
  leukemia, 258
  maternal age risks, 210
  newborn evaluation, 206
  nomenclature, 211
  paternal age risks, 211
  personality, 210
  prenatal testing, 209
  recurrence risks, 211
  simian crease, 210
Droplet precautions, 282
Drug safety in pregnancy, classification by drug
    type, 16–17
Ductal plate, remodeling, 144

Ductus arteriosus. *See also* Patent ductus arteriosus
  closure after birth, 46
  right-to-left shunt in fetus, 32, 45–46
Ductus of Botallo, 31
Dwarfism, types, 213
Dysconjugate gaze, 317
Dysmaturity, 3
Dysplasia, definition, 214

Ear pinna, flexibility and immaturity, 316
EB. *See* Epidermolysis bullosa
ECG. *See* Electrocardiography
Echocardiography
  contractility assessment, 33
  ejection fraction, 33
  patent ductus arteriosus, 46
  pressure differentials, 32
  pulmonary hypertension, fetal diagnosis, 32
  shortening fraction, 33
  ventricular septal defect, 32–33, 34
ECLS. *See* Extracorporeal life support
ECMO. *See* Extracorporeal membrane oxygenation
Edrophonium test, 337
EEG. *See* Electroencephalography
EGD. *See* Esophagogastroduodenoscopy
Electrocardiography (ECG)
  bradycardia differential diagnosis, 62–64
  cyanosis, 36–37
  delta wave in Wolff-Parkinson-White syndrome, 64
  endocardial cushion defect, 45
  hyperkalemia, 65
  hypocalcemia, 65
  hypokalemia, 65
  left axis deviation, 62
  normal neonatal features, 61–62
  QTc calculation, 65
  supraventricular tachycardia, 63
Electroencephalography (EEG), brain death, 22–23
Electrolytes, **115–140**
Electromyography (EMG), indications, 335
EMG. *See* Electromyography
Encephalopathy. *See also* Bilirubin encephalopathy;
    Hypoxic-ischemic encephalopathy
  magnetic resonance imaging, 338
Endemic infection, 282
Endocarditis
  fungal, 68–69
  pathogens in neonates, 68
  risk factors, 68
  signs, 68
Endocrinology, **87–112**
Endotracheal tube
  extubation, 380
  indications, 357
  insertion, 350
  intubation steps, 357
  radiography, 361
  sizes, 350
Energy balance, significance, 147
Epidermolysis bullosa (EB)
  management, 84

Epidermolysis bullosa (EB) *(cont.)*
  types, 84
Epidermolytic hyperkeratosis, 80
Epidural analgesia, infants, 346
Epinephrine, resuscitation administration, 358, 359,
    360
Epstein pearls, presentation, 77
Erb palsy, 341
Erythema infectiosum. *See* Parvovirus B19
Erythema toxicum
  microscopic examination of pustules, 78
  presentation, 78
  resolution, 77, 78
Erythroblastosis fetalis
  definition, 238
  historical perspective, 238
Erythropoietin
  fetal source, 235
  iron supplementation with therapy, 160–161
  laboratory tests of efficacy, 236
  neonatal administration, 235
  pharmacokinetics, 235
  preterm infant use, 236
Esophageal atresia
  causes of dying spells, 164
  incidence, 143
  prognostic factors, 164
  repair complications, 164
  ultrasound, 164
Esophagogastroduodenoscopy, gastroesophageal
    reflux evaluation, 163
Exchange transfusion, hyperbilirubinemia,
    194–195, 197–198
Extracorporeal life support (ECLS), definition, 383
Extracorporeal membrane oxygenation (ECMO)
  definition, 383
  duration, 386
  evidence for efficacy, 384
  inclusion and exclusion criteria, 384
  meconium aspiration syndrome, 368
  monitoring, 386
  oxygen index, 385
  sedation, 346
  vascular access
    venoarterial bypass, 385
    venovenous bypass, 385–386
  weaning, 386
Extremely low birth weight infant, definition, 145

Facial paralysis, peripheral versus central nervous
    system involvement, 319
Familial erythrophagocytic lymphohistiocytosis, 259
Fanconi anemia
  cancer association, 247
  classification, 245
  definition, 245
  diagnosis, 247
  hematologic characteristics, 246
  physical anomalies, 246–247
  prognosis, 247
  severity, 247

Fanconi anemia *(cont.)*
 treatment, 247
Fanconi syndrome, renal tubular acidosis, 127
Fat. *See* Lipid
Fat baby syndromes, 212
Fentanyl, neonatal precautions, 346
Fetal airway obstruction syndromes, 374
Fetal breathing, detection, 1
Fetal circulation
 ductus arteriosus right-to-left shunt, 32, 45–46
 foramen ovale right-to-left shunt, 32
 shunts, 31
 systemic venous return, 31
Fetal development and growth, **1–6**
Fetal distress, 353
Fetal heart rate
 deceleration significance, 13–14
 reactivity assessment, 1
Fetal movement, assessment, 1
Fetal scalp pH, values during labor, 15
Fetal sleep, 1
Fetal surgery
 assessment, 5
 indications, 6
 management considerations, 5–6
Fibronectin, testing, 10
FISH. *See* Fluorescence in situ hybridization
Fluids, **115–140**
 resuscitation of neonates, 359
Fluorescence in situ hybridization (FISH), 208
Fluoride, supplementation, 158
Fontanel, size, 217
Foot, calcaneovalgus deformity, 344
Footprinting, newborns, 22
Formula
 carbohydrate composition, 149
 protein composition, 150
 soy protein-based formula recommendations, 154
Fossa ovalis, closure after birth, 31
Fracture, neonatal management, 344
Fragile X syndrome
 genetic mutation, 221
 mental retardation, 221
Funisitis, 292
Furosemide
 hypercalciuria induction, 121
 nephrocalcinosis association, 132

Galactosemia, screening, 96–97
Galen malformation, 320
Gastroenterology, **143–201**
Gastroesophageal reflux
 evaluation, 162–163
 incidence, 161
 physiologic versus pathologic reflux, 162
 positioning of infants, 163
 referral to specialist, 162
 risk factors, 162
 treatment, 163
Gastrointestinal hemorrhage
 causes, 178

Gastrointestinal hemorrhage *(cont.)*
 management, 178
 swallowed maternal blood test, 178
Gastrointestinal tract
 development, 143
 nervous system development, 144
 villus development, 143
Gastroschisis
 associated syndromes, 172
 delivery, 172
 differential diagnosis, 172–173, 206
 incidence, 171
 management, 172
 prenatal diagnosis, 172
 prognosis, 173
GBS. *See* Group B streptococcus
G-CSF. *See* Granulocyte colony-stimulating factor
Gender reassignment surgery
 accidental penile amputation, 111, 112
 incidence, 112
 problems, 112
 technique, 112
Gene therapy, in utero, **205–224**
 definition, 221
 ethics, 223
 indications, 222–223, 224
 rationale, 222
 risks, 223
General neonatology, **19–29**
Genetics, **205–224**
Genitogram, congenital adrenal hyperplasia, 108
Gentamicin, 271–272, 273
GER. *See* Gastroesophageal reflux
Germ cell tumor, 258
Gestational age, examination, 315, 317
GFR. *See* Glomerular filtration rate
Glomerular filtration rate (GFR)
 neonatal values, 115
 prenatal changes, 115
Glucagon stimulation test, 91
Glucose-6-phosphate dehydrogenase deficiency,
  237, 244
Glucose/galactose malabsorption, 165–166
GM-CSF. *See* Granulocyte-macrophage colony-
  stimulating factor
Gowning, 283
Granulocyte colony-stimulating factor,
  immunotherapy, 280
Granulocyte-macrophage colony-stimulating factor,
  immunotherapy, 280
Graves' disease
 breast-feeding, 104
 maternal effects on fetus and neonate, 103
Group B streptococcus (GBS)
 adverse outcomes, 273
 course, 275
 culture, 273
 early versus late onset disease, 274
 intrapartum antibiotic prophylaxis, 274–275
 management, 10
 osteomyelitis, 275–276

Group B streptococcus (GBS) *(cont.)*
prevention, 274
radiographic features, 349, 362
serotypes, 273–274
sexual transmission, 273
Growth, energy costs, 148
Growth hormone
deficiency
magnetic resonance imaging findings, 107
symptoms in neonates, 107
fetal expression, 106

Handwashing
frequency, 283
infection reduction, 283
reasons for noncompliance, 282
recommendations for perinatal care, 283
skin emollient use, 283
soap and water, 283
Harlequin baby, 80
Harlequin color change, 78
HBV. *See* Hepatitis B virus
hCG. *See* Human chorionic gonadotropin
HCV. *See* Hepatitis C virus
Head, preterm infant growth rate, 3
Head turn, neonatal preference of direction, 317
Hearing loss, etiology, 317
Heart murmur
cyanosis evaluation, 37
innocent murmurs, 34–35
patent ductus arteriosus, 46
Hemangioma
complications, 82–83
incidence, 82
with Kasabach-Merritt phenomenon, 83
lumbosacral hemangioma, 83
multiple hemangiomas, 82
nomenclature, 82
risk factors, 82
treatment, 83
versus vascular malformation, 82
Hematocrit. *See also* Polycythemia
blood volume evaluation, 360
sampling site, 227
Hematology, **227–259**
Hematopoiesis
cell types, 232
fetus, 231
hemoglobin types in fetus, 232–233
Hematuria
causes and evaluation in neonates, 130
definition, 130
Hemoglobin
normal values in neonates, 227
oxygen saturation in fetus versus adult, 234–235
sampling site, 227
types in fetus, 232–233
Hemolytic disease of the newborn, 239–240
Hemophilia
circumcision, 253
factor VIII deficiency, 253

Hemophilia *(cont.)*
factor XIII deficiency, 255
female hemophilia, 254
hemarthrosis, 253
intracranial hemorrhage, 253
PUP trials, 254–255
screening, 254
severe hemophilia, 253
spontaneous cases, 253–254
transfusion, 253, 254
X-linkage, 253
Hemorrhage. *See also* Gastrointestinal hemorrhage;
Intracranial hemorrhage; Vaginal bleeding
extracranial hemorrhage following delivery,
319
Hepatitis B virus (HBV)
complications, 309
prevention of vertical transmission, 309
serologic assay, 308–309
transmission, 308
Hepatitis C virus (HCV)
presentation, 309
transmission, 309
Hereditary spherocytosis
classification, 236–237
differential diagnosis, 237
heredity, 236
incidence, 236
laboratory abnormalities, 237
Hermaphroditism, 109
Hernia uteri inguinalis, 111
Herpes simplex virus (HSV)
acyclovir therapy, 300
delivery, 301
diagnosis, 298–299
differential diagnosis, 299–300
follow-up of neonates, 300
pathogenesis, 300
screening in pregnancy, 299
susceptibility of neonates, 265
treatment, 300
types, 299
High-frequency ventilation
adverse events, 382
definition, 380
factors affecting ventilation, 382
hyaline membrane disease, 383
indications, 383
mean airway pressure, 382
mechanisms, 381
meconium aspiration syndrome, 382
minute ventilation estimation, 381
monitoring, 383
oxygenation variables, 382
respiratory distress syndrome, 365
tidal volume delivery, 381
types, 380, 381
Hip click, 343
Hirschsprung disease
associated disorders, 168
clinical presentation, 168

Hirschsprung disease (cont.)
  counseling of family, 168
  diagnosis, 167
  pathogenesis, 167
  postoperative complications, 168
  risk factors, 167
  screening, 168
  treatment, 167
HIV. See Human immunodeficiency virus
Holoprosencephaly, 331
HSV. See Herpes simplex virus
Human chorionic gonadotropin (hCG), screening,
    205, 206
Human immunodeficiency virus (HIV)
  complications in infancy, 297
  immune dysfunction monitoring, 297
  screening
    neonates, 297
    pregnancy, 296–297
  seroprevalence in pregnancy, 296
  syphilis coinfection, 295
  vertical transmission risks, 296
Hutchinson's triad, 295
Hydrocephalus
  communicating, 331
  etiology, 331
  ex vacuo, 331
  obstructive, 331
  with myelomeningocele, 330
Hydronephrosis, differential diagnosis, 128
17-Hydroxyprogesterone, assay, 109
Hyperbilirubinemia. See Jaundice; Unconjugated
    hyperbilirubinemia
Hypercalcemia
  blue diaper syndrome, 94
  calcium fractions in serum, 92
  differential diagnosis, 93
  etiology, 93
  laboratory tests, 94
  management, 93
  manifestations, 93
  normal calcium levels
    full-term infants, 93
    preterm infants, 93
  treatment, 94
Hypercalciuria, definition, 132
Hyperglycemia, total parenteral nutrition
    association in preterm infants, 152–153
Hyperinsulinism, 91, 92
Hyperkalemia
  definition, 125
  electrocardiography, 65
  preterm infants
    consequences, 126
    incidence, 125
    nonoliguric hyperkalemia, 125–126
    treatment, 126
Hypermagnesemia
  causes, 95
  signs, 95
  treatment, 95–96

Hyperoxia test
  cyanosis differential diagnosis, 36
  indications, 49
  interpretation, 50
  technique, 49–50
Hypertelorism, 217
Hypertension
  blood pressure recording, 133
  causes, 133
  coarctation of the aorta, 134
  definition in neonates, 133
  hormonal effects, 134
  umbilical artery catheter management, 133–134
Hypocalcemia
  calcitropic hormones of mother and fetus, 87
  electrocardiography, 65
  placental transport of calcium, 87
  premature infants
    breast milk rickets, 89
    calcium requirements and feeding, 88–89
    diagnosis, 87
    treatment, 87–88
  risk factors, 87
  seizure differential diagnosis, 89
Hypoglycemia
  adaptation to fasting, 90
  blood sampling, 91
  definition, 90
  diagnostic work-up, 91
  etiology in neonates, 90–91
  fatty acid oxidation disorders, 92
  glucagon stimulation test, 91
  hyperinsulinism, 91, 92
  physical findings, 91–92
  polycythemia association, 252
  resuscitation of neonates, 359
  treatment, 92
Hypogonadotropic hypogonadism, 107
Hypokalemia
  electrocardiography, 65
  treatment, 65
Hypomagnesemia
  calcium homeostasis effects, 95
  etiology, 95
  levels in neonates, 95
  presentation, 95
  treatment, 95
Hypoplastic left heart syndrome, 61
  genetic disorders with, 213
  surgery, 73
Hypospadia
  chromosomal evaluation, 139
  development, 139
  incidence, 140
  surgical correction, 139
Hypotension, neonates
  adrenoreceptors
    cardiac, 39
    renal, 39
    vasopressor actions, 40
  cause in preterm infants, 38–39

Hypotension, neonates *(cont.)*
  corticosteroid management, 42
  dobutamine management, 41
  dopamine management, 40, 41
  fluid resuscitation, 39
  hypovolemia, 39
  pressors versus inotropes, 41–42
Hypothalamic-pituitary-gonadal axis
  fetal development, 106
  malformations with disorders, 107
  tumors with disorders, 107
Hypothalamic-pituitary-thyroid axis, fetal
    development, 99
Hypothyroidism, congenital
  causes, 103
  incidence, 97, 103
  screening, 102
Hypothyroxinemia of prematurity, 101, 102
Hypotonia, differential diagnosis, 335
Hypoxemia, chronic intrauterine, 1
Hypoxic-ischemic encephalopathy
  acute neurologic components, 360
  criteria, 352
  oliguria, 356
  preterm versus full-term infants, 355
  Sarnat classification, 355
  susceptibility sites, 322, 355
  types, 322–323

IgA. *See* Immunoglobulin A
IgG. *See* Immunoglobulin G
Immunity, **261–310**
Immunization, preterm infants, 24
Immunoglobulin A (IgA), types in neonates, 261–262
Immunoglobulin G (IgG), maternal source and
    disappearance following birth, 261
Imperforate anus
  associated anomalies, 176
  classification, 176
  colostomy, 177
  continence outcomes, 177
  diagnosis, 176
  initial management, 177
Impetigo
  bullous, 290–291
  complications, 291
  differential diagnosis, 291
  nonbullous, 290
  organisms, 291
  treatment, 291
Imprinting, 219
Inborn errors of metabolism
  acidosis-associated diseases, 97
  classes and diagnosis, 98
  congenital abnormalities with PKU, 98
  Fanconi syndrome, 98
  initial assessment, 98
  large ketonuria, 97
  neonatal transport, 97
  odors, 97
  seizure-associated diseases, 98

Inborn errors of metabolism *(cont.)*
  signs, 97
Incidence, definition, 281
Incontinentia pigmenti, stages, 334
Indomethacin, patent ductus arteriosus treatment, 47
Infantile acne, 77
Infection, **261–310**
Inferior vena cava, interruption, 58
Insensible water loss (ISL), determinants, 117
Intersex disorders, 107–112
Intestinal atresia
  Down syndrome association, 171
  duodenal atresia, 171
  etiology, 170
  fetal intervention, 170
  ileal atresia, 171
  jejunal atresia, 171
  management, 171
  prenatal diagnosis, 170
  presentation, 170
  prognosis, 171
Intracranial hemorrhage
  aneurysm versus arteriovenous malformation, 320
  intraventricular hemorrhage, 320, 321–322
  posthemorrhagic ventricular dilatation, 321, 322
  subarachnoid hemorrhage, 320–321
  types and pathogenesis, 320
Intrauterine growth restriction
  causes, 145
  complications, 145–146
  delivery considerations, 4
  Doppler flow velocity assessment, 146
  long-term consequences, 146–147
  monitoring, 4
  morbidity, 4
  neonatal evaluation, 207
  versus retardation, 3
  risk factors, 4
  versus small-for-gestational age, 145
  symmetric versus asymmetric infants, 146
  ultrasound, 3
Intravenous immunoglobulin (IVIG),
    immunotherapy, 280
Intraventricular hemorrhage, 320, 321–322
Intubation
  endotracheal tube suctioning, 28–29
  nasotracheal in neonates, 27–28
Intubation. *See* Resuscitation, neonates
Iris coloboma, 217
Iron
  absorption, 160
  anemia with deficiency, 248
  daily requirements, 159
  erythropoietin therapy considerations, 160–161
  hemoglobin content, 160
  placental transport, 161
  preterm infants versus full-term infants, 160, 161
  storage
    infants, 159
    risk factors for low iron stores at birth, 160
  supplementation, 159

Isolette, noise concerns, 21
IVIG. *See* Intravenous immunoglobulin

Jaundice. *See also* Cholestatic jaundice;
    Unconjugated hyperbilirubinemia
  bilirubin measurement, 186
  breast-feeding, 198–199
  causes, 186
  evaluation, 186, 187
  excessive jaundice, 191
  glucose-6-phosphate dehydrogenase deficiency,
      237
  obstructive jaundice causes, 190

Kasabach-Merritt phenomenon, hemangiomas, 83
Kernicterus
  exchange transfusion in prevention, 194–195
  low-bilirubin kernicterus, 192
  preterm infants, 193
KID syndrome, 80
Kidney
  acidification in newborns, 116
  blood supply, 115
  fetal versus neonatal function, 115
  nephrogenesis, 115
  postnatal renal vascular resistance decline, 115
  small kidney causes and diagnosis, 125
  water conservation and excretion in newborns,
      116
Klinefelter syndrome, features, 219–220
Klumke palsy, 341

Labor, **7–17**
  length by sex of baby, 15
Lactase deficiency, 165
Lactation. *See* Breast-feeding
Lactobezoar, 150
Lactose, malabsorption, 149, 164–165
LAD. *See* Leukocyte adhesion deficiency
Ladd's bands, 143
Langerhans histiocytosis, 259
Late metabolic acidosis, 127
Leukemia
  diagnosis, 257
  Down syndrome, 258
Leukocyte adhesion deficiency (LAD)
  omphalitis association, 292
  type I, 265
Limb hemihypertrophy, 213
Linkage map, 218
Lipid
  absorption of fatty acids, 151, 154, 165
  emulsions for premature infants, 151, 152
  energy content, 151
  energy costs of synthesis, 151
  essential fatty acids, 151–152
  long-chain polyunsaturated acids
    depletion effects, 152
    supplementation, 152
  lung disease supplementation, 152
  malabsorption evaluation, 165

Lipid *(cont.)*
  milk composition and sources, 151
  milk content variation, 157
  neonatal ascites nutrition, 185
  triglyceride levels in infants, 152
Liquid ventilation
  clinical trials, 387
  definition, 386
  indications, 387
  lung compliance effects, 387
Listeriosis
  diagnosis, 294
  incidence, 292
  maternal infection
    acquisition, 292
    presentation, 293
  neonatal presentation
    early-onset, 293
    late-onset, 294
  pathogenesis, 294
  treatment, 294
Little, William John, 353
Liver, development, 144
Local anesthesia, caution in infants, 347
Low-birth-weight infant
  caloric requirements, 147
  definition, 145
Low-set ears, 216
Lumbar puncture
  meningitis, 280
  sepsis, 269
Lumbosacral agenesis
  lesion types, 342–343
  maternal diabetes association, 342
Lung, abnormalities, 396–398
Lymph node, palpation in newborns, 21
Lymphangioma, 83

Macrosomia, causes, 146
Magnesium metabolism. *See also*
    Hypermagnesemia; Hypomagnesemia
  absorption and storage, 94
  extracellular reactions, 94
  intracellular reactions, 94
  quantity conversions, 94
Magnesium sulfate, tocolysis, 11
Malformation
  central nervous system, 329–332
  definition, 214
  major versus minor, 214
  oligohydramnios association, 215
  sequences, 215
Malrotation
  bilious vomiting, 170
  definition, 168
  diagnosis, 170
  differential diagnosis, 170
  onset of symptoms, 168
  presentation, 169
MAS. *See* Meconium aspiration syndrome
Masculinization, female fetus, 105

Mean cell volume
    changes in development, 233
    normal values in neonates, 227
Meckel's diverticulum, 143
Meconium
    composition, 144
    passage
        preterm infants, 144–145
        stimuli, 144
        timing, 144
    substance abuse testing, 333
Meconium aspiration syndrome (MAS), 362
    extracorporeal membrane oxygenation, 368
    FDA approval of treatments, 368
    fluid thickness effects, 368
    high-frequency ventilation, 382
    oropharyngeal suctioning, 368
    pathophysiology, 367–368
    persistent pulmonary hypertension of the
        newborn association, 367
    surfactant therapy, 368–369
    veterinary management, 368
Meconium ileus
    complicated condition, 174
    cystic fibrosis association, 171, 173, 175
    features, 173
    plug versus ileus, 173
    surgical management, 174–175
    treatment, 174
Meconium plug
    features, 173
    ileus versus plug, 173
    treatment, 174
Meconium-stained amniotic fluid
    asphyxia association, 367
    duration of exposure, 366–367
    initial postpartum management, 366, 367
Melanocytic nevus, congenital, 84
Meningitis
    antibiotic concentrations in cerebrospinal fluid, 281
    brain injury mechanisms, 281
    cytokine markers, 281
    lumbar puncture, 280
    treatment, 281
Meningocele, 329
Mental retardation, versus developmental delay, 25
Metabolism, 87–112
Methemoglobinemia
    glucose-6-phosphate dehydrogenase deficiency
        association, 244
    oxidants in production, 244
    presentation, 243, 244
    pulse oximetry, 243
    reduction of methemoglobin, 244
    treatment, 245
Microvillus inclusion disease, 165
Midgut volvulus
    bowel necrosis, 170
    diagnosis, 170
    necrotizing enterocolitis differentiation, 184
    symptoms, 169

Milia. See also Prickly heat
    forms, 78
    presentation, 77
    resolution, 77
Milk, breast. See Breast-feeding
Mitochondrial disease, maternal transmission, 212
Mixed gonadal genesis, 111
Moro reflex, 317–318
Mosaicism, 218
Müllerian inhibitory substance (MIS)
    deficiency, 111
    male differentiation, 107
Multiple gestation
    complications, 12
    conjoined twin
        treatment, 13
        types, 13
    delivery order and risks, 13
    identical twins of different sexes, 220
    monozygotic versus dizygotic twin risks, 12–13
Myasthenia gravis
    differential diagnosis, 336
    edrophonium test, 337
    maternal, 336
    permanent versus transient, 336–337
Myelomeningocele
    cerebral disorder association, 330
    delivery, 330
    folic acid deficiency, 329
    mental retardation association, 330
    presentation, 329–330
    prognosis, 331
    stridor etiology, 330
Myoclonic seizure, 328
Myotonic dystrophy
    anticipation, 335
    diagnosis, 335

Naloxone, 358, 359
Natural killer cell, neonatal function, 265
NEC. See Necrotizing enterocolitis
Necrotizing enterocolitis (NEC)
    breast-feeding protection, 179
    definition, 178–179
    differential diagnosis, 178
    infective agents, 179–180
    management case studies, 180–182, 183
    outcomes in preterm versus full-term infants,
        143–144
    risk factors, 179
    staging, 180
    surgical management, 182
    volvulus differentiation, 184
    zinc deficiency, 158
Negative-pressure room, indications for use, 282
Neonatal acne, 77
Nephrocalcinosis
    diagnosis, 132
    furosemide association, 132
    prognosis, 133
    treatment, 132

Neuroblastoma
    diagnosis, 257
    prognostic factors, 258
Neurocutaneous syndromes, 333–334
Neurofibromatosis
    gene mutation rate, 211
    heredity, 78, 333
    NF1 diagnosis, 78–79
    presentation, 334
    types and incidence, 78
Neurology, **315–338**
    neonatal examination, 315–319
Neutropenia
    depletion neutropenia, 262–263
    endotoxemia induction, 249
    kinetic mechanisms, 248–249
    neonatal alloimmune neutropenia, 249
    pregnancy-induced hypertension association, 249
    severe neutropenias, 249
Neutrophil
    defects, 278–279
    factors affecting counts, 270
    neonatal function, 264
    preterm infant function, 278
Nitric oxide (NO)
    congenital diaphragmatic hernia treatment, 373
    hemoglobin binding, 373
    indications for therapy, 373, 374
    persistent pulmonary hypertension of the
        newborn management, 372, 373
    preterm infant use, 374
Nonstress test, principles, 14
Noonan syndrome
    cardiomyopathy, 69
    diagnosis, 207
    Turner syndrome comparison, 221
Nosocomial infection, 282
Nutrition, **143–201**. *See also specific nutrients*
    preterm infants, 24, 154
    total parenteral nutrition. *See* Total parenteral
        nutrition

Obstructive uropathy, 128–129
Olfaction, development, 3, 317
Oligohydramnios sequence. *See* Potter syndrome
Oliguria
    creatinine levels, 123
    definition, 122
    etiology, 122–123
    hypoxic-ischemic encephalopathy, 356
    maternal oligohydramnios association, 123
Omphalitis
    complications, 292
    incidence, 291
    leukocyte adhesion deficiency association, 292
    organisms, 291
    presentation, 291
    risk factors, 291
    treatment, 292
Omphalocele
    associated syndromes, 171–172

Omphalocele *(cont.)*
    delivery, 172
    differential diagnosis, 172–173, 206
    incidence, 171
    management, 172
    prenatal diagnosis, 172
    prognosis, 173
Orthopaedics, **341–347**
Osteogenesis imperfecta, blue sclerae, 216–217
Osteomyelitis
    antibiotic therapy, 289
    blood culture, 288
    candidiasis, 288
    group B streptococcus, 275–276
    incidence in neonates, 287
    laboratory markers in management, 288
    manifestations, 287
    maxillary osteomyelitis, 289
    neonatal susceptibility, 287
    pathogenesis in neonates, 287
    pathogens, 286–287, 344
    radiologic evaluation, 288
Osteopenia of prematurity
    total parenteral nutrition association, 153
    vitamin D supplementation, 158
Ovarian cyst, neonatal management, 200
Oxygen index (OI), 366, 385

PACs. *See* Premature atrial contractions
Pain
    fetal perception, 345
    infant memory, 347
    management in neonates, **341–347**
    neonatal perception, 345
Pancreas divisum, 144
PAPP. *See* Pregnancy-associated plasma protein
Parvovirus B19
    anemia effects, 310
    erythema infectiosum, 310
    fetal risks, 309–310
    immunity, 309
Patent ductus arteriosus (PDA)
    chest film, 47
    clinical manifestations, 46, 47
    echocardiography, 46
    indomethacin treatment, 47
    ligation, 45, 47, 59
    murmurs, 46
        complications, 46
        treatment, 47, 59
    risk factors, 46
PCP. *See Pneumocystis carinii* pneumonia
PCR. *See* Polymerase chain reaction
PDA. *See* Patent ductus arteriosus
Pena-Shokeir phenotype, pulmonary anomalies, 374
Pentoxifylline, sepsis management, 279
Perinatal asphyxia, criteria, 15
Peripheral pulmonary stenosis, cause and findings,
    34
Periventricular leukomalacia (PVL)
    definition, 323

Periventricular leukomalacia (PVL) *(cont.)*
  etiology, 323
  hemorrhage association, 323
  preterm infants, 355
  sequelae, 323
  ultrasound findings, 323
  visual deficits, 324
Persistent pulmonary hypertension of the newborn
  (PPHN)
  causes, 370
  clinical features, 369
  definition, 369
  differential diagnosis, 371–372
  long-term outcome, 372
  management, 372
  meconium aspiration syndrome association,
    367
  nitric oxide treatment, 372, 373
  pathophysiology, 370–371
  prospects for treatment, 372
  vascular remodeling, 371
Phakomatosis, 334
Phlebotomy, blood loss in infants, 228, 231
Phototherapy
  discontinuance, 196
  efficacy variables, 195
  home administration, 197
  irradiance, 197
  mechanisms, 195
  side effects, 195–196
  sunlight, 197
Phrenic nerve injury, causes after cardiothoracic
  surgery, 53–54
Pink tet, 45
Pituitary transcription factors, deficiencies and
  disorders, 107
Placental abruption
  complications, 9
  incidence, 9
  risk factors, 9
Placenta previa
  classification, 8
  complications, 9
  diagnosis, 8
  etiology, 8
  incidence, 8
  risk factors, 8–9
Plantar reflex, competing reflexes, 315
Platelet
  function in neonates, 251
  neonatal counts, 251
  thrombocytopenia management, 251
Pneumatosis intestinalis
  associated conditions, 184
  gas production, 179
Pneumocystis carinii pneumonia (PCP), 297
Pneumonia alba, 295
Pneumothorax
  diagnosis, 362, 388
  renal malformation association, 390
  tension pneumothorax, 38

Pneumothorax *(cont.)*
  ventilation risks, 377, 388–389
Polycythemia
  genitourinary system evaluation, 251–252
  hematocrit evaluation, 252
  hypoglycemia association, 252
  partial exchange transfusion, 253
  risk factors, 252
  screening, 252
  twins, occurrence in, 251
Polyhydramnios
  anencephaly association, 329
  malformations with, 215
Polymerase chain reaction (PCR), 218
Polyuria
  Bartter syndrome, 124
  definition, 124
  management, 124
  renal dysplasia, 123–124
Pompe disease, cardiomyopathy, 69
Port-wine stain
  laser therapy, 83
  location and potential complications, 334
  with Sturge-Weber syndrome, 83
Posterior urethral valve
  consequences, 129
  intervention, 129
  presentation, 129
  prognostic factors, 129–130
  types, 129
Postmature pregnancy, 3
Potassium, neonatal administration, 118
Potter syndrome
  causes, 124, 216
  features, 124
  inheritance patterns, 125
  renal ultrasound of parents, 216
PPHN. *See* Persistent pulmonary hypertension of
  the newborn
PPROM. *See* Preterm premature rupture of
  membranes
Prader-Willi syndrome, 212–213
Preauricular skin tags, 81, 216
Pregnancy-associated plasma protein (PAPP),
  screening, 206
Premature atrial contractions (PACs), 66
Preterm infant
  acid excretion rates, 126–127
  adjusted age, 23
  anetoderma of prematurity, 84
  apnea, 349
  cerebral palsy, 24–25
  clinical manifestations, 46, 47
  counseling of parents, 25
  developmental delay, 25
  fluid and electrolyte requirements, 118
  hyperkalemia
    consequences, 126
    incidence, 125
    nonoliguric hyperkalemia, 125–126
    treatment, 126

Preterm infant *(cont.)*
  hypocalcemia
    breast milk rickets, 89
    calcium requirements and feeding, 88–89
    diagnosis, 87
    treatment, 87–88
  immunization, 24
  intervention services, 25
  nutrition, 24
  patent ductus arteriosus
    complications, 46
    treatment, 47, 59
  potassium excretion, 116
  protein loss, 151
  school-age sequelae, 25
  skin barrier function, 84
  stress in family, 25–26
  weight loss after birth, 116–117
Preterm labor
  inhibitors, 11
  markers, 12
  risk factors, 10, 12
Preterm premature rupture of membranes,
    corticosteroid therapy, 11–12
Prevalence, definition, 281
Prickly heat, treatment, 78
Prolactin, fetal expression, 106
Prostaglandin E$_1$
  hypoplastic left heart syndrome, 61
  indications for neonatal use, 50
  side effects, 50–51
Prostaglandin synthase inhibitors, tocolysis, 11
Protein
  administration routes and requirements, 151
  calorie-to-protein ratio, 151
  conditionally essential amino acids, 150
  essential amino acids, 149–150
  formula composition, 150
  loss in preterm infants, 151
  malabsorption evaluation, 165
  non-nutritive role in human milk, 150
  preterm versus full-term infant requirements, 150
  requirement determination, 150
  utilization factors in neonate, 150
  whey-to-casein ratio of milk, 150
Protein C
  homozygous disease, 257
  plasma levels, 256
Protein S
  homozygous disease, 257
  plasma levels, 256
Proteinuria
  causes, 131
  definition, 131
Prune belly syndrome (PBS)
  definition, 136
  evaluation, 136–137
  extra-genitourinary system anomalies, 136, 137
  nomenclature, 137
  surgical intervention, 137
  urinary tract anomalies, 136

Pseudohypoaldosteronism, 106
  renal tubular acidosis, 127–128
Pulmonary blood flow (PBF), determination, 34
Pulmonary hypertension, fetal diagnosis, 32. *See
    also* Persistent pulmonary hypertension of the
    newborn
Pulmonary interstitial emphysema, treatment, 389
Pulmonary sequestration, 397
Pulmonary stenosis, critical, 61
Pulmonary vascular resistance (PVR)
  changes on birth, 33
  cor pulmonale, 67, 68
  determinants, 31
Pulmonary vasodilatation, postpartum, 363
Pulmonology, **349–398**
Pulse oximetry, site selection, 370
Pupillary reaction, fetal development, 3
Pyelonephritis
  diagnosis, 289
  treatment, 290
Pyloric stenosis, radiographic findings, 166–167

Radius, TAR syndrome, 345
RDS. *See* Respiratory distress syndrome
Red blood cell. *See also* Anemia; Mean cell
    volume; Transfusion
  fetal characteristics, 233
  glucose-6-phosphate dehydrogenase role, 237
  half-life in infants, 227
  indices changes in first months, 233–234
  membrane characteristics in fetus versus adult, 236
  production following birth, 234
Renal cystic dysplasia, 137
Renal disorders, **115–140**
Renal tubular acidosis (RTA)
  associated conditions
    congenital adrenal hyperplasia, 127
    Fanconi syndrome, 127
    pseudohypoaldosteronism, 127–128
  bicarbonate metabolism, 126
  causes, 128
  diagnosis, 127
  presentation, 127
  types, 127
Renal vein thrombosis
  anticoagulant therapy, 136
  fluid and electrolyte abnormalities with, 135
  imaging, 135
  presentation, 134–135
  risk factors, 134
  surgical management, 135
  thrombolytic therapy, 135
Respiratory compromise, causes after
    cardiothoracic surgery, 52–53
Respiratory distress syndrome (RDS)
  bubble collapsing pressure, 362–363
  continuous positive airway pressure, 365
  radiography, 361
  surfactant replacement therapy, 364, 365
Respiratory quotient (RQ)
  definition, 147–148

Respiratory quotient (RQ) *(cont.)*
    values for nutrient classes, 148
Respiratory syncytial virus (RSV), immunization in
        preterm infants, 24
Resting energy expenditure, factors affecting, 148
Resuscitation, neonates
    bicarbonate administration, 358, 359, 360
    cessation, 360
    chest compressions, 359
    endotracheal tube
        indications, 357
        insertion, 350
        intubation steps, 357
        radiography, 361
        sizes, 350
    epinephrine administration, 358, 359
    fluid therapy, 359
    historical perspective, 351
    hypoglycemia, 359
    hypothermia effects, 356
    initial steps, 351
    intubation routes, 352
    lung inflation pressure, 351–352
    naloxone administration, 358, 359
    Neonatal Resuscitation Program, 351
    outcomes, 356
    positive pressure ventilation, indications and
        contraindications, 356
    self-inflating bag oxygen delivery, 350
Reticulocyte count, normal values in neonates,
    227
Retinoblastoma, 258
Retinopathy of prematurity (ROP), 24
    candidiasis association, 278
    cryotherapy, 337
    laser therapy, 337
    oxygen therapy recommendations, 338
    screening indications, 337
    stages, 337
    vitamin E in prevention, 338
Rh blood group
    clinical and laboratory features of
        incompatibility, 240
    follow-up care for incompatibility, 240
    overview, 238
    sensitized fetus, 239
RhoGAM, Rh disease prevention, 238
Riboflavin, supplementation in phototherapy,
    158
Right aortic arch, cardiac lesions, 43
ROP. *See* Retinopathy of prematurity
RTA. *See* Renal tubular acidosis

Sacrococcygeal tumor, 258
Scimitar syndrome, 61
Sclerema neonatorum
    cause, 81
    presentation, 80–81
Scrotum, rugae, 316
Sebaceous gland hyperplasia, resolution, 77
Seborrheic dermatitis, 81

Seizure, neonatal
    causes, 327, 353
    classification, 327–328
    diagnosis, 328
    feeding delay after asphyxia, 328
    significance, 327
    treatment, 238
Sepsis. *See also specific infectious organisms*
    antibiotic therapy, 271–272
    attack rates, 268
    blood culture, 269
    characteristics by age at onset, 267
    C-reactive protein levels, 269–270
    cytokine markers, 271
    epidemiology in preterm infants, 266
    granulocyte transfusion, 279
    intrapartum antibiotic effects, 265
    laboratory tests, 269–270
    lumbar puncture, 269
    maternal fever significance, 268
    nosocomial sepsis
        definition, 267
        glutamine supplementation effects, 279
        incidence, 267
        pathogens, 267
        risk factors, 268
    pentoxifylline therapy, 279
    presentation, 269
    risk factors, 266, 268
    screening, 271
    very-early-onset neonatal sepsis, 267
    white blood cell count, 270
Septic arthritis
    management, 288
    neonatal susceptibility, 287
Sex chromosome disorders, 219–220
Short gut syndrome, diarrhea in, 166
Sickle cell disease
    diagnosis, 228–229
    historical perspective, 241
    infant mortality, 241
    polymerization of sickle hemoglobin, 241
    pregnancy complications, 241
    presentation, 240, 241
    screening, 96, 211, 241
SIDS. *See* Sudden infant death syndrome
Sinus bradycardia, newborns, 66
Sister Ward, 197
Skew gaze, 317
Small left colon syndrome, 174
Sodium
    balance in term versus preterm infants, 115
    neonatal administration, 118, 119
    oliguria, urine concentration, 123
Spina bifida
    occulta, 329
    prevalence, 205
Spinal cord injury, 319
Spinal dysraphism, 319
Spironolactone, 121, 393
Spitzer's laws of neonatology, 19

SSSS. *See* Staphylococcal scalded skin syndrome
Staphylococcal scalded skin syndrome (SSSS), 81, 291
Staphylococcus epidermidis
  prophylaxis, 276
  risk factors for bloodstream infections, 276
  sepsis diagnosis and treatment, 276
Stem cell transplantation, in utero
  barriers to engraftment, 224
  definition, 221
  ethics, 223
  hematopoietic stem cell engraftment, 223–224
  indications, 222, 224
  rationale, 222
  risks, 223
Steroidogenic acute regulatory protein, 105
Stillborn
  autopsy indications, 214
  physical examination, 214
  recurrent pregnancy loss evaluation, 214
Stridor, with myelomeningocele, 330
Sturge-Weber syndrome
  findings, 83
  heredity, 333
Subarachnoid hemorrhage, 320–321
Subcutaneous fat necrosis, 80
Substance abuse. *See* Addiction, neonates
Subtle seizure, 328
Sucking blister, resolution, 77
Sudden infant death syndrome (SIDS)
  child abuse association, 396
  definition, 395
  incidence, 396
  premature infants, 349–350
  risk factors, 396
  trends, 396
Supraventricular tachycardia (SVT)
  electrocardiography, 63
  treatment, 66
Surfactant
  composition, 363
  replacement therapy
    meconium aspiration syndrome, 368–369
    respiratory distress syndrome, 364, 365
  synthesis, 364
Syndactyly, 216
Syphilis
  antibody tests, 296
  human immunodeficiency virus coinfection, 295
  Hutchinson's triad, 295
  incidence trends, 295
  neonatal evaluation, 295, 296
  pneumonia alba, 295
  screening in pregnancy, 295
  substance abuse association, 295
  treatment, 296

Tandrieres, 157–158
TAR syndrome, 345
Tay-Sachs disease, screening, 211

T cell
  antigen response in immunization, 264–265
  cell-mediated immunity maturation, 264
  thymocyte development, 263–264
TEC. *See* Transient erythroblastopenia of childhood
Testes, descent, 316
Testes-determining factor (TDF), gonadal differentiation role, 107
Testosterone
  male differentiation, 107
  sources, 107–108
Tethered cord, 331
Tetralogy of Fallot
  findings, 43, 44
  genetic defects, 43
  tet spell features and management, 52
Thalassemias
  Bart's hemoglobin with α-thalassemia, 241
  Constant Spring hemoglobin, 241
  diagnosis, 228–229, 241
  screening, 211
  types, 228, 241
Thanatophoric dwarfism, 213
Thrombocytopenia. *See also* Alloimmune thrombocytopenia
  diagnosis, 249
  duration, 251
  etiology, 249
  gestational thrombocytopenia, 250
  incidence, 249
  physical findings, 251
  platelet therapy, 250, 251
Thrombolytic therapy
  indications, 256
  stroke, 328
Thymocyte, development, 263–264
Thyroid hormone
  drug effects on fetal function, 103–104
  hypothyroxinemia of prematurity, 101, 102
  maternal effects on fetus, 99
  premature versus full-term infants, 100–101
  sick euthyroid syndrome in preterm infants, 102
  T3, parturition levels in fetus, 100
  T4
    fetal secretion, 99
    gestation role, 100
    triiodothyronine conversion, 99
Thyroid-stimulating hormone (TSH)
  fetal secretion, 99
  neonatal surge, 100, 107
Thyrotoxicosis, neonatal
  management, 103
  signs, 103
Tibia, posteromedial bowing, 344–345
TNPN. *See* Transient neonatal pustular melanosis
Tocolysis
  adverse effects of agents, 11
  contraindications, 10
  efficacy, 11
Tonic seizure, 328

Total parenteral nutrition (TPN)
  complications
    infection, 153
    skin necrosis, 153
  hyperglycemia in preterm infants, 152–153
  intravenous fat emulsion clearance, 153
  neonatal regimens, 152
  osteopenia in preterm infants, 153
  trace element toxicity, 153
Toxoplasmosis, congenital
  evaluation, 302–303
  maternal acquisition, 304
  presentation, 304
  prognosis, 304
  treatment, 304–305
TPN. *See* Total parenteral nutrition
Tracheoesophageal fistula
  causes of "dying" spells, 164
  incidence, 143
Transfusion
  cytomegalovirus transmission, 231
  fresh frozen plasma, 230
  graft-versus-host disease, 230
  hemophilia, 253, 254
  indications, 230
  informed consent, 231
  irradiation of blood, 231
  polycythemia, 253
  random versus single donor platelets, 231
  red blood cell storage, 229–230
  typing and crossmatching, 229
  white blood cell adverse reactions, 230
Transient erythroblastopenia of childhood (TEC)
  definition, 247
  diagnosis, 247–248
  Diamond-Blackfan anemia comparison, 242
  differential diagnosis, 248
  etiology, 247
  treatment, 248
Transient neonatal pustular melanosis, resolution, 77
Transient tachypnea of the newborn, 362
Transposition of the great vessels
  age at diagnosis, 43
  balloon atrial septostomy, 59
  hypoxemia management from D-transposition,
    51
  preoperative management, 59
  prostaglandins, 58
  switch operation, 72
Transpyloric feeding, 154
Tricuspid regurgitation, 352
Triple screen
  conditions detected, 205
  markers, 205
Trisomy 13, features, 209–210
Trisomy 18, features, 209–210
Trisomy 21. *See* Down syndrome
Truncus arteriosus
  findings, 44
  hemodynamics with congestive heart failure, 60
TSH. *See* Thyroid-stimulating hormone

Tuberculosis
  bacterial yield from specimen sampling sites, 307
  diagnosis, 306, 307
  exposure, 307
  infection routes, 306
  infection versus disease, 307
  presentation in neonates, 307
  treatment
    neonates, 307, 308
    pregnancy, 308
Tuberous sclerosis
  cardiac tumors, 71
  complexes and genetics, 79
  cutaneous findings, 79
  diagnosis, 334
  heredity, 333
Turner syndrome
  diagnosis, 207
  features, 219–220
  identical twins of different sexes, 220
  neck webbing, 220
  Noonan syndrome comparison, 221
Twin. *See* Multiple gestation

Ultrasound
  abdominal masses, 200
  cerebral palsy, 325
  cerebrum, 338
  fetal breathing, 1
  growth assessment, 3, 4
  intrauterine growth retardation, 3
  kidney, 128, 135
  periventricular leukomalacia, 323
  prune belly syndrome, 137
Umbilical artery
  catheter
    hypertension management, 133–134
    hypothermia avoidance, 359–360
    positioning, 358
    radiography, 360–361
  single artery screening, 205
Umbilical cord
  catheterization. *See also* Umbilical artery;
    Umbilical vein catheterization
    insertion distance, 20–21
    risks, 21
  handling at birth, 19
  postnatal care, 19
  sloughing and delay, 20
  twisting, 19, 20
Umbilical vein catheterization
  placement, 359
  radiography, 361
Unconjugated hyperbilirubinemia
  albumin administration, 197
  causes, 190–191
  drug displacement of bilirubin from albumin
    binding sites, 194
  encephalopathy
    brain deposition, 191, 192
    kernicterus, 192

Unconjugated hyperbilirubinemia *(cont.)*
  encephalopathy *(cont.)*
    neurotoxicity mechanisms, 191
    presentation of acute disease, 192
    preterm toxicity, 193
    risks, 192
  exchange transfusion, 194–195, 197–198
  fluid therapy, 198
  incidence, 190
  kernicterus
    exchange transfusion in prevention, 194–195
    low-bilirubin kernicterus, 192
    preterm infants, 193
  near-term newborns, 194
  neurotoxic levels
    albumin, 193, 194
    bilirubin, 193
  phototherapy
    discontinuance, 196
    efficacy variables, 195
    home administration, 197
    irradiance, 197
    mechanisms, 195
    side effects, 195–196
    sunlight, 197
  readmission indications, 198
  sepsis evaluation, 198
  severity, 19
  toxicity with asphyxia, 193
Uniparental disomy (UPD)
  associated conditions, 208, 219
  definition, 208, 219
Ureaplasma urealyticum
  diagnosis, 306
  maternal carriage rate, 305
  presentation, 305–306
  treatment, 306
  vertical transmission incidence, 305
Ureterocele, 128–129
Ureteropelvic junction obstruction, 128, 199,
    200
Urinary tract infection
  diagnosis, 289
  imaging studies, 290
  organisms, 289–290
  pathogenesis, 289
  presentation, 289
Urination
  concentrating ability of infants, 122
  fetus, 122
  output determinants, 122
  time of first void, 116
UTI. *See* Urinary tract infection

VACTERL association, 164, 176
Vaginal bleeding
  evaluation, 8
  third trimester causes, 8–10
Vancomycin, 273
Varicella-zoster virus (VZV)
  acyclovir management in pregnancy, 302

Varicella-zoster virus (VZV) *(cont.)*
  chickenpox management in adults, 282
  congenital syndrome, 301
  immunization, 302
  neonatal management, 301–302
Vasa previa
  complications, 10
  definition, 10
Vascular malformation, versus hemangioma, 82
Venous access, neonates, 20, 27
Ventilation. *See also* High-frequency ventilation
  adverse effects, 377
  assist-controlled ventilation
    definition, 378
    indications, 378
    weaning, 379
  carbon dioxide retention causes, 376–378
  deterioration management, 379
  extubation, 380
  factors affecting oxygenation, 375
  liquid ventilation
    clinical trials, 387
    definition, 386
    indications, 387
    lung compliance effects, 387
  manual ventilation, 379
  synchronized mechanical ventilation, 378
  time constant, 378
  time-cycled pressure-limited
    definition, 374–375
    disadvantages, 375
    increasing of ventilation, 375
    mean airway pressure variables, 376
    peak inspiratory pressure selection, 376
  volume-cycled
    definition, 375
    difficulty in neonates, 375
Ventricular septal defect (VSD)
  age at diagnosis, 44
  echocardiography, 32–33, 34
  surgery, 72–73
Very low birth weight infant, definition, 145
Vision, development, 317
Vitamin A, supplementation for bronchopulmonary
    dysplasia, 159
Vitamin D, osteopenia of prematurity,
    supplementation, 158
Vitamin E, in prevention of retinopathy of
    prematurity, 338
von Willebrand disease, heredity, 254
VSD. *See* Ventricular septal defect
VZV. *See* Varicella-zoster virus

Wolff-Parkinson-White syndrome
  electrocardiography findings, 64
  hemodynamic consequences

XX male sex reversal syndrome, 108
Xylose absorption test, 166

Zinc, deficiency causes in preterm infants, 158